Diagnostic and Interventional Ultrasound in Pediatrics and Pediatric Surgery

Stefan Scholz • Marcus D. Jarboe
Editors

Diagnostic and Interventional Ultrasound in Pediatrics and Pediatric Surgery

Springer

Editors
Stefan Scholz
Division of Pediatric General & Thoracic Surgery
Children's Hospital of Pittsburgh of UPMC
University of Pittsburgh School of Medicine
Pittsburgh, PA
USA

Marcus D. Jarboe
Division of Pediatric Surgery
C.S. Mott Children's Hospital
University of Michigan
Ann Arbor, MI
USA

ISBN 978-3-319-79358-0 ISBN 978-3-319-21699-7 (eBook)
DOI 10.1007/978-3-319-21699-7

Springer Cham Heidelberg New York Dordrecht London

Softcover re-print of the Hardcover 1st edition 2016

Printed on acid-free paper

Springer International Publishing AG Switzerland is part of Springer Science+Business Media (www.springer.com)

Preface

Ultrasound (US) has become the radiographic diagnostic method of choice to aid in the diagnosis of medical problems in children, one of the most profound changes in pediatric practice in the past few decades. This is especially true in the realm of pediatric surgical diseases.

Radiation exposure is a recognized problem and a significant concern in the medical community and with the public at large. Many recent studies have highlighted the dangers of radiation exposure in regards to malignancy, especially in children and young adults. Concern among parents has grown to ensure that radiation needed for diagnostic requirements in children is kept at a minimal level.

This concern has been the impetus for change in the world of pediatric imaging, the foremost of which has been increased use of magnetic resonance imaging (MRI) and ultrasound (US). There has been evidence suggesting negative implications of anesthesia on the developing brain. US rarely requires sedation or anesthesia as opposed to other radiation-free techniques such as the MRI. Sonography is a child-friendly nonintimidating imaging technique thriving on the absence of fat with pictures of exquisite clarity, rendering it much more suited to abdominal examinations in children.

The general trend in surgery over the past decades has been toward minimizing the invasiveness of surgical interventions. US used for real-time guidance of needle and catheter placement has resulted in less invasive, safer, and more accurate interventions. The pediatric population is well suited for US with its small body size and, generally, low body fat resulting in tremendous image quality. Given all of these advantages, there is a large impetus to maximize US use to diagnose pediatric surgical diseases. Furthermore, US is often regarded as the modern day equivalent to the stethoscope extending one's physical exam.

Despite these advantages, there are hurdles to overcome to apply US technology successfully. Despite its well-recognized value, education and practice remain the major obstacles in developing expertise in the use of preoperative and intraoperative US limiting its widespread use.

The quality of information gained with US depends largely on the skill and expertise of those scanning the patient and interpreting the dynamic images. Sonography is highly examiner dependent.

In many medical centers, which primarily treat adults, even the radiologists are not comfortable using US in pediatric disease processes. Although the literature has clearly shown that using US for venous access is much safer, US-guided line placement is not the norm. Even though US is not a new technology, there are very few ways outside a radiology residency that you can learn how to use US effectively as a physician or surgeon. In addition, there are very few resources to read with regards to pediatric surgical US.

Because of this, there is a national push to widely implement US in pediatric practice. The American College of Surgery (ACS) offered the very first US course in the USA targeted to pediatric surgeons in fall 2013. This course was so well received by the pediatric surgical community that we were inspired to create a resource and guide for US in pediatric surgical problems to familiarize pediatric practitioners with its possibilities and limitations.

In health care, there is a strong emphasis on safety and quality, and US makes procedures safer and more dependable. There is a demand for less invasive techniques and US provides new minimally invasive options. There is clearly a drive for less cost, and US is relatively inexpensive. There is a push for less radiation and US has none.

Pediatric surgeons and other pediatric subspecialties understand this and are looking for ways to get trained.

Currently, there are no other books dedicated to sonographic applications for pediatric surgical diseases in the English language. Pediatric surgeons and specialists dealing with pediatric surgical disease need a book to read and reference to help them bring US to their practice and use it effectively.

This textbook is designed to present a state-of-the-art guide and review of US applications for children and infants with surgical problems.

The text is meant as a single source to provide information about sonographic application, interpretation, and technique for a diversity of pediatric surgical care providers. The textbook can be a useful tool for the US novice as well as the more advanced ultrasonographer. Initial obstacles faced by a physician starting with US are addressed, such as the scanning techniques, underlying anatomy and normal sonographic findings. The initial chapter provides an introduction and basic overview about US theory and techniques. Subsequent chapters focus on specific body parts and systems and their disease processes as it pertains to pediatric and neonatal patients. The textbook includes a chapter dedicated to abdominal trauma and its evaluation with the focused abdominal sonography for trauma (FAST) exam.

For clarity, the textbook is divided into two separate parts. The first part focuses on US as a tool for diagnosis and monitoring of pediatric surgical and urological problems. The second part will outline interventional procedures routinely performed under US guidance in children. All chapters are written by experts and include the most up to date scientific and clinical information.

For practical purposes, specific details of those chapters include preparation of the patient and technical tips and tricks for safe and effective procedures. Interventional techniques for US-guided vascular access, diagnostic, and therapeutic drainage procedures, core biopsy of masses and solid organs, fine-needle aspiration (FNA) of the thyroid gland, sclerotherapy for vascular malformations, regional blocks for postoperative pain control and intraoperative applications of sonography will be presented. Every chapter is accompanied with extensive illustrations. A brief review of the existing literature of the particular topic follows each chapter.

We hope that this textbook will improve understanding and interpretation of sonographic pictures and reports and serve as a practical guide for a growing number of US users, surgeons, and pediatricians, alike. It is meant to bolster the comfort level for interpretation and performing US themselves for pediatricians, pediatric surgeons, and pediatric radiologists. The aim is to provide the sonographer with a framework to use in diagnosis, so that the maximum amount of information can be gained from the US examination.

As a first edition, the reader may forgive typical "birthing problems" of a newly conceptionalized project. We hope that this text will serve as a natural link between pediatrics, pediatric surgery, and pediatric radiology in a truly collaborative fashion. We are convinced that for US use in pediatric surgical problems, the best is yet to come!

Our book is dedicated to all the sick infants and children and their pediatric practitioners who examine and treat them with the utmost skill and gentility.

Practical tips for performing US:

1. Take a course—US is a valuable tool for diagnosis, management, and therapy. To incorporate it into your toolbox, learning the basics is invaluable: how it works, how to optimize your image, and getting comfortable with all the knobs and buttons of the machine. Many societies and associations are now offering courses, which you should definitely consider as an excellent beginning step.
2. Stay in practice—US is a tool that you should try to use as much as possible. The best use would be to incorporate it in as many cases as possible to develop familiarity and comfort. While you are unlikely to have abdominal and retroperitoneal masses present every day, using US for common cases such as central line insertion is an ideal way of keeping in practice.
3. Learn from experts—Even if you have taken a course, you can always learn from others. Your US technologist and radiologists are great resources. Get into the habit of reviewing all of the images from US that you order and then read the report afterwards—this is a quick way of "testing" yourself to make sure you have seen everything that the experts have. You may even find subtle findings that were not initially identified.
4. Partner with experts—If you are a novice in the use of US, arrange for your radiologist or US technician to be available to help you during your cases. For some of the more difficult cases as described in this chapter, having another set of eyes to interpret, and other hands to adjust images will be invaluable. Additionally, in general, the quality of the US machines from radiology are superior to the smaller mobile ones used in the operating room (OR)—which usually are intended for line insertions and guidance of blocks.
5. Share expenses—The major cost impact of US is the acquisition of probes. Unless you are in a situation where cost is not a concern, and few of us are, you will need to carefully consider which probes you want to purchase. Think about what procedures you want to do now, and in the next 10 years

(about the time that technology will improve). For some probes, such as laparoscopic probes, which you may only use occasionally, it may be best to share the expense with another hospital or borrow their probe on the rare occasion that you will need it. Just be careful about the selection of companies for your US machines and probes, as there are no universal connectors.

Stefan Scholz
Marcus D. Jarboe

Acknowledgments

We would like to gratefully acknowledge the help, stimulation, and advice of all our colleagues at the Children's Hospital of Pittsburgh of UPMC, Pittsburgh, PA, and the C.S. Mott Children's Hospital in Ann Arbor, Michigan, and especially our division chiefs Drs. George Gittes and Ron Hirschl for their encouragement and support.

Our careers in pediatric surgery have been inspired by many teachers and mentors at varying institutions over the years, in Germany and the USA, who served as our role models in the challenging but gratifying care of children.

This book is the result of a team effort and we would like to highlight the hard work and dedication of the pediatric specialists, especially pediatric surgeons, and pediatric radiologists, who have contributed chapters to this text. More importantly, all of them continue their devotion to a career of taking care of infants and children who need our help and who ultimately make it all worthwhile.

Many thanks to Michael Griffin from Springer for his patience, encouragement, and invaluable help in preparing and "fine tuning" the manuscript and all the pictures. My assistant, Pat Fustich, was invaluable in proofreading parts of the manuscripts and providing her moral support. Dr. Ken Gow contributed the practical tips for performing US to the preface.

On a special note, we would like to thank our wives, *Elizabeth and Sarah,* without their support this book would have not been possible. Our wonderful children, *Mischa, Nicholas,* and *Gavin* as well as *Colin, Liam,* and *Katherine,* are the reason we get up early every morning.

I would also like to thank my mother, Birgit Scholz, for her continued support and enthusiasm for my ongoing professional endeavors despite the hurtful distance to another continent.

Stefan Scholz
Marcus D. Jarboe

Contents

Contributors

Justin Barr Department of Surgery, University of Virginia, Charlottesville, VA, USA

Raimondo M. Cervellione Royal Manchester Children's Hospital, Manchester, England, UK

Farokh R. Demehri University of Michigan, Ann Arbor, MI, USA

Alexander Dzakovic Department of Pediatric Surgery, Loyola University Medical Center, Maywood, IL, USA

Guy F. Brisseau Department of Surgery, Division Chief Pediatric Surgery, Sidra Medical and Research Center, Weill-Cornell Medical College, Doha, Qatar

Andre D. Furtado Department of Radiology, Children's Hospital of Pittsburgh of UPMC, Pittsburgh, PA, USA

Samir K. Gadepalli Division of Pediatric Surgery, Department of Surgery, C.S. Mott Children's Hospital, Ann Arbor, MI, USA

Joseph J. Gemmete Department of Radiology, University of Michigan, Ann Arbor, MI, USA

Jan Gödeke Department of Pediatric Surgery, University Medical Center Mainz, Mainz, Germany

Seth Goldstein Department of Surgery, Johns Hopkins Hospital, Baltimore, MD, USA

Kenneth W. Gow Department of General and Thoracic Surgery, Seattle Children's Hospital, Seattle, WA, USA

Judy H. Squires Department of Pediatric Radiology, Children's Hospital of Pittsburgh, Pittsburgh, PA, USA

Juan Carlos Infante Department of Medical Imaging, Ann and Robert H Lurie Children's Hospital of Chicago, Chicago, IL, USA

Marcus D. Jarboe Division of Pediatric Surgery, Department of Surgery, Pediatric Interventional Radiology, Mott Children's Hospital, University of Michigan, Ann Arbor, MI, USA

Nathalie Kremer Department of Pediatric Surgery, Cincinnati Children's Hospital Medical Center, Cincinnati, OH, USA

Stacey Langford Department of Pediatric Radiology, Children's Hospital of Pittsburgh of UPMC, Pittsburgh, PA, USA

Vincent Lee Department of Pediatric Radiology, Children's Hospital of Pittsburgh of UPMC, Pittsburgh, PA, USA

Christine M. Leeper Department of General Surgery, University of Pittsburgh Medical Center, Pittsburgh, PA, USA

Kimberly M. Lumpkins Department of Surgery, University of Maryland School of Medicine, Baltimore, MD, USA

Marcus M. Malek Department of Surgery, Pediatric Surgery Oncology, Children's Hospital of Pittsburgh of UPMC, University of Pittsburgh School of Medicine, Pittsburgh, PA, USA

Oliver J. Muensterer Department of Pediatric Surgery, University Medicine of the Johannes Gutenberg University Mainz, Mainz, Germany

Gary Nace Division of Pediatric General and Thoracic Surgery, Children's Hospital of Pittsburgh of UPMC, Pittsburgh, PA, USA

Kushal Parikh Department of Radiology, University of Michigan, Ann Arbor, MI, USA

Sara K. Rasmussen Department of Surgery, University of Virginia, Charlottesville, VA, USA

Kevin M. Riggle Department of Surgery, University of Washington, Seattle, WA, USA

Oliver L. Sanchez Department of Pediatric Surgery, Children's Hospital Geneva, Geneve, Switzerland

Julia Scholsching Department of Pediatric Surgery, University Medicine of the Johannes Gutenberg University Mainz, Mainz, Germany

Stefan Scholz Division of Pediatric General and Thoracic Surgery, Children's Hospital of Pittsburgh of UPMC, University of Pittsburgh School of Medicine, Pittsburgh, PA, USA

Gayathri Sreedher NEOMED, Rootstown, USA

University of Pittsburgh School of Medicine, Pittsburgh, USA

Department of Pediatric Radiology, Akron Children's Hospital (and Childrens Hospital of Pittsburgh of UPMC), Akron, OH, USA

F. Dylan Stewart Department of Pediatric Surgery, Johns Hopkins Hospital, Baltimore, MD, USA

Sameh Tadros Department of Pediatric Radiology, Children's Hospital of Pittsburgh of UPMC, Pittsburgh, PA, USA

Salmai Turial Department of Pediatric Surgery, University Medicine of the Johannes Gutenberg University Mainz, Mainz, Germany

Ranjith Vellody Department of Radiology, Childrens National Medical Center, Washington, DC, USA

Department of Radiology, University of Michigan, Ann Arbor, MI, USA

Mihaela Visoiu Department of Anesthesiology, Children's Hospital of Pittsburgh of University of Pittsburgh Medical Center, Pittsburgh, PA, USA

Part I
Diagnostic Ultrasound

Overview of Ultrasound Theory and Techniques

1

Seth Goldstein

Introduction

Ultrasound is an increasingly popular and useful diagnostic and interventional imaging modality in contemporary pediatric surgical practice. Among its advantages are portability, real-time instantaneous visualization, wide availability, and lack of ionizing radiation. Relatively unique to ultrasound compared to other imaging is the heavy reliance on the individual skill of the user in determining the quality of the study; thus, a basic understanding of the fundamental theory and techniques of the technology can greatly enhance the practitioner's ability to successfully employ it.

Part I: Technical Principles of Ultrasound Imaging

Medical ultrasound images are created in a pulse-echo manner based on three principal processes: creation of a pulsed ultrasound wave, detection of its echoes, and formation of an image based on the time elapsed between pulse and echo.

Creation of an Ultrasound Wave Ultrasound is an imaging modality based on the piezoelectric effect. Piezoelectricity is the electrical charge that builds up when mechanical stress is applied to certain crystalline structures. Importantly, this is a reversible phenomenon whereby pressure applied to a crystal generates charge, and conversely, charge applied to the crystal creates vibration (Fig. 1.1). An ultrasound transducer is created by applying an alternating current to a row of piezoelectric crystals that cause them to oscillate and produce a beam of acoustic waves. Frequencies used for imaging applications are higher than the upper range of detection by the human ear, hence the name ultrasound. Notably, the bidirectionality of the piezoelectric effect results in a detectable voltage change in the same crystals if they are subjected to vibration. Practically speaking, this means that ultrasound transducers are capable of emitting pulses of sound as well as subsequently detecting the echoes of those waves as they reflect off objects in the beam's path.

Detection of an Ultrasound Echo The physical property that describes the ability of sound to move through an object is called acoustic impedance, which is a function of both density and speed of sound through a substance. When a sound wave reaches a boundary between two entities with different acoustic impedances, a portion of the wave is transmitted and the rest is reflected back to the source as an echo (Fig. 1.2). The degree to which a structure reflects sound pulses during an ultrasound examination is denoted as "echogenicity." Highly echogenic, or hyperechoic, structures typically have relatively

S. Goldstein (✉)
Department of Surgery, Johns Hopkins Hospital, 1800 Orleans St., Tower 110, 21287 Baltimore, MD, USA
e-mail: sgoldstein@jhmi.edu

S. Scholz, M. D. Jarboe (eds.), *Diagnostic and Interventional Ultrasound in Pediatrics and Pediatric Surgery,* DOI 10.1007/978-3-319-21699-7_1

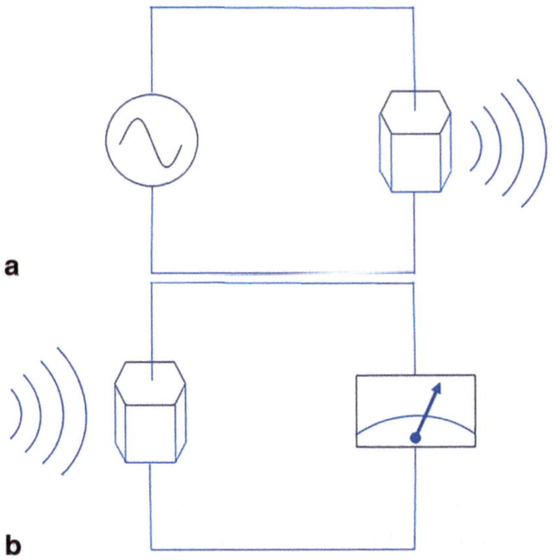

Fig. 1.1 The piezoelectric effect is a bidirectional phenomenon whereby an alternating current applied to a crystal creates vibration *(panel a)*; additionally, oscillation of the crystal by sound waves generates a voltage across the crystal *(panel b)*

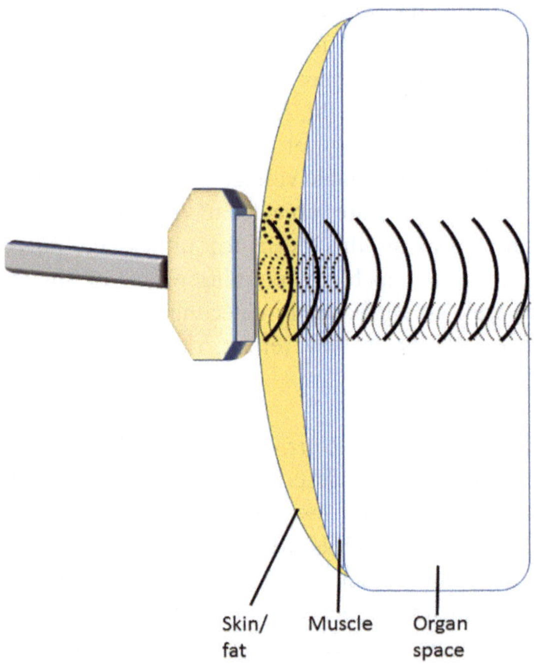

Fig. 1.2 A small portion of the beam created by an ultrasound probe is reflected at each boundary between substances with varying acoustic impedances. The echoed wave is detected by the same transducers within the probe and used to form an image for display

low water content, reflect a large proportion of incoming ultrasound, and are displayed as white on a B-mode image. Commonly seen hyperechoic tissues include cortical bone, tendon, organ and muscle sheaths, nerves, and gallstones. Extremely hyperechoic structures result in an artifact on the image known as acoustic shadowing; since most of thc sound has been reflected to the probe at the structure's surface, the area behind the echogenic material is displayed as a black streak (Fig. 1.3).

Features with low echogenicity are known as hypoechoic or anechoic and are seen on B-mode as dark grey or black, respectively. These include solid organs, muscle bellies, lymph nodes, vasculature, and other structures that are fluid filled or high in water content.

Formation of an Image The simplest mode of ultrasound is known as A-mode (amplitude), in which a single piezoelectric transducer detects the distance to an echogenic structure by precisely measuring the time between emitting a pulse and receiving an echo, utilizing the equation distance=velocity * time. Thus, using the known speed of sound and the detected time to echo, the distance to an object can be calculated. A-mode itself is generally only of historic interest, but can be helpful to understand B-mode (brightness), which is the characteristic mode utilized in modern diagnostic ultrasound. In B-mode imaging, a row of transducers simultaneously act as just described, and the resultant echoes are compiled to produce a two-dimensional image. This is repeated at least 20 times per second to create a real-time effect. An important assumption in creating a B-mode image using the equation above is that the speed of sound through soft tissue is uniform, most frequently assumed to be a constant 1540 m/s, slightly higher than the speed of sound through pure water. However, in reality, the soft tissues encountered in medical ultrasound have a range of acoustic impedances and resultant velocities of sound, which can lead to imprecise localization of an object's depth and is a limiting factor in the axial resolution of the modality in general.

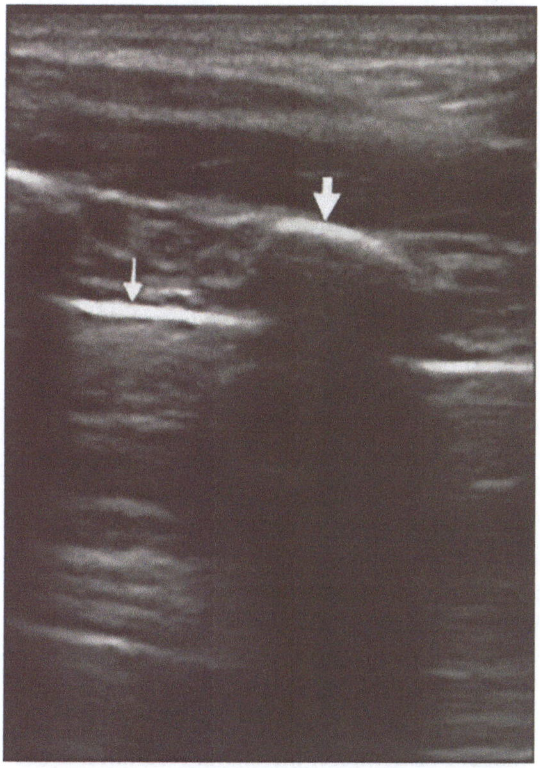

Fig. 1.3 Hyperechoic structures are seen on B-mode ultrasound as bright white. If the object is sufficiently opaque to sound, an acoustic shadow artifact is formed. In this image taken of the chest wall of a 6-year-old boy with a linear probe, both the cortical bone of the rib *(thick arrow)* and the lung pleura *(thin arrow)* appear hyperechoic. The rib does not transmit the ultrasound beam further, thus causing an acoustic shadow

Other commonly employed ultrasound modes are M-mode (movement) and Doppler imaging. M-mode is used to track the movement of an object over time. Initially, a two-dimensional B-mode image is acquired and a scan line is placed along the area of interest. The movement over time of each echogenic interface intersected by that line will then be displayed. M-mode is ideal for characterizing precise temporal events such as the motion of cardiac valves.

Doppler is a mode based on the Doppler effect, by which the frequency of a wave is affected by the movement of the observer and source relative to each other, such as the familiar everyday occurrence when the pitch of a siren or horn changes as a vehicle approaches and passes at high speed. Doppler ultrasound takes advantage of that phenomenon by emitting lower frequency ultrasound waves and detecting the frequency shift of the detected echo. This is often used to interrogate the flow in vasculature and is most effective when the flow is along the same trajectory as the ultrasound beam, since flow perpendicular to the probe has no Doppler effect. Most ultrasound machines will superimpose the relatively low-resolution Doppler signal in color on a B-mode image to facilitate interpretation, this is known as duplex imaging (Fig. 1.4). By convention, movement away from the probe is displayed as blue and movement toward the probe is red (Mnemonic BART: blue away, red toward).

Part II: Practical Considerations of Ultrasound Imaging

The ergonomics of ultrasound are an important component of successful use, not only because visualization of desired structures is user-dependent but also because the cognitive exercise of

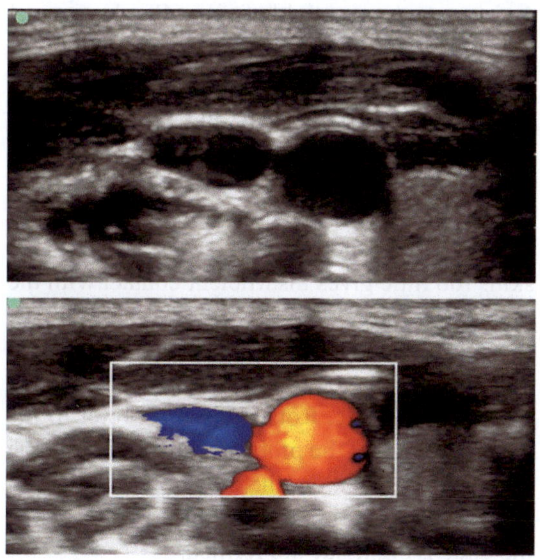

Fig. 1.4 Duplex imaging of the neck of a 6-year-old boy taken with a linear probe. The *top panel* is B-mode, the *bottom panel* is color Doppler overlying the image demonstrating flow toward the probe in the carotid artery at the junction at the internal/external bifurcation *(red)* and flow away from the probe in the internal jugular vein *(blue)*

imagining a three-dimensional object based on a series of two-dimensional screen images is made more difficult if the user is twisted or contorted. Generally, the operator should stand or sit on the ipsilateral side of the patient that is to be examined with the screen on the contralateral side. Occasionally, an examination of the neck of a supine patient is simplified with the user at the head and the screen on the ipsilateral side.

During a purely diagnostic study the probe can be held in either hand. For an ultrasound-guided needle intervention of any sort (venipuncture, abscess drainage, etc.), the probe is grasped with the nondominant hand to facilitate dexterous use of the needle. This is sufficiently common in clinical practice that familiarity with probe use with the nondominant hand is recommended. An assistant could conceivably hold the probe while the needle is inserted, but in actuality, coordination and communication of the proper view and required subtle shifts of the equipment can make that arrangement more difficult than a single user performing the procedure. The probe should be gently held as close to the scanning surface as ergonomically possible to minimize tremor and maintain a constant field of view. Conductive gel should always be applied liberally, as any air interface will greatly diminish the image quality.

The acronym PART (pressure, alignment, rotation, tilt) can be a useful mnemonic to troubleshoot difficulty with an ultrasound exam with respect to probe orientation. Pressure is simply the force with which the probe is pressed onto the skin. Too little gives insufficient contact with the scanning surface, too much can distort or obliterate structures. Alignment is a reminder to keep the object of interest in the middle of the screen whenever possible. Rotation and tilt refer to the positional axis of the probe. By manipulating the transducer orientation, the direction of the beam changes commensurately and different images of the underlying tissue are formed.

Transducer Selection Handheld ultrasound probes are available in a variety of configurations. Users should be familiar with the basics of transducer options in order to choose an appropriate probe for the relevant clinical context, as incorrect selection may preclude the visualization of desired structures. The predominant considerations with respect to probe selection are transducer array arrangement and operating frequency.

The three most common ultrasound transducer types are linear, curvilinear, and phased array (Fig. 1.5). Linear probes comprise an array of transducers in parallel that produce a straight beam of ultrasound and a resultant image width that is equal to the size of the transducer. These are typically used for superficial, vascular, and interventional applications in which high resolution or precise anatomic relationships are important. Curvilinear probes produce a wedge-shaped beam and thus display a cross-section wider than the contact surface. This probe provides a broader view of large internal structures and cavities, and can easily be manipulated to look in directions that are not perpendicular with the skin surface. Users must remember that the determination of depths and distances is imprecise with a curvilinear probe due to widening and distortion of the image. Furthermore, the lateral resolution is sacrificed at greater depths as the scan lines diverge. Finally, phased array probes are constructed as a tightly packed cluster of piezoelectric crystals, which are designed to modulate or "steer" the direction of the ultrasound beam and sweep through a given plane. This allows for a smaller physical footprint than linear and curvilinear probes, and phased array probes are often used for echocardiographic views of the heart that require a small skin contact area in the intercostal spaces.

Usually, smaller sized probes are constructed for high frequency transducers meant for high-resolution imaging of superficial structures. However, it is important to note that the category of transducer array does not solely determine a probe's "footprint," or physical size. Any of the types described above can, in theory, be constructed in any size for various uses.

Typical diagnostic ultrasound probes operate in the frequency range of 2–14 MHz. Higher frequencies permit better spatial resolution but attenuate more rapidly through tissue, yielding a lower depth of penetration. Thus, the characteristic trade-off in any ultrasound examination is that between resolution and depth, with increases in

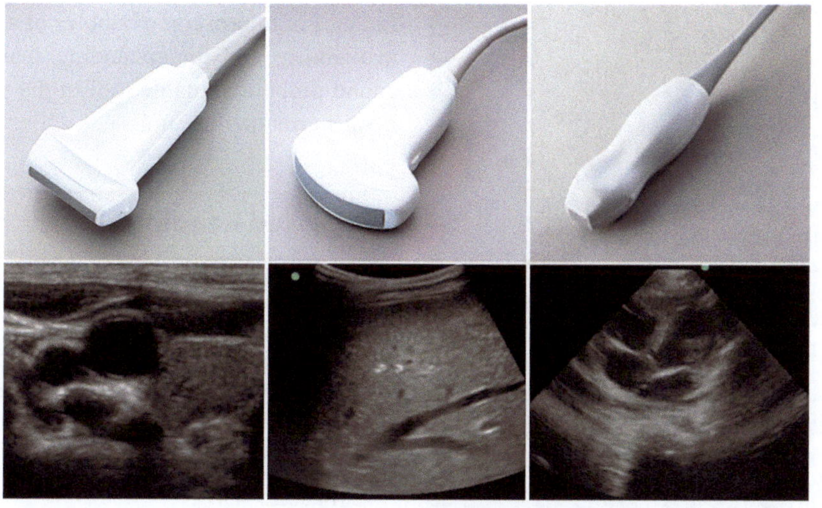

Fig. 1.5 The three most common ultrasound transducer types are *(from left to right)* linear, curvilinear, and phased array. Underneath each probe is an example image. The linear image is of the neck vessels, the image is exactly as wide as the footprint of the probe. The curvilinear probe creates a field of view wider than its contact surface, in this case the liver, and distorts the image slightly. The phased array probe has the smallest footprint and is useful for scanning in between ribs such as this four-chamber view of the heart

either requiring a sacrifice of the other. Generally, any given probe regardless of array configuration will have a fixed bandwidth available based on the physical constraints of the piezoelectric transducers. Commercially these are often denoted with the high end of the range first, such that one could encounter a curvilinear probe with a bandwidth of "8–5 MHz" and a maximum scan depth of 15 cm based on the constraints at the low end of the band.

Basic Knobology The following controls are found as a button, dial, or switch on most modern commercially available ultrasound machines.

Gain Adjusts the intensity of white, gray, and black on the display and is commonly adjusted to improve image quality (Fig. 1.6).

Depth Determines the axial distance of beam penetration and display. This should be adjusted sufficiently deep to include the area of interest, but otherwise minimized to preserve resolution.

Exam type Depending on the manufacturer, there are often a number of machine preset parameters to maximize image quality on the basis of frequency, gain, and frame rate.

Freeze Captures the on-screen image for review, is useful for taking measurements or saving to permanent file.

Summary

In conclusion, the knowledge of basic ultrasound principles has the potential to greatly improve the use of the modality for both diagnostic and interventional applications in pediatric surgical practice. Importantly, there are no identified biologic effects of the frequencies and intensities of sound used in diagnostic ultrasound. Using different, specialized equipment, higher energy ablative ultrasound is possible and has been utilized in some applications; however, the probes and machines described in this chapter are not thought to pose any potential immediate or long-term danger to patients. Future advances in routine ultrasound will likely include probes capable of creating three-dimensional images, as well as exogenous contrast agents employing the echogenic charac-

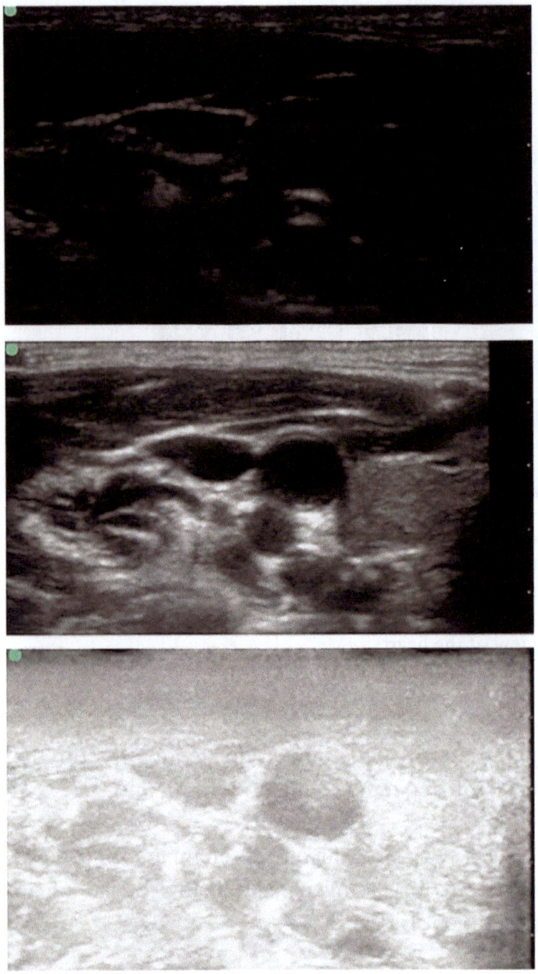

Fig. 1.6 Gain adjustment can be a useful method of improving image quality. The three panels from top to bottom have too low, adequate, and too high gain settings, respectively, of neck vessels with a linear probe in identical position

teristics of microscopic bubbles of air. Increasing availability and understanding make the ultrasound probe a valuable tool in the pediatric surgeon's armamentarium.

Suggested Readings

1. Aldrich JE. Basic physics of ultrasound imaging. Crit Care Med. 2007;35:S131–S7.
2. Chan V, Perlas A. Basics of ultrasound imaging. In: Narouze S, editor. Atlas of ultrasound-guided procedures in interventional pain management. New York: Springer; 2011. p. 13–9.
3. Enriquez JL, Wu TS. An introduction to ultrasound equipment and knobology. Crit Care Clin. 2014;30:25–45.

Pediatric Spinal Sonography

2

Gayathri Sreedher and Andre D. Furtado

Scanning Technique and Anatomy

In the neonate, vertebral ossification is not complete. Hence in the first half of infancy before the spinous processes ossify and fuse, it is possible to image the spinal canal from a dorsal view. Later in life a paramedian approach can be used when the spinous processes are more ossified and lead to posterior acoustic shadowing hence precluding imaging in the midline sagittal plane. A high frequency 7–12 MHz linear array transducer is used. Images are obtained in sagittal/longitudinal and axial/transverse planes. Typically a sagittal and axial cine clip at the level of the conus in rest is obtained to document spinal pulsations due to Cerebrospinal Fluid (CSF) pulsation. Pulsation is restricted in tethered cord. However pulsation is best seen a couple weeks after birth. Typically scanning is done in the prone position in a well-fed infant. Having the caregiver hold the baby in prone position just after feeding increases the chances of an easy motion free exam [1].

The lumbar vertebrae can be labeled by various methods. One method is to assume that the last rib bearing vertebra is T12, another to assign the last square shaped ossified vertebra as S5 and yet another uses the lumbosacral junction as L5-S1 with the vertebra at the end of the lumbar lordosis being L5. When counting the sacral and coccygeal bodies note that the coccygeal vertebras have a central ossification center compared to the square shaped ossification of the sacral vertebrae. All these methods are an approximation. Usually two or more of these criteria are used to determine the lumbar levels.

Normal Sonographic Findings

The cord appears hypoechoic to almost anechoic. The central canal of the spinal cord is visible as two echogenic lines in the center of the cord. Some believe this to be the interface between the anterior white matter commissure and median fissure [2]. The filum terminale, which is the fibrotic continuation of the spinal pia, below the conus may have a small cyst called the filar cyst as a normal variant [3]. The filum terminale is identified as an echogenic line that is thicker and straighter than the surrounding cauda equina nerve roots. The filum terminale is normally 1–2 mm thick and moves with CSF pulsations (Fig. 2.1).

A. D. Furtado (✉)
Department of Radiology, Children's Hospital of Pittsburgh of UPMC, 4401 Penn Avenue, Floor 2, Pittsburgh 15224, PA, USA
e-mail: furtadoad@upmc.edu

G. Sreedher
Department of Pediatric Radiology, Akron Children's Hospital (and Childrens Hospital of Pittsburgh of UPMC), One Perkins Square, Akron 44308, OH, USA
e-mail: doctor.sgayathri@gmail.com

NEOMED, Rootstown, USA

University of Pittsburgh School of Medicine, Pittsburgh, USA

S. Scholz, M. D. Jarboe (eds.), *Diagnostic and Interventional Ultrasound in Pediatrics and Pediatric Surgery,* DOI 10.1007/978-3-319-21699-7_2

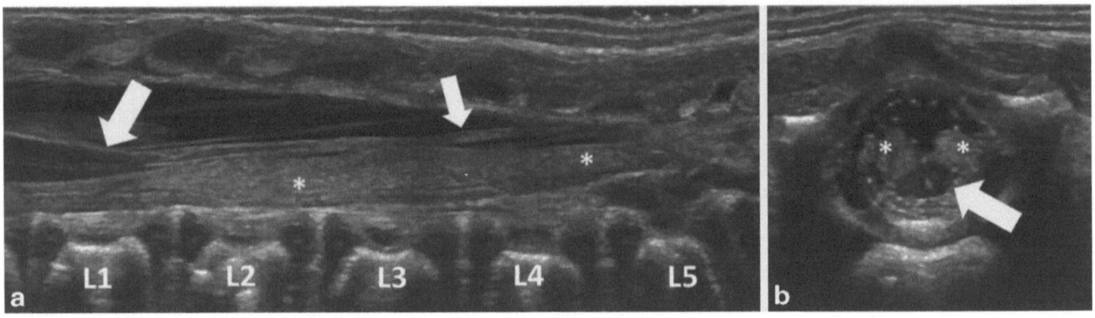

Fig. 2.1 Normal ultrasound of the spine. Sagittal (**a**) and axial (**b**). High-resolution ultrasound image of an infant on prone position. The conus medullaris *(arrow)*, the filum terminale *(small arrow)* and the cauda equina nerve roots (*)

The position of conus is above the L2-3 disc in a normal term infant. Some accept up to the upper border or midbody of L3 to be within normal limits, if the filum is normal. Ventriculus terminalis is persistent focal dilation of the central canal that is limited to the distal cord. It is a normal variant [3]. If there is question about the position of the conus, placing a radiographic skin marker at the level of the conus under ultrasound guidance and taking a subsequent radiograph of the spine to determine the vertebral level can be performed.

Simple coccygeal dimples or pits, which are shallow, 5 mm or smaller in diameter, located within 2.5 cm cephalad to the anal verge and without any associated suspicious skin lesions, are not associated with an increased risk for spinal dysraphism (Fig. 2.2) [4–6]. No imaging is required for simple coccygeal pits.

The craniocervical junction can be imaged using the foramen magnum as a sonographic window. It is rarely performed, however it can be used to image the inferior cerebellum and proximal cervical cord [1].

Spinal Dysraphism

Spinal dysraphism is the term used for incomplete fusion of the posterior arch of the vertebrae. Closed spinal dysraphism is covered by skin and in open spinal dysraphism the spinal canal contents are exposed without overlying skin.

Open spinal dysraphism can be of two major types: (1) Myelocele with a flat neural placode (distal end of the cord) exposed and flush with the surrounding skin; (2) Myelomeningocele where the placode is associated with herniated subarachnoid space and meninges. In both the defect is repaired with approximation of the skin within the first 72 h of birth (Fig. 2.3).

Myelomeningocele is virtually always associated with Chiari II malformation. Chiari II malformation involves a small posterior fossa with downward herniation of cerebellar tonsils. In fetal life ultrasound demonstrates the bifrontal skull narrowing called lemon sign and crowding of cerebellum around the brainstem, called banana sign. In the neonate sonographic scanning of the posterior fossa and via the foramen magnum at the craniocervical junction can demonstrate the herniated cerebellar tonsils lying posterior to the upper

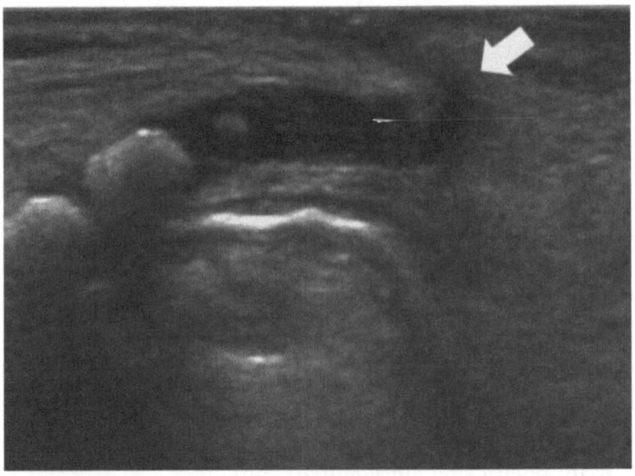

Fig. 2.2 Simple coccygeal dimple. Sagittal ultrasound image of the coccygeal region. Hypoechoic line extending from the skin dimple to the distal coccyx. This finding is considered a normal variant and is not associated with spinal dysraphic anomalies

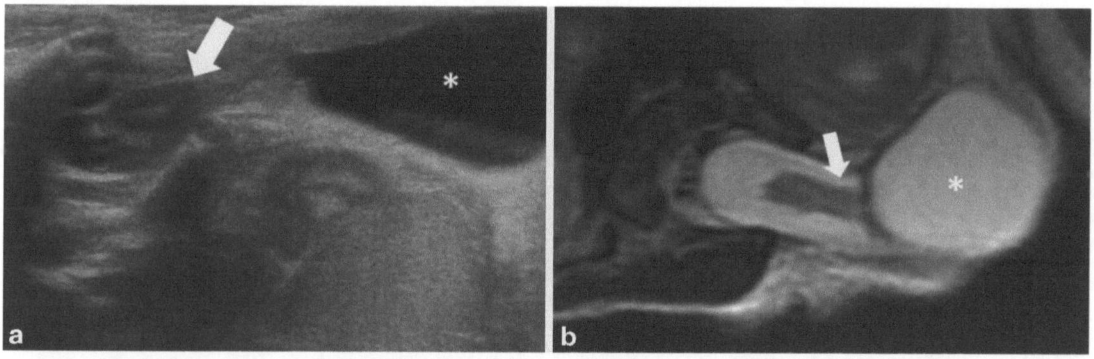

Fig. 2.3 Myelomeningocele. Axial ultrasound (**a**) and axial T2 MRI weighted image (**b**). The neural placode *(arrows)* and the meninges (*) protruding through the spinal dysraphism

cervical cord. Repair of the cerebellar herniation is only rarely performed in infancy [3]. The cord remains low in position after tethered cord release and closure of the myelomeningocele. It is very difficult to diagnose secondary tethering due to adhering scar tissue after surgery as the imaging findings overlap normal postoperative appearance. Clinical assessment is of utmost importance when re-tethering is suspected.

A meningocele, whether in the cervical or more commonly lumbosacral region, contains only CSF-filled sac of dura mater without any neural elements. The cord can be tethered to the periphery of the sac. It is not associated with Chiari II malformation. A terminal myelocystocele is a rare condition where the herniated CSF space communicates with the distal spinal canal. It is associated with more proximal cord syrinx. Terminal myelocystoceles are associated with omphalocele, cloacal exstrophy, imperforate anus, and spinal anomalies (OEIS) complex [7].

Closed spinal dysraphism is covered by skin. Also called as occult spinal dysraphism it is not associated with an increase in maternal serum and amniotic fluid Alpha-feto Protein (AFP) levels. Most commonly it manifests as a midline spinal abnormality on physical examination in the newborn. Bifurcation or asymmetry of the superior gluteal crease, skin covered hairy patch, skin tag, subcutaneous mass or lump (lipoma), abnormally pigmented patch, telangectasias, hemangiomas, and high sacral dimples may herald an underlying spinal dysraphic anomaly [4, 8].

Spinal lipoma is the term given to a variety of spinal dysraphisms associated with a fatty component. Lipomyelocele is akin to a myelocele, except that the neural placode is covered by a lipoma that is contiguous with the subcutaneous fat. The neural elements lie within the confines of the vertebral canal (Fig. 2.4). In a lipomyelomeningocele the subarachnoid spaces bulges out of the vertebral canal and pushes the

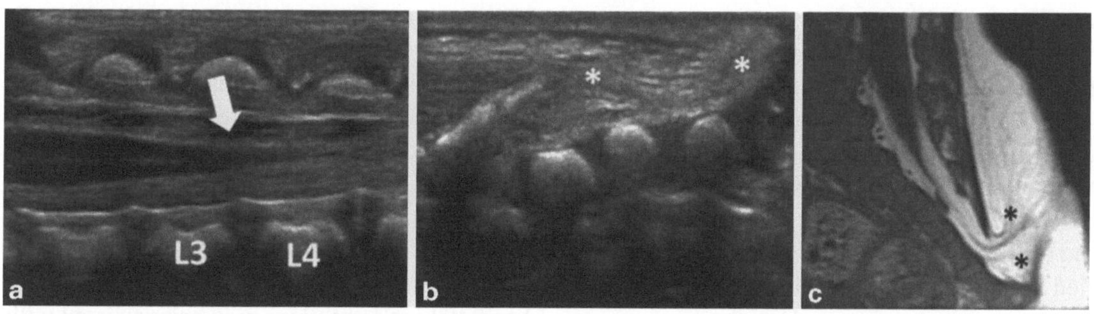

Fig. 2.4 Lipomyelocele. Sagittal ultrasound image (**a, b**) and sagittal MRI T1 weighted image (**c**). Low-lying conus medullaris terminating at the level of L4 *(arrow)* with the distal spinal dysraphism covered by a lipoma that is contiguous with the subcutaneous fat (*)

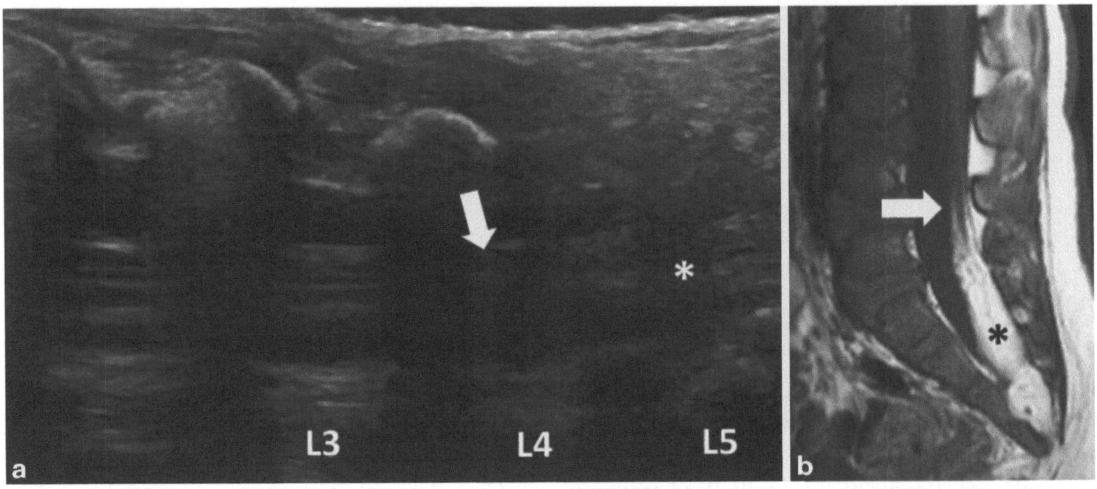

Fig. 2.5 Terminal lipoma. Sagittal ultrasound images of the lumbosacral junction (**a**) and the sagittal MRI T1 weighted image (**b**). Tethered cord terminating at the level of the lumbosacral junction *(arrow)* inseparable from an echogenic mass, consistent with the terminal lipoma seen on MRI T1-weighted image (*)

neural placode and the overlying lipoma as well. The nomenclature of these defects can be easily understood as it represents the layer that is first encountered from the dorsal aspect [1].

Intradural lipoma is a lipoma in the subpial location that is typically attached to the dorsal spinal cord. Intradural lipomas occur more commonly in the thoracic spine, followed by the cervicothoracic junction, and may cause symptoms related to cord compression. The intradural lipomas located in the lumbosacral region, intimately related to the filum terminale, are named terminal lipomas and are often associated with tethered cord (Fig. 2.5). Terminal lipomas are frequently associated with sacral hypoplasia, anorectal malformations, genitourinary malformations, and dorsal dermal sinus.

Lumbosacral dimple: High lumbosacral dimples that are located higher than the gluteal cleft, more than 2.5 cm cephalad to the anal verge, have a higher risk of underlying spinal anomalies and tethered cord. They may represent the opening of dorsal dermal sinuses, which communicate with the underlying spinal canal and dura via a stratified squamous epithelial-lined sinus tract and dysraphic spinous process. Dimples may or may not be associated with hair tufts or hemangiomas.

Tethered Cord

The caudal fixation of spinal cord which leads to stretching of the lower spinal cord and associated neurological dysfunction is the essence of tethered cord (Fig. 2.6). When not treated, the neurological disability may progressively become irreversible. The cord can be tethered in a variety of conditions associated with occult and open spinal dysraphisms. In addition diastematomyelia, filar lipoma, and dorsal dermal sinus may lead to tethering of the cord [3].

Diastematomyelia

Diastematomyelia can be recognized as a split cord which usually reunites distally and may be separated by a bony or fibrous septum. Scanning the entire cord can identify the level of the split and reunited cord.

Findings in Anorectal Malformation

Anorectal malformations may be associated with a variety of spinal anomalies.

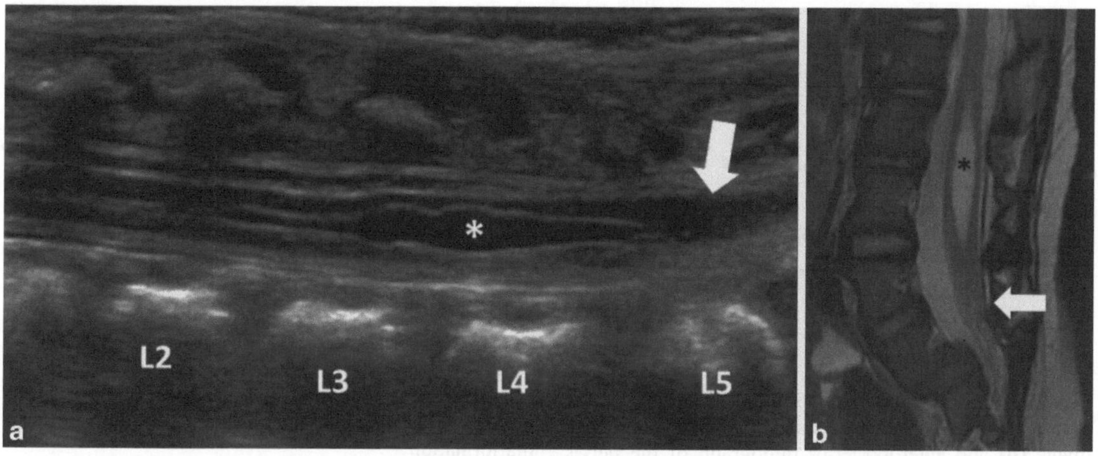

Fig. 2.6 Tethered cord with hydromyelia. Sagittal ultrasound images of the lumbosacral region (**a**) and the sagittal MRI T2 weighted image (**b**). Tethered cord terminating at the level of L5-1 *(arrow)* with dilation of the distal ependymal canal, consistent with hydromyelia (*)

Caudal regression syndrome is characterized by insult to the caudal cell mass that gives rise to the coccyx, distal sacrum and the lower lumbar spine. It is more common in infants of diabetic mothers [9]. Anorectal anomalies such as imperforate anus are typically associated. Bladder and renal anomalies may also be present. The spinal cord in caudal regression type 1 is high ending and blunted (Fig. 2.7). In type 2 caudal regression, which is less common, the cord is low lying and tethered to a fibrolipoma.

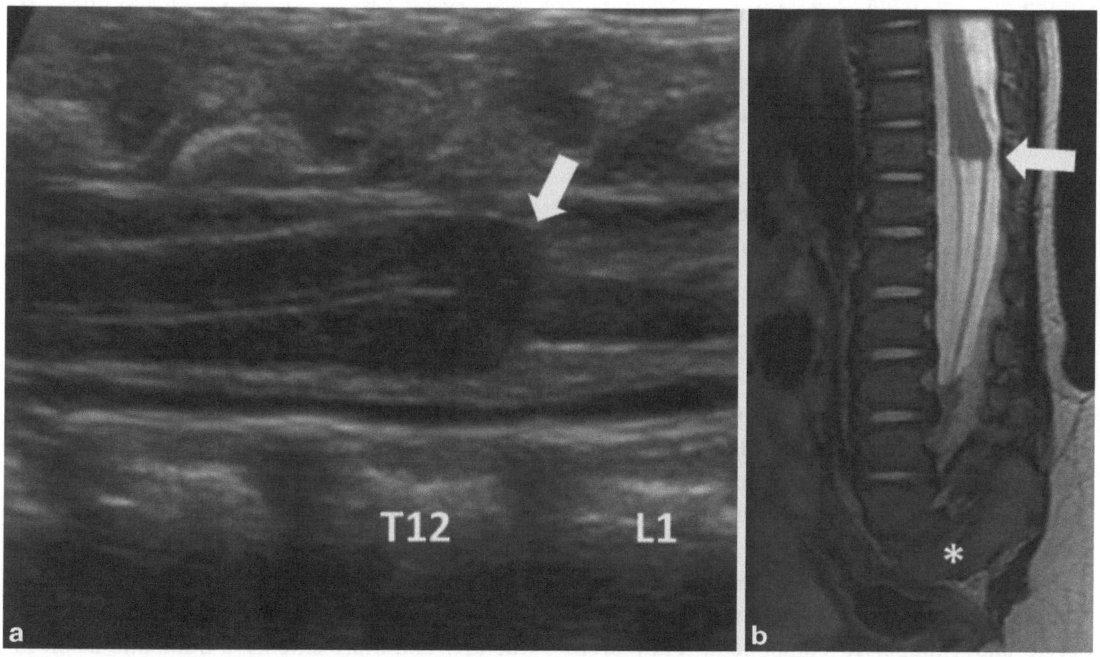

Fig. 2.7 Caudal regression syndrome. Sagittal ultrasound image of the thoracolumbar junction (**a**) and sagittal MRI T2-weighted image (**b**). High ending, blunted distal spinal cord *(arrow)* and dysplastic sacrum (*)

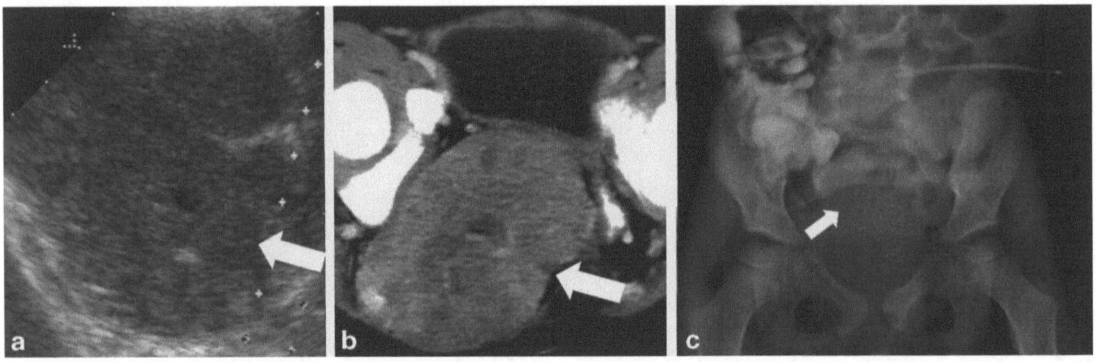

Fig. 2.8 Currarino syndrome. Sagittal ultrasound image of the lumbosacral region (**a**), axial contrast enhanced CT image (**b**) and anteroposterior radiograph of the pelvis (**c**). Heterogeneous presacral mass *(arrow)* and dysplastic sacrum *(small arrow)* in an infant with the anorectal malformation

The syndrome of Currarino is a rare congenital disorder that comprises a triad of dysplastic sacrum, anorectal malformation, and presacral mass (Fig. 2.8). Infants with Currarino syndrome may also have urogenital malformation. The presacral mass is commonly a teratoma, although anterior sacral meningocele or duplication cysts are also possible. The dysplastic sacrum is typically partial and one sided leading to a scimitar shaped sacrum. Agenesis, scalloping, and sacral hypoplasia are also described. Inheritance is autosomal dominant [10].

The presence of cloacal anomalies, such as extrophy, cloacal malformations and, imperforate anus and ectopic anus are highly associated with spinal cord anomalies and dysraphism. OIES syndrome is associated with cloacal extrophy and terminal myelocystocele (vide supra).

Neoplasm

The most common spinal tumor of infancy is intraspinal extension of a neuroblastoma. Ultrasound can be used to evaluate the extent of intraspinal tumor and may demonstrate the extent of cord compression [1].

Sacrococcygeal teratomas form the next most common spinal tumors. They can have an intrapelvic and extrapelvic component. They were classified by Altman into four types that progressively have an increase in the intrapelvic component, with minimal intrapelvic extension in type I to predominantly intrapelvic in type IV. Up to 50% are of type I (Fig. 2.9). Saccrocoocygeal teratomas may be mature or immature on pathology and the level of differentiation determines the malignant potential. These masses are typically heterogeneous in echotexture with solid and cystic components. Many are now diagnosed in prenatal life and up to 70% are evident on neonatal exam as a lump or exophytic extrapelvic mass. Diagnosis may be delayed with Type IV sacrococcygeal teratomas. Delayed diagnosis is associated with a more complex surgery as well as higher incidence of malignant elements on pathology [11].

In adults and older children intraoperative guidance with ultrasound can be useful to delineate tumor from the spinal cord. Sonography is performed after laminectomy is done. A high frequency transducer is used.

Spinal Trauma

Intraspinal hemorrhage after lumbar puncture may be seen as echogenic debris in the subarachnoid space in infants. An epidural or subdural hemorrhage may occasionally be seen as a fluid collection posterior to the cord. For bony fractures and more extensive traumatic insult including traumatic infarcts of the cord, an MRI is more useful. Beyond infancy the value of spinal

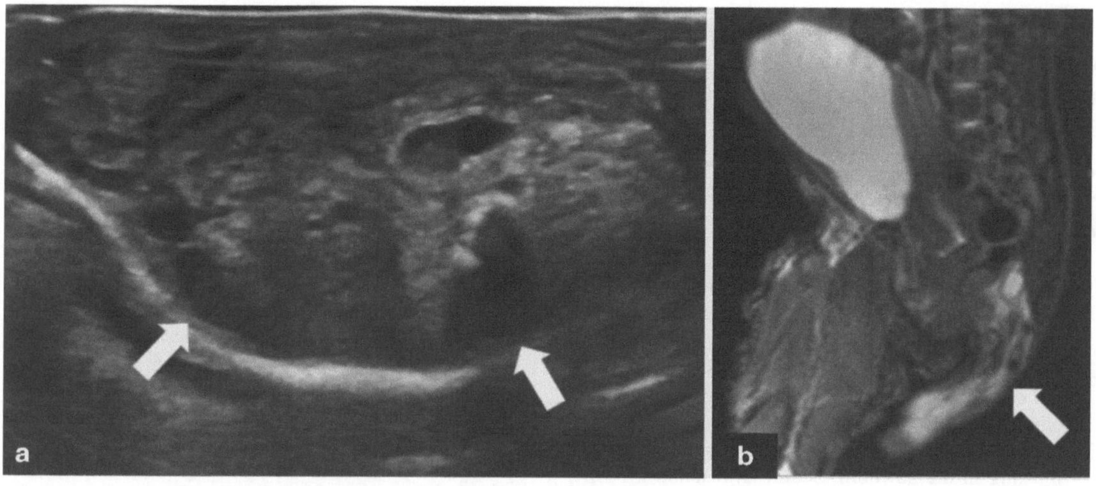

Fig. 2.9 Sacrococcygeal teratoma. Sagittal ultrasound image (**a**) and sagittal MRI T2-weighted (**b**) of the perineal region. Exophytic, heterogeneous mass with solid and cystic components *(arrows)*, consistent with type I sacrococcygeal teratoma

sonogram is rapidly reduced. It remains useful for evaluating posterior spinal collections and seromas after surgery [1].

With the recent focus on child abuse, a study by Edelbauer et al. suggests use of spine sonography in less than 6-month-old infants for evaluating subdural collections. Spinal trauma with ligamentous injuries and cord insult are described with non-accidental trauma. Spinal subdural collections are also common in the presence of subdural haemorrhage in the cranium. Ultrasound may in future prove to be a valuable adjunct in evaluating extra-axial collection in the spinal canal in this patient group [12].

Prenatal Diagnosis

During second trimester routine screening fetal ultrasound scans the skin overlying the spine is evaluated for integrity. The spinous processes form a linear echogenic line. The absence of skin and the spinous process herald the presence of an open neural tube defect. The splayed ossification centers lateral to the defect is seen on axial imaging. When the defect is covered by a thick sac, it may represent skin covering of a closed neural tube defect. Indirect signs of a myelomeningocele in the brain in the form of frontal notching and small posterior fossa can be seen. Closed spinal dysraphisms are generally occult and difficult to diagnose prenatally unless associated with a lipomyelomeningocele that protrudes significantly away from the canal. Sporadically some of these have been diagnosed prenatally. Visualizing the level of the conus prenatally is challenging, however a significantly low-lying conus below L3 may point towards underlying occult spinal dysraphism. Anterior sacral meningocele and sacrococcygeal teratomas are diagnosed prenatally in a large percentage of patients. Smaller defects, particularly closed spinal dysraphisms and intradural lipomas may not be apparent on prenatal scanning [13].

Summary

Vertebral ossification is not complete in the first half of infancy and sound beam transmits through the cartilage. This combination makes imaging the spinal canal with sonography possible. Sonography is usually the first imaging exam to be performed in infants because of its simplicity, low cost, and lack of deleterious effects. Another advantage of sonography over most imaging modalities is its capacity to visualize the motion of the filum terminale, which is restricted in tethered cord. In this chapter, the ultrasound techniques, the indications and the imaging findings of the most common disorders involving the infant's spine are reviewed.

References

1. Levin D. The pediatric spinal canal. Diagnostic ultrasound, Barnewolt and Rumack. 4th ed. Philadelphia: Elsevier Mosby; 2011.p. 1733–67.
2. Nelson MD, Jr., Sedler JA, Gilles FH. Spinal cord central echo complex: histoanatomic correlation. Radiology. 1989;170:479–81.
3. Ladino Torres MF, DiPietro MA. Spine ultrasound imaging in the newborn. Semin Ultrasound CT MR. 2014;35:652–61.
4. Drolet BA, Chamlin SL, Garzon MC, Adams D, Baselga E, Haggstrom AN, Holland KE, Horii KA, Juern A, Lucky AW, Mancini AJ, McCuaig C, Metry DW, Morel KD, Newell BD, Nopper AJ, Powell J, Frieden IJ. Prospective study of spinal anomalies in children with infantile hemangiomas of the lumbosacral skin. J Pediatr. 2010;157:789–94.
5. Kriss VM, Desai NS. Occult spinal dysraphism in neonates: assessment of high-risk cutaneous stigmata on sonography. AJR Am J Roentgenol. 1998;171:1687–92.
6. Weprin BE, Oakes WJ. Coccygeal pits. Pediatrics. 2000;105:E69.
7. Drolet BA. Cutaneous signs of neural tube dysraphism. Pediatr Clin North Am. 2000;47:813–23.
8. Badve CA, Khanna PC, Phillips GS, Thapa MM, Ishak GE. MRI of closed spinal dysraphisms. Pediatr Radiol. 2011;41:1308–20.
9. Nievelstein RA, Valk J, Smit LM, Vermeij-Keers C. MR of the caudal regression syndrome: embryologic implications. AJNR Am J Neuroradiol. 1994;15:1021–9.
10. Lynch SA, Wang Y, Strachan T, Burn J, Lindsay S. Autosomal dominant sacral agenesis: currarino syndrome. J Med Genet. 2000;37:561–6.
11. Kocaoglu M, Frush DP. Pediatric presacral masses. Radiographics: Rev Publ Radio Soc North Am. Inc. 2006;26:833–57.
12. Edelbauer M, Maurer K, Gassner I. Spinal subdural effusion—an additional sonographic sign of child abuse. Ultraschall Med. 2012;33:E339–43.
13. Ben-Sira L, Garel C, Malinger G, Constantini S. Prenatal diagnosis of spinal dysraphism. Child's nerv syst: ChNS: Off J Int Soc Pediatr Neurosurg. 2013;29:1541–52.

Surgical Ultrasound of the Pediatric Head and Neck

3

Guy F. Brisseau

Introduction

Ultrasound of the pediatric head and neck has allowed clinicians to more quickly diagnose and manage their patients. In the office, real-time ultrasound has also allowed demonstration of pathology, or normality to the parents. Biopsies, should you wish to perform them, can also be performed more accurately and safely. Together these contemporarily performed procedures save both the patient's and parent's time [12]. Timely, efficient care of the highest quality are key components of patient and family-centered care.

In the clinical setting, such as a hospital, the capabilities of pediatric ultrasound are further enhanced by the addition of anesthesia and sedation. These adjuncts enhance our diagnostic and therapeutic options in our pediatric patient since fear, anxiety, and pain are no longer factors for the clinician to have to struggle with.

In order to perform a high-quality ultrasound of the neck, one must have an intimate knowledge in many aspects of the diseases and use of technology. These include the clinical areas such as normal anatomy, clinical diseases, and anatomic pathology. Surgeons, and others, have this knowledge given the nature of their clinical practice. While necessary, this knowledge is insufficient to perform pediatric head and neck ultrasound. The clinician's knowledge must also extend to the ultrasound technology being used. This includes physics, use of equipment, settings, and interpretation of images and artifacts. Finally, the technical aspects of performing the ultrasound examination must be mastered. The technical aspects must further be reinforced when procedures are planned under ultrasound guidance. When all knowledge and skills are correctly applied, interpretation of the images becomes possible and with sufficient experience fairly straightforward.

This chapter discusses the general approach to the ultrasound of the pediatric head and neck. We then discuss and illustrate different uses of ultrasound in the pediatric patients.

General Approach

Examination of any pediatric patient can be challenging and this can be associated with a significant degree of anxiety. Approaches to relieve the anxiety will go a long way to making the examination experience better for the child, parents, and the clinician. As with all procedures, preparation is a key to success. In the office, establishing a rapport with the patient before the ultrasound exam is key. This involves building trust and often involves letting the patient see you perform part of the examination on yourself or the parents. The setting should be warm and the light dimmer, should ideally be located close to

G. F. Brisseau (✉)
Department of Surgery, Division Chief Pediatric Surgery, Sidra Medical and Research Center, Weill-Cornell Medical College,
26999, Doha, Qatar
e-mail: guybrisseau@me.com

S. Scholz, M. D. Jarboe (eds.), *Diagnostic and Interventional Ultrasound in Pediatrics and Pediatric Surgery*, DOI 10.1007/978-3-319-21699-7_3

your examination station. Distraction equipment is sometimes quite helpful [11]. Some offices have a dedicated ultrasound room while others move the machine. Either is acceptable so long as the quality of the imaging is not compromised.

After preparation, the patient is positioned for the examination. Ideally, this would be in the supine position or slight reverse Trendelenburg. The neck should be extended by placing a small roll under the shoulders. This position allows the best access to the neck. The cooperative patient will allow this and will also move as needed to access all aspects of the neck. Unfortunately, pediatric patients do not read the same text you are reading now. A well laid out room and building trust can go a long way to achieving your goal of cooperation, however, this sometimes is not enough. In these cases, alternatives can be used such as having a parent hold the child in a parent's arm for comfort rather than restraint. This is followed by a limited examination that is necessary to decide on care. In the end, the office-based examination may have to be abandoned and repeated at another time or in another setting. The hospital or clinic setting that affords sedation and anesthesia allows for a more thorough examination. This also allows procedures to be done more easily.

Equipment

The equipment today is relatively inexpensive and can be very portable. When selecting your equipment several factors must be considered. These are the particular machine and the transducer. Characteristics to consider for head and neck ultrasound are the portability and computing power of the machine. The selection of transducers that are available for that machine must also be considered. The portability is important for the utility in both the clinic and the hospital setting. Unless you have a dedicated room and do not need to move your machine often, portability must be considered. The portability is balanced against the image quality. Image quality is generated by the computing power of the machine and the transducers used. Today's portable machines, though small, give excellent computing power to meet the needs of pediatric head and neck ultrasound. Other characteristics of the machine to consider include the ability to carry out high-quality Doppler and color flow analysis. Again, most commercial machines allow these features, although the quality can vary. Figure 3.1 shows a portable ultrasound in an operating room.

The transducer must have several important characteristics. These include the frequency, the array, and the footprint. The most common transducer used for head and neck ultrasound is a linear array probe. Occasionally, a curvilinear probe may be used for wider field visualization but this is rarely needed in children. The footprint of the transducer must be appropriate to the patient. Given the varied size of the pediatric age group, generally two linear probes are used with different footprints (Fig. 3.2a). This must be balanced against the price of the probes ranging from US $ 5–10,000. If only one probe is possible, then the small "hockey stick" type probe is the most versatile (Fig. 3.2b). Finally, the transducer

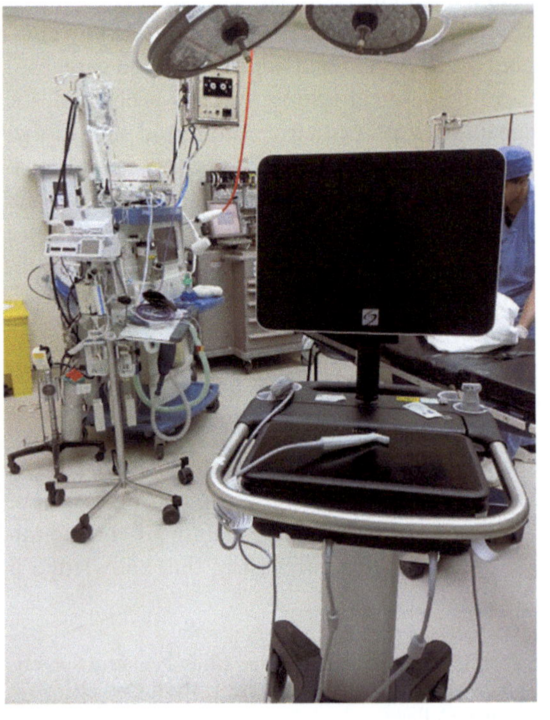

Fig. 3.1 A portable ultrasound machine in the operating room

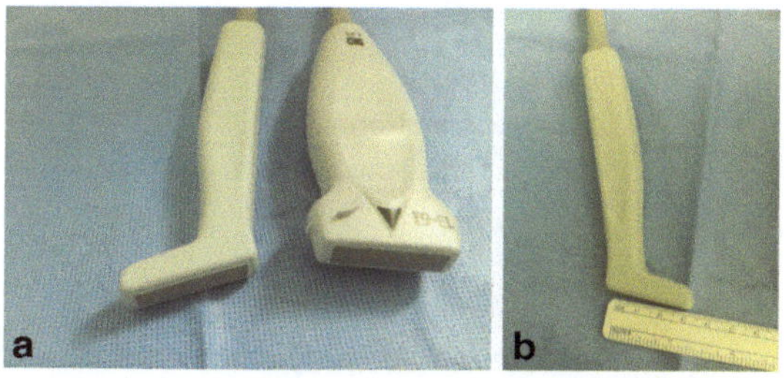

Fig. 3.2 **a** and **b**. Two linear probes with different configurations. The "hockey stick" probe

must have a high frequency for the most detailed pictures. Given the thinness of the neck, a high-frequency probe should be used to optimize the picture. This probe would ideally be 10–15 MHz although some use probes down to 7.5 MHz.

The final, and often overlooked, piece of equipment to be decided upon and used is the documentation system. Without documented images and an interpretation, the highest quality of care is not being ensured. This is both for the individual care and for the quality assurance methodology used in your practice. The capture and documentation may be part of an electronic picture archiving and communication system (PACS) within a hospital or a printer and a handwritten interpretation in an office chart. The principles, however, are the same. Representative images and an interpretation are needed to provide excellent patient care. Figure 3.3a, b demonstrates a patient with thyroiditis showing an enlarged and hypervascular gland. Documentation of these images in the chart is critical for this patient's ongoing care.

Once the equipment and the patient are prepared, an approach to the patient is necessary. The first fundamental question to be asked is what is the purpose of the ultrasound examination? Are you doing a complete head and neck ultrasound or do you want a limited scan? What is the clinical indication? Is it to assess a mass? Is it to assess the patency of a vein? Is it to assess the thyroid gland? Each of these studies will have a different approach.

A complete examination of the head and neck must cover all anatomic structures and a general screen of the head and neck. There is no standard sequence within the profession [1]. Institutions or individuals must develop their own approach. However, an internal systematic approach must be done the same way every time. This systematic approach ensures that all organs and areas of the head and neck are examined. The complete examination is often done is an ultrasound department as part of a comprehensive examination.

While clinicians can do a comprehensive ultrasound examination, they often perform a focused examination to answer a clinical question and obtain any specific information. Further information may be obtained on ultrasound depending on the initial findings. An example of this is assessment of the lymph nodes when a thyroid mass

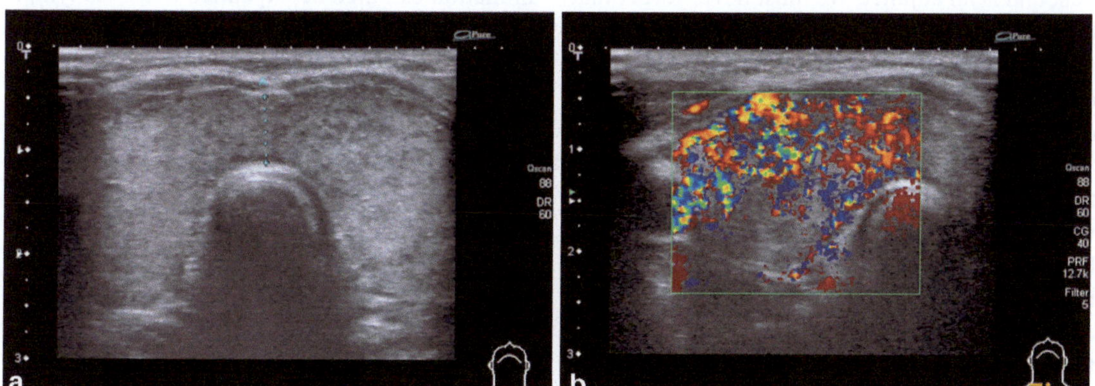

Fig. 3.3 **a** A 4-year-old girl with a thyroid gland scanned in the transverse plane demonstrating coarse echotexture and edema suggestive of thyroiditis. **b** The same patient with color Doppler demonstrating hypervascularity

Table 3.1 Differential diagnosis of neck masses based on location

	Anterior neck	Lateral triangle
Congenital	Lymphatic malformation	Lymphatic malformation
	Vascular malformation/hemangioma	Vascular malformation/hemangioma
	Thyroglossal duct cyst	–
	Brachial cleft cyst	–
Acquired	Lymphadenopathy	Lymphadenopathy
	Thyroid mass	Lipoma
	Parathyroid mass	Paraganglioma
	Thymus (ectopic or mass)	Torticollis

is detected. Thus, clinicians are able to make a decision of further examination or intervention based on the data obtained real time. Beyond the technical aspects, more timely use of the new information is possible since the performing clinician is often the primary clinical decision-maker for this patient. The scanning technique between a complete and focused examination is the same, it is merely a decision to focus the examination to answer a specific clinical question, such as what is this mass?

One of the most common conditions asked about in pediatric patients is the lump in the neck. The assessment of this involves a detailed history and physical examination, and ultrasound is used to confirm the diagnosis or to answer a specific question such as what is this mass or does lymphadenitis have a liquefied center?

In this chapter, we discuss some of the ultrasound characteristics that are helpful in diagnosing these masses. However, as a clinician the ultrasound is an adjunct. We must never forget that the history and physical examination give us a plethora of information that will guide us to our differential diagnosis. The ultrasound adds more data to this clinical decision-making process.

Following the history and physical examination, one easy approach is to anatomically decide what region the lesion is in. Some lesions are in both. The anatomic location helps differentiate the possible lesions. Table 3.1 presents a differential diagnosis of neck masses based on location being in the anterior neck (medial to the sternocleidomastoid muscle (SCM)) or lateral neck (lateral to the SCM and including the SCM).

The anterior neck contains three normal structures; we will assess as we look at a mass. Masses can come from all three. These organs are the thyroid gland, parathyroid gland, and thymus. The thyroid gland is the easiest of the three to visualize. This bi-lobar structure curves over the trachea in the lower neck. It has an isthmus that projects superior in the midline. Scanning of the thyroid should be assessed in two planes. The probe is easily slid over the lobes and simple maneuvers can allow scanning of the entire gland (Fig. 3.4).

Lesions of the thyroid are easily seen and can be solid or cystic. Often, there are multiple masses. No one characteristic is pathognomonic for neoplasia. However, size greater than 2 cm, microclacifications, and a completely solid lesion were predictive of neoplasia [15]. Given that neoplasia is much higher in the pediatric population, these findings warrant further investigations. If this was the lesion in question, examination can then be expanded to assess lymph nodes in both the anterior and lateral neck, as this is where regional spread would occur. This decision to further scan is made real time given your new information. Further, if the patient was old enough and cooperative, a fine needle aspiration under ultrasound control could be contemplated. The approach to interventional procedures will be discussed below.

The parathyroid glands are more difficult to identify and commonly are not seen. They are 6×4 mm in adults and smaller in pediatric patients. The identification of parathyroid glands on ultrasound is suggestive of a pathologic process [13].

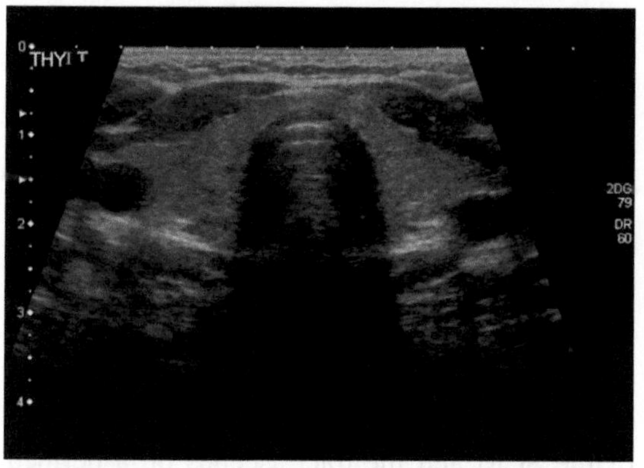

Fig. 3.4 A normal thyroid scanned in the transverse plane

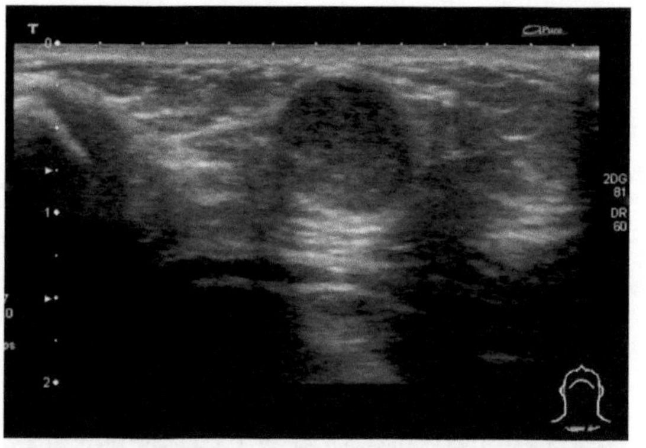

Fig. 3.5 A midline oval thyroglossal cyst in a 1-month-old infant. Note the increased posterior acoustic enhancement deep to the cyst confirming the fluid contents

The thymus can be found in the inferior–anterior neck. The thymus is normally 2.5 × 3 cm in newborn babies. Its relative size dissipates as the child grows. However, abnormality of organ migration can lead to ectopic thymus. This mass will live in the anterior neck. Ultrasound can easily assess this mass. Thymic tissue has a course echostructure similar to liver. It is easily delineated from the surrounding structures and has normal flow. It can have tissue going into the superior mediastinum. Besides ectopic normal thymus, cysts and occasionally masses will develop. These masses appear markedly different compared to the normal surrounding thymus. They may be solid or cystic.

Besides the three normal organs, a common mass is found in the midline. This midline anterior mass is a thyroglossal duct cyst. This superior cyst comes from the descent of the thyroid in the neck from the foramen cecum at the base of the tongue. Failure of obliteration of the thyroglossal duct can lead to cyst formation. Ultrasound has two roles in this disease process. The first is the diagnosis of the thyroglossal duct cyst. The second is to prove the existence of a normal thyroid since this midline mass may represent an ectopic thyroid and failure of decent. The thyroglossal duct cyst is a thin-walled midline cyst that is anechoic to hypoechoic. There is posterior enhancement present. This enhancement is an artifact from the fluid-filled cyst and is helpful in diagnosing fluid-filled structures (Fig. 3.5).

If the cyst has been infected, the wall is often thicker and the fluid may be more turbid. The location of the cyst is infrahyoid in up to 65 % of the cases; however, it can also be suprahyoid. A small percentage can be intralingular [13]. Movement of the tongue outward causes an upward movement of the cyst both on physical and ultrasound examination. Ultrasound when compared to computed tomography (CT) and magnetic resonance imaging (MRI) is the best imaging modality to diagnose thyroglossal duct cysts [7].

Another common cystic mass in the neck is lymphatic malformations. These are also known as cystic hygromas and lymphangiomas. These lesions can be in any part of the body including in all aspects of the head and neck. They are congenital in nature but may present well after birth with an increase in size due to infection or bleeding. Ultrasound of the neck presents an ideal modality for both diagnosis and treatment of these complex lesions. These lesions present in a continuum from a microcystic relatively solid mass, to a macrocystic fluid-filled and typically multi-septated mass. The ultrasound characteristics vary accordingly; however, some common features do prevail. The cyst of a lymphatic malformation typically demonstrates a hypoechoic or anechoic nature with a simple wall (Fig. 3.6). If bleeding or infection has occurred, the individual or multiple cysts may show debris within rather than a simple anechoic fluid. In the case of

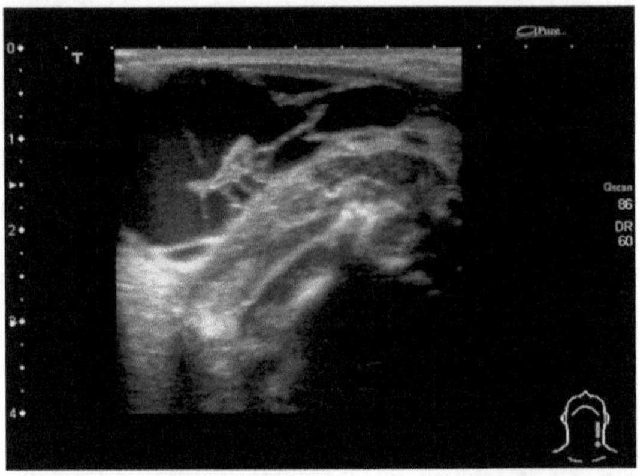

Fig. 3.6 Lymphatic malformation in a 3-day-old female on the left neck scanned in the sagittal plane. Ultrasound demonstrates an anechoic fluid collection with septations and is compressible with minor pressure. Posterior enhancement is also present

bleeding as a presentation, layering of the clotted blood within the cyst may be seen.

After diagnosis of the lymphatic malformation, appreciation of the lesion in relation to the organs of the head and neck is important to plan therapeutic interventions. Therapeutically, ultrasound allows for aspiration and injection of a sclerosing agent into the cysts. Multiple agents have been used including sodium dodecyl sulfate (SDS) [5], tetracycline [5], OK-432 [8], and bleomycin [17]. All sclerosing agents have a similar outcome and elicit an inflammatory response. All appear safe when used properly.

Our protocol involves aspiration of a near total volume from the cyst while leaving the needle in place. Bleomycin at a dose of 0.3–0.6 mg/kg (maximum 30 mg) is diluted into 30 cc of normal saline (NS). This solution is then injected into the cyst or multiple cysts. The patient is then observed for 3 months, assessed and if necessary another session of sclerotherapy is planned. These procedures can be done on an outpatient basis with same day discharge. Inflammation typically appears 1–5 days later and is treated with analgesia. The cysts then slowly dissipate over several months. Several factors appear to effect outcomes. Macrocystic disease is most effectively managed with this therapy. There is 50% complete resolution and 15–40% significant improvement [5, 8]. Often multiple sessions are needed to achieve success in a patient with multiple lesions and should be planned for. Microcystic disease is less amenable to sclerotherapy but larger cysts can be considered for sclerotherapy.

Besides lymphatic abnormalities, another cyst can be located in the anterior neck at the border of the SCM, a branchial cleft cyst. This can be confused with a lymphatic abnormality. The most common is the second branchial cleft cyst. This solitary cyst is on the anterior border of the SCM and the tract ascends on a defined tract going through the bifurcation of the carotid vessels, then ending within the palatine tonsil. The third and fourth branchial cleft cysts are much rarer and may involve the thyroid. They are also called pyriform sinus fistulas. Real-time ultrasound again proves useful in these disease processes. A solitary cyst in the neck in the typical location differentiates this from a lymphatic malformation. The second brachial cleft cyst is located anterior to the SCM and lateral to the carotid vessels. The third or fourth branchial cleft cysts are located more inferior and often in proximity to the thyroid. The cyst is often anechoic or hypoechoic with a thin wall. In this case, there is posterior enhancement (Fig. 3.7). If there has been infection, the fluid may be more turbid and the walls may be more heterogeneous. Thus, real-time ultrasound can help differentiate between cystic masses that can appear identical in history and physical examination.

The final structures to talk about in the anterior neck are the vessels, both arterial and venous. Vascular access, thrombosis, and ultrasound approaches will be discussed in a chapter dedicated to this common issue. Vascular diseases of the great vessels are rare in the pediatric age group. The classic arterial pathology is a carotid body tumor or paraganglioma, a rare tumor in the pediatric age group. This is typically a lesion of the carotid bifurcation that is solid and about 1–5 cm in size. Color Doppler demonstrates high flow and hypervascularization [3, 18].

Carotid body tumors when discovered need a more extensive workup than can be provided by ultrasound alone.

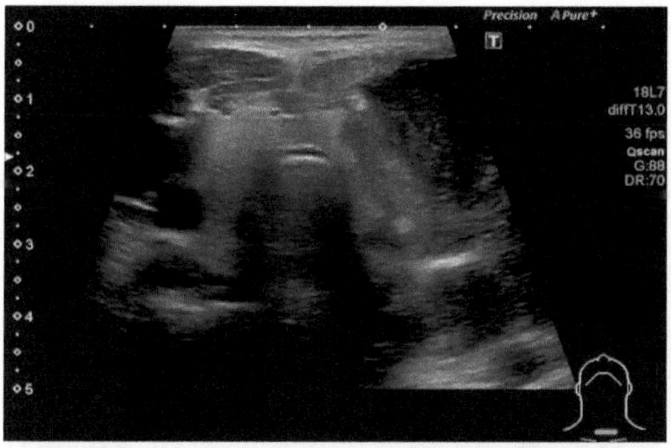

Fig. 3.7 A 9-year-old female presents with recurrent left neck abscesses. A fourth branchial cleft cyst is identified. Note the location to the thyroid gland thus requiring a hemithyroidectomy

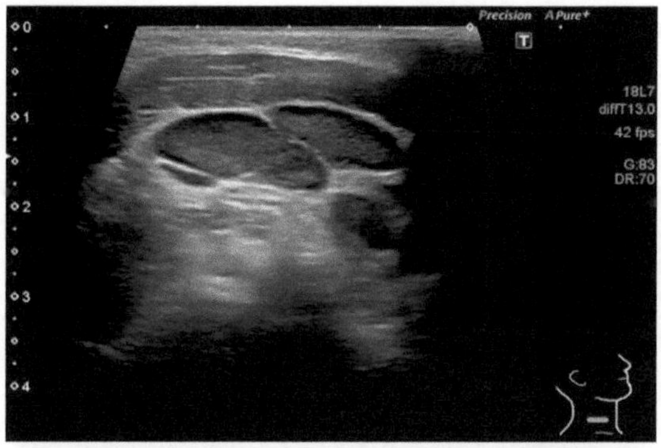

Fig. 3.8 Reactive lymphadenopathy in the right side of the neck in a 4-year-old child. Note the oval configuration and the fatty echogenic center of the nodes

Vascular malformations of the head and neck are much more common and are the most common tumor of the head and neck in infancy. They can be found in all areas of the head and neck. Ultrasound features of vascular malformations are fairly classic. These lesions are heterogeneous and are either hypo- or echogenic. Proliferative hemagiomas are more solid, while vascular malformations have more prominent vascular structures. Vascular flow on color Doppler demonstrates multiple internal vessels. The velocity of flow is proportional to the amount of arteriovenous fistulization. As with lymphatic malformations assessing the relationship to other structures is critical [6].

Lateral Neck

Lymphatic malformations can be present in both the anterior and lateral neck. Another organ that can be present in both with a greater predominance in the lateral neck is pathologies of the lymph nodes. These lymphadenopathies can be infectious, immunologic, metabolic as well as neoplastic.

Lymphadenopathies are one of the most common reason for a pediatric head and neck ultrasound examination. Examination involves multidimensional scanning in grey scale as well as assessment of flow with Doppler. For very superficial lymph nodes, a stand off gel pad will help bring the lesion into the focal zone of the ultrasound field. Multiple characteristics have been studied to try to distinguish neoplasia from inflammatory causes. These include number, size, shape, echogenicity, and the border characteristics. Unfortunately, no characteristics are proven to be a distinguishing feature. These characteristics must also be used along with the clinical symptoms of the patient to decide about a diagnosis or next step. One unique but uncommon finding is calcifications in an abnormal lymph node. This finding is predictive of papillary thyroid cancer [10, 14].

With respect to the ultrasound findings, lymphadenitis from infectious causes typically appears as homogenous, hypoechoic, and round masses (Fig. 3.8). They may be matted together. They have an echogenic hilum and individually they are greater than 5 mm. The individual size can often be difficult as the mass of nodes becomes matted. As this inflammatory phlegmon of matted nodes progresses, the center can liquefy and need drainage. The ultrasound is superior at diagnosing liquefaction compared to physical exam especially in large edematous masses. The ultrasound characteristics of liquefaction demonsrate a change from a homogeneous mass to a heterogeneous one. In the beginning of this process, there are multilocular heterogeneous areas with debris and septations. Over time, these multiple locules often coalesce into one single large

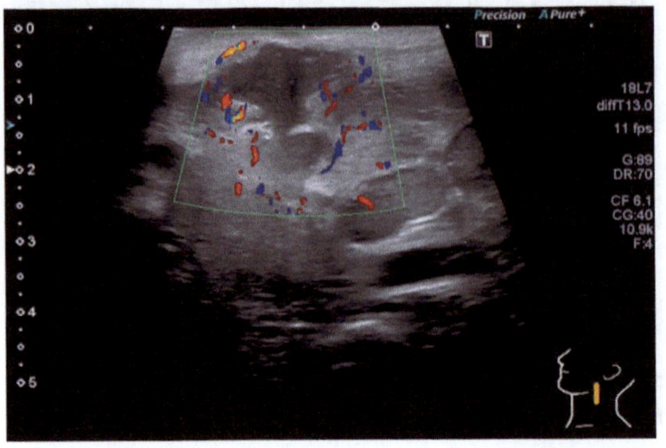

Fig. 3.9 Sagittal view of the left neck in a 5-year-old boy with fever, tenderness, erythema, and swelling of the left neck. The ultrasound demonstrates an area of low echogenicity with no Doppler signal. This area extends to the surface and is within an area of adjacent enlarged lymph nodes

abscess (Fig. 3.9). As the abscess forms, there is no flow in the center and a variable thickness of rim can develop. The ultrasound can then be used to facilitate needle aspiration for microbiologic diagnostic or therapeutic interventions.

Ultrasound unfortunately cannot differentiate neoplastic from inflammatory and infectious causes of lymphadenopathy. Neoplastic lymph nodes may be multiple and separate or matted as a single mass. They are homogeneous and often do not have an echogenic hilum. Necrosis and liquefaction within the lymph node mass is rare.

Other than a site of primary tumor, the cervical lymph node may also be a site for metastatic spread of neoplasia. The most common of these is thyroid cancer, but the differential also include neurogenic tumors, rhabdomyosarcoma, and nasopharyngeal carcinoma. These lesions are often discreet and can be in multiple lymph nodes. Metastatic lymph nodes are homogeneous, echogenic, and nontender. If multiple lymph nodes are identified, the thyroid gland as well as the neck in general should be assessed for primary pathology. Further imaging and possible biopsy may be necessary.

Ultrasound can also be used to confirm other diagnoses in the clinic that, in prior decades, we may have felt that an ultrasound is not really needed given the requirement for another visit.

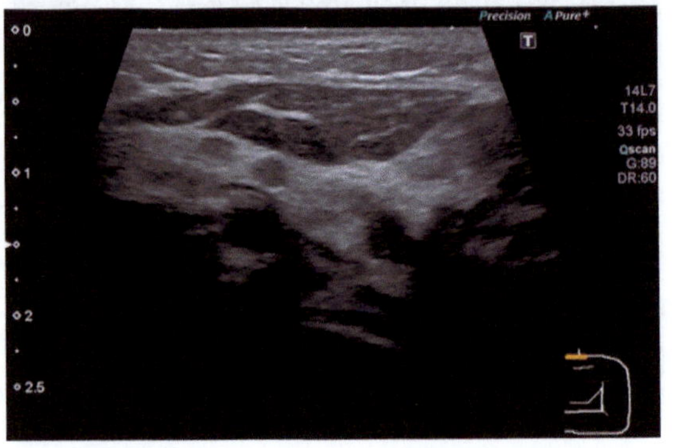

Fig. 3.10 Normal sternocleidomastoid muscle in a 1-month-old boy

An example of this is the sternocleidomastoid "tumor" of congenital torticollis. Congenital torticollis is a fibrotic process with shortening and thickening of the sternocleidomastoid (SCM) muscle. Babies with torticollis present in the first few months of life with a turned head and a thick and hard mass in the SCM muscle. The history often is characterized by prolonged or traumatic delivery. Physical examination demonstrates a thickened SCM muscle with a mass. Parents present worried and often have been told there is a suspicious mass in their young child's neck. The diagnosis and treatment were often made in the past with no imaging. Many parents remain frightened, and cervical MRI under general anesthesia is a common modality requested by pediatricians in this setting. The real time use of ultrasound has aided in care of the patients and family. This SCM tumor is characterized by its location within the body of the SCM and its borders fade into the normal muscle. It is echogenic and often heterogeneous depending on the fibrosis and stage of the mass. Figure 3.10 demonstrates a normal SCM, while Fig. 3.11 shows the SCM tumor. The lesion can be anywhere in the SCM but often is in the lower half of the muscle. Once diagnosed, nonoperative management with active and passive stretching exercises guided by a physical therapist is needed, which almost always resolves the problem over time. This therapy does not result in immediate resolution of the mass and the ultrasound further reassures parents that their persistence is warranted.

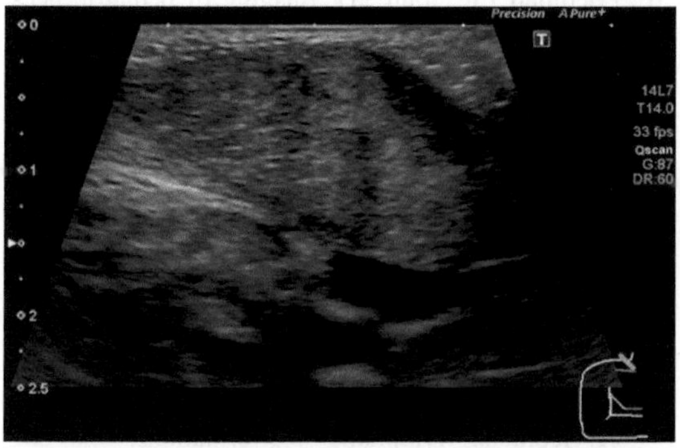

Fig. 3.11 The same child has an enlarged SCM muscle compared to the normal side with increased enchogenicity on the effected side. *SCM* sternocleidomastoid muscle

Several other miscellaneous masses can arise in the neck in the pediatric age group. These are teratomas and neurogenic tumors. Teratomas contain all three germ cell layers. Thus, the teratoma can have a variety of tissue types. The ultrasound features show a mass that is typically round. It is located in both, the anterior or lateral neck. It is heterogenous given the solid and cystic nature of the tumor. Depending on the makeup of the particular mass there are often both, echogenic as well as hypoechoic areas. Sometimes, calcifications can be seen within the cyst.

Neurogenic tumors in children are most commonly neuroblastomas and neurofibromas. They are hypoechoic solid masses located in the paraspinal area typically behind the vessels of the neck. The ultrasound cannot distinguish the two or the neoplastic process. Therefore, further imaging is required.

Interventions of the Neck

Until now we have primarily discussed the use of ultrasound as a diagnostic adjunct for the head and neck. There is an interventional use for ultrasound in the pediatric patient with head and neck pathology. Vascular access is discussed in another chapter. However, the technique of vascular access is not different than that of accessing any lesion, either for biopsy or therapeutic intervention. The concepts of in-plane (parallel) and out of plane (perpendicular) scanning approaches are the same. For biopsy purposes, a decision of a core biopsy or fine needle aspiration must be decided depending on the differential diagnosis. Most lesions, other than lymphoma, can be diagnosed with fine needle aspiration. Fine needle aspiration gives cytologic, while core biopsy give pathologic diagnosis with tissue architecture. Both, fine needle aspiration and core biopsy should be carried out under real-time ultrasound control. Fine needle aspiration is relatively safer since the core biopsy needles take a larger piece of tissue and can damage nearby structures. This is especially important in the neck where many vital structures such as large vessels and nerves are very close together. Other than diagnostic biopsy, ultrasound can also allow aspiration of liquid for diagnostic testing such as culture.

Therapeutic interventions can also be carried out including aspiration of lymphadenitis that is liquefying as well as sclerotherapy for lymphatic malformations. We have discussed the effectiveness of ultrasound guided sclerotherapy for lymphatic abnormalities [8, 9]. There is also a developing body of literature that ultrasound aspiration of neck abscesses may be a superior therapy compared to traditional open drainage [2].

All of these procedures, while possible under local anesthesia, most frequently are carried out under sedation. In the vast majority of pediatric patients, this is best done under general anesthesia since sudden movement during the procedure can be catastrophic.

Besides pure interventional work with the ultrasound and a needle, this technology has allowed for hybrid surgical approaches. Hybrid approaches use ultrasound to guide the open operations on neck lesions. With the use of intraoperative ultrasound, the incisions are directed to the lesion and an extended neck incision and dissection can be avoided. This technique is useful in selected cases such as biopsy of a deep lymph node or removal of a lesion that is hard to palpate. In parathyroid surgery, this approach has changed an entire approach to a disease process. Ultrasound and other localizing techniques have eliminated mandatory four gland exploration for primary hyperparathyroidism. Selective parathyroid exploration for parathyroid adenoma is the gold standard with ultrasound having the most utility. After localizing studies demonstrate a solitary lesion ultrasound guidance with solitary parathyroidectomy can eliminate a significant operation with potential complications and make it into the technical equivalent of a lymph node biopsy [4, 16].

Summary

Pediatric surgical ultrasound of the head and neck allows the clinicians real-time access to data that can aid in their care of the patient. It improves timeliness of care and is an integral part of office- and hospital-based practice. Expertise in medical knowledge as well as the performance and interpretation of imaging is critical for the clinician to have optimal patient outcomes. Ultrasound represents one modality of imaging and is part of a continuum. Ultrasound has limitations and other modalities may be essential. The best care for these patients require all physicians involved in imaging of our patients to collaborate more than ever before.

References

1. AIUM. AIUM practice guideline for the performance of ultrasound examinations of the head and neck. J Ultrasound Med (Official Journal of the American Institute of Ultrasound in Medicine). 2014;33(2):366–82. doi:10.7863/ultra.33.2.366.
2. Biron VL, Kurien G, Dziegielewski P, Barber B, Seikaly H. Surgical vs ultrasound-guided drainage of deep neck space abscesses: a randomized controlled trial: surgical vs ultrasound drainage. J Otolaryngol Head Neck Surg (Le Journal D'oto-Rhino-Laryngologie Et De Chirurgie Cervico-Faciale). 2013;42(1):18. doi:10.1186/1916-0216-42-18.
3. Derchi LE, Serafini G, Rabbia C, De Albertis P, Solbiati L, Candiani F, et al. Carotid body tumors: US evaluation. Radiology. 1992;182(2):457–9. doi:10.1148/radiology.182.2.1310163.
4. Dimas S, Michas S, Christakis I, Augoustis C, Alevizaki M. Minimally invasive parathyroidectomy in patients with previous neck surgery. Hormones (Athens). 2012;11(2):160–5.
5. Farnoosh S, Don D, Koempel J, Panossian A, Anselmo D, Stanley P. Efficacy of doxycycline and sodium tetradecyl sulfate sclerotherapy in pediatric head and neck lymphatic malformations. Int J Pediatr Otorhinolaryngol. 2015;79(6):883–7. doi:10.1016/j.ijporl.2015.03.024.
6. Friedman ER, John SD. Imaging of pediatric neck masses. Radiol Clin North Am. 2011;49(4):617–32,v. doi:10.1016/j.rcl.2011.05.005.
7. Huoh KC, Durr ML, Meyer AK, Rosbe KW. Comparison of imaging modalities in pediatric thyroglossal duct cysts. Laryngoscope. 2012;122(6):1405–8. doi:10.1002/lary.23262.
8. Kim DW. OK-432 sclerotherapy of lymphatic malformation in the head and neck: factors related to outcome. Pediatr Radiol. 2014;44(7):857–62. doi:10.1007/s00247-014-2889-0.
9. Kim SY, Lee S, Seo J-M, Lim SY. Postoperative adjuvant OK-432 sclerotherapy for treatment of cervicofacial lymphatic malformations: an outcomes comparison. Int J Pediatr Otorhinolaryngol. 2015;79(4):570–5. doi:10.1016/j.ijporl.2015.01.030.
10. Lee YS, Hong SW, Chang H-S, Park CS. Scattered psammomatous calcifications around papillary thyroid carcinoma. World J Surg. 2014;38(7):1738–42. doi:10.1007/s00268-014-2460-z.
11. Lim SH, Kim M-J, Lee M-J. Use of animated cartoons with children's songs to increase compliance with ultrasonography in young children. Yonsei Med J. 2013;54(6):1533–7. doi:10.3349/ymj.2013.54.6.1533.
12. Matt BH, Woodward-Hagg HK, Wade CL, Butler PD, Kokoska MS. Lean six sigma applied to ultrasound guided needle biopsy in the head and neck. Otolaryngol Head Neck Surg (Official Journal of American Academy of Otolaryngology-Head Neck Surgery). 2014;151(1):65–72. doi:10.1177/0194599814528659.
13. Policeni BA, Smoker WRK, Reede DL. Anatomy and embryology of the thyroid and parathyroid glands. Semin Ultrasound CT MR. 2012;33(2):104–14. doi:10.1053/j.sult.2011.12.005.
14. Pyo J-S, Kang G, Kim D-H, Park C, Kim JH, Sohn JH. The prognostic relevance of psammoma bodies and ultrasonographic intratumoral calcifications in papillary thyroid carcinoma. World J Surg. 2013;37(10):2330–5. doi:10.1007/s00268-013-2107-5.
15. Smith-Bindman R, Lebda P, Feldstein VA, Sellami D, Goldstein RB, Brasic N, et al. Risk of thyroid cancer based on thyroid ultrasound imaging characteristics: results of a population-based study. JAMA Intern Med. 2013;173(19):1788–96. doi:10.1001/jamainternmed.2013.9245.
16. Soon PSH, Delbridge LW, Sywak MS, Barraclough BM, Edhouse P, Sidhu SB. Surgeon performed ultrasound facilitates minimally invasive parathyroidectomy by the focused lateral mini-incision approach. World J Surg. 2008;32(5):766–71. doi:10.1007/s00268-007-9436-1.
17. Yang Y, Sun M, Ma Q, Cheng X, Ao J, Tian L, et al. Bleomycin A5 sclerotherapy for cervicofacial lymphatic malformations. J Vasc Surg. 2011;53(1):150–5. doi:10.1016/j.jvs.2010.07.019.
18. Zaupa P, Höllwarth ME. Carotid body paraganglioma: rare tumor in a 15-year-old adolescent boy. J Pediatr Surg. 2007;42(4):E13–7. doi:10.1016/j.jpedsurg.2007.01.059.

The Thorax

4

Christine M. Leeper, Jan Gödeke and Stefan Scholz

Introduction

With limitations imposed by bone and air, the thorax at first seems to be an unforgiving place to perform ultrasound. Although the thoracic sonography provides no overview of the entire thorax, it may provide valuable information in addition to other studies such as plain radiograph, computed tomography (CT), and Magnetic resonance (MR) imaging or alone. Ultrasound is without radiation exposure, noninvasive, inexpensive, and portable. Indications for thoracic ultrasound include opacities or other abnormality on chest radiograph, detection and characterization of pleural effusion, a widened mediastinum or suspicion for mediastinal mass, in the workup of pleural, juxta-diaphragmatic, and peripheral chest lesions as well as the evaluation of diaphragmatic mobility [1].

S. Scholz (✉)
Division of Pediatric General and Thoracic Surgery, Children's Hospital of Pittsburgh of UPMC, University of Pittsburgh School of Medicine, One Children's Hospital Drive, 4401 Penn Avenue, Pittsburgh, PA 15224, USA
e-mail: stefan.scholz@chp.edu

C. M. Leeper
Department of General Surgery, University of Pittsburgh Medical Center, 200 Lothrop Street, Pittsburgh, PA 15213, USA
e-mail: leepercm@upmc.edu

J. Gödeke
Department of Pediatric Surgery, University Medical Center Mainz, Mainz 55101, Germany
e-mail: jan.goedeke@unimedizin-mainz.de

Technical Requirements

For the ultrasound examination of the thorax, probes used in sonography of the abdomen, thyroid, or the vasculature can be suitable. Basic B-mode real-time ultrasound is generally all that is required. Probe selection varies by target anatomic structure. A high-resolution linear transducer is required for the examination of superficial structures such as the chest wall and pleura as well as for neonates and young children. For deeper lung lesions in older patients, a lower frequency probe is required. Sector transducers with small contact areas can be used intercostally, but these investigations are also possible with convex transducers. It should be noted that device settings that are used for echocardiography are not suitable for the rest of the mediastinum; the contrast, the frame rate, and the grayscale depth compensation must be adjusted for mediastinal structures. In these cases, one should use linear or convex transducers, especially if there are near-field processes [2, 3].

The use of M-mode imaging has proved helpful in the evaluation of pneumothorax and quantification of diaphragmatic motion [4, 5]. Doppler and color flow imaging should be used for all lesions close to the diaphragm. For instance, anomalous feeding vessels may be demonstrated

S. Scholz, M. D. Jarboe (eds.), *Diagnostic and Interventional Ultrasound in Pediatrics and Pediatric Surgery,* DOI 10.1007/978-3-319-21699-7_4

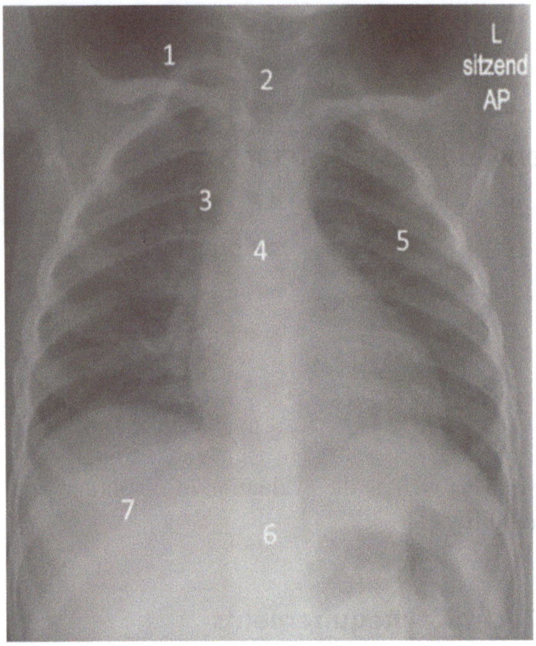

Fig. 4.1 Acoustic windows for thoracic sonography: 1. supraclavicular, 2. suprasternal, 3. parasternal, 4. transsternal, 5. intercostals, 6. subxyphoid, and 7. subdiaphragmatic

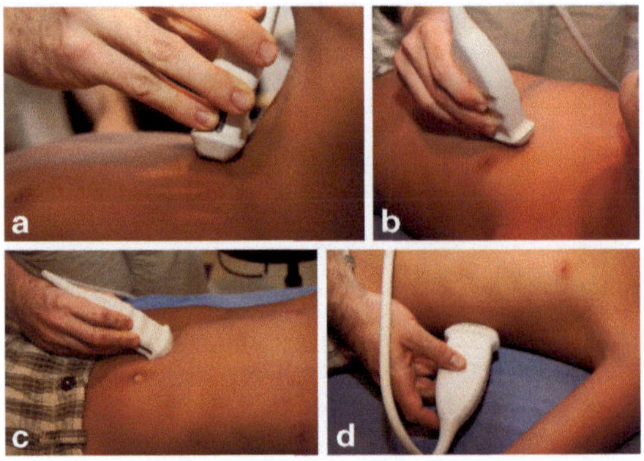

Fig. 4.2 Demonstration of select acoustic windows for assessment of the pediatric chest. **a** Suprasternal, **b** Parasternal, **c** Subxiphoid, and **d** Transdiaphragmatic. [2]

arising from the aorta in the abdomen in a suspected pulmonary sequestration.

Ultrasound Examination

If the patient's condition or cooperation permits, the investigation should be performed in a seated position by inspiration and expiration optionally combined with respiratory maneuvers such as coughing or "sniffing." Respiratory excursions may help to evaluate subpleural structures behind the ribs. Additionally, placing the hands behind the head may lead to an expansion of the intercostal spaces and may facilitate the access window.

Intrathoracic pathology is systematically examined using the longitudinal lines on the thorax as a guide. Acoustic windows may include: (1) supraclavicular, (2) suprasternal, (3) parasternal, (4) transsternal, (5) intercostals, (6) subxyphoid, and (7) subdiaphragmatic (Fig. 4.1 and Fig. 4.2), though this will be dictated by the pathology. In addition, the examination should follow oblique thoracic lines along the intercostal spaces from dorsal to ventral. Intercostal scanning allows imaging of the lung and pleura throughout the thorax and of the posterior mediastinum. The posterior chest must always be examined in suspected pleural effusions, as fluid tends to accumulate posteriorly whenever the patient lies supine in bed. Ventilated intensive care unit patients should be turned slightly to the side, so that both dorsal thorax sides become alternately accessible.

To evaluate the diaphragm and the inferior thoracic cavity, subdiaphragmatic and subxiphoid should be obtained using the liver, the spleen, or the fluid-filled stomach as an acoustic window. The examination of the thoracic inlet starts at the base of the lateral cervical triangle. The apex of the lungs and parts of the subclavian vessels can be evaluated via supraclavicular and transaxillar windows. For this examination, the patient's shoulders are positioned on a pillow to help extend the neck for better access. With higher resolution probes (>5 MHz) even branches of the brachial plexus can be evaluated [6]. The anterior mediastinum is examined with the suprasternal and parasternal views in the left and right lateral position. Suprasternal or supraclavicular approaches may also be useful in examining the anterior mediastinum and thoracic vessels [3].

The Mediastinum

The contents of the mediastinum are organized into three compartments: anterior (thymus, vessels, lymphoid structures, and nerves), middle (trachea, mainstem bronchi, the heart and great vessels, and the hilar lymph nodes), and posterior (aorta, esophagus, and the sympathetic nerve chains). Particularly suitable sonographic windows to the mediastinum are the parasternal plane, suprasternal plane, and transsternal plane, especially in babies, as the bones are not yet well ossified, which allows for improved ultrasound access to the chest. The anterior-superior mediastinum up to the aortopulmonary window is easily visible via transjugular ultrasound examination. As a supplement, transesophageal and transbronchial ultrasonography may offer valuable information.

Anterior Mediastinum

Thymus

The thymus is the dominant structure within the upper pediatric chest and is critical in the development of the immune system. It is located in the anterior superior mediastinum and consists of two lobes that are fused in the midline. The size, shape, and imaging finding of the normal thymus changes with age. The thymus appears largest relative to patient size at birth and may extend into the neck or down to the cardiac apex. It increases in weight through puberty, achieving maximal weight between 12 and 19 years. After puberty, the thymus slowly involutes [7].

The thymus is easily accessible for ultrasound examination. The normal thymus has a triangular shape in the longitudinal section, while in cross section it generally shows a trapezoidal or horseshoe like shape (Fig. 4.3a and 4.3b). The thymus is located in the anterior to the great vessels; caudally it sits on the heart and sometimes extends to the diaphragm. Sonographically, a normal thymus has a homogeneous and reticular echotexture and is slightly less echogenic than the liver, spleen, and thyroid gland. It is hypovascular on Doppler imaging and has well-defined margins, as it is surrounded by a demarcating capsule. The abnormal sonographic thymus, therefore, will have an irregular or lobular margin, heterogeneous echogenicity, coarse echotexture, and calcifications [8].

Thymic Aplasia/Hypoplasia

Thymic aplasia is a condition where no thymic tissue can be detected due to underdevelopment or involution of the organ. The ultrasound examination is the diagnostic method of choice and is superior to the chest radiograph. A diminished thymic size is seen in infants and children during physiologic stress; however, most of the times it is a pathologic state. Etiology may be a primary congenital defect as in DiGeorge syndrome or ataxia telangiectasia, or may be a secondary to long-term glucocorticoid therapy or human immunodeficiency virus (HIV) [9].

Thymic Hyperplasia

Thymic hyperplasia is a disorder whereby there is an increased production of the normal thymic tissue. It is usually a benign process related to a stress situation or disease, for example, burns, other severe systemic illness, chemotherapy, or radiation therapy. It is important to distinguish this from thymic or other mediastinal mass or neoplasm, which ultrasound is able to do readily. Sonographically, the thymus maintains an echotexture and echogenicity which is identical compared to the normal thymus. The position of the thymus is normal in most cases, although the shape may be changed.

Thymic Masses

Primary thymic neoplasms in children are rare and usually incidental findings [10]. Thymomas occur in older children and adolescents who may present with paraneoplastic syndromes or myasthenia gravis [11]. These can be heterogeneous tumors with areas of necrosis and calcification (Fig. 4.4a, 4.4b, 4.4c), in contrast with thymolipomas which are homogeneously echogenic due to their high fatty content.

Secondary neoplastic thymic infiltration is more common and occurs with leukemia, lymphoma, and Langerhans cell histiocytosis.

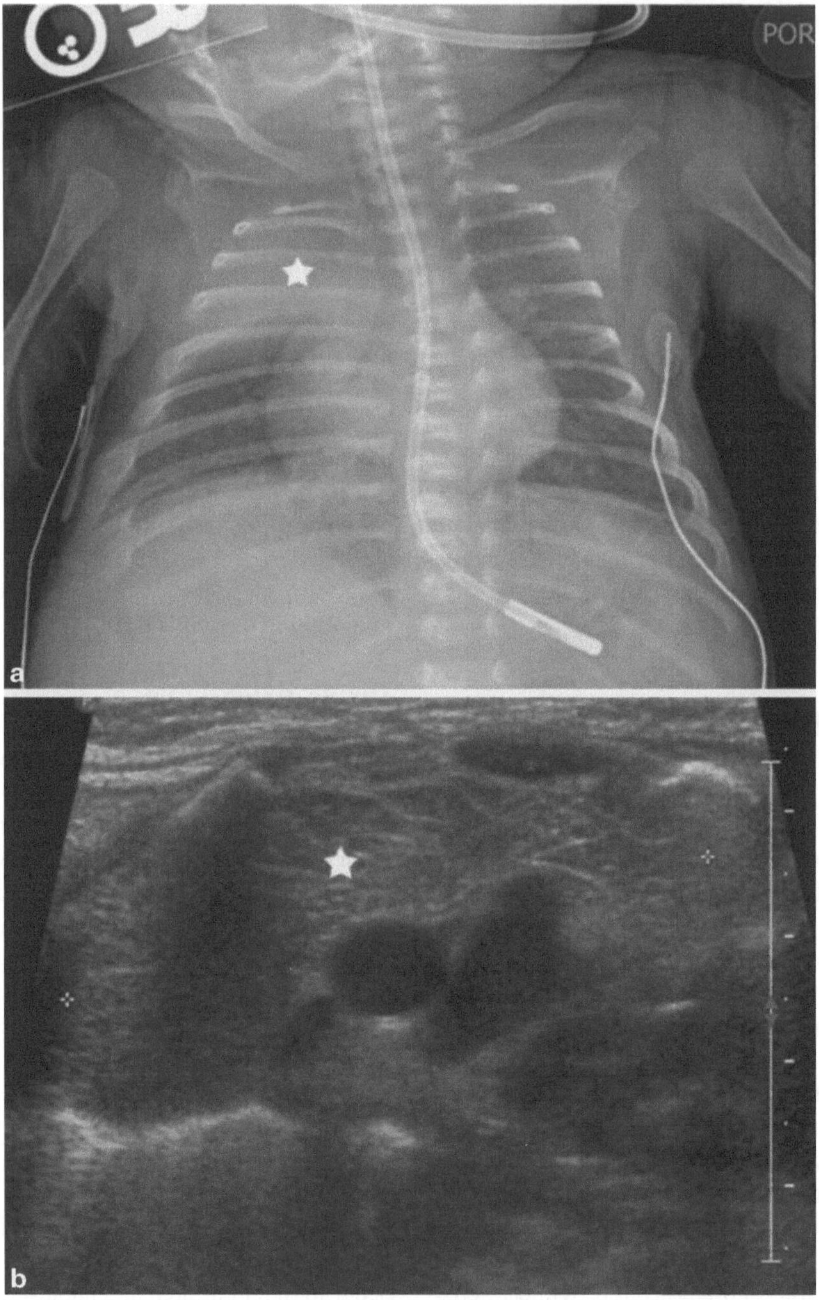

Fig. 4.3 Images of normal thymic tissue. **a** Chest radiograph demonstrates opacity in the right upper lobe *(star)*. **b** Ultrasound reveals normal thymic tissue *(star)*. [2]

In these cases, the normal sonographic thymic pattern is replaced with variably echogenic and heterogeneous soft tissue and associated abnormal lobulation of the thymic capsule (Fig. 4.5). An infiltrated thymus loses its normal compliance and may be seen to displace and distort adjacent structures instead of conforming to their shape [9].

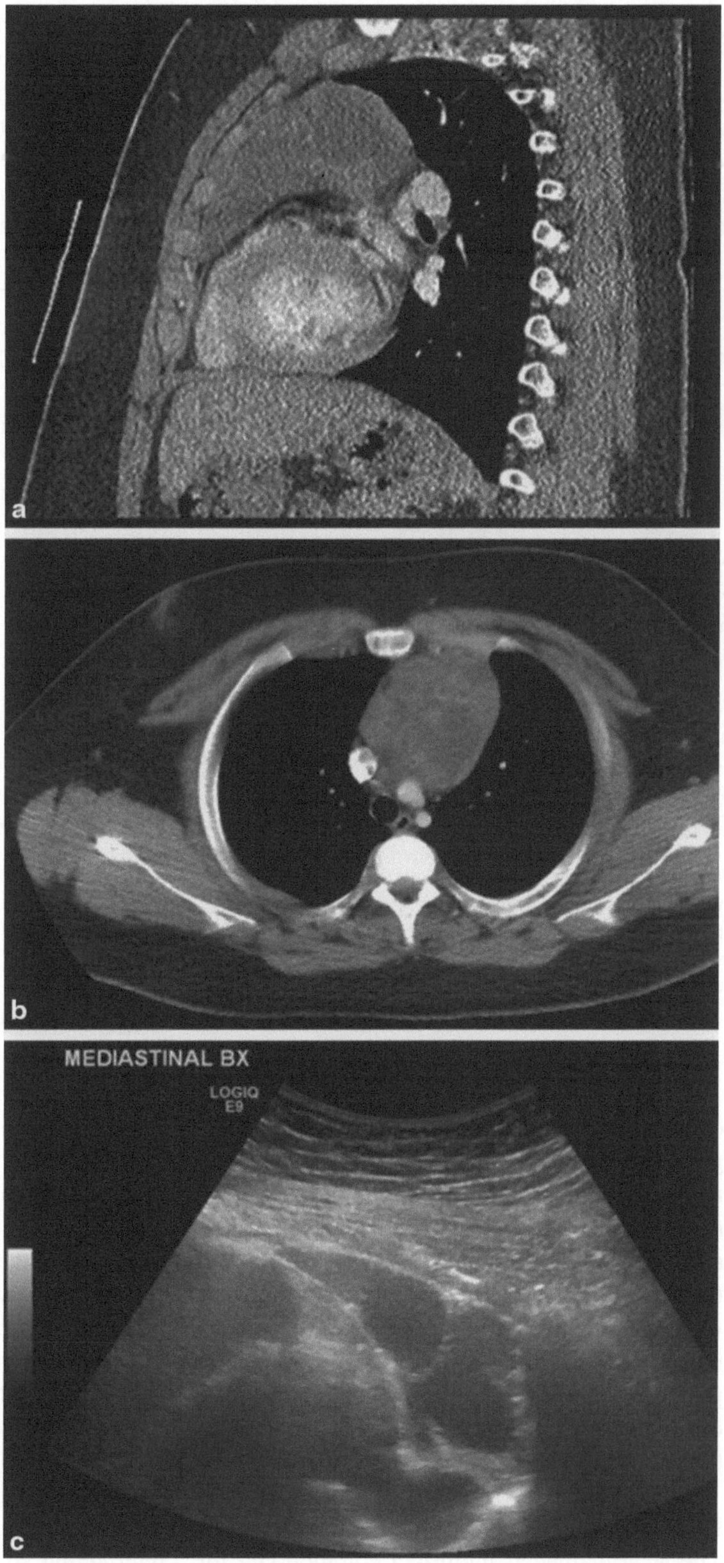

Fig. 4.4 Thymoma. **a** Ultrasonography shows a large mediastinal mass consisting of complex, septate, partly hyperechoic solid areas, and partly hypoechoic cystic areas. **b** and **c** CT scan confirms large mediastinal mass and heterogeneous nature

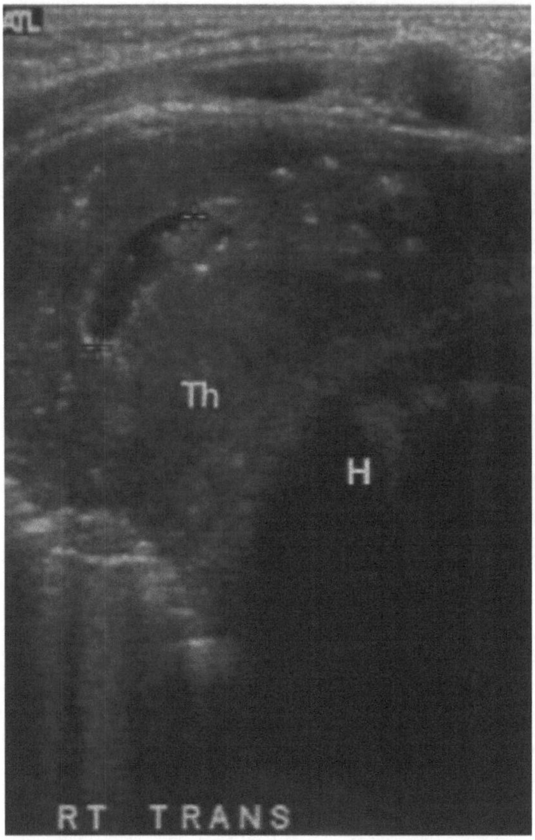

Fig. 4.5 Langerhans' cell histiocytosis with thymic involvement. Transverse ultrasound scan demonstrates disruption of normal thymic anatomy with cystic area and strongly echogenic irregular foci, which proved to be calcifications on CT (*Th*—thymus, *H*—heart). [40]

Benign thymic cysts can arise from remnants of the thymopharyngeal ducts or result from degeneration of the thymus itself after mediastinal trauma or surgery. Most congenital cases of thymic cysts are diagnosed in childhood, presenting as slowly enlarging masses that may extend into the neck. Thymic cysts typically are unilocular with imperceptible walls and anechoic contents, though superimposed hemorrhage or infection produces cyst contents of variable echogenicity or even debris [8]. Sonographic demonstration of their continuity with the thymus allows diagnosis.

Lymphoma

The anterior mediastinum is a common site for neoplasms, in particular, lymphoma. The majority of children with lymphoma have anterior mediastinal involvement, more frequent with Hodgkin's lymphoma than with non-Hodgkin lymphoma. Patients may present with constitutional symptoms such as fever or weight loss, respiratory complaints. Sonographically, lymphomas may appear as discrete masses, nodal enlargement (Fig. 4.6), or with diffuse thymic infiltration. They tend to be hypoechoic and hypovascular compared with inflammatory processes and other neoplasms [9].

Germ Cell Tumor

Teratomas and other germ cell tumors may arise in the anterior (Fig. 4.7a, 4.7b, 4.7c) or posterior (Fig. 4.8) mediastinum. The ultrasound appearance of germ cell tumors is variable, ranging from purely soft tissue masses to heterogeneous masses containing fat, bone, and cystic elements. Tissue diagnosis is required before chemotherapy. Compression of the airways often associated with large anterior mediastinal masses is a contraindication for general anesthesia due to the danger of airway collapse [12]. Ultrasound-guided percutaneous biopsy is an excellent alternative in these patients and can be done safely under local anesthesia and mild sedation, even in critically ill patients.

Middle Mediastinum

Middle mediastinal lesions include cystic (bronchogenic, enteral duplication, pericardial, and lymphatic) and solid (lymphadenopathy) masses. Bronchogenic cysts are the most common intrathoracic cysts. They are thin-walled structures found around the carina that may compress or communicate with the trachea, resulting in collapse of a lobe. Esophageal duplication cysts may have a hypoechoic muscular rim typical of gastrointestinal duplications. Pericardial cysts have a typical appearance on plain radiographs and ultrasound can confirm their cystic nature. Lymphatic malformations are usually comprised of multiple loculated cysts with thin bands of intervening soft tissue. Normally hypovascular,

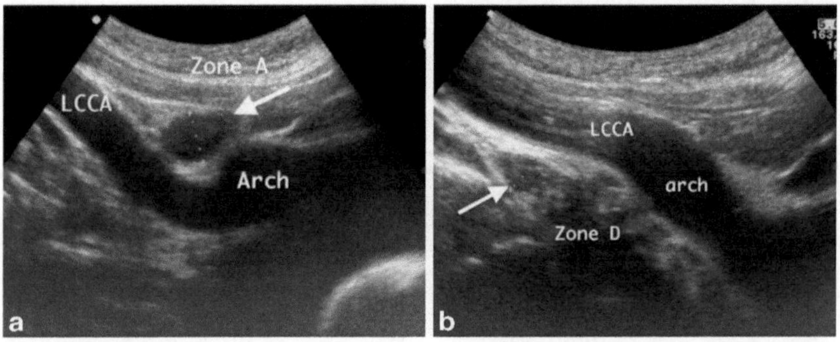

Fig. 4.6 Lymphadenopathy: Sagittal suprasternal ultrasound imaging in two children demonstrates lymphadenopathy. **a** A 3-year-old female lymphadenopathy *(arrow)* in *zone A* and **b** A 13-year-old male lymphadenopathy in *zone D*, which is echogenic in the center as compared to the echo-free vascular structures in recognized anatomical positions, that is, the aortic arch *(Arch)* and the left common carotid artery *(LCCA)*. [41]

lymphatic malformations may contain hemangiomatous components that demonstrate flow on color Doppler. Lymphatic malformations are frequently found in the vicinity of the great vessels and may cause compression of these vessels. Lymphadenopathy can arise from underlying neoplasia or infections, such as tuberculosis and fungal infections. Nodes appear abnormally enlarged and hypoechoic, often with hyperemia on color Doppler [2].

Posterior Mediastinum

Posterior mediastinal masses can often be best visualized via a posterior thoracic or paraspinal approach. Most of these are solid masses that arise from neural crest cells within the sympathetic ganglions. In order of decreasing malignancy, these include neuroblastoma, ganglioneuroblastoma, and ganglioneuroma [13]. The sonographic appearance of these tumors is nonspecific although calcifications can be seen; CT and MR imaging are more commonly used and more sensitive than ultrasound in this setting. Teratoma or other germ cell tumors can also be seen in the posterior mediastinum [14]. Less common are neurenteric cysts, hypoechoic thin-walled structures that have failed to separate from the neural canal during development [2].

Large Vessels

Vessels close to the heart are major arteries (aorta, pulmonary artery, and brachiocephalic trunk) and major veins (superior and inferior vena cava, internal jugular, and subclavian veins). Color Doppler ultrasound remains the principle method of investigation of vascular disease particularly within the subclavian and jugular vessels. Deep structures, such as the superior vena cava and the thoracic aorta, are difficult to evaluate sonographically in older pediatric patients and in these cases MR or CT angiography may be favored.

Vessel stenosis, aneurysms, and arteriovenous fistulae may occur from trauma, vascular access complications, or one of the arteritides. Diagnosis is made with color Doppler ultrasonography of the vessels. Arteriovenous fistulas demonstrate high diastolic arterial flow with elevated and turbulent venous flow. Stenoses demonstrate elevation of peak systolic flow through the narrowing, delayed systolic upstroke distal to the narrowing, and elevated diastolic flow due to downstream vasodilatation. Vascular malformations, intimal dissections, and other vascular anomalies can also be visualized directly by sonography.

The venous vessels are best visualized suprasternally. The most common indication for venous ultrasound is the evaluation of a suspected venous thrombosis. Acute thrombosis appears on ultrasound as hypoechoic material expanding the

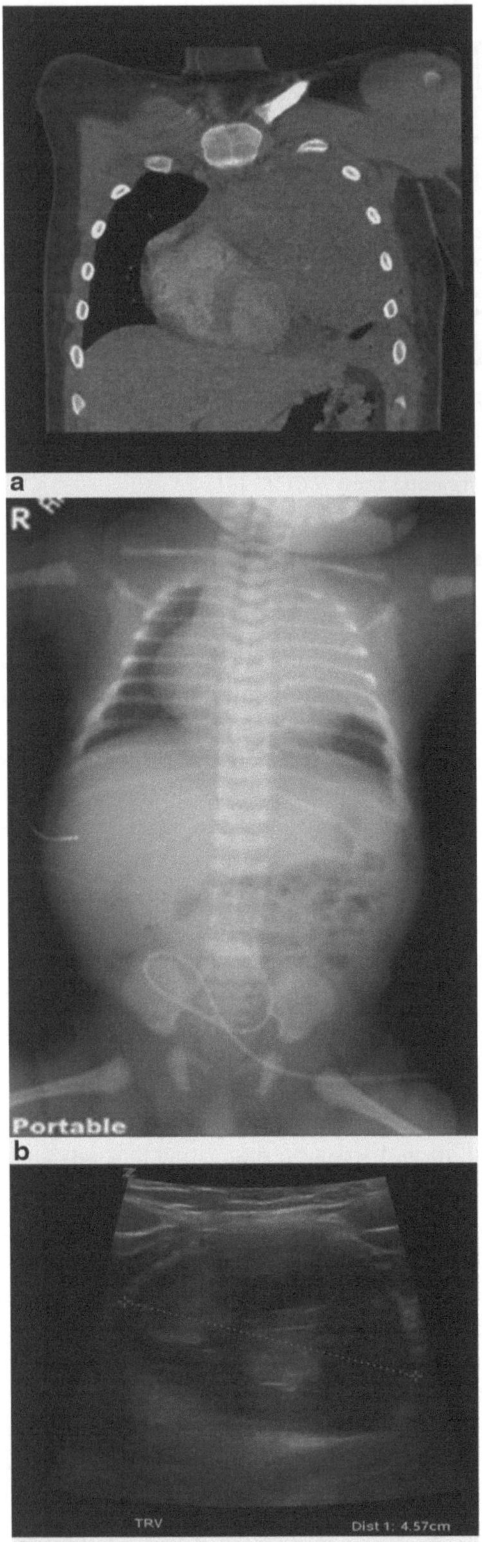

Fig. 4.7 Germ cell tumor, anterior mediastinal mixed germ cell. **a** CT scan and **b** chest radiograph demonstrate anterior mediastinal mass. Ultrasound **c** shows mass with mixed echogenicity, solid and cystic components

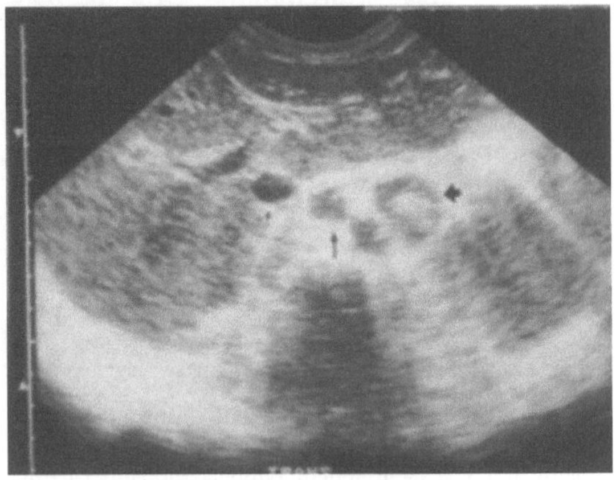

Fig. 4.8 Germ cell tumor, posterior mediastinal teratoma—42-mm wide mass of mixed echotexture in the posterior mediastinum displacing the inferior vena cave *(arrow)* and the aorta *(arrow)* anteriorly. [14]

vessel lumen (Fig. 4.9a, 4.9a, 4.9c, 4.9d, 4.9e). Since compression of the subclavian and deeper thoracic veins is not possible, color Doppler investigation of both sides is helpful in uncovering subtle flow differences to identify proximal venous thrombosis.

Thoracic Outlet Syndrome

Thoracic outlet syndrome produces neurologic or vascular symptoms from compression of neurovascular structures in the upper chest. Anomalous cervical or first thoracic ribs, the anterior scalene muscle, and vascular variants may all contribute and may be seen by ultrasound. MR imaging provides exquisite anatomic detail of the thoracic outlet, but duplex ultrasound may provide important physiologic information by demonstrating alterations in arterial and/or venous flow, especially during reproduction of the position in which symptoms occur. Arterial flow may show acceleration or dampening of flow, depending on the proximity to the stenotic segment. Venous flow is more commonly affected, and there may be engorgement of the lateral subclavian and axillary veins and loss of transmitted cardiac waveforms [15]. Thrombosis may complicate repetitive venous compression, a typical finding in

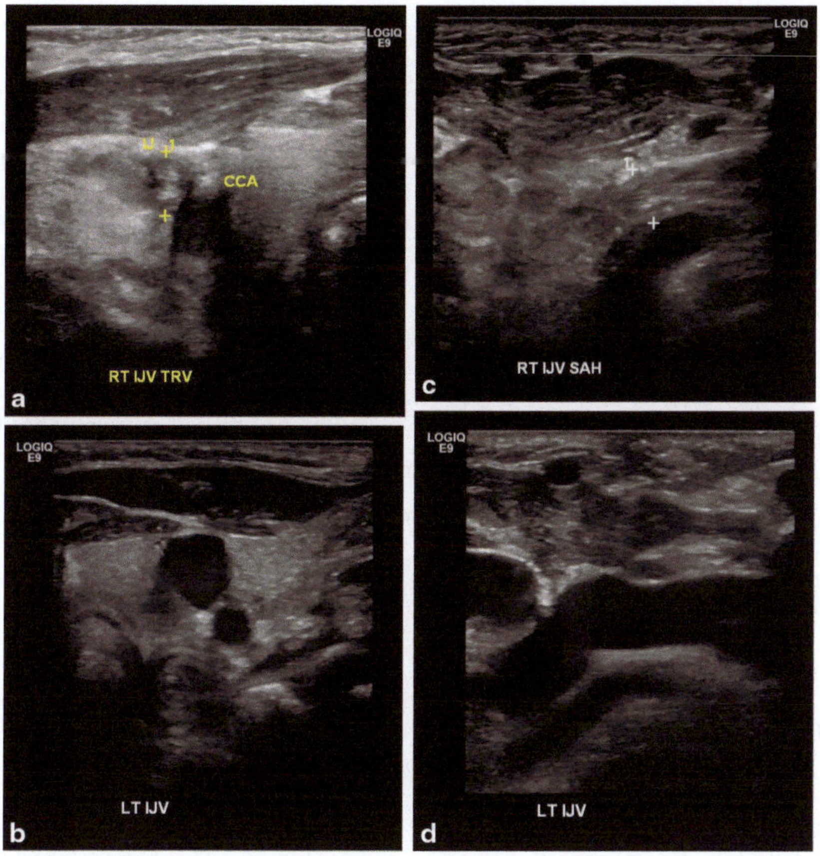

Fig. 4.9 Deep vein thrombosis of right internal jugular vein. Bilateral internal jugular veins are seen on sagittal (**a** and **b**) and transverse views (**c** and **d**)

Paget–von-Schrötter syndrome, which is readily diagnosable by duplex ultrasound [16].

Chest Wall

The chest wall consists of skin, subcutaneous tissue, muscles, bone, and cartilage. Pathology involving these superficial structures is often clinically apparent and is easily evaluated with high-frequency linear ultrasound transducers.

Ultrasound can be used in the diagnosis of many infectious or inflammatory pathologies. Osteomyelitis is seen as fluid adjacent to bone signifying exudative reaction (Fig. 4.10). Cellulitis appears as diffusely increased echogenicity while defined fluid collections secondary to abscess can be diagnosed and drained under ultrasound guidance [17]. Rib fractures are identified by ultrasound in victims of non-accidental trauma by demonstrating disruption of the rib's cortical surface as well as adjacent hematoma or callous formation depending on the age of the injury ([18], Fig. 4.11a and 4.11b). Traumatic separation of the costochondral cartilage from rib ends is visible sonographically but missed on plain radiographs.

Ultrasound reliably details the important variables for chest wall masses, including the location, size, contour, architecture, echographic pattern, compressibility, and relationship to other structures. Benign tumors, including hemangioma, lymphangioma, desmoid tumor, mesenchymal hamartoma, and lipoma, occur more commonly than malignant tumors [19]. Hemangioma can be diagnosed with a specificity of 98% using the criteria of vessel density greater than 5 vessels/cm^2 combined with a maximum

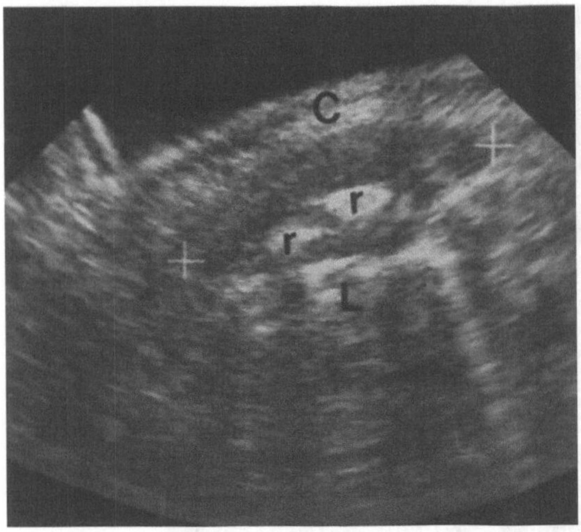

Fig. 4.10 Osteomyelitis. Longitudinal ultrasound scan of the right chest wall at the site of the soft tissue swelling. There is an obvious ovoid medium level echogenic structure around the ribs *(r)* indicating pericostal edema. *C*—chest wall, *L*—lung. [42]

systolic Doppler shift of greater than 2 kHz [20]. Lipomas are generally well-circumscribed echogenic masses usually located within the subcutaneous tissues. A lymph node can be identified by its echogenic fatty hilum containing the central nodal blood supply.

Other benign chest wall masses might not be easily diagnosed; tumors such as hemangioendotheliomas, tufted angiomas, and infantile myofibromatosis may share characteristics with hemagioma such that evaluation with CT, MRI, or biopsy is warranted for definitive diagnosis [8, 19, 21].

Venous malformations appear as a spongy, bluish deformable mass beneath the skin. Blood flow may be too slow to produce pulsed or color Doppler signal but with gentle compression and release the slow inflow of blood can be detected. Arteriovenous malformations are seen as jumbles of arteries and veins without associated mass. Lymphatic malformations have variably sized septated cystic components without flow on color Doppler most commonly found in the axillary region [22].

Malignant tumors of the chest wall most likely originate from bony structures, and may include Ewing sarcoma, rhabdomyosarcoma, and lymphoma [19]. Echogenicity of these malignant chest wall lesions is variable, and the margins may be distinct or infiltrative. Color Doppler flow of malignant chest wall lesions is usually increased. Chest wall and rib invasion can be detected as interruption of the normal muscular layers of the chest wall and loss of the normally smooth bony cortical surface. As with most other imaging, ultrasound is not histologically specific, and some benign lesions (such as abscesses and hematomas) may have aggressive sonographic appearances. Tissue sampling, often via ultrasound-guided biopsy, is usually needed for a definitive diagnosis.

Pleura

The healthy visceral and parietal pleura are poorly visualized on ultrasound examination, and evaluation of these structures relies on sonographic artifacts. For instance, the acoustic interface of the chest wall with normal aerated lung provides a strong reflective surface and produces a characteristic reverberation within the ultrasound image. This horizontal artifact is called an A-line and indicates the normal lung surface. The thin chest wall of infants and small children, however, may not demonstrate this artifact. In addition, aerated lung is also seen to move along the parietal pleural surface with respiration, termed the gliding sign [2].

Pleural Effusion

Ultrasound is able to demonstrate pleural effusions as small as 2–5 ml; therefore, it is much more sensitive in detecting pleural fluid than chest radiographs. The literature suggests that in most cases CT scan does not offer any advantage, and ultrasound may in fact be superior to CT for identifying debris or septated collections [23, 24] and in one study was associated with reduced need for VATS procedures and decreased readmission rates [25]. Ultrasound is a reasonable first-line modality for most patients with effusion, and CT scan should be reserved for complicated cases or preoperative planning.

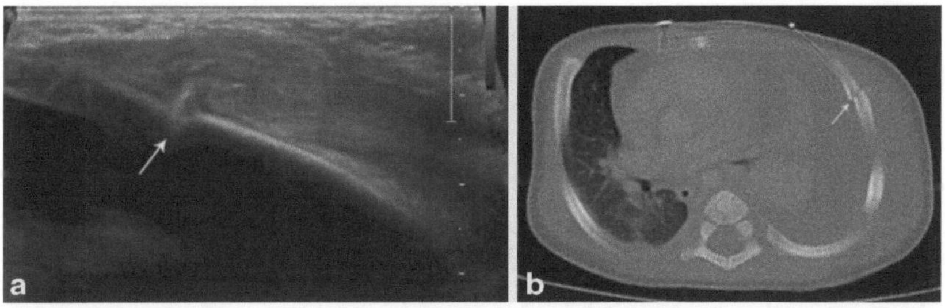

Fig. 4.11 Images in a 2-month-old boy with non-accidental trauma. Ultrasound **a** demonstrates a lateral left rib fracture *(arrow)* confirmed with CT **b** *(arrow)*. [2]

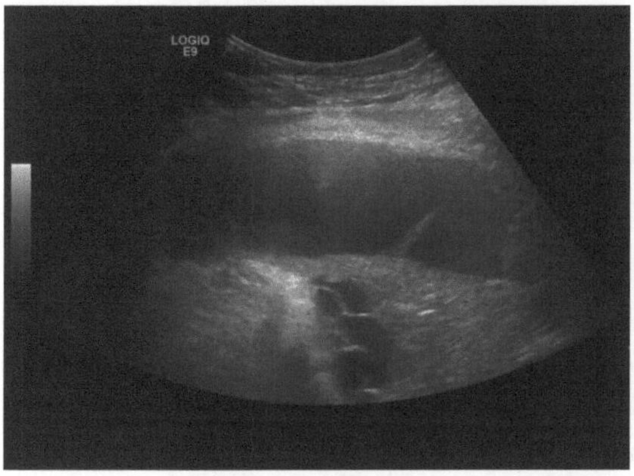

Fig. 4.12 Pleural effusion. Ultrasound demonstrates a mostly simple fluid collection with a few septations

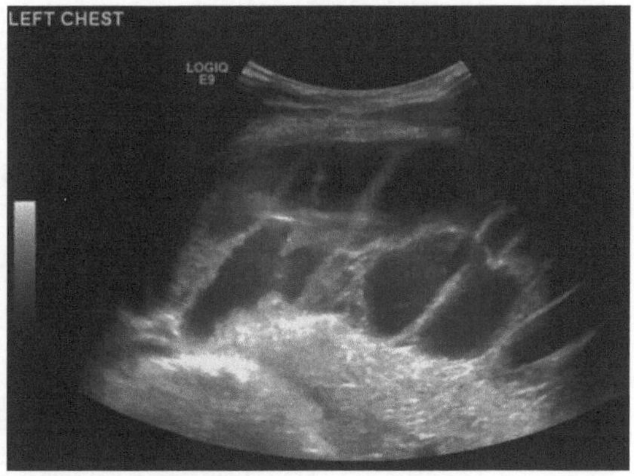

Fig. 4.13 Pleural empyema. Ultrasound demonstrates complex fluid collection with debris, loculation, and septations

The normal pleural space contains a tiny amount of fluid, but fluid is seen with ultrasound in less than 50% of normal healthy children. Small effusions may be visualized better while the patient is in an upright position. This tends to collect the fluid in the posterior costophrenic recess. The most suitable transducer positions are the cranially angulated subxiphoid cross section and the longitudinal section of the middle and posterior axillary line.

The most common etiology of a pleural effusion is a reaction to an adjacent pneumonia, but other causes may include reaction to thoracic surgery or trauma, reaction to a subphrenic abscess, or extension of mediastinal, retropharyngeal, or paravertebral infections [26]. An important characteristic of effusion that will dictate management is the fluid composition or whether the collection looks simple (Fig. 4.12) or complex (Fig. 4.13). There are three stages of organization for pleural effusion: exudative (simple, clear fluid), fibrinopurulent (loculations, fibrin strands, and empyema), and organized (thick rind) [26]. The sonographic appearance of pleural fluid changes depending on the stage and may range from completely anechoic, in the case of simple transudative collections, to collections with mobile echogenic debris in cases of infection and hemorrhage, to septated and more solid appearing collections with organizing infection. Simple non-loculated collections can be seen to change shape with patient breathing or change in position, while organizing fluid no longer changes with patient position or respiration. The distinction between echogenic fluid collections from more solid collections can be aided by the fluid color sign: With color Doppler, mobile de-

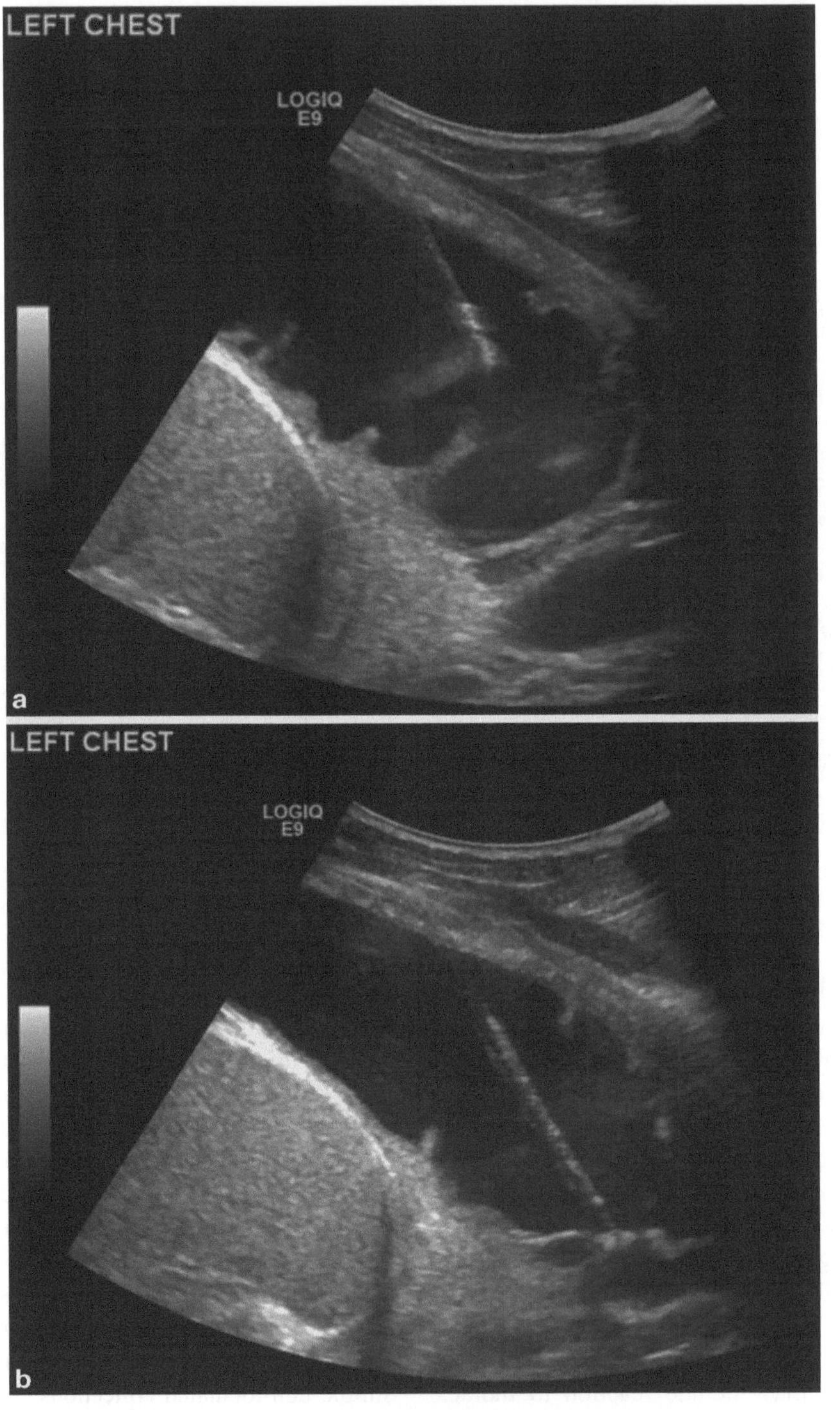

Fig. 4.14 **a** and **b** Ultrasound is utilized for image-guided percutaneous drain placement

bris will produce color signal whereas nonmobile solid material does not [27].

In addition to establishing the diagnosis of pleural effusion as well as the extent and position of the fluid, ultrasound may help to assess the exact position for fluid aspiration or drainage (Fig. 4.14a and 4.14b). Management of pleural effusion may range from drainage to fibrinolysis to operative decortication depending on the stage.

Solid Pleural Masses

Malignant disease involving the pleural space is much less common in children than in adults. It can occur for instance with Wilms tumor, neuroblastoma, leukemia, and sarcomas. Primary chest wall neoplasms and pleural metastases are often accompanied by hemorrhagic pleural effusions, which appear as echogenic debris-filled fluid in sonography. The presence of pleural fluid aids in detection of solid masses adherent to the parietal or visceral pleura.

Diaphragm

The diaphragm is a thin muscle that separates the thoracic cavity from the abdominal cavity. The diaphragm presents best next to the cardia (sternal section) and one may also visualize the diaphragm with high-resolution transducers cranial to the liver and spleen. Ultrasound is a valuable tool in assessing the diaphragm allowing delineation of juxta-diaphragmatic masses, contour abnormalities and hernias, and evaluation of diaphragmatic motion.

Diaphragmatic Hernia

A diaphragmatic hernia is a defect of the diaphragm that permits displacement of abdominal contents into the chest (Fig. 4.15a, 4.15b, 4.15c, 4.15d, 4.15e). Diaphragmatic hernias in infants are generally congenital, representing the most common intrathoracic anomaly seen in the fetus. In older children, they may also be acquired as a result of trauma.

Congenital diaphragmatic hernias (CDHs) (incidence 2.4:10,000) are located on the left in 80 % of patients, are more common in males, and are often associated with other congenital anomalies. Survival ranges from 50 to 90 % with major morbidity resulting from pulmonary hypoplasia [26].

Approximately 50–70 % of CDH are diagnosed antenatally by obstetric ultrasound. Fetal ultrasound features include polyhydramnios, intrathoracic bowel loops or stomach, an echogenic chest mass or mediastinal shift. The diagnosis can be made as early as 11 weeks, but most may not be evident until 16 weeks or later [28]. Postnatally, the diagnosis of CDH is often evident on chest radiograph with intestine visualized in the chest cavity. In cases that are equivocal, especially with right-sided hernias, ultrasound (sagittal and coronal scanning) becomes a useful modality for confirmation and further characterization. Ultrasound will demonstrate abdominal tissue extending into the thoracic cavity. While a herniation of liver or spleen is easily identifiable, the reliable detection of air-filled bowel or stomach might be more challenging.

Diaphragmatic Eventration/ Diaphragmatic Paresis

Eventration is an abnormal elevation of the diaphragm resulting from the incomplete development of the central tendon; this results in paradoxical motion during respiration which inhibits normal pulmonary function. This defect may be a congenital lesion or may be a complication of a birth trauma, mediastinal tumor, or cardiothoracic surgery [26].

The movement of the diaphragm has traditionally been examined by fluoroscopic screening, however, the use of ultrasound for this purpose in children is increasing due to the many advantages it affords [29]. The ultrasound must be performed with the child in quiet respiration. Difficulties arise for the sonographer when the child is on a ventilator as the ventilator fills the lungs with air causing the diaphragms to move down with inspiration even when paralyzed. In this case, it is best to assess the diaphragms for a short period of spontaneous breathing.

Sagittal or coronal imaging of the upper abdomen provides information about that particular hemidiaphragm, whereas transverse imaging allows comparison of both hemidiaphragms and evaluation for paradoxic motion with unilateral

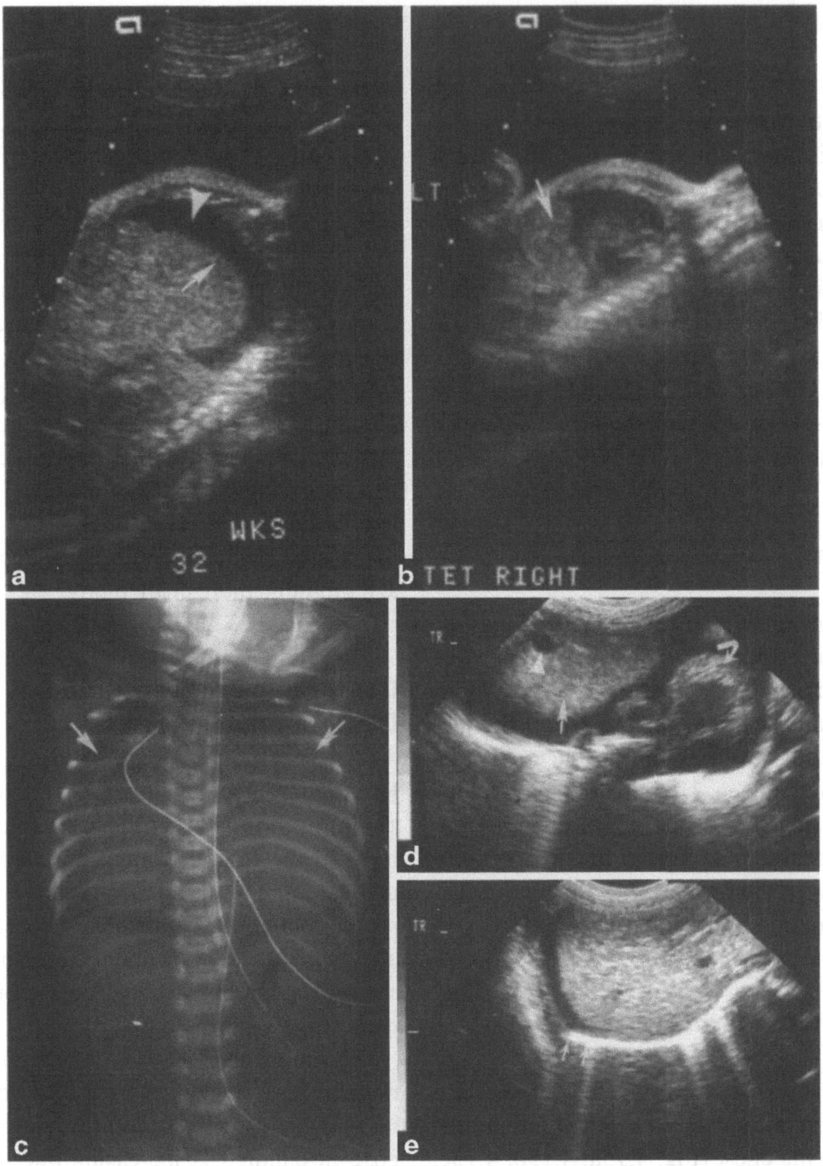

Fig. 4.15 Congenital diaphragmatic hernia, prenatal and neonatal ultrasound. **a** Sagittal ultrasound image of the right fetal chest; dome of the liver *(arrow)* was adjacent to the thoracic apex, with a small crescent of pleural fluid in the intervening space *(arrowhead)*. **b** Sagittal ultrasound image of the left fetal chest; left lobe of the liver *(arrow)* was herniated into the thoracic cavity, although not as severely as the right lobe. Pleural effusion was present. **c**. X-ray of the chest and abdomen reveals a large central intrathoracic mass *(arrows)*. **d** Transverse ultrasound image of the neonatal chest demonstrated bilateral pleural fluid which extended around the heart *(curved arrow)* and communicated with ascitic fluid. The liver *(arrow)* and gallbladder fundus *(arrowhead)* were identified at this level. **e** Transverse neonatal ultrasound of the right upper quadrant of the abdomen; a small rim of diaphragm was seen posterolateral to the liver, with an abrupt termination *(arrows)*. [43]

paralysis. With M-mode recording, ultrasound can provide quantitative information about diaphragmatic excursion as diaphragmatic movement appears as a sinusoidal curve (Fig. 4.16). Diaphragmatic excursion is normal when greater than 4 mm and symmetric between the leaflets of

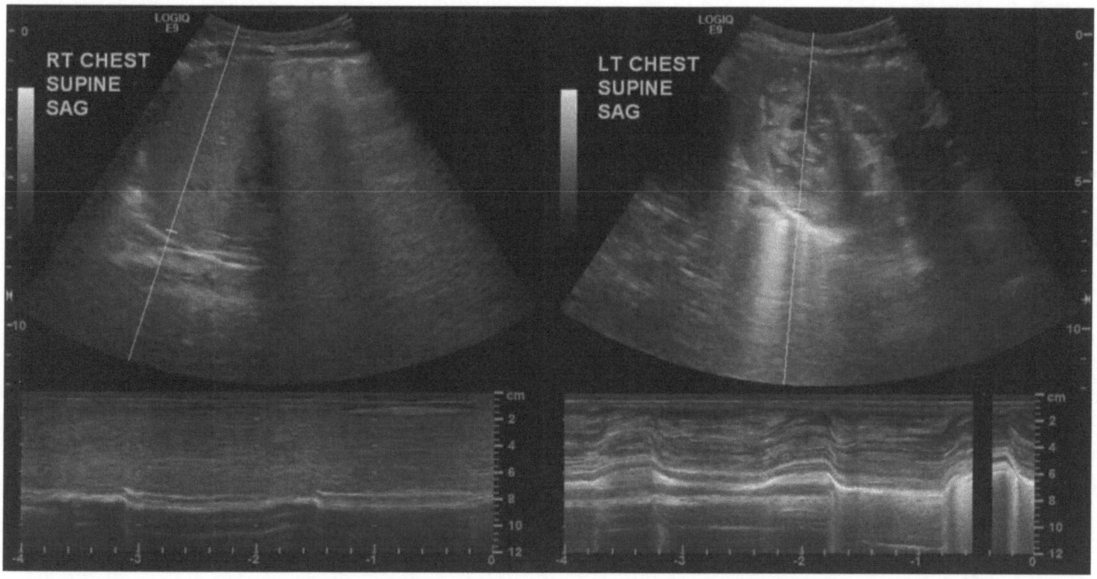

Fig. 4.16 Right eventration. Excursion of the diaphragm is reduced on dynamic imaging, and amplitude is greatly decreased in M-mode

the diaphragm (less than a 50 % difference). Normal excursion will be toward the transducer with a subxiphoid approach [30]. Intraindividual comparisons in the course of a disease can be very useful. Typical sonographic signs of diaphragmatic paresis are: (1) limited or lack of mobility in the longitudinal and cross-sectional view, (2) reduced or zero amplitude in M-mode, and (3) in cross section, greater distance between the transducer and the diaphragm line on the affected side [28].

Lung

Consolidation—Atelectasis, Pneumonia, Abscess

Airless lung can appear sonographically similar to liver (hepatization) (Fig. 4.17) [31]. Despite the lack of air in the consolidated lung, the underlying internal architecture of the lung is preserved, allowing differentiation from masses or other processes.

In pneumonia, branching linear echogenicities representing air bronchograms are often seen [32] (Fig. 4.17). Entrapped fluid or mucoid material within bronchi in necrotizing or postobstructive pneumonias produces hypoechoic branching structures— the sonographic fluid bronchogram [33]. Pulmonary vascular flow is preserved in simple pneumonic consolidation and is readily demonstrated with color Doppler. If there is an effusion present, the diagnosis of consolidation can be aided by the presence of an effusion; an aerated lung lobe will float over the effusion, while a consolidated lobe will swim within the effusion (the jellyfish sign) [34].

In atelectatic lung, air bronchograms are also present. Blood vessels become crowded together and display an orderly linear and branching structure that distinguishes this entity from the more irregular vasculature found in neoplasms.

Distinguishing pneumonic consolidation from simple atelectasis can be difficult radiographically. It has been suggested that ultrasound can be more specific than CT scan in this situation. If there is movement of the air within bronchi, this usually indicates pneumonia, whereas the air bronchograms in atelectasis are most often static. In one study, this dynamic air bronchogram had a sensitivity of 61 % and a positive predictive value of 97 % in distinguishing pneumonia from atelectasis [35].

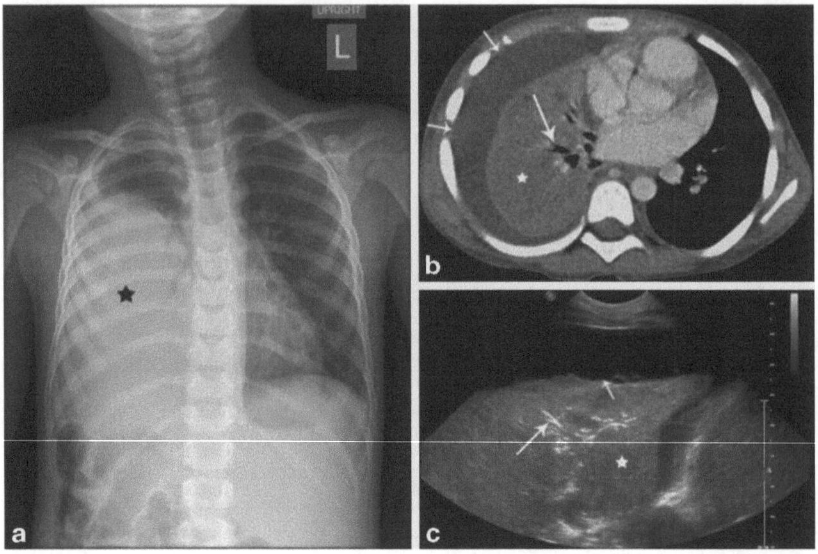

Fig. 4.17 Images in a 4-year-old boy with pneumonia. **a** Frontal radiograph of the chest shows opacity at the right lung base *(star)*. **b** CT and **c** US images show hepatization of the right lower lobe *(star)* with air bronchograms *(long arrow)* and surrounding pleural effusion *(short arrows)*. [2]

Abscesses form as a complication of lung infection. Parenchymal necrosis, indicated by decreased echogenicity with lack of color Doppler flow within a region of pulmonary consolidation, is a characteristic finding of early abscess. Developed abscesses display a thick wall and air fluid levels. If abutting the pleura, lung abscesses are sonographically visible, and ultrasound-guided aspiration and drainage can play an important role in diagnosis and treatment [26].

Pneumothorax

Ultrasound is popular for the diagnosis of pneumothorax in trauma patients, ventilated patients, and those undergoing lung procedures amongst others [36]. Characteristic signs such as lung sliding [37], comet tail artifacts (Fig. 4.18a and 4.18b) [38], the A-line sign [38], and lung point [39] have been described for the sonographic diagnosis of pneumothorax. Sensitivity and specificity of this diagnosis is operator dependent, with some reports as high as 100 % in one study of 285 patients.

Tumors

Primary lung neoplasms are very rare in children. Pulmonary blastoma is the most common and usually starts as a peripheral lesion, often attaining large size before becoming clinically apparent. Other less common tumors include mucoepidermoid carcinoma, hemangiopericytoma, leiomyosarcoma, rhabdomyosarcoma, and bronchogenic tumors. If the tumor is fully surrounded by aerated lung tissues, it might be sonographically invisible; a reliable sonographic evaluation of intrathoracic tumors is only possible if they are next to the chest wall or diaphragm or if they are surrounded by a pleural effusion. As with pleural lesions, if a lung mass is sufficiently peripheral and abuts the lung surface, percutaneous ultrasound-guided biopsy is a safe and effective method for obtaining a tissue diagnosis.

Bronchopulmonary Malformations (BPM)

Congenital parenchymal masses include congenital pulmonary airway malformation (CPAM)

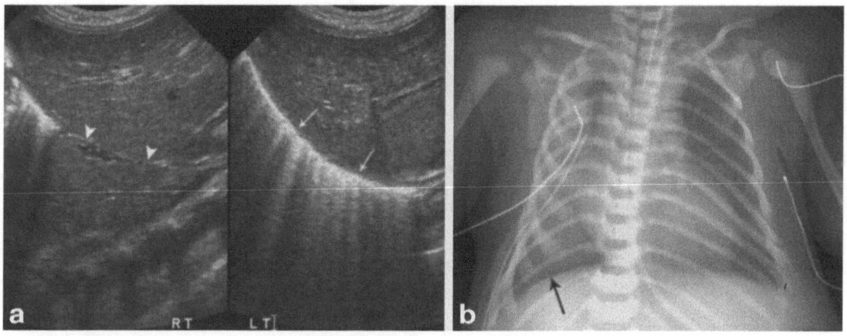

Fig. 4.18 **a** and **b** US images of the right and left lung bases demonstrate absence (*arrowheads*) and presence (*arrows*) of comet tail sign, indicating right-sided pneumothorax. [2]

and sequestration. Although often regarded as separate entities, these malformations are part of a spectrum of CPAMs and may have overlapping imaging and histologic features. These masses may be detected prenatally by ultrasound or MR imaging, appearing as variably solid or cystic structures. Postnatally, plain radiographs usually show the lesion as incidental finding or on images taken for respiratory symptoms.

CPAM

CPAM is the most common BPM (incidence 0.66:10,000) [26]. CPAM is a congenital hamartomatous lesion of the lung resulting in a mass of disorganized lung tissue that is localized to a single bronchial tree segment. CPAMs can be classified into two categories: (1) macrocystic lesions containing single or multiple cysts that are at least 5.0 mm in diameter and (2) microcystic lesions presenting as a solid echogenic mass. Most CPAMs derive their blood supply from the pulmonary artery and drain via the pulmonary veins, with the exception of hybrid lesions, which can have a systemic blood supply. Importantly, they normally communicate with bronchial tree [26].

CPAMs are typically diagnosed antenatally on fetal ultrasound or in the early postnatal period with chest radiograph. Ultrasound will usually demonstrate an area of hyperechogenic tissue with or without hypoechoic cysts that vary in number and size (Fig. 4.19a, 4.19b, 4.19c). Signs of mass effect may be seen, such as mediastinal shift, diaphragmatic eversion, and polyhydramnios. With very large lesions, heart failure (hydrops) due to mediastinal shift and cardiac compression can occur [26]. Ultrasound can also contribute to the evaluation of these patients when there is a suspected sequestrated segment in association with the CPAM.

Pulmonary Sequestration

Pulmonary sequestration is a segment of lung which does not function, has an anomalous arterial blood supply from the systemic circulation, and has no communication with the tracheobronchial tree. It is due to a developmental abnormality in which there is an accessory tracheobronchial foregut bud. There are two types of pulmonary sequestration: intralobar, which shares visceral pleural investment with normal lung and drains into the pulmonary venous system, and extralobar, which has a separate pleural investment and may have either systemic or pulmonary venous drainage [26].

Many pulmonary sequestrations are diagnosed prenatally but some are diagnosed in children with the typical clinical presentation of a lower lobe consolidation that never clears completely. In those patients, color Doppler sonography is diagnostically reliable. Due to the typical location, one will be able to visualize the sequestration best from subxiphoidal or subcostal in most patients. It has an echogenicity similar to liver tissue with occasional central hypoechoic areas.

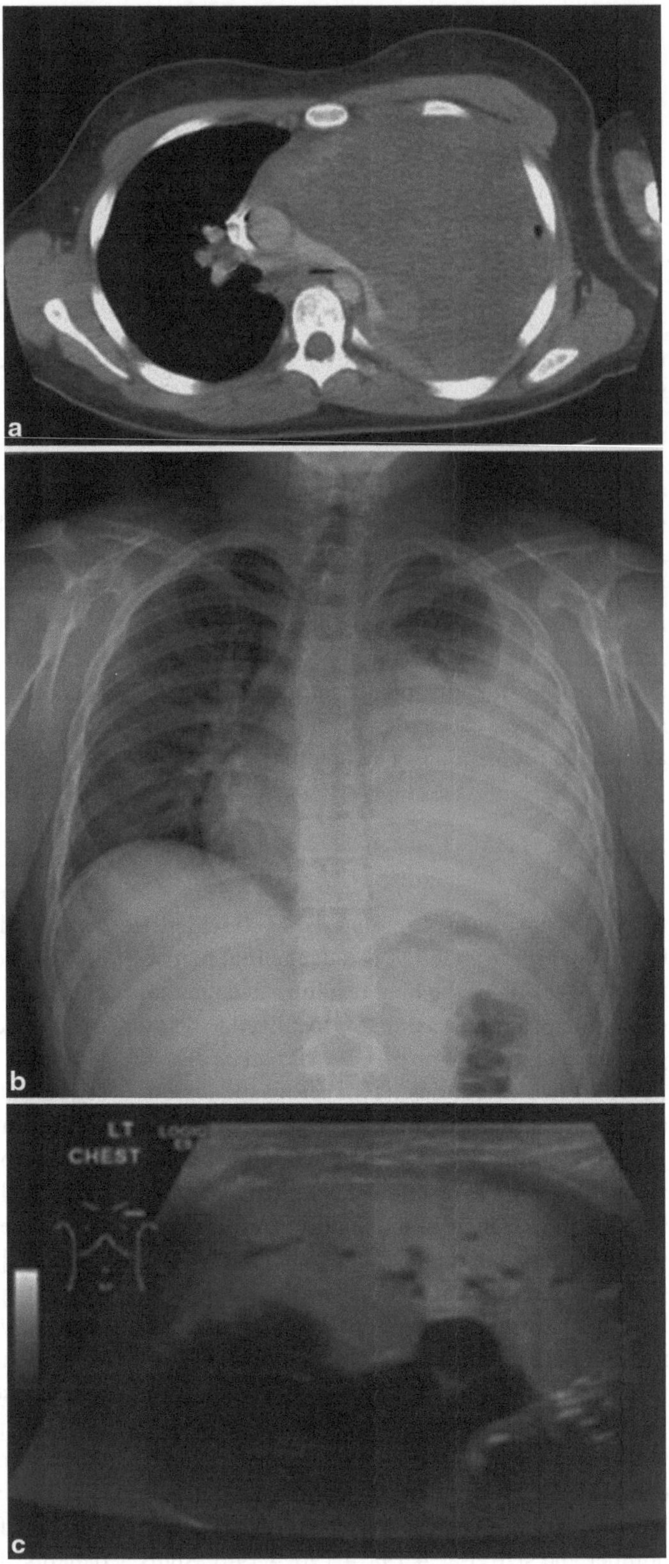

Fig. 4.19 Congenital pulmonary airway malformation *(CPAM)*. **a** CT scan and **b** chest radiograph demonstrate intrathoracic mass. **c** Ultrasound shows hyperechogenic tissue with cysts

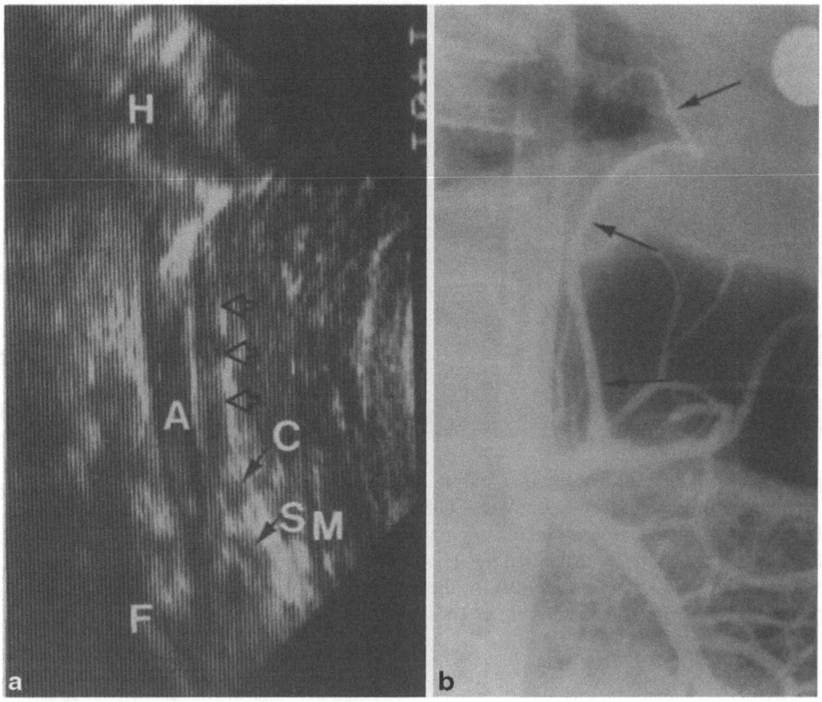

Fig. 4.20 Extralobar sequestration. Longitudinal, oblique ultrasound scan of the mid-abdomen. Aberrant vessel (*arrows*) anterior to the abdominal aorta **a** for better comparison, the scan is presented in the same position as the lateral angiogram (*SM*—superior mesenteric artery, *C*—celiac axis, *H*—head, *F*—feet), **b** Abdominal aortogram, lateral view demonstrating the aberrant artery (*arrows*) supplying the sequestration (compare with **a**). [44]

Since the sequestration has no connection to the bronchial system, it does not show reflexes with high echogenicity. The key diagnostic feature of sequestration is demonstrating systemic arterial supply, usually from the descending aorta. In cases of blood supply originating from the abdominal aorta, the visualization of the feeding vessel is often possible (Fig. 4.20a and 4.20b). Contrast-enhanced CT and MR imaging are often required in unclear cases or in older patients with limited acoustic windows.

Intralobar sequestrations have pulmonary venous drainage and variable degrees of hyperechogenicity by ultrasound. They are always associated with the lower lobes and are distinguishable by the absence of pulmonary arterial inflow. Extralobar sequestrations (Fig. 4.21) occur more commonly in males and are four times more common on the left. Over 60 % of patients have associated anomalies (e.g., diaphragmatic defect, CPAM). They appear as homogeneous hyperechoic masses at any level in the pleural space and can be found within or beneath the diaphragm [26] (Fig. 4.22). They are found in a

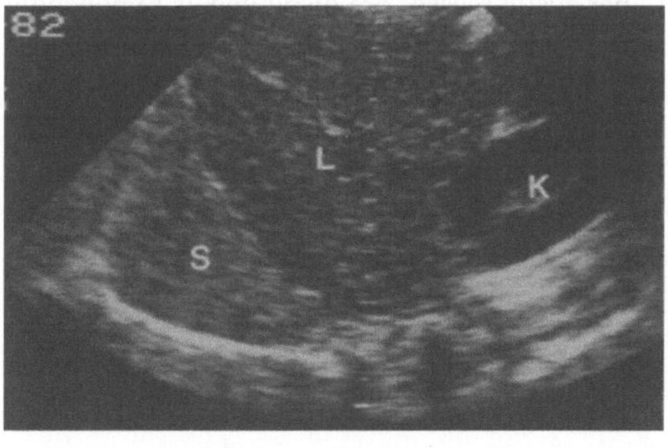

Fig. 4.21 Extralobar sequestration. Longitudinal view of solid triangular mass *(S)* in the chest, separated from the liver *(L)* *(K*—right kidney*)*. [44]

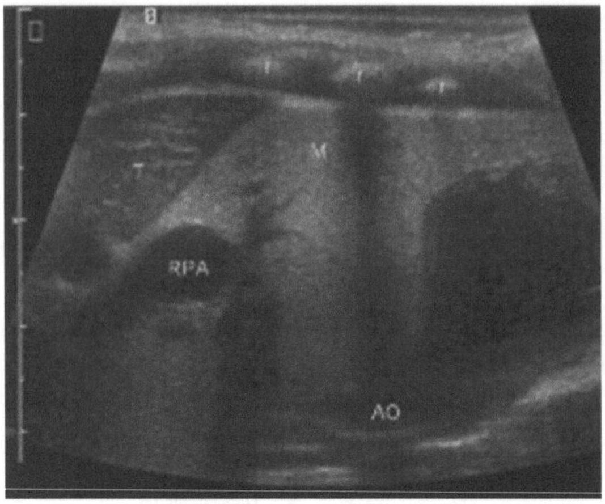

Fig. 4.22 Inptrapericardial extralobar sequestration. Sagittal right parasternal ultrasound scan showing the thymus *(T)* and the mass *(M)* in the superior mediastinum. The acoustic shadows are caused by rib cartilage *(r)*. The mass abuts the aorta *(AO)*, and vessels arising from the right pulmonary artery *(RPA)* could be demonstrated. [45]

paraspinal location with systemic blood supply and systemic venous drainage identified by color Doppler.

Cysts

Other cystic masses are displayed as hypoechoic areas. They can be visualized by ultrasound if they are located peripherally, but reliable identification may require additional imaging modalities in many cases. Differential diagnoses include abscesses in the final stage, bronchogenic cysts, echinococcal cysts, pericardial cysts, and arteriovenous fistulas. The latter can be distinguished using color Doppler sonography.

Summary

Ultrasound is the most important imaging modality in children and can play an important role in evaluation of the pediatric chest. It can be used as an adjunct or the sole diagnostic modality for a variety of congenital and acquired conditions. The mediastinum, lungs, chest wall, diaphragm, and the major intrathoracic vessels can all be evaluated with ultrasound imaging. Ultrasound permits dynamic, real-time assessment of these structures without risk or radiation exposure.

References

1. Ben-Ami TE, O'Donovan JC, Yousefzadeh DK. Sonography of the chest in children. Radiol Clin North Am. 1993;31(3):517–31.
2. Mong A, Epelman M, Darge K. Ultrasound of the pediatric chest. Pediatr Radiol. 2012;42(11):1287–97.
3. Coley BD. Chest sonography in children: current indications, techniques, and imaging findings. Radiol Clin North Am. 2011;49(5):825–46.
4. Volpicelli G. Sonographic diagnosis of pneumothorax. Intensive Care Med. 2011;37(2):224–32.
5. Barillari A, Kiuru S. Detection of spontaneous pneumothorax with chest ultrasound in the emergency department. Intern Emerg Med. 2010;5(3):253–5.
6. Lapegue F, Faruch-Bilfeld M, Demondion X, Apredoaei C, Bayol MA, Artico H, et al. Ultrasonography of the brachial plexus, normal appearance and practical applications. Diagn Interv Imagin. 2014;95(3):259–75.
7. Francis IR, Glazer GM, Bookstein FL, Gross BH. The thymus: reexamination of age-related changes in size and shape. AJR Am J Roentgenol. 1985;145(2):249–54.
8. Kim OH, Kim WS, Kim MJ, Jung JY, Suh JH. US in the diagnosis of pediatric chest diseases. Radiographics: a review publication of the Radiological Society of North America Inc. 2000;20(3):653–71.
9. Ja T. Mediastinal Tumors. In: Gw H, Editor. Ashcraft's pediatric surgery. Miamisburg: Elsevier; 2014. p. 341–50.
10. Fonseca AL, Ozgediz DE, Christison-Lagay ER, Detterbeck FC, Caty MG. Pediatric thymomas: report of two cases and comprehensive review of the literature. Pediatr Surg Int. 2014;30(3):275–86.
11. Castro D, Derisavifard S, Anderson M, Greene M, Iannaccone S. Juvenile myasthenia gravis: a twenty-year experience. J Clin Neuromuscul Dis. 2013;14(3):95–102.
12. Azizkhan RG, Dudgeon DL, Buck JR, Colombani PM, Yaster M, Nichols D, et al. Life-threatening airway obstruction as a complication to the management of mediastinal masses in children. J Pediatr Surg. 1985;20(6):816–22.
13. Kawashima A, Fishman EK, Kuhlman JE, Nixon MS. CT of posterior mediastinal masses. Radiographics: a review publication of the Radiological Society of North America. Inc. 1991;11(6):1045–67.
14. Sidani AH, Oberson R, Deleze G, Barras MH, Genton N, Laurini R. Infected teratoma of lower posterior mediastinum in a six-year-old boy. Pediatr Radiol. 1991;21(6):438–9.

15. Demondion X, Herbinet P, Van Sint JS, Boutry N, Chantelot C, Cotten A. Imaging assessment of thoracic outlet syndrome. Radiographics. 2006;26(6):1735–50.
16. Farrar TA, Rankin G, Chatfield M. Venous thoracic outlet syndrome: approach to diagnosis and treatment with focus on affected athletes. Curr Sports Med Rep. 2014;13(2):81–5.
17. Abiri MM, Kirpekar M, Ablow RC. Osteomyelitis: detection with US. Radiology. 1989;172(2):509–11.
18. Kelloff J, Hulett R, Spivey M. Acute rib fracture diagnosis in an infant by US: a matter of child protection. Pediatr Radiol. 2009;39(1):70–2.
19. Faber LP, Somers J, Templeton AC. Chest wall tumors. Curr Probl Surg. 1995;32(8):661–747.
20. Dubois J, Patriquin HB, Garel L, Powell J, Filiatrault D, David M, et al. Soft-tissue hemangiomas in infants and children: diagnosis using Doppler sonography. AJR Am J Roentgenol. 1998;171(1):247–52.
21. Dubois J, Garel L, David M, Powell J. Vascular soft-tissue tumors in infancy: distinguishing features on Doppler sonography. AJR Am J Roentgenol. 2002;178(6):1541–5.
22. Paltiel HJ, Burrows PE, Kozakewich HP, Zurakowski D, Mulliken JB. Soft-tissue vascular anomalies: utility of US for diagnosis. Radiology. 2000;214(3):747–54.
23. Yang PC, Luh KT, Chang DB, Wu HD, Yu CJ, Kuo SH. Value of sonography in determining the nature of pleural effusion: analysis of 320 cases. AJR Am J Roentgenol. 1992;159(1):29–33.
24. Lomas DJ, Padley SG, Flower CD. The sonographic appearances of pleural fluid. Br J Radiol. 1993;66(787):619–24.
25. Pillai D, Song X, Pastor W, Ottolini M, Powell D, Wiedermann BL, et al. Implementation and impact of a consensus diagnostic and management algorithm for complicated pneumonia in children. J Investig Med. 2011;59(8):1221–7.
26. St. Peter S. Acquired lesions of the lung and pleura. In: GW. H, editor. Ashcraft's pediatric surgery. Miamisburg: Elsevier Inc; 2014. p. 302–14.
27. Wu RG, Yang PC, Kuo SH, Luh KT. "Fluid color" sign: a useful indicator for discrimination between pleural thickening and pleural effusion. J Ultrasound Med. 1995;14(10):767–9.
28. Tsao K, Lally K. Congenital diaphragmatic hernia and eventration. In: GW. H, editor. Ashcraft's pediatric surgery. Miamisburg: Elsevier Inc; 2014.
29. Bih LI, Wu YT, Tsai SJ, Tseng FF, Lin CY, Ding H. Comparison of ultrasonographic renal excursion to fluoroscopic diaphragmatic excursion for the assessment of diaphragmatic function in patients with high cervical cord injury. Arch Phys Med Rehabil. 2004;85(1):65–9.
30. Epelman M, Navarro OM, Daneman A, Miller SF. M-mode sonography of diaphragmatic motion: description of technique and experience in 278 pediatric patients. Pediatr Radiol. 2005;35(7):661–7.
31. Durant A, Nagdev A. Ultrasound detection of lung hepatization. West J Emerg Med. 2010;11(4):322–3.
32. Weinberg B, Diakoumakis EE, Kass EG, Seife B, Zvi ZB. The air bronchogram: sonographic demonstration. AJR Am J Roentgenol. 1986;147(3):593–5.
33. Yang PC, Luh KT, Chang DB, Yu CJ, Kuo SH, Wu HD. Ultrasonographic evaluation of pulmonary consolidation. Am Rev Respir Dis. 1992;146(3):757–62.
34. Lichtenstein DA. Ultrasound in the management of thoracic disease. Crit Care Med. 2007;35(5 Suppl):S250–61.
35. Lichtenstein D, Meziere G, Seitz J. The dynamic air bronchogram. A lung ultrasound sign of alveolar consolidation ruling out atelectasis. Chest. 2009;135(6):1421–5.
36. Ding W, Shen Y, Yang J, He X, Zhang M. Diagnosis of pneumothorax by radiography and ultrasonography: a meta-analysis. Chest. 2011;140(4):859–66.
37. Lichtenstein DA, Menu Y. A bedside ultrasound sign ruling out pneumothorax in the critically ill. Lung sliding. Chest. 1995;108(5):1345–8.
38. Lichtenstein D, Meziere G, Biderman P, Gepner A, Barre O. The comet-tail artifact. An ultrasound sign of alveolar-interstitial syndrome. Am J Respir Crit Care Med. 1997;156(5):1640–6.
39. Lichtenstein D, Meziere G, Biderman P, Gepner A. The "lung point": an ultrasound sign specific to pneumothorax. Intensive Care Med. 2000;26(10):1434–40.
40. Han BK, Suh YL, Yoon HK. Thymic ultrasound. I. Intrathymic anatomy in infants. Pediatr Radiol. 2001;31(7):474–9.
41. Moseme T, Andronikou S. Through the eye of the suprasternal notch: point-of-care sonography for tuberculous mediastinal lymphadenopathy in children. Pediatr Radiol. 2014;44(6):681–4.
42. Bar-Ziv J, Barki Y, Maroko A, Mares AJ. Rib osteomyelitis in children. Early radiologic and ultrasonic findings. Pediatr Radiol. 1985;15(5):315–8.
43. Gross BR, D'Agostino C, Coren CV, Petrikovsky BP. Prenatal and neonatal sonographic imaging of a central diaphragmatic hernia. Pediatr Radiol. 1996;26(6):395–7.
44. Kaude JV, Laurin S. Ultrasonographic demonstration of systemic artery feeding extrapulmonary sequestration. Pediatr Radiol. 1984;14(4):226–7.
45. de Vreede I, Bilardo CM, van Rijn RR, Clur SA, Heij HA. Intrapericardial extralobar pulmonary sequestration presenting as a prenatal intrathoracic mass. Pediatr Cardiol. 2008;29(5):980–2.

The Liver

5

Juan Carlos Infante and Alexander Dzakovic

Introduction

The use of ultrasonography during the initial evaluation of a child with a liver mass allows the pediatric surgeon to instantly narrow the differential diagnosis and determine the next line of imaging or interventional modality. Based on anatomical findings, resectability is determined and the operative strategy developed. However, many of our patients have a limited ability for meaningful cooperation during an ultrasound examination and hence a combination of patience and skills is required to obtain adequate images.

Normal Anatomy and Hepatic Variants

Intimate knowledge of the segmental anatomy of the liver is essential to the pediatric hepatobiliary surgeon not only to plan a resection but also to precisely document and communicate findings. The French anatomist *Couinaud* first described the hepatic segmental anatomy based on its vascular watershed in 1957 [1]. The currently most widely accepted nomenclature based on this description was defined at a consensus meeting in Brisbane, Australia, in 2000 [2]. The plane along the gallbladder fossa and the middle hepatic vein known as *Cantlie's line* divides the liver into a left and right hemi-liver. The caudate lobe represents segment 1. The umbilical fissure divides the left hemi-liver or left hepatic lobe into the left lateral section or sector (segments 2 and 3) and the left medial section (segment 4), which is subdivided into a superior segment 4A and inferior segment 4B. The right hepatic lobe is divided by the right hepatic vein into the right anterior section (segments 5 and 8) and the right posterior section (segments 6 and 7) (Fig. 5.1). Hepatic venous drainage is rather consistent via the right, middle, and left hepatic veins into the inferior vena cava (IVC). The left hepatic vein often joins the middle hepatic vein before entering the IVC which can be a critical detail when assessing for resectability of masses near the confluence. The proper hepatic artery (HA) divides into left and right artery supplying the respective lobes. The left HA enters the umbilical fissure where it gives off a branch supplying segment 4 before terminating in the left lateral section. The right HA divides into right anterior and posterior sections as well as a cystic artery branch [3]. The hepatic arterial anatomy has several rather common variants of great importance for surgical planning. A completely replaced right HA arises directly from the superior mesenteric artery and traverses behind the head of the pancreas and posterior and right lateral to the common bile

A. Dzakovic (✉)
Department of Pediatric Surgery, Loyola University Medical Center, 2160S. First Ave, Maywood, IL 60153, USA
e-mail: ADZAKOVIC@lumc.edu

J. C. Infante
Department of Medical Imaging, Ann and Robert H Lurie Children's Hospital of Chicago, 225 E Chicago Ave, Chicago, IL 60611, USA
e-mail: juan.infante.md@gmail.com

S. Scholz, M. D. Jarboe (eds.), *Diagnostic and Interventional Ultrasound in Pediatrics and Pediatric Surgery,* DOI 10.1007/978-3-319-21699-7_5

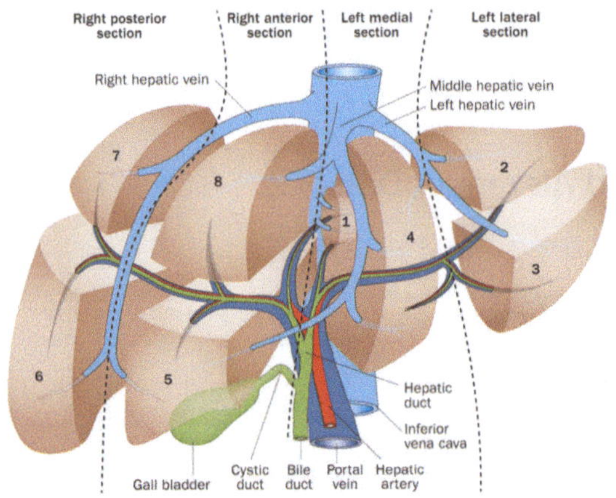

Fig. 5.1 Segmental anatomy of the liver based on vascular supply (inferior vena cava, right hepatic vein, middle hepatic vein, left hepatic vein, portal vein *(PV)* (http://www.siopel.org)

duct into the porta hepatis and is the sole supply to the right lobe. This configuration is called accessory right HA if it is in addition to a right sided branch arising from the proper HA. A replaced or accessory left HA arises from the left gastric artery before it traverses the gastrohepatic ligament and enters the umbilical fissure as either the sole or additional blood supply to the left lobe. Anomalous right or left hepatic arterial configurations are present in up to 40% of individuals and have to be recognized prior to any liver resection [4].

Scanning Technique

A systematic approach will be presented which will cover the required components of a sonographic liver examination. It is crucial that the operator or sonographer establishes a routine by conducting the examination in the same sequence every time to avoid missing any critical findings.

Porta Hepatis

Structures of interest include:

- Portal vein—deepest of the three structures and usually most prominent (unless there is underlying pathology)
- HA proper and right and left branches
- Common bile duct

Technique

The transducer should first be oriented transversely over the right upper quadrant. Because a large portion of the liver is usually situated posterior to the ribs and the lung base, one must ask the patient to hold a deep inspiratory breath. The transducer must then be angled parallel to the structures of the porta hepatis, usually accomplished by rotating it clockwise from the transverse position (so that the part of the transducer previously pointing to the right side of the patient, or 9 o'clock, then points roughly at 10–11 o'clock).

At this point, the three main portal structures should be readily identifiable. The portal vein is the deepest of the structures and usually the most prominent unless there is underlying disease such as stenosis or chronic thrombosis. Activating color and spectral Doppler will allow confirmation of monophasic or nonphasic waveforms in the portal vein. In contradiction, the adjacent HA is normally characterized by pulsatile waveforms, characteristic for any healthy systemic artery. Finally, the common bile duct is void of any flow with Doppler interrogation.

Systematic Evaluation

Grayscale

The caliber of the main portal vein, HA, and their right and left branches should be assessed. While Doppler evaluation will allow for confirmation of blood flow through a vessel, the more rapid frame rate of grayscale images is helpful to point out caliber changes. If there is a caliber change, a potentially significant hemodynamic effect can be assessed with Doppler.

Color Doppler

The main portal vein should fill with color if it is patent and should fill with the same color as the HA (Fig. 5.2). If colors on opposite sides of the color spectrum (e.g., red and blue with many vendors) are seen in the same segment of a vessel within

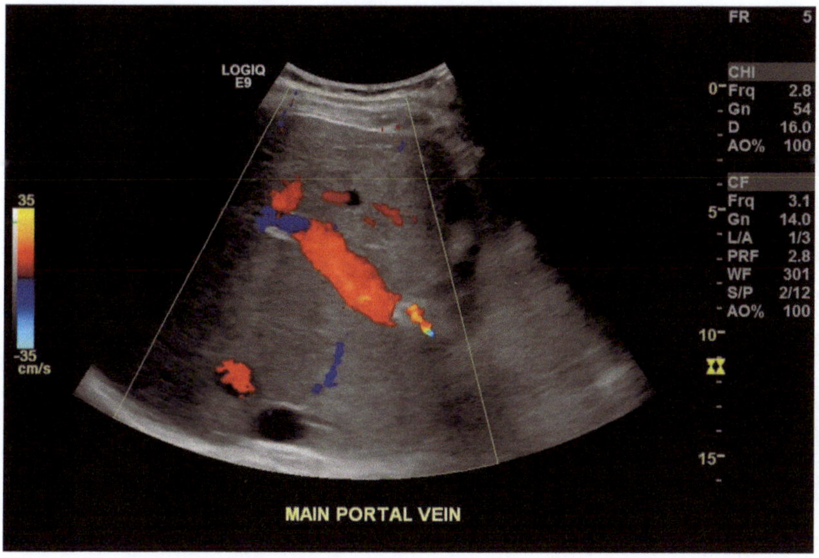

Fig. 5.2 Normal filling of the portal vein with color Doppler. The adjacent hepatic artery *(HA)* is also *red* in color indicating that flow is in the same direction, as normally expected, in both vessels

one heart beat, then this means that blood is moving towards and away from the transducer during the cardiac cycle—in other words, portal flow is not unidirectional. This can be further detailed with spectral Doppler as below. Please note that it is normal to find colors on the opposing side of the spectrum even in contiguous vessels; this occurs when they physically point in different directions as in the example where one may see "blue" flow (away from the transducer) in the main portal vein and "red" flow in the right portal vein (or towards the transducer). This is simply the product of the main portal vein pointing away and the right portal vein pointing towards the transducer and does not imply bidirectional flow (Fig. 5.3).

The HA, in contradistinction to the portal vein, will appear pulsatile with color Doppler, and this will also be further characterized with spectral Doppler.

Spectral Doppler

Waveforms are helpful for identifying structures and including and excluding disease.

Main portal vein waveforms should be unidirectional and therefore on only one side of the baseline on the displayed color graph (Fig. 5.4). The wave should be monophasic (synonymous with nonphasic), but some degree of phasicity is allowed. Pressure is partially transmitted to the portal venous branches from the right atrium and hepatic veins across the hepatic parenchyma. However, a portal vein wave, which reaches baseline or crosses baseline (i.e., hepatofugal flow) should raise concern for portal hypertension. Unidirectional flow with increased phasicity or pulsatility raises concern for right-sided cardiac disease, shunting as can be seen in cirrhosis, or potentially arteriovenous fistula in the appropriate setting. Finally, absent flow is concerning for occlusion whether by bland or tumor thrombus; again, a confirmatory study (such as computed tomography (CT) or magnetic resonance imaging (MRI)) should be considered before definitely diagnosing complete occlusion because slow flow can remain occult even with power Doppler.

HA waveforms are normally pulsatile and low resistance. That is, a sharp upstroke is seen during systole, and the end-diastolic velocity should be well above baseline with some leeway in post-surgical cases where parenchymal edema may increase the resistance in vascular circuit. The cited normal range of resistive index (RI) varies from publication to publication, but a reasonable range of normal can be considered 0.55–0.70 [5]. An

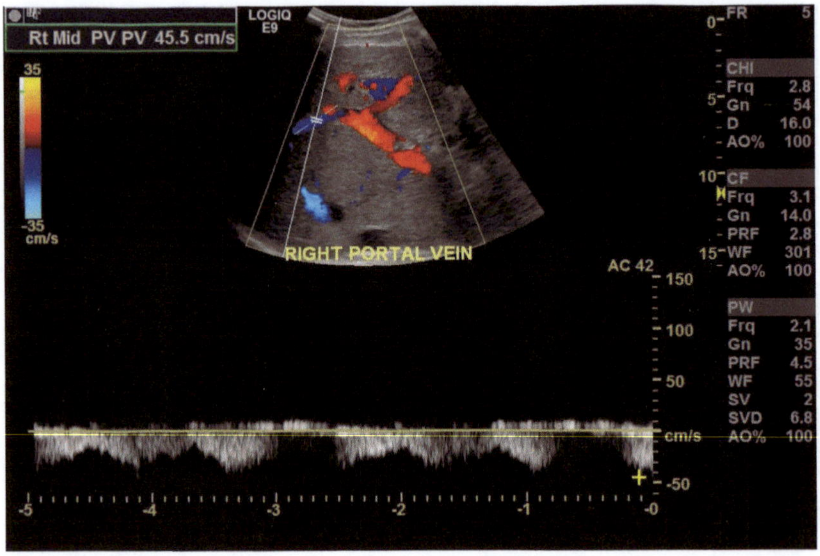

Fig. 5.3 Normal color Doppler appearance of the main, right, and left portal vein branches. Notice that the *blue* flow of the *right* portal vein with waveforms below baseline should not be mistaken for flow reversal. This is antegrade flow and is explained by the direction of the *right* portal vein towards the transducer, whereas the *left* and main portal veins are physically pointing away from the transducer. Incidentally, the right portal vein waveforms show increased phasicity due to increased pressure transmitted from the inferior vena cava *(IVC),* hepatic veins and liver parenchyma in this cardiac patient

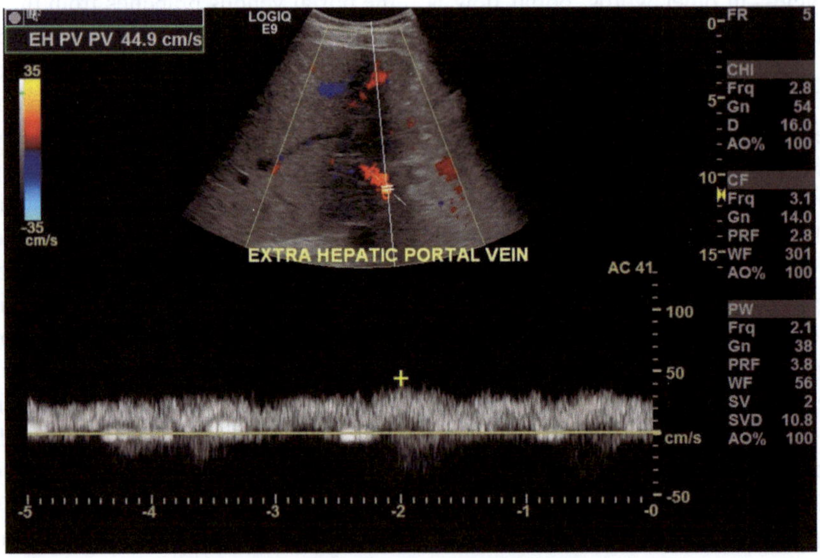

Fig. 5.4 Main portal vein waveforms stay on one side of the baseline and are thus termed monophasic, synonymous with nonphasic. The blood flow is antegrade moving away from the transducer and is represented with "red" flow in the color spectrum and waveforms above the baseline. Please refer to comments in Fig. 5.3 and note that the color and position of the waveforms relative to baseline represent the direction of flow relative to the transducer (and not direction of flow relative to the liver). In Fig. 5.3, antegrade flow in the right portal vein is moving towards the transducer, while in this figure antegrade flow moves away from the transducer.

RI below 0.55 is said to be related to decreased resistance which can be caused by upstream stenosis or atherosclerosis. An RI above 0.70 is said to be high resistance and can be caused by downstream stenosis; parenchymal disease (which results in microvascular compression or disease) including cirrhosis, hepatitis, and rejection; and hepatic venous congestion such as, in cardiac disease or occlusive disease such as Budd-Chiari Syndrome [6].

Color Versus Power Doppler

Compared to power Doppler, color Doppler has the distinct advantage of depicting directionality of flow in real time. Power Doppler is more sensitive to flow and is therefore particularly advantageous in areas where flow is not depicted with color Doppler but flow nonetheless suspected. In such cases, the direction of flow is less important and therefore sacrificed in power Doppler to gather evidence for complete occlusion. If flow is seen with power Doppler but not with color Doppler, this is usually said to be related to "slow flow." If no flow is seen with either technique, then this speaks heavily for complete occlusion and a confirmatory imaging study such as computed tomography angiogram (CTA) may be considered.

Hepatic Veins and IVC

Moving the transducer cranially and oblique along the subcostal margin will allow visualization of this region.

Grayscale

This mode of imaging will allow for rapid assessment of the anatomy. After the right, middle, and left hepatic veins are identified, they should be followed to the confluence with the IVC.

Color Doppler

Unlike in the main portal vein and HA system described above, it is normal to find colors on both sides of the color spectrum in the hepatic veins within one cardiac cycle. This is because hepatic vein and IVC flow is bidirectional and directly related to the cardiac cycle as detailed below.

Spectral Waveforms

Hepatic vein and IVC flow can be characterized four different waveform components, namely, A, S, D, and V waves (shown in Fig. 5.5a, b) and are therefore called triphasic or tetraphasic (depending on whether or not the V wave crosses the baseline). Triphasic and tetraphasic waveforms are both characteristic in normal cases. Rather, it

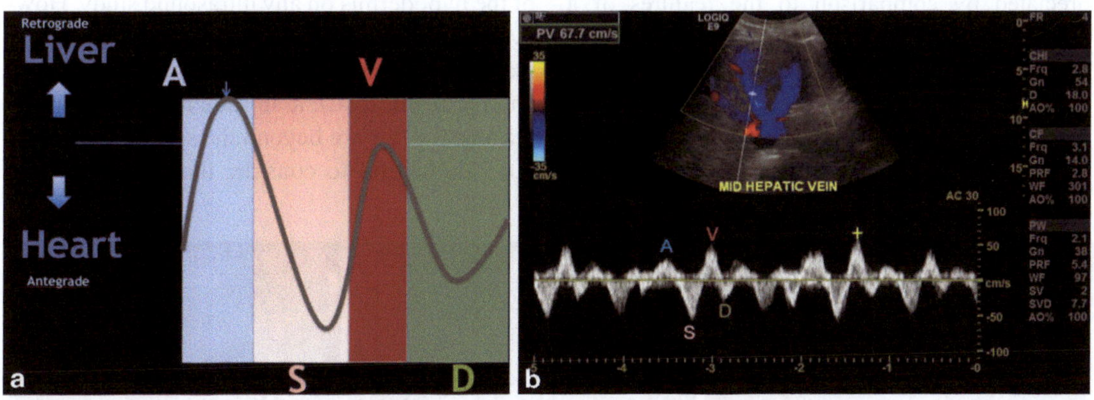

Fig. 5.5 **a** *A*, *S*, *D*, and *V* waves represented in diagrammatic fashion. The *A* wave represents a small amount of flow towards the liver during the atrial kick. The *S* wave represents flow towards the heart due to decrease in pressure in the atrium during ventricular contraction. The *V* wave represents atrial overfilling as the ventricle starts to relax; this wave can be below, at, or above baseline in normal patients, but if its amplitude is greater than the *S* wave, consider *right* heart or valvular disease. Finally, the *D* wave represents flow towards the heart during passive filling of the right atrium and ventricle after the tricuspid valve opens. **b** Normal *A, S, D* and *V* waves in a *middle* hepatic vein

is the individual characteristics of the waveforms which point towards the possibility of disease, but this topic is beyond the scope of this text [6, 8]. A description of these waves in the normal condition is as follows:

The A wave is seen during early systole as the result of the "atrial kick." Although the atrial kick serves to propel blood into the right ventricle, a small amount of retrograde flow is directed towards the liver and thus towards the transducer. The S wave lies on the opposite side of the baseline relative to the A wave and is related to antegrade flow of blood (towards the heart). This wave represents the relative decreased pressure generated by the contraction of the right ventricle and movement of the tricuspid annulus [7, 8]. The V wave is the result of atrial overfilling as the right ventricle starts to relax and the relative pressure in the right atrium begins to increase as the tricuspid annulus begins to return towards its resting diastolic position. The D wave represents antegrade passive filling of the right atrium and ventricle during diastole (see Fig. 5.5a and b).

Diffuse Parenchymal Changes/Metabolic Disorders

Diffuse parenchymal changes can be best appreciated by comparison to the features of a normal liver noticing anomalies. A normal liver will allow the fibrofatty tissues around the portal veins to appear echogenic, and detail in the posterior aspect of the liver will be preserved (Fig. 5.6a). Chronic parenchymal disease such as fatty infiltration from obesity or alcoholism will usually cause the liver parenchyma to become more echogenic thus reducing the contrast between the parenchyma and the echogenic borders of the portal structures (Fig. 5.6b). In addition, the increased acoustic attenuation in the more echogenic tissues will cause the parts of the liver furthest from the transducer (often the posterior liver with routine scanning technique) to appear more hypoechoic (Fig. 5.6c).

The liver's response to insult is often similar regardless of the insult, and the resultant fibrosis/cirrhosis will appear the same regardless of the underlying cause. For example, it should not be surprising that there is no consistent imaging feature that would allow one to distinguish diffuse hepatic disease from Wilson's disease from other types of hepatocyte injury.

Benign Focal Changes

When evaluating a focal mass, it is useful to keep a few principles in mind. Fluid is anechoic; thus, fluid containing structures such as cysts or cystic components of complex masses will also be anechoic. Fatty tissue, despite what one may read elsewhere, is anechoic to hypoechoic to soft tissue; for proof, simply notice the low echogenicity of the hypodermis on any ultrasound study. However, when fat is encountered as a component of a mass or connective tissue (i.e., angiomyolipoma and perinephric fat), it appears hyperechoic. The reasons for this are beyond the scope of this text, but it is helpful to consider that the ultrasound

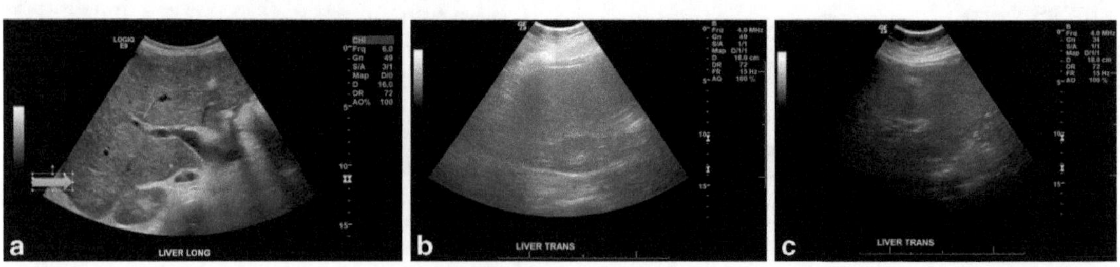

Fig. 5.6 **a** Normal liver parenchyma. Notice how the parenchymal detail can be seen and nicely contrasts against the echogenic periportal fibrofatty tissues *(small arrow)*. Also, the detail in the posterior liver parenchyma is preserved *(large arrow)*. **b** Hepatic steatosis. The liver detail is lost and the periportal fibrofatty echogenic tissue contrasts less with the surrounding parenchyma. **c** Hepatic steatosis. The liver at the posterior aspect of the scan field is hypoechoic due to increased sound attenuation throughout the parenchyma

does not interpret echogenicity simply based on tissue type but rather the speed of sound in the path of the sound wave which is altered by complex tissue interfaces. Because a mixture of fat and other tissue create complex echoes, such fat-containing areas will appear echogenic.

Cysts

Cysts are circumscribed structures which are predominantly anechoic with posterior acoustic enhancement. A simple cyst will be completely anechoic. Any septations or solid components within a cyst will usually appear anything but anechoic and probably obvious against the background of the anechoic fluid in the cyst and such findings expand the differential beyond the simple cyst. We defer to other more detailed sources for further description of cystic lesions, but the following brief synopsis may prove helpful:

- Simple cyst—completely anechoic with posterior acoustic enhancement and usually not overtly numerous.
- Biliary hamartoma (von Meyenburg complex)—numerous and small, less than 1.5 cm in diameter [9, 10].
- Polycystic disease—larger and multiple cysts.
- Biliary cystadenocarcinoma—thick septations in an anechoic background.
- Abscess—thick walls with internal echoes and/or septations.
- Biloma—associated with a history of trauma or surgery. Otherwise, it is virtually identical to a simple cyst on sonography.

Liver Tumors

Primary liver tumors are rare in pediatric patients occurring in less than three per million children in the USA. Approximately two thirds of these tumors are malignant with hepatoblastoma (HB) and hepatocellular carcinoma (HCC) being the most common (Fig. 5.7). Abdominal ultrasonography is the imaging modality of choice to confirm a clinical suspicion for a liver mass and screen for involvement of major vessels or biliary dilatation.

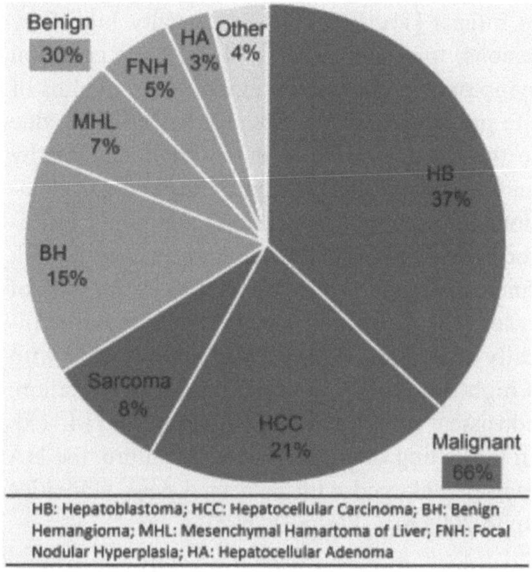

Fig. 5.7 Tumors of the liver. (Lopez-Terrada D. and Finegold M.J. In Suchy F.J., and Sokol R.J. (eds): Liver Disease in Children, (ed 4). Cambridge, UK: Cambridge University Press, 2014. pp. 728–729)

While the vast majority of cases will require additional CT or MRI imaging for definitive diagnosis, proper oncologic workup and preoperative planning, intraoperatively ultrasonography is the dominating imaging tool to guide successful and safe anatomic and nonanatomic resections. Following liver resection, diagnosis and treatment of bile collections or hematomas as well as evaluation of vascular patency can efficiently and reliably be accomplished by ultrasound.

Benign Tumors

Benign liver tumors are often incidental findings in asymptomatic patients. Generally, they have distinct delineation, increased echogenicity, and are often hypervascular.

Hemangioendothelioma

The infantile hemangioendothelioma (IH), also known as simply the infantile hemangioma, is a benign mesenchymal lesions and represents the most common benign vascular tumor of the liver in infants [11, 12]. They are usually high-flow lesions, true neoplasms, and the most common symptomatic liver tumor in the first 6 months of life presenting with congestive heart failure due to the rapid growth, consumptive coagulopathy and thrombocytopenia. On ultrasound examination, the lesions appear most commonly multifocal, hypoechoic, and inhomogeneous. Small, fine calcifications may be seen in up to 36% of cases [13]. Color and spectral Doppler will typically show a pulsatile waveform consistent with a high-flow lesion with little diastolic variation, consistent with arteriovenous shunting [14, 15]. In the setting of congestive heart failure, the HA may be enlarged with increased peak velocities up to 200 cm/s (Fig. 5.7a, b, c).

Cavernous Hemangioma

Hepatic cavernous hemangiomas of infancy and childhood, also known as capillary hemangiomas, are venous malformations that mostly occur in association with their superficial or deep cutaneous counterpart within the first few weeks of life [16]. Unlike the IH, this is not a true neoplasm and considered a venous malformation (a slow-flow lesion). The cavernous hemangioma appears well defined, variably echogenic, homogeneous with posterior enhancement in the parenchyma periphery. Calcifications are atypical and reported in larger lesions [17], although nonhepatic counterparts will often have calcifications in the way of phleboliths. Small cystic or dilated sinusoidal areas give it a more heterogeneous appearance. Generally, low flow characteristics make blood flow difficult to detect with Doppler ultrasound, but blood flow may be seen peripherally on power if not color Doppler studies [18] (Fig. 5.8).

Focal Nodular Hyperplasia (FNH) and Adenoma

Focal nodular hyperplasia (FNH) is a benign hyperplastic hepatic proliferation believed to arise from circulatory abnormality with predominantly arterial supply and limited portal flow. It may be seen in association with congenital porto-systemic shunt which is why patency of the portal vein and hepatopetal flow should be confirmed whenever a FNH is detected, and vice versa. FNH is composed of elements found in the normal hepatic parenchyma. Thus, a common sonographic presentation of this entity is that one will not be able to see it at all because it will blend in with the surrounding liver tissue. However, ultrasound may be able to find a solitary mass, rather hyperechoic and heterogeneous (Fig. 5.9a). Doppler US may demonstrate a characteristic "spoke and wheel pattern" around a hyperechoic central scar. While a well-published feature in the literature, the central scar is not entirely sensitive or specific. That is, many FNH lesions do not demonstrate a central scar, and many other types of lesions have also been described with a central scar including large hemangiomas and malignancies [19, 20]. Some institutions especially in Europe have contrast-enhanced ultrasound available, and this may be a viable option to those so fortunate to have access to this modality. Ultimately, the appearance of FNH on ultrasound is most often nonspecific, and other cross-sectional imaging such as CT and MR are needed to differentiate FNH from a hemangioma based on contrast-enhancement characteristics (Fig. 5.9b, c).

Hepatic adenomas are very rare during childhood and are usually associated with a high-estrogen environment in teenage females or predisposing conditions such as glycogen storage disease Type 1 or Fanconi's anemia. On ultrasound, hepatic adenomas may appear hypo-, iso-, or hyperechoic [11]. Areas of increased echogenicity may reflect fat, hemorrhage, or calcifications (the latter may present with or without posterior acoustic shadowing depending on the size of the calcifications with larger, calcified foci more prone to exhibit posterior shadowing). Hypo- to anechoic areas suggesting fluid may reflect necrosis.

Mesenchymal Hamartoma

Mesenchymal hamartomas (MH) are the second most common benign liver tumors typically presenting in patients less than 2 years of age. They are considered malformations rather than true

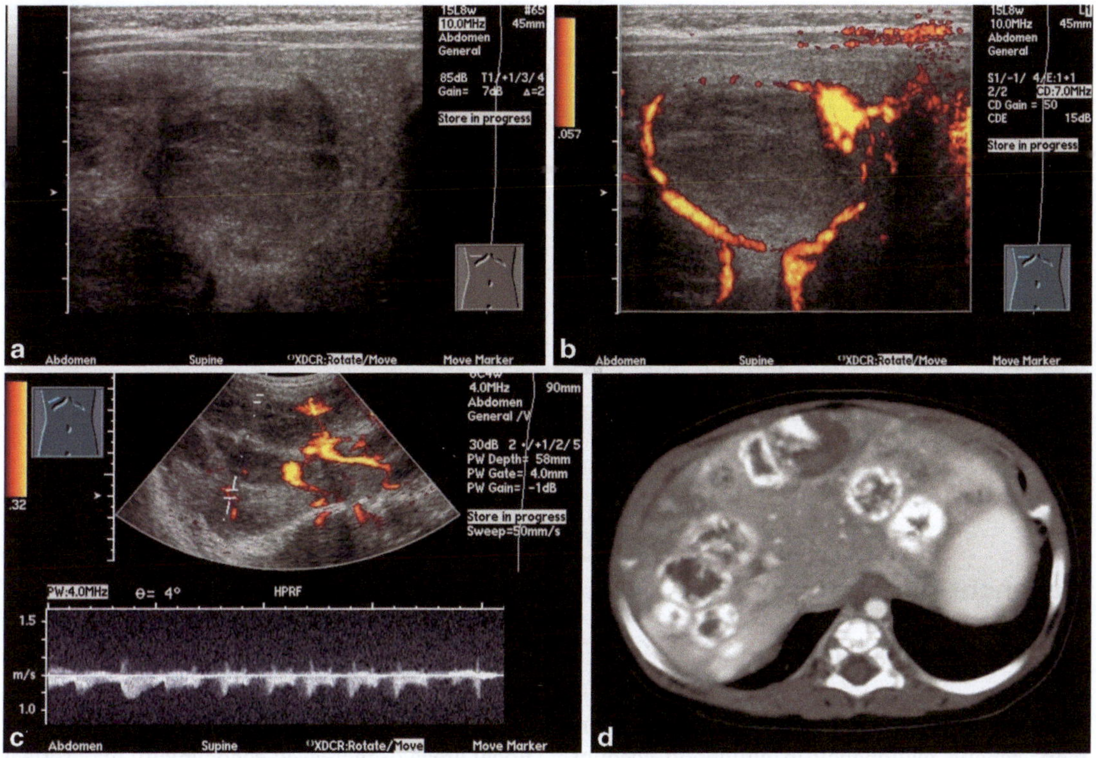

Fig. 5.8 **a** Infantile hemangioma (hemangioendothelioma). This mass presents as a heterogeneously hypoechoic mass relative to the surrounding liver with linear echogenic structures. **b** Flow around but not clearly within this lesion was observed although this entity can present with sonographically detectable internal blood flow. **c** A separate lesion in the same liver as in 5.6a demonstrates pulsatile (arterial) flow within the lesion. **d** For comparison, the same patient and liver containing the multiple infantile hemangiomas in 5.8**a**, **b** **c** care shown on this arterial phase CT image. Notice the characteristic uninterrupted centripetal enhancement of the lesions

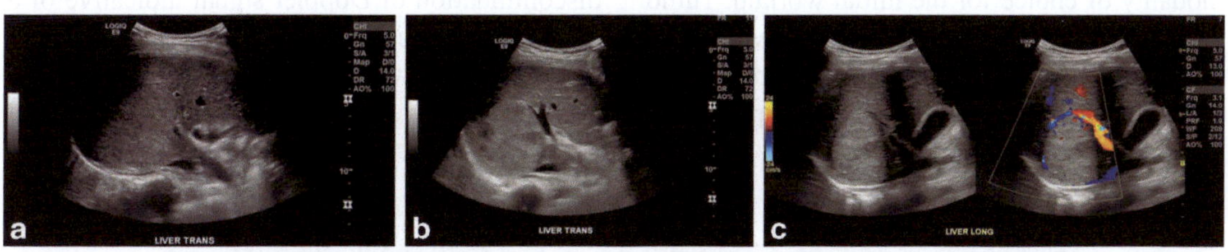

Fig. 5.9 **a** The Focal nodular hyperplasia *(FNH)* is easy to dismiss on this particular image. **b** On a separate image, the echogenicity of this FNH allows it to contrast against the normal hepatic parenchyma. **c** No flow is detectable by ultrasound in this particular FNH lesion

neoplasms and may go through phases of growth and regression. On ultrasound the mass typically appears heterogeneous, septated, and multicystic with a well-defined margin. However, less commonly a predominantly solid lesion with only few cysts seen [10] (Fig. 5.10). These appear more hyperechoic than the surrounding hepatic parenchyma. MH are most often confined to one hepatic lobe which is more commonly the right [21, 22]. Although generally benign lesions, several cases of HB and sarcoma after non-oncologic resection have been reported. Complete surgical resection is the widely accepted standard of care for MH.

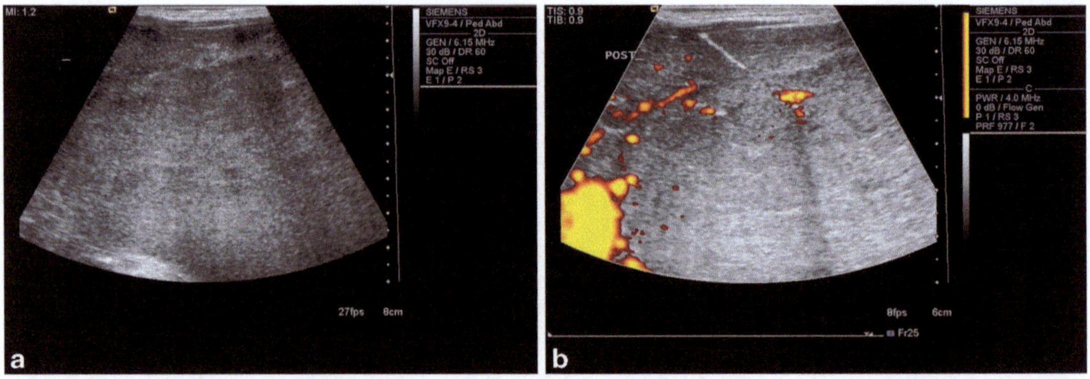

Fig. 5.10 **a** Mesenchymal hamartoma. Although usually predominantly cystic, these lesions contain a preponderance of stromal components and they present as solid masses. **b** No intrinsic flow is seen within this lesion during ultrasound-guided biopsy

Malignant Tumors

Hepatoblastoma (HB)

Hepatoblastoma (HB) is the most common primary hepatic malignancy in childhood accounting for almost half of all pediatric liver tumors. Most patients present with an abdominal mass before the age of three but non-specific symptoms such as vague abdominal symptoms, failure to thrive, anemia, or emesis may be associated as well. Abdominal ultrasonography is the imaging modality of choice for the initial workup. Tumor extent and caval, portal, and hepatic venous involvement can be assessed. Most lesions are solitary but can be multifocal. Margins appear well delineated, heterogeneous with slightly increased echogenicity compared to normal hepatic parenchyma (Fig. 5.11a, b). Calcifications causing acoustic shadows can be seen in up to half of the patients. Cystic and/or necrotic areas will appear anechoic with varying levels of internal echoes. Focal areas of increased echogenicity may reflect hemorrhage into the lesion although very early hemorrhage can appear hypoechoic. Color Doppler often shows increased vascularity. Intrahepatic portal and hepatic vein branches structures often are "wrapped" around the mass but may demonstrate tumor invasion, thrombus and abrupt discontinuation of Doppler signal indicative of a malignancy. While oncologic treatment strategies for HB differ between Europe and North America, assessment for resectability is uniformly the first step of the surgical algorithm. The PRETreatment

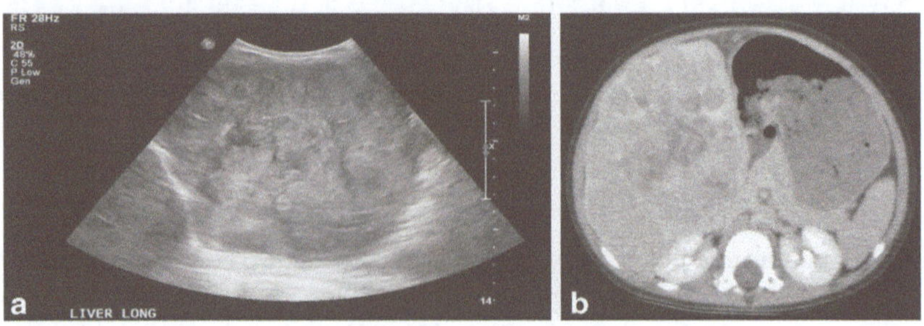

Fig. 5.11 **a** Hepatoblastoma. This grayscale ultrasound image shows a heterogeneously echogenic mass. **b** Corresponding delayed contrast-enhanced CT image shows heterogeneous attenuation including fluid density areas suggestive of necrosis

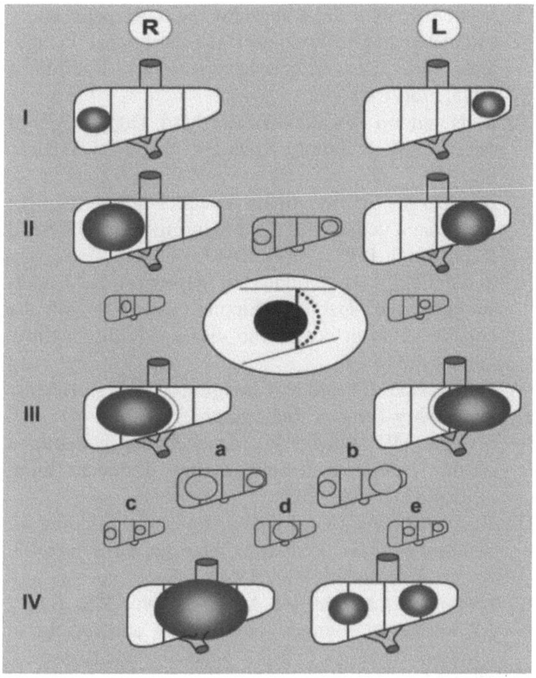

Fig. 5.12 **PRE**Treatment **EXT**ent of disease **PRETEXT** I-IV staging system for liver lesions. (http://www.siopel.org)

EXTent of disease (PRETEXT) is a staging system using the number of involved liver sections ([23], Fig. 5.12) CT scan or MRI of the chest and abdomen is the most widely utilized preoperative imaging modality of choice but thorough hepatic ultrasound can provide adequate PRETEXT information as well [24].

Hepatocellular Carcinoma (HCC)

Hepatocellular carcinoma (HCC typically affects teenage children and is associated with conditions predisposing to cirrhosis such as biliary atresia, hemochromatosis, hereditary tyrosinemia, infantile cholestasis, glycogen storage disease, and hepatitis B. Sonographically, HCC has imprecise delineation with a heterogeneous structure. A fine network of blood vessels surrounding the tumor nodule resembling a "basket pattern" may be observed. The vessels cling to the tumor and develop many fine branches around and within the tumor nodule. [25].

Intraoperative Ultrasound (IOUS)

The advantage of intraoperative use of ultrasound during liver resections has been established in the adult literature [26, 27] and some evidence is published in the pediatric patient population in very small case series [28, 29]. IOUS can provide additional detail on tumor extent, margins and vascular involvement. Preoperative MRI and CT have limitations in smaller patients and subcentimeter lesions [30]. IOUS has been shown to correct the preoperative resection strategy based on real time intraoperative assessment and lead to more accurate and liver sparing resections [31]. In addition, it is the authors preference after nonanatomic resection to confirm portal and hepatic arterial inflow and assess adequate hepatic venous drainage in bordering segments to recognize the risk for postoperative tissue necrosis or venous congestion.

Transplantation

Ultrasonography is an integral part of pre-, intra-, and postoperative management of pediatric liver transplant patients. Preoperatively, patency and size of the portal vein and anatomic variations of the cava and HA can accurately be assessed by ultrasonography and allow the surgeon to determine an appropriate graft and possible need for vascular conduits. Portal vein thrombosis without sizable and patent superior mesenteric vein is a contraindication for transplant. IOUS is frequently used during the transplant procedure particularly when using technical variant grafts or complex vascular reconstructions (Fig. 5.13). Confirming adequate portal venous and arterial duplex signals in all parts of the graft can help differentiate arterial spasm from technical anastomotic error and lead to immediate revision. Postoperative vascular complications, particularly arterial thrombosis have devastating consequences and may require retransplantation if uncorrectable. Early recognition is paramount and scheduled postoperative bedside ultrasonography is part of every transplant protocol. Besides assessment of graft perfusion and vascular patency, presence of a biloma or hematoma can also be detected.

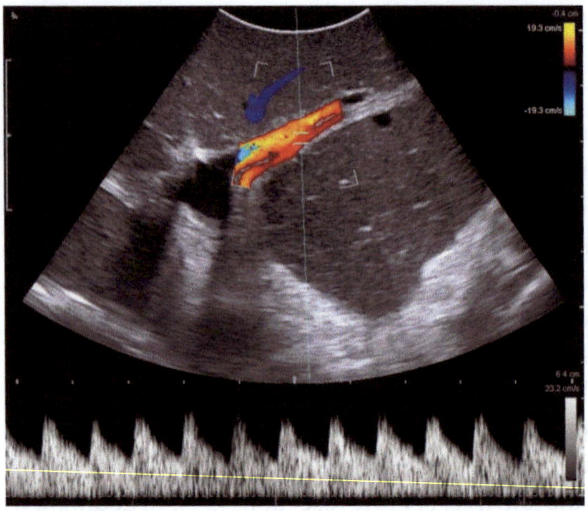

Fig. 5.13 Intraoperative image of 6-year-old confirming arterial flow signals in segment four after left lobe split liver transplant with reconstructed arterial supply

Summary

Ultrasonography is an essential tool in the hands of a pediatric hepatobiliary and transplant surgeon. It is an integral part of the preoperative workup of liver lesions and prospective transplant candidates. Intraoperatively, it guides resection margins and detects potential vascular anastomotic compromise or graft hypoperfusion. Following surgery ultrasonography is an ideal noninvasive screening modality for post resection complications as well as vascular patency.

References

1. Couinaud C. Liver lobes and segments. Notes on the anatomical architecture and surgery of the liver. Presse Med. 1954;62(33):709–12. (Article in French).
2. Strasberg SM. Nomenclature of hepatic anatomy and resections: a review of the Brisbane 2000 system. J Hepatobiliary Pancreat Surg. 2005;12(5):351–5.
3. Blumgart LH, Hann LE. Surgical and radiologic anatomy of the liver, biliary tract, and pancreas. In: Blumgart LH, Belghiti J, Jarnagin W, DeMatteo R, Chapman W, Buchler M et al. editors. Surgery of the Liver, Biliary Tract, and Pancreas. Philadelphia: Saunders; 2007. p. 3.
4. D'Angelica M, Fong Y. The liver. In: Beauchamp D, Evers M, Mattox K, editors. Sabison's Textbook of Surgery. 18th ed. Philadelphia: Saunders; 2008.
5. Joynt LK, Platt JF, Rubin JM, et al. Hepatic artery resistance before and after standard meal in subjects with diseased and healthy livers. Radiology. 1995;196(2):489–92.
6. McNaughton DA, Abu-Yousef MM. Doppler US of the Liver Made Simple. Radiographics. 2011;31:161–88.
7. Abu-Yousef MM. Duplex Doppler sonography of the hepatic vein in tricuspid regurgitation. AJR Am J Roentgenol. 1991;156(1):79–83.
8. Scheinfield MH, Ardiana B, Mordecai K. Understanding the spectral Doppler waveform of the hepatic veins in health and disease. Radiographics. 2009;29:2081–98.
9. Horton KM. CT and MR Imaging of Benign Hepatic and Biliary Tumors. Radiographics. 1999;19:431–51.
10. Stringer MD, Alizai NK. Mesenchymal hamartoma of the liver: a systematic review. J Pediatr Surg. 2005;40(11):1681–90.
11. Jha P, Chawla SC, Tavri S, Patel C, Gooding C, Daldrup-Link H. Pediatric liver tumors–a pictorial review. Eur Radiol. 2009;19(1):209–19.
12. Kochin IN, Miloh TA, Arnon R, Iyer KR, Suchy FJ, Kerkar N. Benign liver masses and lesions in children: 53 cases over 12 years. Isr Med Assoc J. 2011;13(9):542–7.
13. Boon LM, Burrows PE, Paltiel HJ, Lund DP, Ezekowitz RA, Folkman J, Mulliken JB. Hepatic vascular anomalies in infancy: a 27 year experience. J Pediatr. 1996;129(3):346–54. Review.
14. Kassarjian A, Zurakowski D, Dubois J, Paltiel HJ, Fishman SJ, Burrows PE. Infantile hepatic hemangiomas: clinical and imaging findings and their correlation with therapy. AJR Am J Roentgenol. 2004;182(3):785–95.
15. Keslar PJ, Buck JL, Selby DM. From the archives of the AFIP. Infantile hemangioendothelioma of the liver revisited. Radiographics. 1993;13(3):657–70.
16. Dickie B, Dasgupta R, Nair R, Alonso MH, Ryckman FC, Tiao GM, Adams DM, Azizkhan RG. Spectrum of hepatic hemangiomas: management and outcome. J Pediatr Surg. 2009;44(1):125–33.
17. Mirk P, Rubaltelli L, Bazzocchi M, et al. Ultrasonographic patterns in hepatic hemangiomas. J Clin Ultrasound. 1982;10:373–8.
18. Choi BI, Kim TK, Han JK, Chung JW, Park JH, Han MC. Power versus conventional color Doppler sonography: comparison in the depiction of vasculature in liver tumors. Radiology. 1996;200(1):55–8.
19. Kim T, Hori M, Onishi H. Liver masses with central or eccentric scar. Semin Ultrasound CT MR. 2009;30(5):418–25.
20. Chung EM, et al. From the archives of the AFIP: Pediatric liver masses: radiologic-pathologic correlation part 1. Benign tumors. Radiographics. 2010;30(3):801–26.
21. Meyers RL. Tumors of the liver in children. Surg Oncol. 2007;16(3):195–203. Review.

22. Srouji MN, Chatten J, Schulman WM, Ziegler MM, Koop CE. Mesenchymal hamartoma of the liver in infants. Cancer. 1978;42(5):2483–9. Review.
23. Roebuck DJ, Aronson D, Clapuyt P, et al. PRETEXT: a revised staging system for primary malignant liver tumours of childhood developed by the SIOPEL group. Pediatr Radiol 2007. 2005;37:123.
24. Smith D, Downey D, Spouge A, Soney S. Sonographic demonstration of Couinaud's liver segments. J Ultrasound Med. 1998;17(6):375–81.
25. Tanaka S, Kitamura T, Fujita M, et al. Color Doppler flow imaging of liver tumors. AJR Am J Roentgenol. 1990;154:509e14.
26. Torzilli G, Montorsi M, Donadon M, et al. "Radical but conservative" is the main goal for ultrasonography-guided liver resection: prospective validation of this approach. J Am Coll Surg. 2005;201:517.
27. Donadon M, Torzilli G. Intraoperative ultrasound in patients with hepatocellular carcinoma: from daily practice to future trends. Liver Cancer. 2013;2:16.
28. Thomas BL, Thomas MK, Parker GA, et al. Use of intraoperative ultrasound during hepatic resection in pediatric patients. J Pediatr Surg. 1989;24:690.
29. Vaos G. Segmental liver resection in a child using intraoperative ultrasound-guided radiofrequency energy. J Pediatr Surg. 2007;42:E5.
30. Felsted AE, Shi Y, Masand PM, Nuchtern JG, Goss JA, Vasudevan SA. Intraoperative ultrasound for liver tumor resection in children. J Surg Res. 2015;198(2):418.
31. Hammerstingl R, Huppertz A, Breuer J, et al. Diagnostic efficacy of gadoxetic acid (Primovist)-enhanced MRI and spiral CT for a therapeutic strategy: comparison with intraoperative and histopathologic findings in focal liver lesions. Eur Radiol. 2008;18:457.

Gallbladder and Biliary Tract

6

Christine M. Leeper, Gary Nace and Stefan Scholz

Introduction

Ultrasound is the preferred initial imaging modality for investigating right upper quadrant pain, jaundice, and any suspected pathology of the gallbladder and the biliary system. It is noninvasive, portable, relatively inexpensive, and does not carry the risk or radiation burden that accompanies computed tomography (CT) scan or general anesthesia for infants and children undergoing magnetic resonance imaging (MRI). Ultrasound has high sensitivity, specificity, and predictive value for many abnormal findings within the hepatobiliary tree. Many clinicians rely upon ultrasound as an adjunct or the definitive diagnostic tool in the workup of pediatric gallbladder and bile duct pathology.

S. Scholz (✉)
Division of Pediatric General and Thoracic Surgery, Children's Hospital of Pittsburgh of UPMC, University of Pittsburgh School of Medicine, One Children's Hospital Drive, 4401 Penn Avenue, Pittsburgh, PA 15261, USA
e-mail: stefan.scholz@chp.edu

C. M. Leeper
Department of General Surgery, University of Pittsburgh Medical Center, 200 Lothrop Street, Pittsburgh, PA 15213, USA
e-mail: leepercm@upmc.edu

G. Nace
Division of Pediatric General and Thoracic Surgery, Children's Hospital of Pittsburgh of UPMC, 4401 Penn Avenue, Pittsburgh, PA 15224, USA
e-mail: nacegw@upmc.edu

Scanning Technique and Anatomy and Normal Sonographic Findings

Similar to the liver, the gallbladder is typically scanned in a supine position with the addition of prone and upright in selective cases. The edge of the right lobe of the liver and the liver hilum can be used as landmarks during the examination. Asking the child to take a deep breath may bring the gallbladder down below the liver edge for better visualization [1]. The patient should have fasted for 4–6 h to fill the gallbladder, which contracts and empties after a fatty meal. Using the liver as a sonographic window, the gallbladder can easily be found on ultrasound and is a good point of orientation for scanning the upper abdomen and the liver. After fasting, the normal size of the gallbladder measures >2 cm in a neonate, about 4 cm at 4 years of age, and about 6 cm at 10 years.

As part of a complete gallbladder evaluation, the wall thickness should always be measured (normally <3 mm when fasted and filled). Thickening of the gallbladder wall is nonspecific and is caused by gallbladder or surrounding inflammation (cholecystitis, hepatitis, and pancreatitis) and other acute or chronic diseases such as hepatic cirrhosis, mucoviscidosis, or right heart failure. Importantly, the normal gallbladder wall thickness may measure more than 3 mm when contracted and empty.

In the right subcostal plane, the gallbladder can be seen as a round or oval hypoechoic structure seemingly within the liver parenchyma.

S. Scholz, M. D. Jarboe (eds.), *Diagnostic and Interventional Ultrasound in Pediatrics and Pediatric Surgery,* DOI 10.1007/978-3-319-21699-7_6

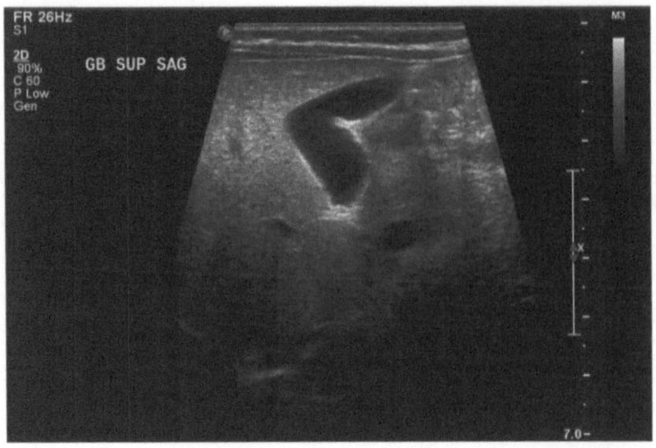

Fig. 6.1 Normal gallbladder shaped as a Phrygian cap

Moving the probe cranio-caudally, the gallbladder turns toward a ventro-lateral direction. The longitudinal view can be obtained by turning the probe into an almost sagittal direction. The probe is slightly moved medially and laterally and angled to scan the complete gallbladder lumen not to miss any intraluminal structures such as polyps or echogenic sludge or stones. For better visualization of small stones, a high frequency probe (>5 MHz) may be used. Folds of the gallbladder wall are commonly seen and normal, but may be confused with intraluminal polyps. A Phrygian cap is a relatively common inversion of the distal fundus into the body of the gallbladder [2] (Fig. 6.1).

Next, the cystic and common bile ducts (CBD) are identified, which runs parallel to the portal vein as an anechoic tube with hyperechoic borders. Intrahepatic ductal dilatation is indicative of distal obstruction (Fig. 6.2). Color Doppler aids in differentiation of vascular structures and extra- and intrahepatic bile system. When dilated in the setting of choledocholithiasis, pancreatitis or type 1 choledochal cyst, the common bile duct can be easily followed into the pancreatic head and to the duodenum with the ultrasound probe. The size of the CBD is age-dependent; in adults, the upper limit of 6 mm is frequently used, but a study of healthy pediatric patients less than 13 years of age found that all had a CBD size less than 3.3 mm, and children less than 3 months had a CBD size less than 1.2 mm [3]. After cholecystectomy, the bile duct tends to enlarge by a few millimeters.

The intrahepatic bile system is examined as part of the liver scan. The fine ducts follow the intrahepatic arterial system and may be differentiated by color Doppler. When not dilated, the ducts are hard to follow into the periphery of the liver. Segmental or general lobular or cystic dilatation is reported and may be caused by acquired distal or intrahepatic obstruction or congenital anomalies such as type 4 and 5 choledochal cysts [2].

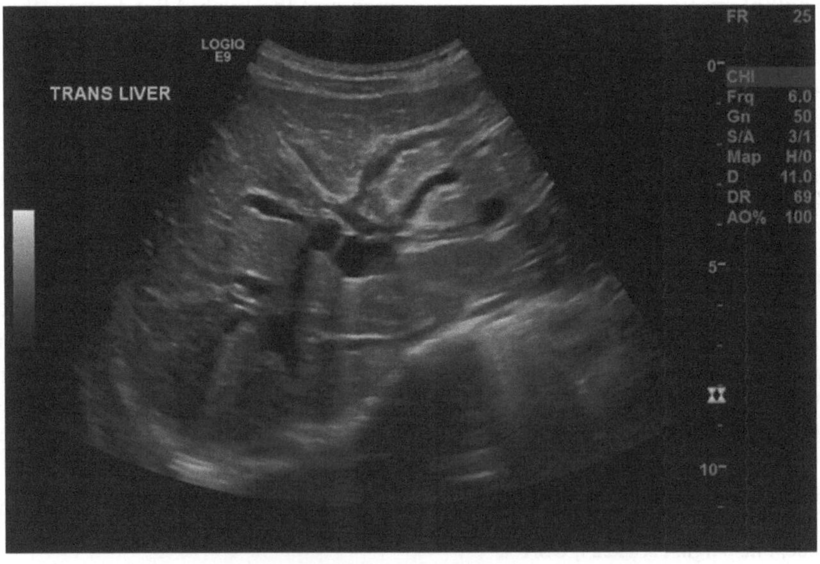

Fig. 6.2 Intrahepatic biliary ductal dilatation as a sign of distal bile duct obstruction

Malformation of the Biliary System

Biliary Atresia

Biliary atresia is an obstructive condition caused by progressive sclerosis of the extrahepatic bile ducts that, if untreated, leads to cirrhosis, liver failure, and eventually death. It is a relatively rare condition (incidence 1:15,000) with a variable incidence based on ethnicity and a slight female preponderance. The etiology of this entity remains unknown, though some postulate intrauterine viral infection, genetic mutation, vascular or metabolic insult, or dysfunctional immune response. There are three main types of biliary atresia: atresia of the CBD (type I), atresia of the common hepatic duct (type IIa) or atresia of the CBD and the common hepatic duct (type IIb), and atresia of all extrahepatic bile ducts up to the porta hepatis (type III). A great majority of patients have type III. A cystic form of biliary atresia can be confused with a type 1 choledochal cyst.

First described in the literature in 1891, biliary atresia was a universally fatal disease until the development of the Kasai hepatic portoenterostomy procedure in the 1950s, which allowed for drainage of the biliary system. The Kasai procedure continues to be the primary operation with liver transplant being the secondary option if the Kasai is unable to reverse the bile stasis and thereby suspend the cirrhosis progression. Early intervention within the first 2 months of life improves patient outcomes, with overall 5-year patient survival currently approaching 90 % [4].

The clinical presentation for biliary atresia is a jaundiced infant with hepatomegaly and pale stools. The diagnosis of biliary atresia is made with a battery of tests that includes liver function tests, hepatitis serologies, tissue biopsy and hepatobiliary ultrasonography, as well as transcystic cholangiogram. Ultrasound demonstrates several characteristic features of biliary atresia. In a study of 30 neonates, absence of the common bile duct had an 83 % sensitivity, 71 % specificity, positive predictive value of 90 %, and negative predictive value of 56 % [5]. However, this criterion should not be used in isolation as a patent distal CBD can be found in up to 20 % of biliary atresia cases [6]. A study of 56 infants evaluated the diagnostic value of the "triangular cord," a triangular or bandlike periportal echogenicity (3 mm or greater in thickness), which corresponds clinically to a cone-shaped fibrotic mass cranial to the portal vein bifurcation (Fig. 6.3a and b). This finding has a diagnostic accuracy of 94 %, with 84 % sensitivity, and 98 % specificity [7]. In patients with biliary atresia, the gallbladder is absent or shrunken and

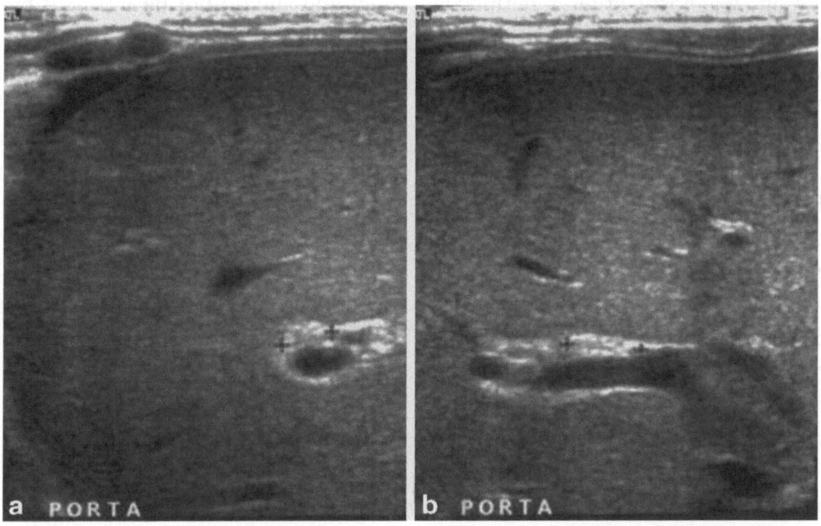

Fig. 6.3 (**a**) and (**b**) "Triangular cord" sign in an infant with biliary atresia, a triangular or bandlike periportal echogenicity (3 mm or greater in thickness), which represents a cone-shaped fibrotic mass cranial to the portal vein bifurcation. Transverse (**a**) and longitudinal (**b**) views (with permission from Poh et al. Biliary atresia: making the diagnosis by the gallbladder ghost triad. Pediatr Radiol 2003; 33:311–315, license number 3637101328502)

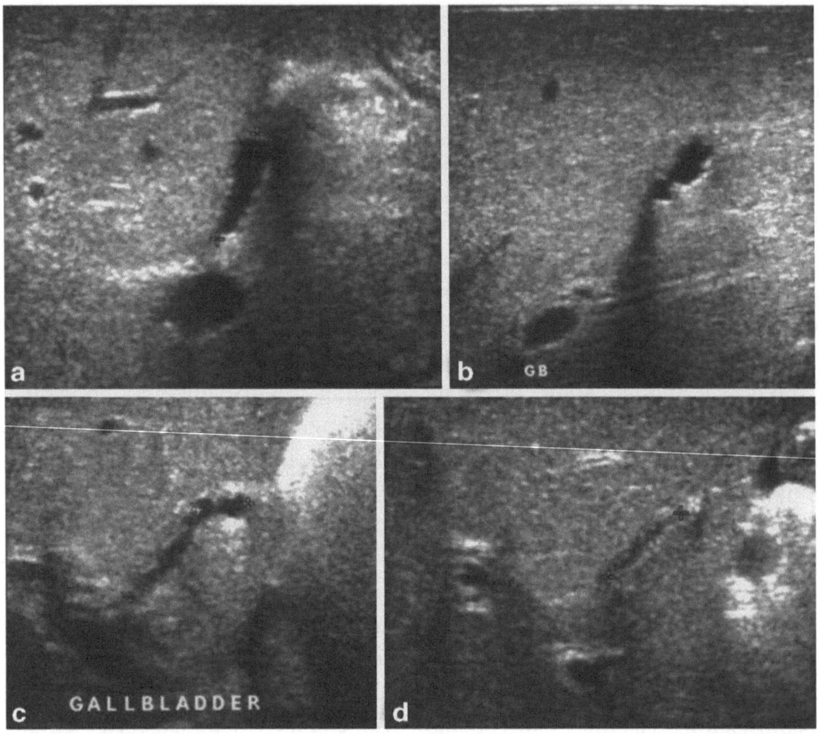

Fig. 6.4 (**a**–**d**) The "gallbladder ghost triad" in patients with biliary atresia. Longitudinal scans of the gallbladder in a (**a**) 2-week-old male, (**b**) 3-week-old female, (**c**) 5-week-old male, and (**d**) 6-week-old male, demonstrating a short gallbladder length, an irregular or lobular contour, and a relatively indistinct lining and wall (with permission from Poh et al. Biliary atresia: making the diagnosis by the gallbladder ghost triad. Pediatr Radiol 2003; 33:311–315, license number 3637101328502)

irregular. Tan and colleagues describe the "gallbladder ghost triad" diagnostic criteria, defined as gallbladder length <1.9 cm, lack of smooth/complete echogenic mucosal lining with an indistinct wall, and irregular/lobular contour (Fig. 6.4a, b, c and d). Out of 31 patients with biliary atresia, 30 met all three sonographic criteria [8].

After the Kasai procedure, ultrasound is utilized to monitor the patency of the hepatic vessels and health of the native liver. The sonographic finding of the bile lakes (Fig. 6.5), or clusters of fused damaged bile ducts that form as a result of bile stasis and inflammatory destruction of the bile ducts [9], is thought to be associated with poor prognosis. In one study, the presence of bile lakes predicted a greater number of episodes of cholangitis in the long term [10]. This finding can also be seen in Caroli's disease, or Type 5 choledochal cyst.

Ultrasound is a vital component in the workup of patients with biliary atresia yielding valuable information in this challenging patient population, and should not be replaced by liver biopsy or hepatobiliary iminodiacetic acid (HIDA) scan only. Ten percent of children with biliary atresia can have associated anomalies, including polysplenia, azygous continuation of the inferior vena cava, preduodenal portal vein, hepatic arterial anomalies, and bilaterally bilobed lungs—these diagnoses would be missed with a more limited imaging modality [11]. Ultrasound also has the benefit of excluding other causes of jaundice such as choledochal cyst or inspissated bile syndrome.

Choledochal Cyst

A choledochal cyst is a congential or acquired dilation of the bile duct. Infants typically present with jaundice or an abdominal mass, while older children can present with abdominal pain and

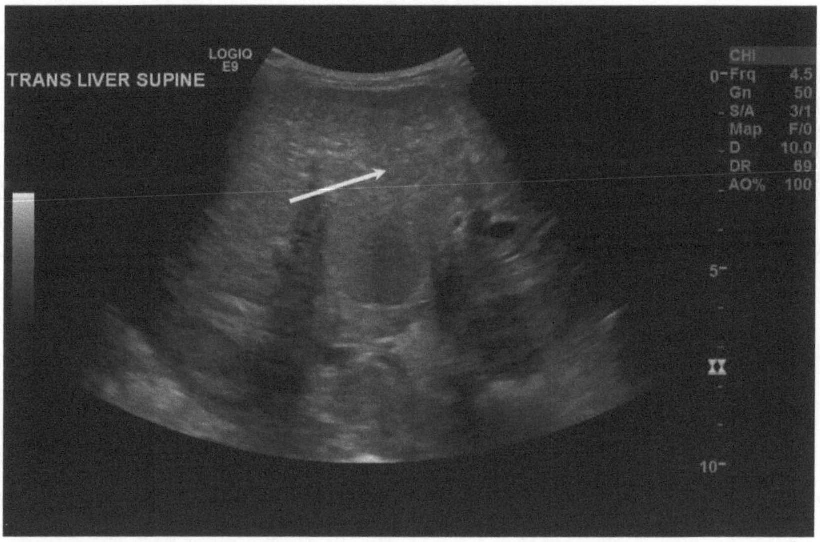

Fig. 6.5 Bile lakes (*arrow*) in the *left* lobe of a patient with biliary atresia after Kasai procedure

vomiting. The most commonly utilized classification schema by Todani includes five types of choledocal cyst—Type I: dilation of the CBD, Type II: diverticulum of the CBD, Type III: choledochocele (dilatation of the terminal CBD within the duodenal wall), Type IV: multiple cysts of the extrahepatic and intrahepatic ducts, and Type V: single or multiple intrahepatic duct cysts (Caroli disease). Type I is by far the most common, followed by Type IV. Pancreatitis and cholangitis are known complications of choledochal cysts; malignant transformation has been described but is rare and typically limited to adults. Surgical management involves complete cyst excision with a bilio-enteric anastomosis [12].

Ultrasound is the first-line imaging study of choice for diagnosis and description of choledochal cysts (Figs. 6.6 and 6.7). It permits com-

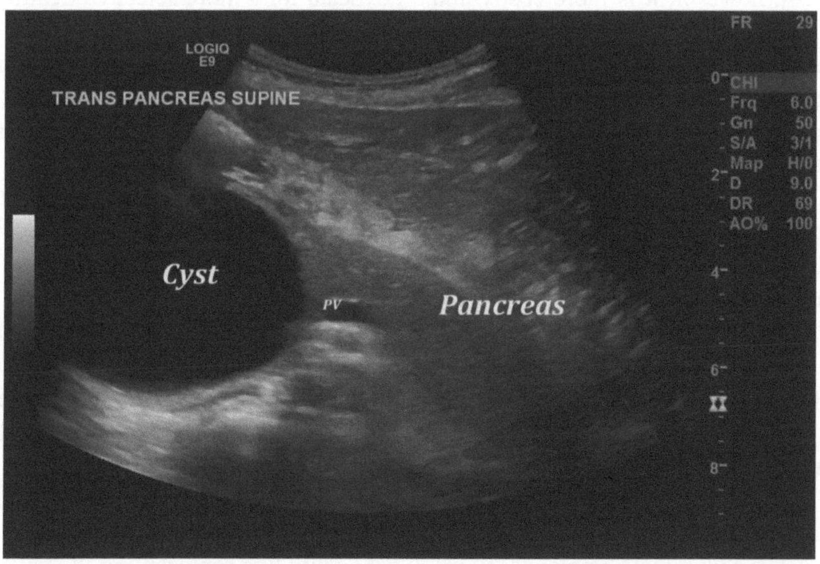

Fig. 6.6 Choledochal cyst, Type 4, adjacent to head of the pancreas (*portal vein* = *PV*) (the intrahepatic dilated bile system is not well pictured here)

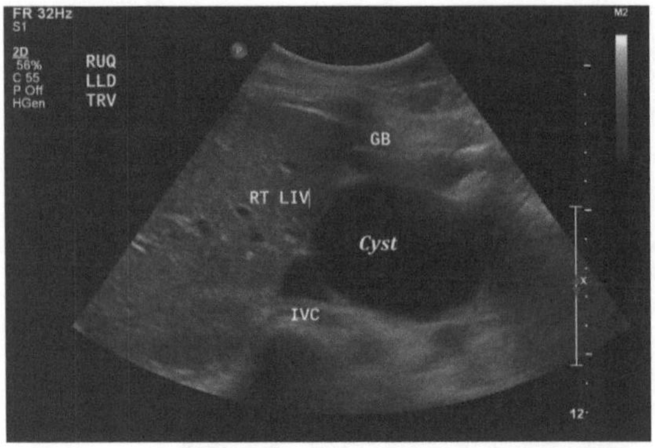

Fig. 6.7 Choledochal cyst, Type 1

plete assessment of the shape, size, and position of the cyst, as well as an evaluation of the proximal ducts, vascular anatomy, and hepatic parenchyma [12]. Ultrasound can accurately classify the type of choledochal cyst in a cost-effective and reliable manner. Some literature suggests that ultrasound may be the only imaging modality needed in cases where no intrahepatic biliary ductal dilatation is visualized [13]. However, when dilated intrahepatic ducts are encountered on ultrasound, additional imaging by magnetic resonance cholangiopancreatography (MRCP) should be performed in order to distinguish between Type I and Type IV choledochal cysts, as this distinction may alter the operative approach. MRCP is accurate and noninvasive [14]; however, it is more costly and requires the patient to be still and cooperative and has to performed under general anesthesia in young children. Endoscopic retrograde cholangiopancreatography (ERCP) offers complete characterization of the cyst and ductal anatomy, though it is invasive and can be complicated by perforation, pancreatitis, and hemorrhage [15]. Contrast-enhanced CT may be considered in some patients if an associated tumor is suspected [12].

Disorders of the Gallbladder

Cholelithiasis

With the wide use of abdominal ultrasound in the workup of pediatric abdominal complaints, symptomatic and asymptomatic cholelithiasis are increasingly common diagnoses in pediatric patients. Older studies report an estimated incidence of cholelithiasis in children between 0.13 and 0.22% [16, 17]. A more recent study, however, reports an incidence of 1.9%, with an additional 1.5% having gallbladder sludge [18]. Cholelithiasis can be idiopathic or secondary to known contributing factors. In infants, stones are usually secondary to a variety of factors, such as obstructive congenital anomalies of the biliary tract, total parenteral nutrition, furosemide treatment, phototherapy, dehydration, infection, hemolytic anemia, and short-gut syndrome. In older children, gallstones can be associated with sickle cell disease, bowel resection, hemolytic anemia, and choledochal cyst [19].

The incidence of pediatric gallbladder disease is increasing, due in large part to the rising childhood obesity epidemic. Previously, hemolytic disease was the most common risk factor for gallbladder disease in children. However, recent data demonstrates that obesity is associated with 39% of gallstone disorder [20]. The cholecystectomy rate in children without the diagnosis of hemolytic anemia has doubled in the USA in recent years, with an increased percentage undergoing a laparoscopic procedure [21]. Laparoscopic cholecystectomy enjoys a low complication rate in pediatric patients. It is the treatment of choice for symptomatic cholelithiasis, and at some centers even for asymptomatic gallstones [22, 23]. However, many advocate for a more selective treatment approach given the fact that many children will continue to be asymptomatic without intervention [18].

Ultrasound is the gold standard for detecting cholelithiasis. The diagnosis is made by visualizing an echogenic focus within gallbladder lumen, typically with prominent posterior acoustic shadowing (Figs. 6.8 and 6.9). A change in patient position will frequently result in gravity dependent movement of the stone. One ultrasound finding associated with cholelithiasis is the "twinkle artifact," which refers to an artifact on color Doppler demonstrating alternating colors behind a gallstone that mimic turbulent blood flow. Another possible finding is the "wall-echo-shadow" sign, which refers to the layered appearance of a gallbladder filled with stones (hyperechogenic line representing the gallbladder wall, hypoechoic space representing a small amount of bile, hyperechogenic line representing the near

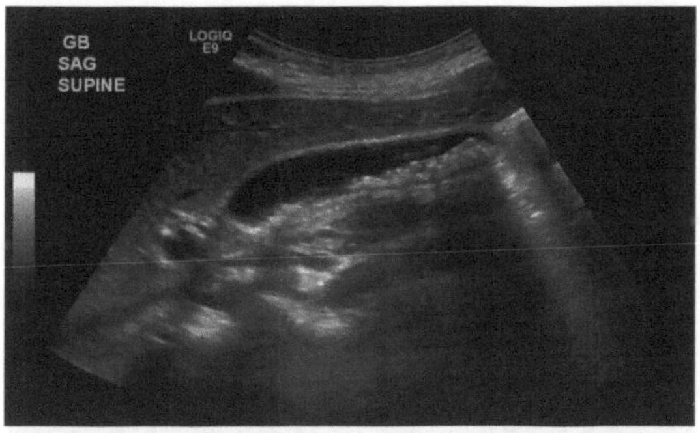

Fig. 6.8 Cholelithiasis with posterior acoustic shadowing (*longitudinal view*)

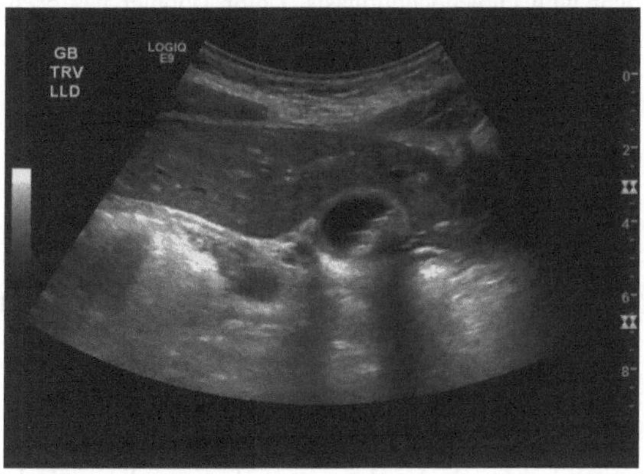

Fig. 6.9 Cholelithiasis (*transverse view*)

surface of gallstones, acoustic shadowing distal to the surface of the gallstones).

Cholecystitis

Cholecystitis may be a challenging diagnosis to make in children. This inflammatory condition occurs secondary to gallbladder outlet obstruction, often caused by a stone impacted in the cystic duct neck, and the resulting increased intraluminal pressure. Pediatric patients often do not present with the "classic" symptoms of fever, right upper quadrant pain, and leukocytosis [24]. Especially in younger children, abdominal pain may be vague and diffuse [12]. Calculous cholecystitis is more common, as acalculous cholecystitis is almost exclusively associated with postoperative complications, sepsis, burns, trauma, transfusion, or infection [16].

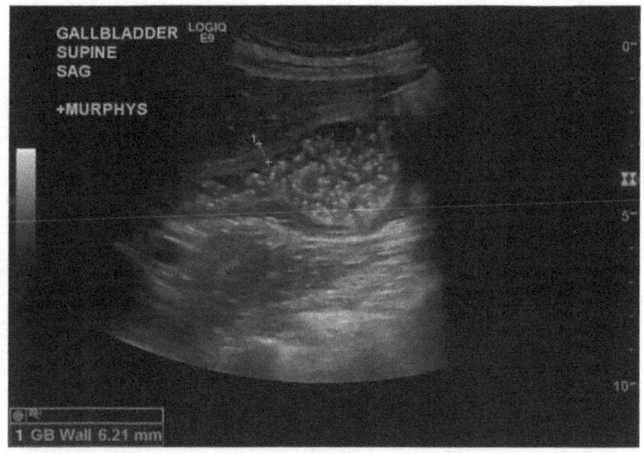

Fig. 6.10 Acute cholecystitis—distended sludge-filled gallbladder with wall thickening (6.2 mm). Notation indicates positive sonographic Murphy's sign during the exam

Ultrasound is a first-line modality for diagnosing acute cholecystitis. There are no mandatory criteria, rather the diagnosis relies on a combination of nonspecific signs including wall thickness >3 mm, dilation of the gallbladder, pericholecystic fluid, wall hyperemia on color Doppler, and a positive sonographic Murphy's sign (point of maximal tenderness over the visualized gallbladder), which should be always reported with the ultrasound report (Fig. 6.10). In advanced cholecystitis, ultrasound may demonstrate emphysema (hyperechoic intramural air), gangrene (thick streaky gallbladder wall or sloughed membranes), or frank perforation (disruption of the gallbladder wall) [25]. In adults, the best predictor is the Murphy's sign [26], however in children this may be more difficult to elicit and signs such as cholelithiasis and gallbladder sludge (Fig. 6.11) may be more reliable indicators of cholecystitis. All

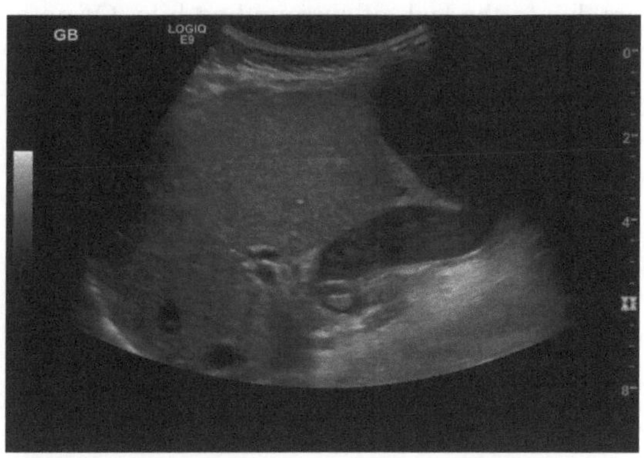

Fig. 6.11 Gallbladder sludge in a patient on TPN

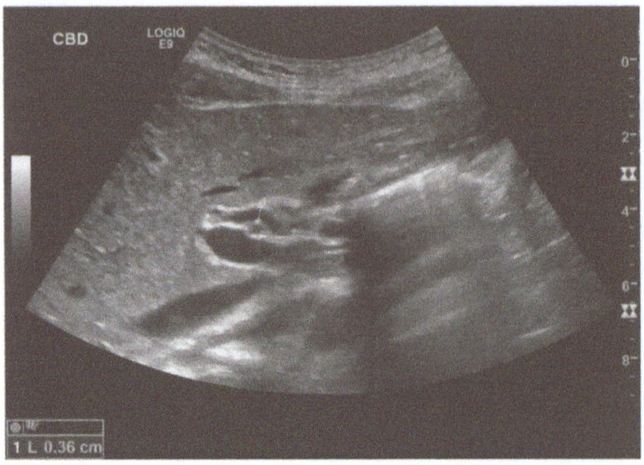

Fig. 6.12 Normal common bile duct (0.36 cm)

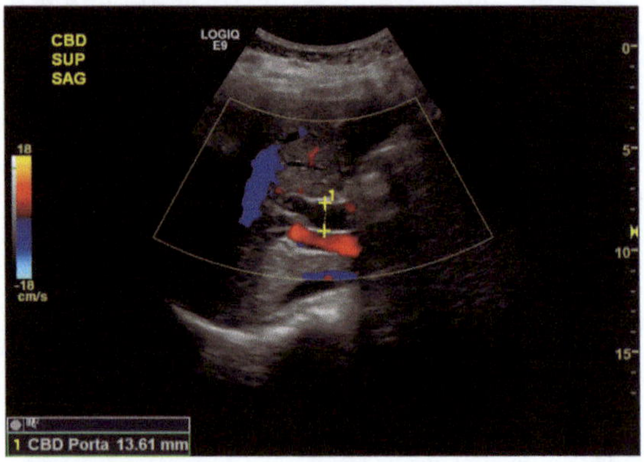

Fig. 6.13 Dilated common bile duct (1.36 cm) in a patient with choledocholithiasis. Color Doppler has been applied to clarify portal structures

sonographic indicators of pediatric cholecystitis have lower sensitivities and predictive values as compared to those for adults [27], therefore nuclear medicine studies are important adjuncts. In a HIDA scan that is positive for acute cholecystitis, the radioactive tracer is excreted in the liver, but does not accumulate in the gallbladder due to obstruction of the cystic duct by stone or edema.

Choledocholithiasis

Ultrasound can also diagnose dilation of the CBD secondary to an obstructing stone, or choledocholithiasis. Choledocholithiasis is uncommon in children with an incidence of 2–7% [16, 28]. The CBD may be followed distally toward the duodenum to evaluate for impacted stones as the underlying pathology. Intraductal stones are hyperechoic and immobile. Shadowing is evident in some cases but may be absent in others due to the lack of surrounding bile. Of note, a dilated CBD can be confused with the portal vein, in which case color Doppler may be helpful to clarify whether the structure contains vascular flow [25] (Figs. 6.12 and 6.13). The management of choledocholithiasis includes antibiotics and ERCP for biliary tree decompression followed by cholecystectomy.

Cholangitis

Cholangitis is a rare entity in children with typical hepatobiliary anatomy; diagnosis may be challenging as pediatric patients who present with this disease may not meet all criteria of the classic Reynold's pentad (right upper quadrant pain, jaundice, fever, hypotension, and altered mental status). In the case of ascending cholangitis caused by distal obstruction, ultrasound may demonstrate dilation of the common bile duct and possibly visualize the impacted stone. Of note, biliary dilatation is not always present in the early stages of bile duct obstruction and MRCP may be required to diagnose the cause and level of biliary tree obstruction [29]. Cholangitis in pediatric patients is also an uncommon complication of hepaticoenterostomy that has been performed after choledochal cyst excision, liver transplant, or treatment for another hepatobiliary pathology [30]. Cholangitis after portoenterostomy for biliary atresia is a clinical diagnosis and carries no sonographic correlate.

Summary

Ultrasound is an important diagnostic tool in the pathology of the gallbladder and biliary system. It is reliable and accurate in the detection of hepatobiliary malformations such as choledochal cysts, as well as gallbladder disease including cholelithiasis, cholecystitis, choledocholithiasis, and cholangitis. It plays an important role in the evaluation of biliary atresia. Abdominal ultrasound should be used as a first-line imaging modality in the workup of suspected gallbladder or biliary disease.

References

1. Soto JA, Castrillon G. Gallbladder and biliary tree imaging techniques. In: Hamm B, editor. Abdominal imaging. Heidelberg: Springer; 2013. p. 1229–40.
2. Marvin M, Jones CM, Byam JA, Iannitti DA. Hepatobiliary ultrasound. In: Schrope B, editor. Surgical and interventional ultrasound. New York: McGraw-Hill Education; 2014.
3. Hernanz-Schulman M, Ambrosino MM, Freeman PC, Quinn CB. Common bile duct in children: sonographic dimensions. Radiology. 1995;195(1):193–5.
4. Yamataka ACJ, Miyano T. Biliary Atresia. In: Holcomb GWMJ, Ostlie DJ, editors. Ashcraft's pediatric surgery. Philadelphia: Elsevier Inc; 2014. p. 580–92.
5. Azuma T, Nakamura T, Nakahira M, Harumoto K, Nakaoka T, Moriuchi T. Pre-operative ultrasonographic diagnosis of biliary atresia–with reference to the presence or absence of the extrahepatic bile duct. Pediatr Surg Int. 2003;19(6):475–7.
6. Farrant P, Meire HB, Mieli-Vergani G. Ultrasound features of the gall bladder in infants presenting with conjugated hyperbilirubinaemia. Br J Radiol. 2000;73(875):1154–8.
7. Park WH, Choi SO, Lee HJ. The ultrasonographic 'triangular cord' coupled with gallbladder images in the diagnostic prediction of biliary atresia from infantile intrahepatic cholestasis. J Pediatr Surg. 1999;34(11):1706–10.
8. Tan Kendrick AP, Phua KB, Ooi BC, Tan CE. Biliary atresia: making the diagnosis by the gallbladder ghost triad. Pediatr Radiol. 2003;33(5):311–5.
9. Tainaka T, Kaneko K, Nakamura S, Ono Y, Sumida W, Ando H. Histological assessment of bile lake formation after hepatic portoenterostomy for biliary atresia. Pediatr Surg Int. 2008;24(3):265–9.
10. Inoue Y, Kato Y, Tamura T, Kobayashi H, Ichikawa S, Lane GJ, et al. Prognostic implications of bile lakes after surgery for biliary atresia. J Pediatr Surg. 2008;43(12):2165–8.
11. Abramson SJ, Berdon WE, Altman RP, Amodio JB, Levy J. Biliary atresia and noncardiac polysplenic syndrome: US and surgical considerations. Radiology. 1987;163(2):377–9.
12. Liem N, Holcomb GW. Choledochal cyst and gallbladder disease. In: Holcomb GWMJ, Ostlie DJ, editors. Ashcraft's Pediatric Surgery. Philadelphia: Elsevier Inc.; 2014. p. 593–606.
13. Murphy AJ, Axt JR, Crapp SJ, Martin CA, Crane GL, Lovvorn HN 3rd. Concordance of imaging modalities and cost minimization in the diagnosis of pediatric choledochal cysts. Pediatr Surg Int. 2012;28(6):615–21.
14. Huang CT, Lee HC, Chen WT, Jiang CB, Shih SL, Yeung CY. Usefulness of magnetic resonance cholangiopancreatography in pancreatobiliary abnormalities in pediatric patients. Pediatr Neonatol. 2011;52(6):332–6.
15. Otto AK, Neal MD, Slivka AN, Kane TD. An appraisal of endoscopic retrograde cholangiopancreatography (ERCP) for pancreaticobiliary disease in children: our institutional experience in 231 cases. Surg Endosc. 2011;25(8):2536–40.
16. Rescorla FJ. Cholelithiasis, cholecystitis, and common bile duct stones. Curr Opin Pediatr. 1997;9(3):276–82.
17. Palasciano G, Portincasa P, Vinciguerra V, Velardi A, Tardi S, Baldassarre G, et al. Gallstone prevalence and gallbladder volume in children and adolescents: an epidemiological ultrasonographic survey and relationship to body mass index. Am J Gastroenterol. 1989;84(11):1378–82.
18. Wesdorp I, Bosman D, de Graaff A, Aronson D, van der Blij F, Taminiau J. Clinical presentations and predisposing factors of cholelithiasis and sludge in children. J Pediatr Gastroenterol Nutr. 2000;31(4):411–7.
19. Gubernick JA, Rosenberg HK, Ilaslan H, Kessler A. US approach to jaundice in infants and children. Radiographics: a review publication of the Radiological Society of North America. Inc. 2000;20(1):173–95.
20. Mehta S, Lopez ME, Chumpitazi BP, Mazziotti MV, Brandt ML, Fishman DS. Clinical characteristics and risk factors for symptomatic pediatric gallbladder disease. Pediatrics. 2012;129(1):e82–8.
21. Balaguer EJ, Price MR, Burd RS. National trends in the utilization of cholecystectomy in children. J Surg Res. 2006;134(1):68–73.
22. Herzog D, Bouchard G. High rate of complicated idiopathic gallstone disease in pediatric patients of a North American tertiary care center. World J Gastroenterol. 2008;14(10):1544–8.
23. Tannuri AC, Leal AJ, Velhote MC, Gonlcalves ME, Tannuri U. Management of gallstone disease in children: a new protocol based on the experience of a single center. J Pediatr Surg. 2012;47(11):2033–8.
24. Gruber PJ, Silverman RA, Gottesfeld S, Flaster E. Presence of fever and leukocytosis in acute cholecystitis. Ann Emerg Med. 1996;28(3):273–7.
25. Poffenberger CM, Gausche-Hill M, Ngai S, Myers A, Renslo R. Cholelithiasis and its complications in children and adolescents: update and case discussion. Pediatr Emerg Care. 2012;28(1):68–76; quiz 7–8.
26. Ralls PW, Halls J, Lapin SA, Quinn MF, Morris UL, Boswell W. Prospective evaluation of the sonographic Murphy sign in suspected acute cholecystitis. J Clin Ultrasound. 1982;10(3):113–5.
27. Tsai J, Sulkowski JP, Cooper JN, Mattei P, Deans KJ, Minneci PC. Sensitivity and predictive value

of ultrasound in pediatric cholecystitis. J Surg Res. 2013;184(1):378–82.
28. Lugo-Vicente HL. Trends in management of gallbladder disorders in children. Pediatr Surg Int. 1997;12(5–6):348–52.
29. Gallix BP, Aufort S, Pierredon MA, Garibaldi F, Bruel JM. [Acute cholangitis: imaging diagnosis and management]. J Radiol. 2006;87(4 Pt 2):430–40.
30. Yamataka A, Ohshiro K, Okada Y, Hosoda Y, Fujiwara T, Kohno S, et al. Complications after cyst excision with hepaticoenterostomy for choledochal cysts and their surgical management in children versus adults. J Pediatr Surg. 1997;32(7):1097–102.

The Pancreas

7

Julia Scholsching and Oliver J. Muensterer

Introduction

Obtaining high-quality sonographic images of the pancreas in children is challenging in many aspects. Most importantly, the retroperitoneal location of the pancreas makes it difficult to visualize without good respiratory cooperation of the patient. Furthermore, pathologies of the pancreas in children are rare and may be misinterpreted easily. However, with high-resolution modern ultrasound devices, the resulting images have improved, and sonographic examination of the pancreas has become somewhat more routine. This chapter describes instructions for choosing the appropriate equipment, preparing the patient, and systematically scanning the pancreas in order to obtain clinically relevant pictures.

Scanning Techniques

Position of the Patient

Imaging of the pancreas is achieved with the curvilinear and linear array transducer. A sector transducer can be useful in neonates. Fasting of 4–6 h in older children or 3 h in neonates is mandatory for best results since air in the colon or bowel may limit visualization. It is advisable, however, to have non-carbonated water or other clear liquids available on-site to fill the stomach as an acoustic window.

Usually, ultrasound imaging of the pancreas starts in a supine position but can be changed throughout the examination for best results. A slight left lateral decubitus angulation of the patient facilitates imaging of the body and tail, whereas a right lateral position enhances the view on the pancreatic head.

In a compliant child, locating the pancreas is best achieved during maximum inspiration, which places the left hepatic lobe over the pancreas to act as an acoustic window. Gentle pressure with the probe can be used to disperse any overlying intestinal gas.

A useful adjunct for creating an acoustic window is to fill the stomach with non-carbonated clear liquids. This should be done at the end of a complete abdominal scan, and it is advisable to postpone imaging for 15 min to allow air bubbles ingested when swallowing the liquids to resolve. Changing the position of the patient thereafter leads to a shift of liquid from the gastric antrum to the duodenum and can thereby improve visualization of the pancreatic head.

Anatomical Features/Sonographic Neighborhood/Probe Placement

The pancreas is located in the retroperitoneum extending from the duodenum to the splenic

O. J. Muensterer (✉) · J. Scholsching
Department of Pediatric Surgery, University Medicine of the Johannes Gutenberg University Mainz, Langenbeckstraße 1, 55131 Mainz, Germany
e-mail: oliver.muensterer@unimedizin-mainz.de

J. Scholsching
e-mail: julia.scholsching@unimedizin-mainz.de

S. Scholz, M. D. Jarboe (eds.), *Diagnostic and Interventional Ultrasound in Pediatrics and Pediatric Surgery*, DOI 10.1007/978-3-319-21699-7_7

hilum. Closest to the duodenum is the pancreatic head (Latin, *caput*). Overlying the vertebral column is the body *(corpus),* and the tail *(cauda)* extends towards the spleen. Vessels dominate the sonographic "neighborhood" of the pancreas and serve as important landmarks. The pancreatic head is surrounded by duodenum laterally, with the superior mesenteric artery and vein running along the posterior aspect of the head, anterior to the uncinate process. The splenic vein accompanies the posterior wall of body tail in a mostly parallel fashion, joining the superior mesenteric vein forming the portal vein in a retropancreatic location between the head and body. The superior margin of the corpus and cauda is marked by the splenic artery. Left to the spine is the aorta, which is typically round on transverse sections and gives off the two renal arteries at this level. In contrast, the vena cava is usually teardrop shaped and located to the right of the spine.

These landmarks are used to localize the pancreas: Initially, the probe is placed beneath the xhiphoid process, starting with a transverse epigastric view. By angulating the probe downward slightly, the celiac trunk is seen superior to the pancreas and the splenic vein running along in parallel to the gland. With the probe in transverse position, the splenic vein appears like a hockey stick, whereas the celiac trunk often impresses with a dove-like shape. The pancreas can be fully visualized by moving the probe slowly from the upper transverse epigastric view downward to a subgastric angulation. In addition, the longitudinal depiction—a "head to tail" survey—should be performed with the probe in sagittal orientation, completed by an oblique subcostal view with slow rotation of the probe in a clockwise manner.

The main pancreatic duct is displayed parallel to the splenic vein, but is often hard to visualize if not dilated. Changes in diameter related to obstruction due to a tumor, postinflammatory stenosis, or choledocholithiasis should be noted on the ultrasound report. Normal age findings of the diameter of the main pancreatic duct in children have been poorly investigated, but the upper limit for a non-dilated duct range from 1 mm in 1–6-year-olds up to 2 mm in teenagers [1], see Table 7.1. Everything above 2 mm, particularly when associated with an elevation of serum amylase and clinical findings of abdominal pain, should be considered highly suspicious for acute or chronic pancreatitis.

Table 7.1 Average approximate age-dependent sonographic measurements of the pancreatic duct in millimeters. (Adapted from [1])

Age (years)	Normal	Acute pancreatitis	Chronic pancreatitis
1–3	1.13	1.9	n.a.
4–6	1.35	2.07	n.a.
7–9	1.67	2.13	2.42
10–12	1.78	2.34	2.77
13–15	1.92	2.56	2.91
16–18	2.05	2.63	3.15

Examination of the pancreas should always be considered as an integral part of a comprehensive evaluation of the hepatobiliary system, in addition to the mandatory examination of the bile duct, gallbladder, and liver parenchyma.

Age-Dependent Size and Echogenicity

The size of the pancreas is age dependent, with a high interindividual variability [2, 3]. Measurements of the pancreas, particularly during routine scans in otherwise healthy children without pancreatic disorders, are optional and usually have no clinical significance. The corpus of the pancreas is usually the easiest part to assess. When taking measurements, the anterior–posterior diameters of all parts of the pancreas should be obtained and reported (see age-depending dimensions in Table 7.2). The most substantial growth of the

Table 7.2 Average approximate age-dependent sonographic measurements of the pancreas in centimeters. (Adapted from [1])

Age (years)	Normal	Acute pancreatitis	Chronic pancreatitis
1–3	0.98	1.15	n.a.
4–6	1.01	1.22	n.a.
7–9	1.04	1.30	1.05
10–12	1.06	1.35	1.15
13–15	1.11	1.37	1.15
16–18	1.18	1.43	1.20

pancreas occurs in the first year of life [2, 3]. Pathologic increase in size at a young age mostly occurs in cases of acute pancreatitis or congenital hyperinsulinism (formerly known as nesidioblastosis). Patients with chronic pancreatitis often have normal or decreased pancreatic caliber due to fibrosis [1]. In cases of insulin-dependent diabetes mellitus (IDDM), studies have shown that long duration of the disease was associated with a reduction in the size of the pancreas at all ages. Furthermore, the decrease in the size was correlated with the severity of insulin deficiency due to fibrosis [4].

In healthy children, the echo structure of the pancreas appears "cobblestone-like" on high-resolution ultrasound imaging. In infants, the echogenicity initially appears similar to liver, becoming more hyperechogenic with increasing age (Fig. 7.1a, b). In newborns, however, the pancreas may also be transiently slightly hyperechoic [5]. Reasons for diffuse hyperechoicity include fibrosis, fatty degeneration, long-term corticosteroid or cytostatic therapy, Shwachman–Diamond syndrome, congenital hyperinsulinism, chronic pancreatitis, edematous pancreatitis, hemosiderosis, parenteral nutrition, Cushing's disease, and obesity. Focal alterations of the size and echogenicity are described separately below.

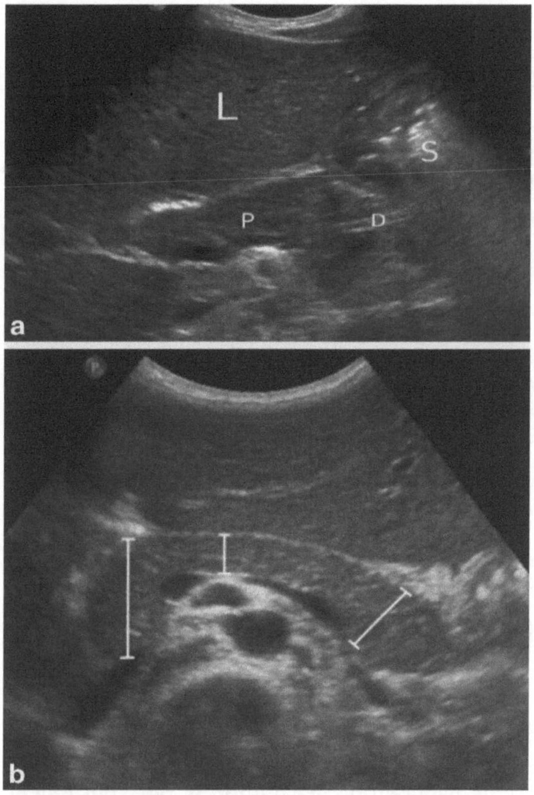

Fig. 7.1 **a** Normal pancreas *(P)* imaged through the left lobe of the liver *(L)*. The pancreatic duct is partially visible *(D)*, while the tail is obscured by the gas-containing stomach *(S)*. **b** Transverse ultrasonography (US) image shows the measurements of the head, body, and tail of the pancreas in a child. [6]

Sonographic Pathology of the Pancreas

Pancreatic Embryology and Related Anomalies

The embryological fusion of the pancreas from a ventral and dorsal bud gives rise to a certain variance in the anatomy of the major and minor pancreatic duct. Note that in 60 %, the two ducts insert separately into the duodenum, whereas in about 30 %, the individual ducts unite before the main pancreatic duct drains into the duodenum in a single location. Pancreatic duct anomalies can predispose to recurrent pancreatitis.

Pancreas divisum is the most common anatomical variant and occurs if no or only incomplete fusion of the ventral and dorsal bud takes place. The major portion of the pancreatic secretion drains into the duodenum through the minor papilla via the dorsal duct. It can be a reason for recurrent pancreatitis due to relative obstruction, but the need of therapy in asymptomatic cases is still controversial. Ultrasound is the first diagnostic tool to rule out pancreatitis or pancreatic pseudocysts as a manifestation of pancreas divisum. In order to clearly evaluate the ductal anomaly, ultrasound should be complemented by endoscopic retrograde cholecystopancreatography (ERCP) or magnetic resonance cholecystopancreatography (MRCP). However, new ultrasound techniques, including secretin-stimulated ultrasonography (US) [7] or endoscopic ultrasonography (EUS) [8], have also been employed and may be more accurate.

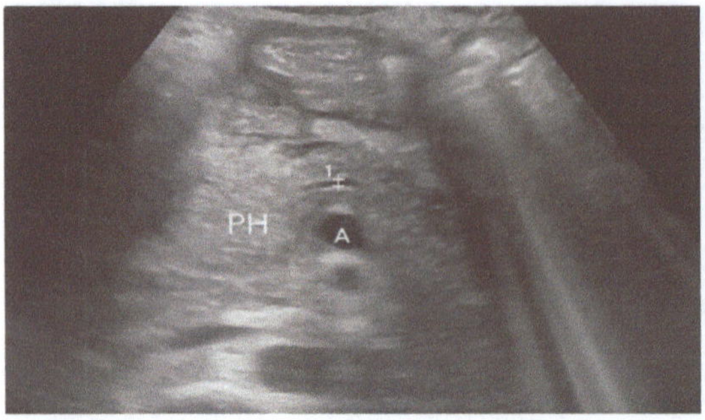

Fig. 7.2 Gallstone pancreatitis. The pancreatic head *(PH)* is echogenic and swollen. The pancreatic duct *(1)* is mildly dilated. The mesenteric artery is visible *(A)* as a landmark

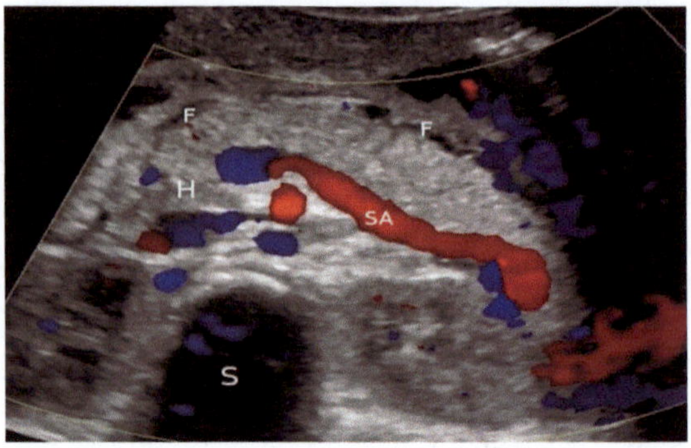

Fig. 7.3 Doppler study of acute pancreatitis. The head *(H)* and body of the pancreas are visible, with the splenic artery *(SA)* serving as a landmark. The spine is in the background *(S)*. There is peripancreatic fluid *(F)* visible as a sign of inflammation

Annular pancreas can cause congenital duodenal obstruction, seen on ultrasound as the typical "double bubble" appearance as an indirect sign of the diagnosis.

Acute Pancreatitis

Acute pancreatitis in children is rare, but recent studies found that the prevalence is increasing, possibly due to improved diagnostic tools or higher awareness [9]. It is associated with a high mortality and morbidity [10]. While idiopathic in 23 % of cases, the most common causes are trauma (22 %), structural anomalies (15 %), multisystem disease (14 %), drugs and toxins (12 %), as well as viral infections (10 %). Cholelithiasis causing pancreatitis due to obstruction has previously been considered unusual [11], but lately the incidence has been increasing, in part due to a rise in pediatric and adolescent obesity (Fig. 7.2) [12].

Acute pancreatitis is defined by an acute onset of symptoms (abdominal pain, vomiting, paralytic ileus, rebound tenderness, jaundice), elevated levels of serum/urine amylase, and a pathological ultrasound with compromise of pancreatic structure and function. Factors secondary to the pancreatitis itself may obscure the sonographic diagnosis, particularly in children. For example, increased intestinal gas due to paralytic ileus or lack of compliance due to pain can negatively impact the examination.

Ultrasound may show an increase in anterior–posterior diameter of the pancreas, usually because of edematous swelling with diffuse or focal-elevated echogenicity. Organ enlargement, however, can be absent in up to 50 % of cases. Peripancreatic fluid is another typical finding (Fig. 7.3). As mentioned beforehand, dilation of the pancreatic duct greater than 1.5 mm in children between 1 and 6 years, 1.9 mm at ages 7–12 years, 2.2 mm at ages 13–18 years is significantly associated with the presence of acute pancreatitis [1].

In summary, diagnostic accuracy of acute pancreatitis by native ultrasound depends on severity, the presence of complications such as paralytic ileus, typical associated findings, including a pancreatic pseudocysts, as well as operator experience. Increased diagnostic accuracy can be achieved with contrast-enhanced ultrasound, which is particularly useful to detect ischemic areas seen with pancreatic necrosis [13]. Using ultrasound elastography to gain information about organ stiffness not accessible to exterior palpation could also increase the rate of correct diagnosis in the future, but is currently mostly experimental [14].

When in doubt, the diagnostic tools can be extended to MRCP with full imaging of the pancreatic duct system, discovering structural anomalies. In most young children, sedation or full anesthesia is needed for this study, and visu-

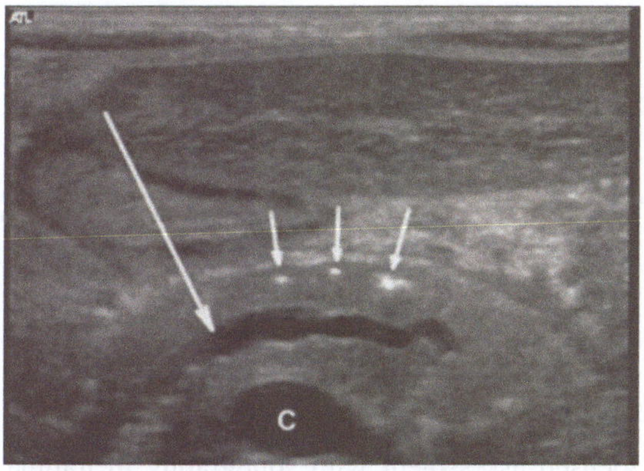

Fig. 7.4 Transverse ultrasonography (US) image in a 5-year-old boy with chronic hereditary pancreatitis shows the typical features of chronic pancreatitis: calcifications *(small arrows)* and dilatation of the pancreatic duct *(large arrow)*. *C* confluence of the superior mesenteric and splenic veins [19]

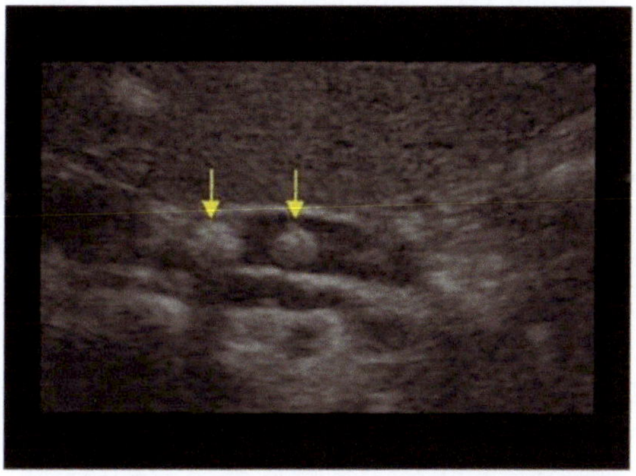

Fig. 7.5 Transverse ultrasound of the pancreas in an older with chronic pancreatitis. The liver is used as a sonographic window. Note the two large stones obstructing the dilated pancreatic duct *(arrows)*. (Case courtesy of Dr Maulik S. Patel, radiopaedia.org)

alization of ducts with a diameter less than 1 mm is still difficult [15].

Chronic Pancreatitis

In chronic pancreatitis—which is rather rare in children—the etiology includes cystic fibrosis, fibrosing pancreatitis, hereditary chronic pancreatitis, inborn errors of metabolism, or structural anomalies (Fig. 7.4). Chronic pancreatitis is defined as a combination of clinical symptoms such as abdominal pain, exocrine (malabsorprion, steatorrhea, etc.) and endocrine dysfunction (diabetes mellitus), along with imaging findings characteristic of the irreversible morphologic damage of the pancreatic parenchyma [10, 16–18].

The sonographic examination of chronic pancreatitis may show inhomogeneous echogenicity and prominent margins caused by progressive fibrosis and fatty injections of the gland. The size of the pancreas can be normal or reduced. The duct appears dilated and sometimes irregular in its course, with intermittent dilation and stenosis. Ultrasound-guided fine needle aspiration biopsy to confirm the diagnosis has been found to have a lower complication rate (1 %) than ERCP [15]. Potential complications of chronic pancreatitis are pseudocystformation, focal calcifications, and recurrent intraductal stones (Fig. 7.5).

Cystic Fibrosis

Pancreatic involvement in patients with cystic fibrosis occurs more often than liver disease (85–90 %) with progressive fatty tissue replacement and atrophy resulting in exocrine insufficiency [17]. In most cases, the pancreas appears as a homogeneous hyperechoic band representing the lipomatosis and overall decreased size due to progressive atrophy. The pancreatic duct can be dilated or inhomogeneous in size because of cell debris, scarring, and obstruction. Multiple small pancreatic cysts, calcifications, and focal hypoechoic areas representing fibrosis can be present. Detection of very small cysts with diameters of less than 1–3 mm can be difficult. Contrast-enhanced US or EUS may increase detection of very small lesions. Despite the mentioned risk factors, pancreatitis is actually rarely (1.2 %) seen sonographically in patients with cystic fibrosis [15].

Pseudocysts

In children, pancreatic cysts are usually secondary to pancreatitis caused by blunt abdominal trauma but can also occur in pancreatitis of other origin or genetic diseases such as cystic fibrosis. Solitary, congenital cysts are rare and may be related to ductal anomalies with a higher incidence in patients with von Hippel–Lindau syndrome or polycystic kidney disease [20].

Sonographically they appear as anechoic, round, thin-walled structures which are well distinguishable from the surrounding tissue.

Pancreatic Neoplasms

The most common pancreatic tumors in children are adenomas, insulinoma, and so-called solid pseudopapillary (or Frantz) tumors (Fig. 7.6). On ultrasound, the two former entities usually present as round areas of uniform echogenicity. The latter are usually well marginated with solid and cystic areas surrounded by a well-demarcated, fibrous capsule [21]. Solid pseudopapillary tumors are more common in girls and usually behave like a very low-grade malignancy [23]. Therefore, complete removal is the treatment of choice. Ultrasound is an ideal modality for postoperative follow-up to rule out local recurrence.

Other, but much less common tumors of the pancreas in children are pancreatoblastoma and adenocarcinoma. The sonographic imaging features are those of a large heterogeneous tumor that invades into adjacent tissues and is not well demarcated. A sonographer who discovers a pancreatic tumor in a child should think of the possible association with Type 1 multiple endocrine neoplasia (MEN).

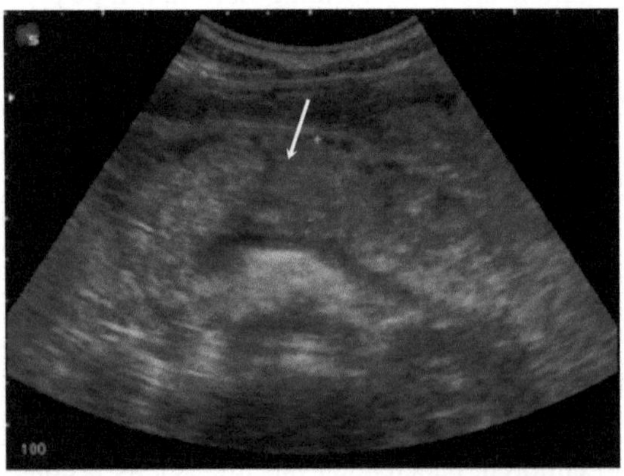

Fig. 7.6 Heterogenous mass at the junction of the pancreatic head and the caudate lobe of the liver [22]

Intraoperative ultrasound may be useful to detect pancreatic tumors during surgery and to determine resection margins more accurately [24].

Blunt Pancreatic Trauma

The pancreas itself is not assessed during the focused assessment with sonography in trauma (FAST) scan. A comprehensive ultrasound exam, however, in a stable pediatric trauma victim can aid in the diagnosis, although the sensitivity for traumatic injuries of the pancreas may be lower than that of computed tomography [25].

Pancreatic lacerations may present as a low-echogenic gap in the continuity of the organ. Free fluid may be visible in the retroperitoneum as a sign of ductal disruption (Fig. 7.7a, b). Moore et al. have proposed a grading system of blunt pancreatic trauma [26], which is adaptable to sonographic findings (Table 7.3).

Traumatic injuries of the pancreas that involve the duct may lead to pseudocyst formation (Fig. 7.8a, b, c, d; [27]). Ultrasound is an ideal modality for the follow-up of these sequellae since size, wall thickness, and surrounding tissue reaction can be assessed. Once formed, pediatric pseudocysts are drainable under endoscopic ultrasound guidance with a high success rate [28, 29].

Future Tools and New Horizons in Pancreatic Sonography

Endoscopic Ultrasound

In recent years, endoscopic ultrasound has been employed and established for a variety of pediatric indications, including pancreatitis, pancreatic masses, cystic lesions, suspected annular pancreas, suspected common bile duct stones, abdominal pain, and ampullary adenoma [31].

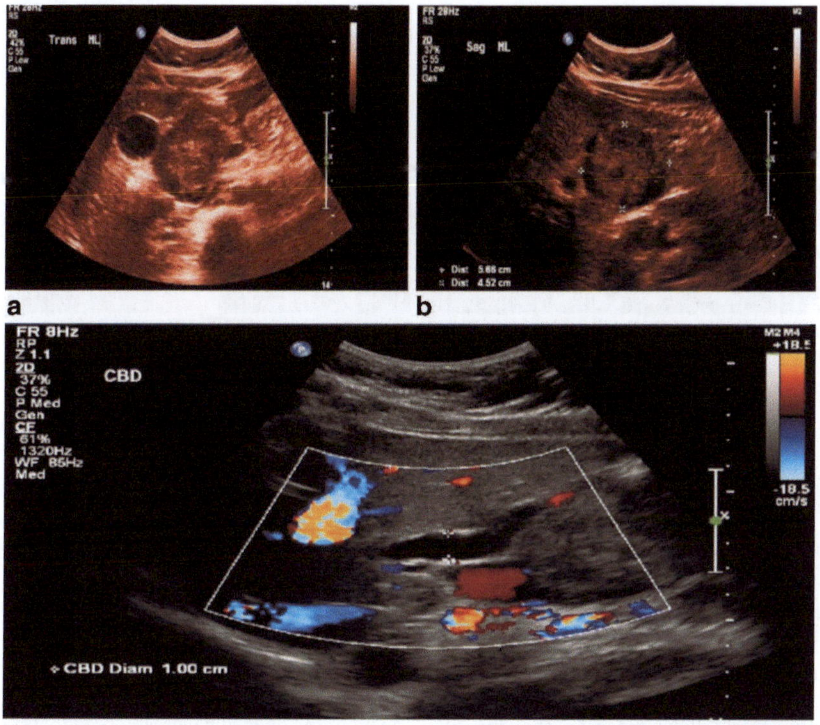

a b c

Fig. 7.7 **a** Young boy with history of blunt abdominal trauma showing bulky and heterogenous pancreas with linear anechoic laceration in the region of body of pancreas *(arrow)* with minimal free fluid around pancreas [22]. **b** Typical location for pancreatic trauma due to the underlying spine. (Courtesy of S. Ledbetter and R. Smithuis, Acute Abdomen—Role of computed tomography (CT) in Trauma. www.radiologyassistant.nl)

Furthermore, therapeutic interventions guided by endoscopic ultrasound, and sometimes combined with ERCP, have been performed successfully in children [32]. The technique entails placement of the ultrasound probe endoscopically into the stomach or duodenum to obtain high-resolution real-time ultrasound pictures of the pancreas. The main disadvantage is that the intervention is more invasive than transabdominal ultrasound and mostly requires sedation or even general anesthesia in children.

Table 7.3 Grading of blunt pancreatic injuries. (Adapted from [25])

Grade	Description
1	Minor contusion or superficial laceration without duct injury
2	Deep contusion or laceration without duct injury or tissue loss
3	Distal transection or parenchymal injury with duct injury
4	Proximal (right of the superior mesenteric vein) transection
5	Complete disruption of the pancreatic head

Ultrasound Elastography

As mentioned above, ultrasound elastography is currently being investigated to add tissue elasticity to the conventional morphologic and flow information acquired during the sonographic exam. In children, elastographic techniques have been used to assess for pancreatic fibrosis in patients with cystic fibrosis [33] and the degree of inflammation in patients with acute pancreatitis [19], some of which were children as young as 6 years old.

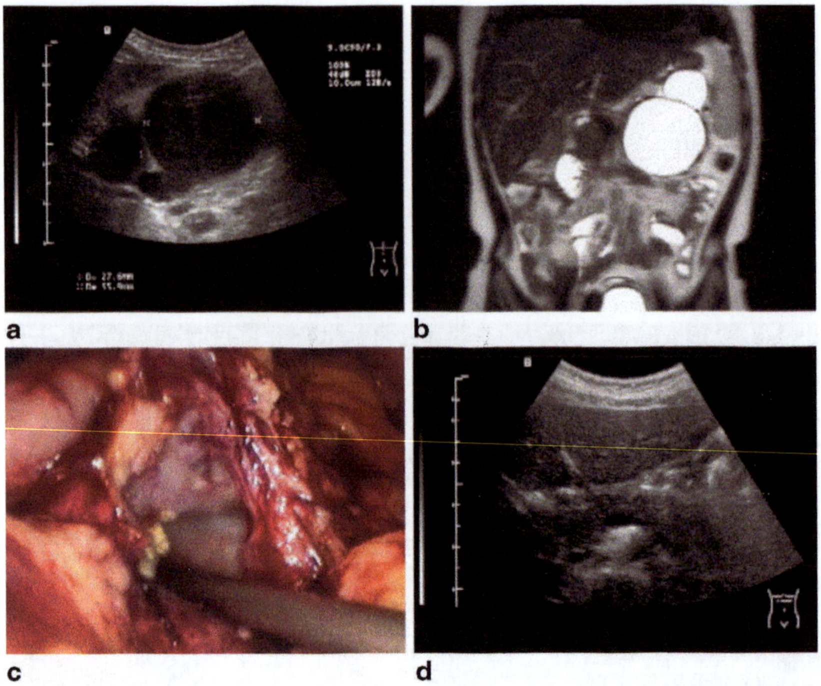

Fig. 7.8 **a** Longitudinal ultrasound scan showing two pancreatic pseudocysts at the tail of the pancreas. **b** Magnetic resonance cholangiopancreatography image showing two pancreatic pseudocysts with no sign of dilated bile ducts or injury of the pancreatic duct. **c** Intraoperative view of the opened pancreatic pseudocyst during laparoscopy (clamp inserted into cyst). **d** Transverse ultrasound scan 1 week after laparoscopic cystojejunostomy revealing a completely drained pancreatic pseudocyst [30]

Summary

Sonographic imaging of the pancreas in a child is challenging. Although computed tomography may be the more accurate imaging modality for pancreatic pathology in children, the lack of radiation and universal availability make sonographic imaging an attractive alternative. Certain preparatory steps can increase the accuracy of pancreatic sonography, and it is applicable for a wide variety of pathology. New developments such as endoscopic ultrasound and ultrasound elastography may enhance the applicability for diagnostic and therapeutic applications regarding the pancreas in children in the future.

References

1. Chao HC, Lin SJ, Kong MS, Luo CC. Sonographic evaluation of the pancreatic duct in normal children and children with pancreatitis. J Ultrasound Med. 2000;19:757–63.
2. Siegel MJ, Martin KW, Worthington JL. Normal and abnormal pancreas in children: US studies. Radiology. 1987;165:15.
3. Ueda D. Sonographic measurement of the pancreas in children. J Clin Ultrasound. 1989;17:417–23.
4. Altobelli E, Blasetti A, Verrotti A, Giandomenico V D, Bonomo L, Chiarelli F. Size of pancreas in children and adolescents with Type I (insulin-dependent) diabetes. J Clin Ultrasound. 1998;26:391–5.
5. Worthen NJ, Beabeau D. Normal pancreatic echogenicity: relation to age and body fat. AJR Am J Roentgenol. 1982;139:1095–8.
6. Nievelstein RAJ, Robben SGF, Blickman JG. Hepatobiliary and pancreatic imaging in children—techniques and an overview of non-neoplastic disease entities. Pediatr Radiol. 2011;41: 55–75.

7. Warshaw AL, Simeone JF, Schapiro RH, Flavin-Warshaw B. Evaluation and treatment of the dominant dorsal duct syndrome (pancreas divisum redefined). Am J Surg. 1990;159:59–64.
8. Rana SS, Bhasin DK, Sharma V, Rao C, Singh K. Role of endoscopic ultrasound in the diagnosis of pancreas divisum. Endosc Ultrasound. 2013;2:7–10.
9. Joergensen M, Brusgaard K, Cruger DG. Incidence, prevalence, etiology, and prognosis of first-time chronic pancreatitis in young patients: a nationwide cohort study. Dig Dis Sci. 2010;55:2988–98.
10. Morinville VD, Husain SZ, Bai H, Barth B, Alhosh R, Durie PR, Freedman SD, Himes R, Lowe ME, Pohl J, Werlin S, Wilschanski M, Uc A. INSPPIRE Group. Definitions of pediatric pancreatitis and survey of present clinical practices. J Pediatr Gastroenterol Nutr. 2012;55(3):261–5.
11. Benifla M, Weizman Z. Acute pancreatitis in childhood: analysis of literature data. J Clin Gastroenterol. 2003;37:169–72.
12. Ma MH, Bai HX, Park AJ, Latif SU, Mistry PK, Pashankar D, Northrup VS, Bhandari V, Husain SZ. Risk factors associated with biliary pancreatitis in children. J Pediatr Gastroenterol Nutr. 2012;54: 651–6.
13. Ardelean M, Şirli R, Sporea I, Bota S, Martie A, Popescu A, Dănila M, Timar B, Buzas R, Lighezan D. Contrast enhanced ultrasound in the pathology of the pancreas - a monocentric experience. Med Ultrason. 2014;16:325–31.
14. Ohno E, Kawashima H, Hashimoto S, Goto H, Hirooka Y. Current status of tissue harmonic imaging in endoscopic ultrasonography (EUS) and EUS-elastography in pancreatobiliary diseases. Dig Endosc. 2015;27:68–73.
15. Anupindi SA, Darge K. Pancreatitis and the role of US, MRCP and ERCP. Pediatr Radiol 2009;39 (Suppl 2):S153–7.
16. Nydegger A, Couper RT, Oliver MR. Childhood pancreatitis. J Gastroenterol Hepatol. 2006;21:499–509.
17. Haber HP. Cystic fibrosis in children and young adults: findings on routine abdominal sonography. AJR Am J Roentgenol. 2007;189:89–99.
18. van Rijn RR, Nievelstein RA. Paediatric ultrasonography of the liver, hepatobiliary tract and pancreas. Eur J Radiol. 2014;83:1570–81.
19. Mateen MA, Muheet KA, Mohan RJ, Rao PN, Majaz HM, Rao GV, Reddy DN. Evaluation of ultrasound based acoustic radiation force impulse (ARFI) and eSie touch sonoelastography for diagnosis of inflammatory pancreatic diseases. JOP. 2012;13:36–44.
20. Auringer ST, Ulmer JL, Sumner TE, Turner CS. Congenital cyst of the pancreas. J Pediatr Surg. 1993;28:1570–1.
21. Ozcan HN, Oguz B, Sen HS, Akyuz C, Haliloglu M. Imaging features of primary malignant pancreatic tumors in children. AJR Am J Roentgenol. 2014;203:662–7.
22. http://www.radrounds.com/photo/pancreatic-laceration/prev?context=user. Accessed 28 July 2015.
23. Peranteau WH, Palladino AA, Bhatti TR, Becker SA, States LJ, Stanley CA, Adzick NS. The surgical management of insulinomas in children. J Pediatr Surg. 2013;48:2517–24.
24. Browning JG, Wilkinson AG, Beattie T. Imaging paediatric blunt abdominal trauma in the emergency department: ultrasound versus computed tomography. Emerg Med J. 2008;25:645–8.
25. Moore EE, Cogbill TH, Malangoni MA, Jurkovich GJ, Champion HR, Gennarelli TA, McAninch JW, Pachter HL, Shackford SR, Trafton PG. Organ injury scaling, II: Pancreas, duodenum, small bowel, colon, and rectum. J Trauma. 1990;30:1427–9.
26. Sheikh F, Fallon S, Bisset G, Podberesky D, Zheng J, Orth R, Zhang W, Falcone RA Jr, Naik-Mathuria B. Image-guided prediction of pseudocyst formation in pediatric pancreatic trauma. J Surg Res. 2015;193:513–8.
27. Ramesh J, Bang JY, Trevino J, Varadarajulu S. Endoscopic ultrasound-guided drainage of pancreatic fluid collections in children. J Pediatr Gastroenterol Nutr. 2013;56:30–5.
28. Jazrawi SF, Barth BA, Sreenarasimhaiah J. Efficacy of endoscopic ultrasound-guided drainage of pancreatic pseudocysts in a pediatric population. Dig Dis Sci. 2011;56:902–8.
29. Seitz G, Warmann SW, Kirschner HJ, Haber HP, Schaefer JW, Fuchs J. Laparoscopic cystojejunostomy as a treatment option for pancreatic pseudocysts in children—a case report. J Pediatr Surg. 2006;41:e33–5.
30. Attila T, Adler DG, Hilden K, Faigel DO. EUS in pediatric patients. Gastrointest Endosc. 2009;70:892–8.
31. Scheers I, Ergun M, Aouattah T, Piessevaux H, Borbath I, Stephenne X, De Magnée C, Reding R, Sokal E, Veyckemans F, Weynand B, Deprez PH. The diagnostic and therapeutic role of endoscopic ultrasound in pediatric pancreaticobiliary disorders. J Pediatr Gastroenterol Nutr 2015, in press.
32. Friedrich-Rust M, Schlueter N, Smaczny C, Eickmeier O, Rosewich M, Feifel K, Herrmann E, Poynard T, Gleiber W, Lais C, Zielen S, Wagner TO, Zeuzem S, Bojunga J. Non-invasive measurement of liver and pancreas fibrosis in patients with cystic fibrosis. J Cyst Fibros. 2013;12:431–9.
33. Shuja A, Alkimawi KA. Solid pseudopapillary tumor: a rare neoplasm of the pancreas. Gastroenterol Rep. 2014;2:145–9.

The Spleen

8

Julia Scholsching and Oliver J. Muensterer

Introduction

Except when grossly enlarged, the spleen is usually non-accessible in the clinical examination. Ultrasound, however, offers a very sensitive and specific noninvasive imaging tool for a variety of pathological conditions in the pediatric population of every age group, from trauma to tumors. Hence, examination of the spleen should be an integral part of every standardized abdominal scan.

Obtaining high-quality sonographic images of the spleen is no easy task, due to its location high in the left upper quadrant under the ribs. This chapter offers hints to produce optimal ultrasound pictures of the most common pediatric splenic pathologies.

Scanning Techniques

Position of the Patient

Imaging of the spleen should be done with a curvilinear or linear transducer of lower frequency (2–5 MHz) capable of color-flow Doppler imaging. The spleen is best accessed through the 9th–11th intercostal space, between the anterior and posterior axillary lines. A first overview of the spleen can be obtained with the child in a supine position. Individual anatomical variation requires that the operator search for the best acoustic window in a dynamic, flexible fashion.

Often it is helpful to angle the patient left side up which facilitates a more posterior access. This can be accomplished by having the patient roll sideways actively, or by placing a roll or a pillow under the left flank.

Elevation of the left arm maximizes the intercostal space. If the patient can follow instructions, having the patient raise the arm behind their head is sufficient. In nonverbal patients, parents can manipulate the arm gently, according to the scanner's instructions.

Another point to remember is that the probe needs to be angled slightly along the intercostal spaces to prevent shadows of the ribs. Again, the amount of angulation is highly variable and patient dependent.

Patient Preparation and Coaching

It is helpful to have the patient inhale or exhale to provide different views of the spleen. Naturally, breathing is hard to control in young and nonverbal children, but an experienced sonographer will sense and benefit from their natural respiratory cycle. Older children should be appropriately coached to inhale or exhale in a way to offer a

O. J. Muensterer (✉) · J. Scholsching
Department of Pediatric Surgery, University Medicine of the Johannes Gutenberg University Mainz, Langenbeckstraße 1, 55131 Mainz, Germany
e-mail: oliver.muensterer@unimedizin-mainz.de

J. Scholsching
e-mail: julia.scholsching@unimedizin-mainz.de

S. Scholz, M. D. Jarboe (eds.), *Diagnostic and Interventional Ultrasound in Pediatrics and Pediatric Surgery,* DOI 10.1007/978-3-319-21699-7_8

good view of the spleen. It can be helpful to show schoolchildren and teenagers a live image of their scan during the process as feedback, to let them participate actively in the process.

Table 8.1 Approximate age-dependent normal splenic lengths [1]

Age	Mean (cm)	Standard deviation
0–3 months	4.5	0.7
3–6 months	5.5	0.7
6–12 months	6.5	0.7
3 years	7.5	0.9
7 years	8.5	0.9
11 years	9.5	0.9
15 years	10.5	1.0

Normal Sonographic Findings

Age-dependent Splenic Size

Splenic length is measured as the largest diameter of the organ independent of hilum location with a convex transducer via an intercostal window (Fig. 8.1). Splenic width is measured perpendicular to this line at the level of the hilum.

Nomograms for splenic length as a function of age, height, weight, and body surface area have been published [1]. These show a complex, nonlinear relationship. Splenic dimensions are highly variable, but the average length ranges from 4.5 cm in 0–3-month-old to 10.5 cm in 14–17-year-old children (Table 8.1).

Echogenicity

In routine sonographic evaluation, healthy children demonstrate homogenous splenic echogenicity that is slightly lower than that of healthy liver tissue. Detailed discrimination between red and white splenic pulp can be accomplished by using a higher-frequency linear transducer (10–13 MHz). The white pulp is typically lower in echogenicity. It is important to remember that the lymphatic system and lymphatic follicles are not completely formed in newborns and infants, so the volume of the white pulp increases with age.

Blood Supply

A complete ultrasonographic evaluation of the spleen should always include Doppler flow studies of the surrounding and intraparenchymatous vessels. The architecture of the spleen is predominantly determined by the vascular structure. The

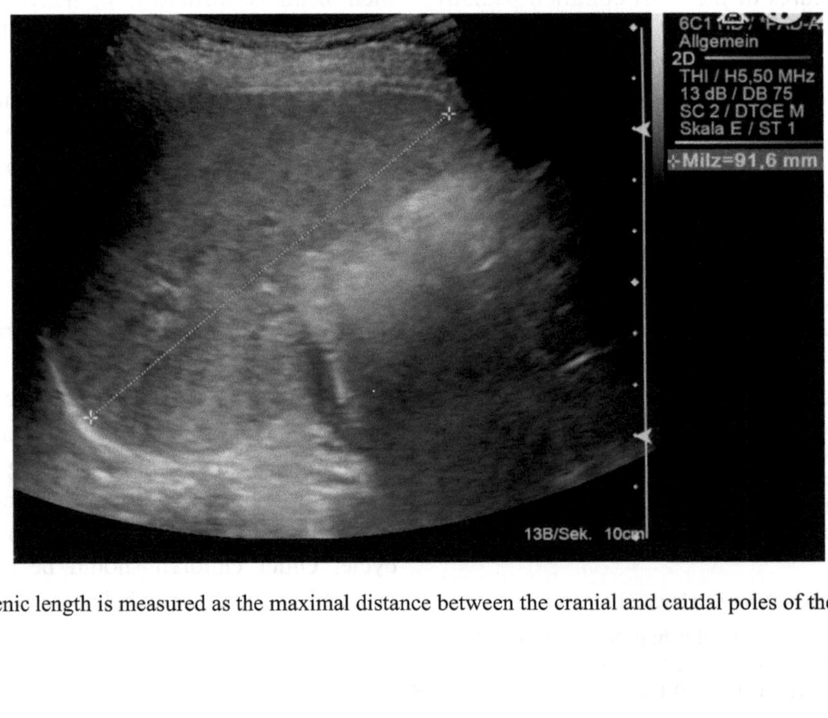

Fig. 8.1 Splenic length is measured as the maximal distance between the cranial and caudal poles of the spleen

Table 8.2 Common reasons for splenomegaly

Reason	Example
Increased hemolysis	Spherocytosis, thalassemia, sickle cell anemia
Cancer	Leukemia, lymphoma, histoplasmosis
Autoimmune diseases	Rheumatoid arthritis, lupus erythematosus, autoimmune hemolytic anemia, sarcoidosis
Infectious	Mononucleosis, leishmaniasis, malaria, tuberculosis, abscess, ehrlichiosis, echinococcosis
Portal hypertension	Liver cirrhosis, hepatic vein obstruction (Budd–Chiari syndrome), portal vein obstruction
Storage diseases	Gaucher, Hurler, Hunter, Niemann–Pick disease
Benign tumors	Hemangioma, hamartoma, epidermoid cyst

spleen is mainly supplied by the splenic artery, which arises from the celiac trunk and in most (80 %) cases traverses along the upper border of the pancreas. Close to the hilum, it separates into two (80 %) or three (20 %) lobar arteries. These lobar arteries supply segments that typically do not form any collaterals between each other, which are important for spleen-preserving surgery. The spleen also obtains some blood from the short gastric vessels arising from the gastroepiploic artery.

Venous drainage is accomplished via the hilum into the splenic vein, which joins the mesenteric vein to form the portal vein. Therefore, splenomegaly may result from portal hypertension. Normal spleen size, however, does not rule out portal hypertension. Therefore, evaluation of the splenic drainage should always include a careful evaluation of the liver as well.

Contrast Enhanced Ultrasound

Contrast enhanced ultrasound for splenic indications has not been well studied in children. In a study that included some children, contrast enhancement increased the sensitivity for detection of splenic lacerations after blunt abdominal trauma from 59 to 96 % [2]. The main disadvantage is that intravenous microbubbles of sulfur hexafluoride gas must be infused shortly before imaging.

Anomalies

Splenomegaly

In general, the spleen must increase in size at least twofold to be clinically palpable [3]. Clinical splenomegaly is defined by the organ being palpable under the left costal angle in the midclavicular line. However, the spleen may be palpable in healthy newborns in up to 17 % of cases [4]. A good indicator for splenomegaly is the spleen–kidney ratio. The length of the spleen should not surpass the length of the kidney by 125 % [5]. Another age-independent criterion for splenomegaly is caudal extension of the spleen beyond the lower pole of the kidney. The most common reasons for splenomegaly are listed in Table 8.2.

Asplenia, Polysplenia, and Topographic Anomalies

Asplenia/polysplenia, as well as the single right-sided spleen, belong to a very heterogeneous group of laterality defects including extreme variants such as total situs inversus. The exact cause remains widely unknown, but chromosomal aberrations are sometimes identified (i.e., Kartagener syndrome). Laterality defects are usually accompanied by congenital heart defects and major other anomalies such as biliary atresia, intestinal malrotation with microgastria, or isomerism of the lungs (bilateral left or right lung).

Accessory Spleen

Accessory spleens can be found in 7–20 % of patients at autopsy or in computed tomography series [6, 7]. The most common location is the splenic hilum (75 %; Fig. 8.2) and pancreatic tail but accessory tissue can be found anywhere in the abdomen. Ultrasound usually shows an oval mass of the same parenchymal structure and

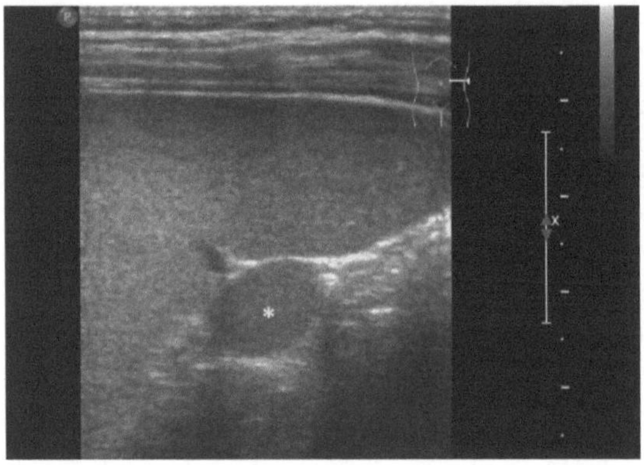

Fig. 8.2 An accessory spleen is identified at the splenic hilum (*). The mass has an oval shape and is similar in echotexture to the spleen itself

echogenicity as the spleen, sometimes with a visible feeding artery from the splenic arteria. In cases of torsion, the ultrasound shows a homogeneous hypoechoic mass without evidence of perfusion or, in cases of recurrent torsion, signs of infarction with inhomogenic parenchyma. Free intra-abdominal fluid can be a sign of rupture.

Wandering Spleen

The ectopic location of the spleen occurs either in missing ligamental fixation, laxity, or maldevelopment of the splenic ligaments. In very rare cases, the absent ligamental fixation can lead to torsion of the wandering spleen. This may manifest as an acute abdomen with no detectable spleen in the typical location, and an abdominal mass with spleen-like echostructure on the initial ultrasound instead. Lack of perfusion of the abdominal mass in Doppler imaging, as well as an elevated resistive index in the proximal splenic artery is highly suspicious for torsion of the wandering spleen.

In all cases of splenic ectopia, ultrasound remains a noninvasive, easily accessible imaging method. In symptomatic unclear cases, however, further imaging with magnetic resonance imaging or computed tomography should be considered before surgical exploration.

Diffuse Changes of the Splenic Parenchyma

Diffuse parenchymal changes (Fig. 8.3) may be a sign of hematopoietic diseases, storage disorders, infections, autoimmune disorders, sequellae of trauma, or portal hypertension (Table 8.2). Further investigation with cross-sectional radiographic or nuclear scans may be indicated in these cases.

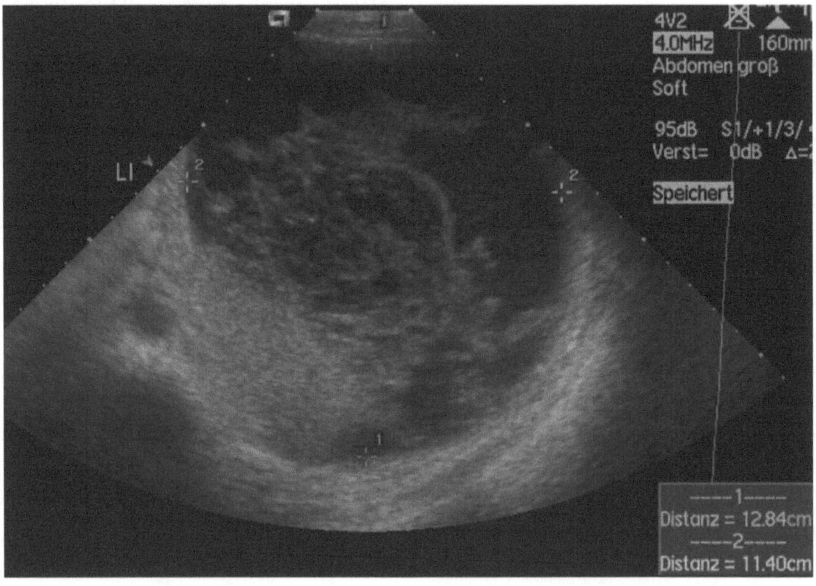

Fig. 8.3 Diffuse complex parenchymatous changes may result from a variety of disorders. They can also appear as sequellae to trauma, as in this case

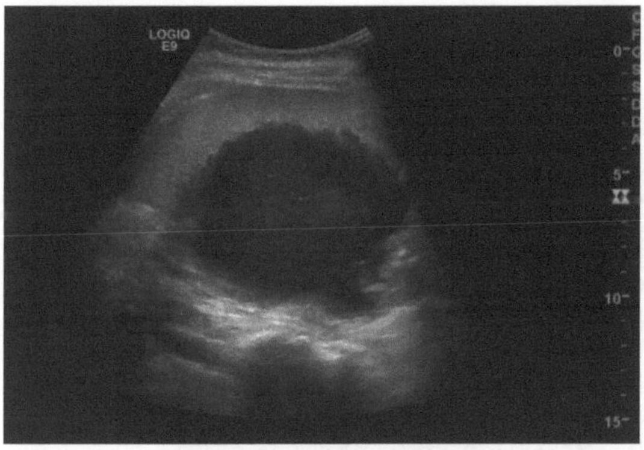

Fig. 8.4 Splenic cysts may be congenital or acquired. Epidermoid splenic cysts have typical trabeculation in the cyst wall

Cysts, Abscesses, Tumors

Fluid-filled anomalies are readily visible on ultrasound examination. They include cysts (Fig. 8.4), abscesses (Fig. 8.5), and post-traumatic pseudocysts (Fig. 8.6). Solid and mixed tumors are also easily picked up because their structural appearance contrasts sharply to the even echogenicity of the spleen in most of the cases (Fig. 8.7). If indicated, cysts and masses can be accessed percutaneously under sonographic guidance to aid in diagnosis [8], but simple percutaneous drainage of most cysts almost always results in recurrence [9].

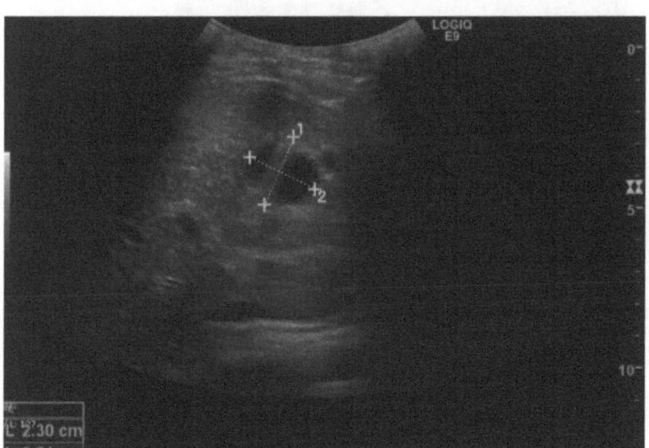

Fig. 8.5 Abscesses are usually smaller than primary splenic cysts and may be loculated. They also may contain echogenic debris

Traumatic Injury

Focused assessment with sonography in trauma (FAST) has become a standard practice in the adult setting and is increasingly used in children as well. It comprises taking standardized ultrasound images of the hepatorenal recess, the bladder, the pericardium, and the perisplenic space (Fig. 8.8). A positive FAST implies the detection of free peritoneal or pericardial fluid or obvious solid organ injury, but is not used for solid organ injury staging. The sensitivity and specificity of FAST in children ranges from 33 to 93 % and 85 to 97 %, respectively [10–12]. In cases of known splenic laceration or avulsion, ultrasound in general is a very good diagnostic tool for further monitoring, especially in the pediatric population, because there is no need for sedation and no exposure to ionizing radiation.

Splenic Laceration and Avulsion

Splenic laceration is the second most common solid organ injury in blunt pediatric trauma. Careful scanning of the spleen is quite sensitive to pick up splenic lacerations (Fig. 8.9), although sonography has never been validated for grading the injury. Besides splenic morphology, indirect signs of trauma such as perisplenic or free intraperitoneal fluid, as well as focal pain during the examination itself should be taken into consideration. It is also mandatory to perform a color Doppler examination of the organ (Fig. 8.10), since avulsion of the spleen can be picked up by the lack of perfusion.

Post-traumatic Arteriovenous Fistula

Splenic lacerations close to the hilum may result in a post-traumatic arteriovenous fistula (Fig. 8.11). These usually heal spontaneously, but in some refractory cases with pronounced blood flow, transarterial embolization may be indicated. Ultrasound is an ideal method to follow such changes over time.

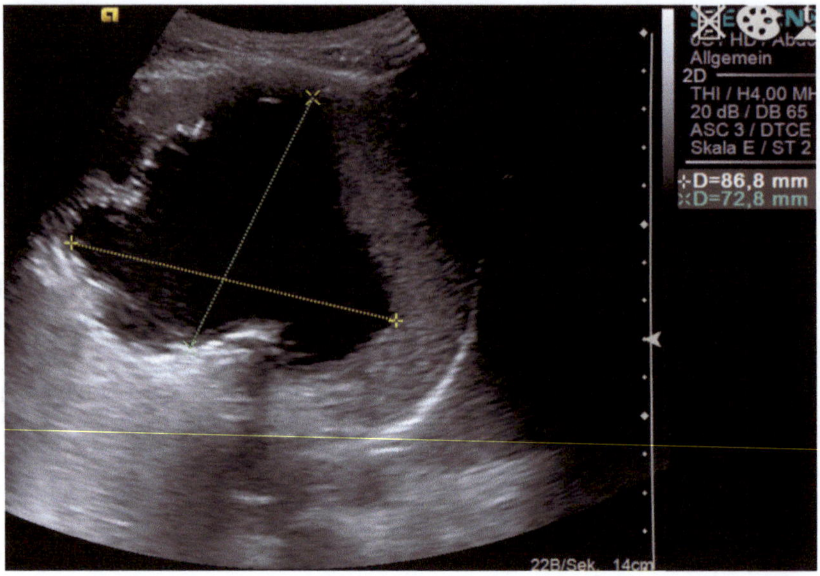

Fig. 8.6 Post-traumatic splenic cysts are common. Most of them can be observed, but persistent ones may require resection

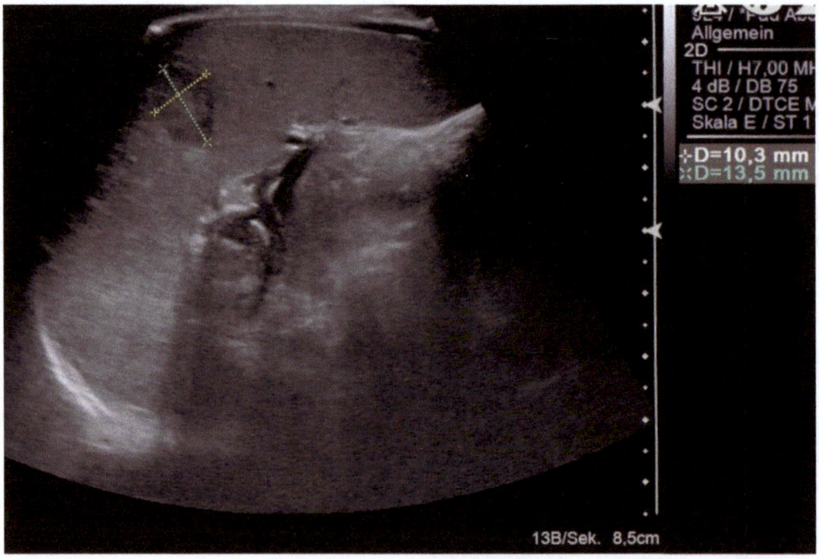

Fig. 8.7 Solid and mixed tumors of the spleen include hemangiomas and vascular malformations. Doppler studies may be useful to differentiate them from malignancies such as lymphoma

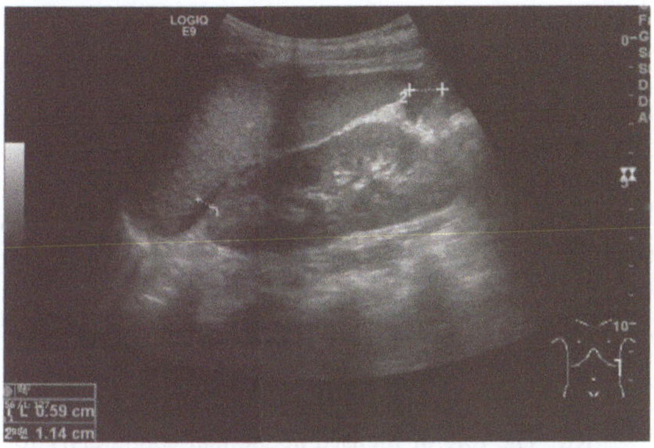

Fig. 8.8 Positive FAST scan with fluid in the splenorenal fossa (1) and around the lower pole of the spleen (2)

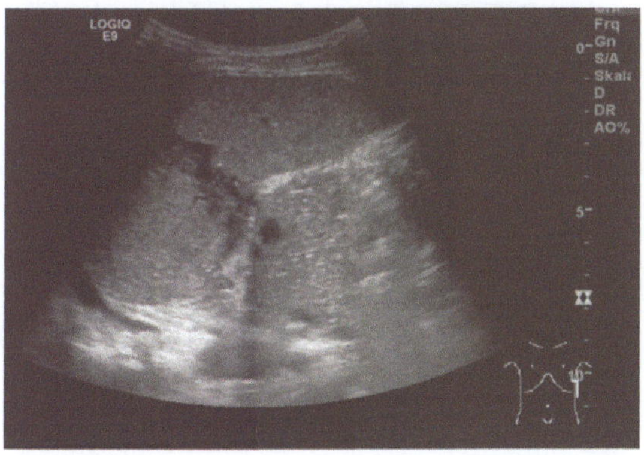

Fig. 8.9 B-mode ultrasound of the spleen after blunt abdominal trauma. The laceration in this case is hypoechoic and extends from the hilum to the periphery

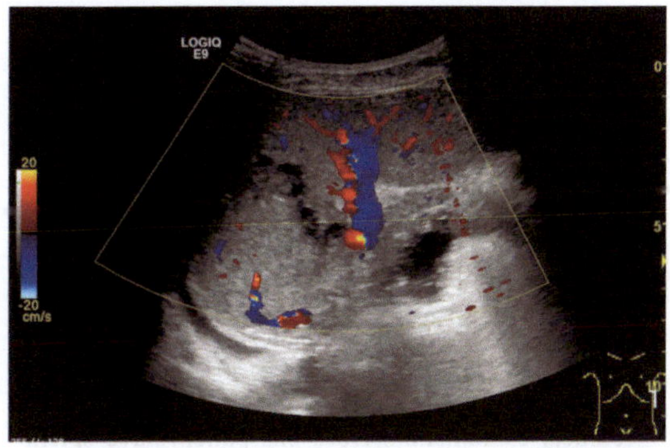

Fig. 8.10 Doppler imaging of the same patient as in Fig. 8.9 shows the relationship of the laceration *(dark line)* to the left of the vessels. Free fluid is also seen at the hilum, and below the diaphragm *(lentiform dark line in the lower left corner of the scan)*

Summary

Ultrasound is an ideal modality to image the pediatric spleen, although obtaining high-quality images can be challenging due to location and lack of patient cooperation. Splenomegaly is easily picked up on ultrasound, as are cystic and solid lesions, as well as trauma. Comprehensive imaging of the spleen should always include color Doppler studies.

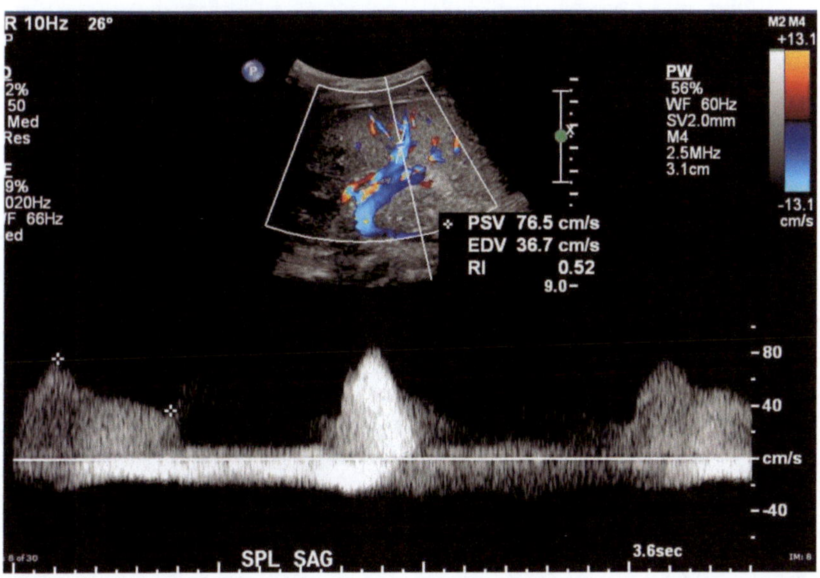

Fig. 8.11 This Doppler study shows a large, hemodynamically important post-traumatic arteriovenous fistula that did not improve with time. It was eventually coiled by interventional radiology

References

1. Megremis SD, Vlachonikolis IG, Tsilimigaki AM. Spleen length in childhood with US: normal values based on age, sex, and somatometric parameters. Radiology. 2004;231:129–34.
2. Sessa B, Trinci M, Ianniello S, Menichini G, Galluzzo M, Miele V. Blunt abdominal trauma: role of contrast-enhanced ultrasound (CEUS) in the detection and staging of abdominal traumatic lesions compared to US and CE-MDCT. Radiol Med. 2015;120:180–9.
3. Grover SA, Barkun AN, Sackett DL. The rational clinical examination. Does this patient have splenomegaly? JAMA. 1993;270:2218–21.
4. Mimouni F, Merlob P, Ashkenazi S, Litmanovitz I, Reisner SH. Palpable spleens in newborn term infants. Clin Pediatr (Phila). 1985;24:197–8.
5. Loftus WK, Metreweli C. Ultrasound assessment of mild splenomegaly: spleen/kidney ratio. Pediatr Radiol. 1998;28:98–100.
6. Unver Dogan N, Uysal II, Demirci S, Dogan KH, Kolcu G. Accessory spleens at autopsy. Clin Anat. 2011;24:757–62.
7. Quah C, Ayiomamitis GD, Shah A, Ammori BJ. Computed tomography to detect accessory spleens before laparoscopic splenectomy: is it necessary? Surg Endosc. 2011;25:261–5.
8. Singh AK, Shankar S, Gervais DA, Hahn PF, Mueller PR. Image-guided percutaneous splenic interventions. Radiographics. 2012;32:523–34.
9. Wu HM, Kortbeek JB. Management of splenic pseudocysts following trauma: a retrospective case series. Am J Surg. 2006;191:631–4.
10. Patel JC, Tepas JJ. The efficacy of focused abdominal sonography for trauma (FAST) as a screening tool in the assessment of injured children. J Pediatr Surg. 1999;34:44–7.
11. Scaife ER, Rollins MD, Barnhart DC, Downey EC, Black RE, Meyers RL, Stevens MH, Gordon S, Prince JS, Battaglia D, Fenton SJ, Plumb J, Metzger RR. The role of focused abdominal sonography for trauma (FAST) in pediatric trauma evaluation. J Pediatr Surg. 2013;48:1377–83.
12. Soudack M, Epelman M, Maor R, Hayari L, Shoshani G, Heyman-Reiss A, Michaelson M, Gaitini D. Experience with focused abdominal sonography for trauma (FAST) in 313 pediatric patients. J Clin Ultrasound. 2004;32:53–61.

9 Abdominal Vessels

Justin Barr and Sara K. Rasmussen

Abdominal Vessel Anatomy

Every abdominal organ and its vascular supply can be assessed using ultrasound. Color and spectral Doppler can be employed to measure flow characteristics and detect or monitor pathologies or postoperative results.

The aorta supplies arterial blood to the abdominal viscera and has several feeding vessels supplying the structures in the abdomen. The first major trunk is the celiac artery, which usually gives rise to the left gastric, splenic, and common hepatic arteries, although there is wide anatomic variation (Fig. 9.1a, b). The common hepatic artery gives off the right gastric artery and the gastroduodenal artery before it becomes the proper hepatic artery. It then divides into the left and right hepatic branches. The cystic artery commonly branches off the right hepatic artery. The gastroduodenal artery gives rise to the supraduodenal artery, the right gastroepiploic artery, and the superior pancreaticoduodenal artery. The right and left gastric arteries join along the lesser curve of the stomach. The splenic artery gives rise to the short gastric arteries and the left gastroepiploic arteries that supply the stomach.

The superior mesenteric artery (SMA) is the next major trunk off the aorta (Fig. 9.2a, b). This artery supplies the midgut with blood. The SMA first gives rise to the middle colic artery and then the right colic artery as well as the ileocolic artery. The SMA also gives rise to the several arcuate arteries that provide most of the blood to the small intestine. The middle colic artery gives rise to the marginal artery of Drummond, which supplies the transverse and the left colon.

The left and right renal arteries also originate from the aorta, most commonly inferior to the SMA and superior to the inferior mesenteric artery (IMA), though there is wide anatomic variation here as well. Most often the renal arteries are single, but they can be double or have early and varied branching. The adrenal glands receive their blood supply from suprarenal arteries that branch directly off of the aorta as well, usually superior to the main renal arteries.

Inferior to the SMA are the gonadal arteries, which supply the testicle or ovary, and the IMA. The IMA arises proximal to the bifurcation of the aorta. The main branches of the IMA are the left colic artery, which anastomoses with the aforementioned marginal artery of Drummond, and the colosigmoid artery. Distal to the take off of the colosigmoid is the origin of the rectosigmoid artery. The superior rectal arteries are the final branches of the IMA.

S. K. Rasmussen (✉) · J. Barr
Department of Surgery, University of Virginia,
P.O. Box 800709, 1215 Lee Street, Charlottesville,
VA 22908, USA
e-mail: Skr3f@virginia.edu

J. Barr
e-mail: jnb9k@virginia.edu

S. Scholz, M. D. Jarboe (eds.), *Diagnostic and Interventional Ultrasound in Pediatrics and Pediatric Surgery,* DOI 10.1007/978-3-319-21699-7_9

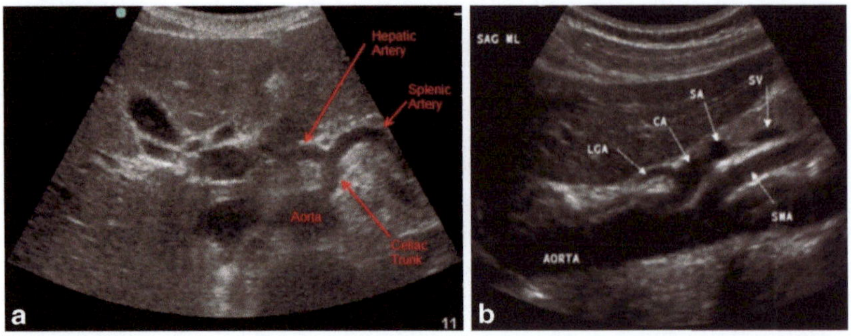

Fig. 9.1 **a** During sonography, look for the vertebral body in the transverse plane. The aorta and inferior vena cava *(IVC)* will be anterior to it. The *IVC* is compressible. The aorta will be anechoic with a pulsating circle. In the proximal aorta, the celiac trunk can be seen with its branches (seagull sign—hepatic and splenic arteries are the wings). **b** Sagittal epigastric view of the aorta and its branches, celiac artery *(CA)*, splenic artery *(SA)*, left gastric artery *(LGA)*, and the superior mesenteric artery *(SMA)*. The splenic vein *(SV)* is visualized below the transverse cut of the pancreas (https://carmenwiki.osu.edu/display/10337/AAA)

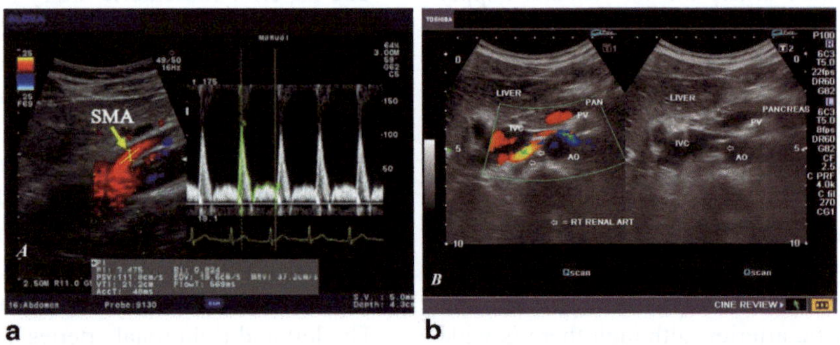

Fig. 9.2 **a** Color Doppler image of the aorta and the *SMA*. **b** *Grayscale* and color Doppler images show the origin of the normal right renal artery from the abdominal aorta *(Ao)*, just below the origin of the superior mesenteric artery. It takes careful adjustment of the wall filter settings to remove the motion artifacts from the aortic pulsations, with appropriate pulse repetition frequency (PRF) settings to get a good color flow image of the right renal artery. The right renal artery is seen coursing behind the *IVC* after an antero-lateral origin from the aorta *(Ao)*. The left renal vein *(LRV)* is also seen traversing anterior to the abdominal *Ao* and between it and the *SMA*. The above images are transverse sections through the epigastrium. The liver provides a good window to view these vessels (http://www.ultrasound-images.com/vascular.htm)

The main venous drainage systems of the abdomen are the inferior vena cava (IVC) and portal vein (PV). The superior and inferior mesenteric veins drain the intestines; the superior mesenteric vein (SMV) merges with the splenic vein to form the PV. This confluence usually occurs just dorsal to the pancreas. The gonadal veins have an asymmetric drainage, with the left gonadal vein draining into the left renal vein (LRV) and the right gonadal vein draining into the IVC directly. Similarly, the left suprarenal vein drains into the LRV, and the right suprarenal vein drains directly into the IVC above the renal veins.

Scanning Technique

For best results, exams should be done in the morning when possible. The patient should not have eaten since the previous midnight and refrain from chewing gum to reduce the amount

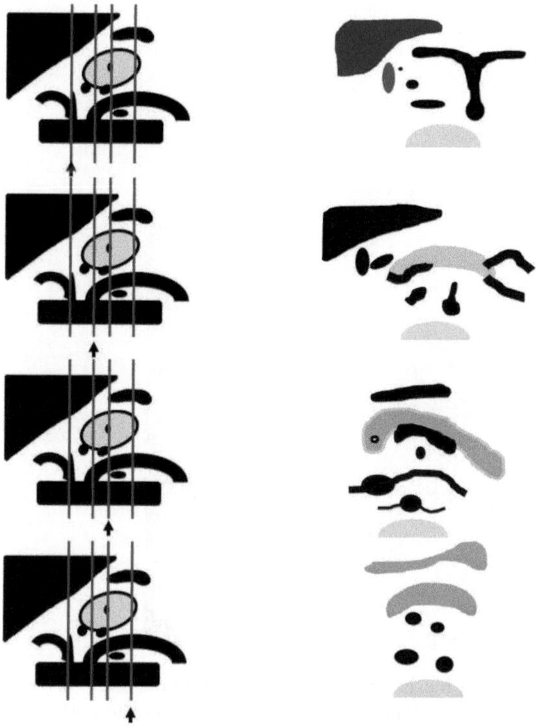

Fig. 9.3 Schematic representation of the abdominal vessels and their relationships to abdominal viscera. *Left*: Sagittal view of abdominal aorta, celiac, *SMA*, and renal artery origins and the pancreas, liver, and spleen with splenic artery and vein. *Right*: Each panel from top to bottom corresponds with a schematic of the ultrasound images that would be seen with the probe positioned in the line marked with the *arrow* in the *left* panel

of gaseous distention of the intestine, which can limit ultrasonography of the abdominal vessels. To reduce bowel gas further, the patient can be asked to drink some water immediately prior to the exam.

Abdominal vessels are typically imaged in several planes (Fig. 9.3). By switching the orientation of the probe, it is possible to measure the diameter of the vessels, the origin of vessels, and their angles as they take off from the abdominal aorta. Use of pulse-wave and color Doppler ultrasound allows measurement of flow in the vessels, with the measurement of velocity, resistive index, and turbuluence of flow. Color Doppler waveforms can provide information about the direction and quality of blood flow through the vessels. Waveforms can distinguish between the arterial and venous blood flow.

Malrotation and Midgut Volvulus

Intestinal malrotation refers to the incomplete rotation of the small intestine in utero. It can result in midgut volvulus, or the complete torsion of the small bowel around the SMA axis, causing acute obstruction requiring prompt surgical intervention. Early recognition of symptoms—bilious emesis—and appropriate, prompt imaging can lead to earlier diagnosis and operation, improving outcomes. The anatomical repositioning of the SMA and SMV during malrotation lends itself to sonographic and especially Doppler diagnosis. Normally, the SMV lies right and ventral to the SMA; in malrotation, that positioning is switched. A large study of 337 patients demonstrated that left/right reversal had a higher sensitivity and specificity for malrotation than ventral/dorsal switching [1–6]. It is possible to have malrotation of the intestines without SMA/SMV reversal, and SMA/SMV reversal can exist without malrotation. In addition this SMA/SMV reversal can be persistent after a Ladd's procedure [7, 8]. The best early study, a prospective comparison of US versus UGI in 427 children, found SMA/SMV reversal to have a 70 % sensitivity, 96 % specificity, 62 % positive predictive value, and 97 % negative predictive value [9].

An additional sonographic sign consistent with malrotation is the "Whirlpool sign" [10]. This finding reflects the clockwise rotation of the SMV around the SMA axis as a part of the malrotation. A subsequent study confirmed both the importance of the clockwise orientation (with counterclockwise orientation commonly reflecting nonspecific hemorrhagic enteritis) and the value of this finding [11]. Early reports documented sensitives in the 90th percentiles and specificities approaching 100 % [12, 13]. While specificities remain high, reports of whirlpool sign in patients without malrotation have also emerged [14]. Figure 9.4 contains an example illustration [15].

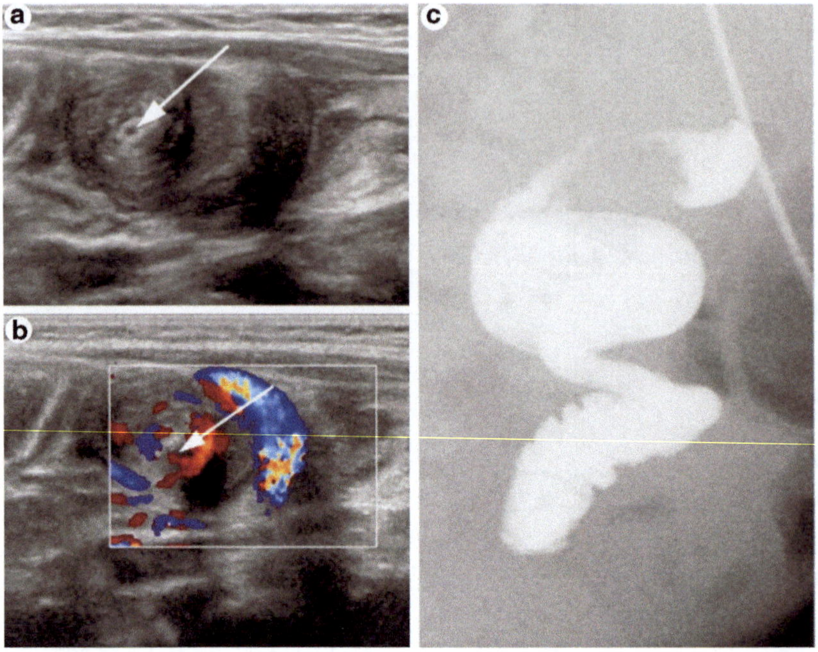

Fig. 9.4 Midgut volvulus diagnosed using ultrasound *(US)* in an 83-day-old boy evaluated for hypertrophic pyloric stenosis. Gray-scale (**a**) and Doppler US (**b**) demonstrate the "whirlpool sign" of the peripheral swirling superior mesenteric vein *(SMV)* around the *SMA* (*arrow*). *UGIs* (**c**), which followed the US, shows the corkscrew sign of midgut volvulus, which was confirmed during surgery [15]

An alternative strategy for diagnosing malrotation with ultrasound involves assessing the position of the third portion of the duodenum (D3). Normally, D3 rests in the retroperitoneum. In malrotation, D3 will be intraperitoneal and anterior to the mesenteric vessels [16]. Sonographic demonstration of a retroperitoneal D3 effectively excludes the diagnosis of malrotation and thus that of midgut volvulus [17–19]. This technique is simple and efficient for diagnosis of malroatation in newborns.

Ultrasound has some limitations. Bowel gas can be problematic. Most series report an inability to perform sonography on around 15% of the patients due to bowel gas interference [20]. Multiple studies have demonstrated a significant false-negative rate with ultrasound, corresponding to sensitivities in the 70–80% range [21]. Given these detractions and the serious consequences of a volvulus diagnosis, clinicians strongly suspicious of malrotation with volvulus should continue to order upper gastrointestinal radiological studies (UGIs), even after a negative ultrasound. However, the low-cost, noninvasiveness, lack of radiation, and strong specificity of several sonographic features—especially whirlpool sign—make ultrasound an excellent screening modality where positive findings may allow the surgeon to skip additional diagnostic steps and proceed directly to the operating room.

Compression Syndromes

Compression syndromes are products of anatomic variants in abdominal vasculature that result in compression of intra-abdominal organs to produce a pattern of symptoms. The difficult evaluations for these conditions have been simplified by the use of abdominal US of the vessels in question.

Median Arcuate Ligament Syndrome

Median arcuate ligament syndrome (MALS), also called the celiac artery compression syndrome and Dunbar syndrome, occurs when the median arcuate ligament compresses the celiac axis and celiac ganglion, typically producing abdominal pain. It was first identified by Harjola in 1963 [22]. The median arcuate ligament connects the right cura and the left cura of the diaphragm, forming the anterior border of the aortic hiatus.

Inexpensive, noninvasive, rapid, and without the risks of contrast and radiation, Doppler ultrasound provides an effective alternative to the angiography and CT-angiography. Two prospective trials in adults comparing the Doppler Ultrasound to the lateral abdominal aortography confirmed the accuracy of this modality in diagnosing the condition. The more recent investigation confirmed 100 % sensitivity of the Doppler ultrasound for identifying clinically significant (> 70 %) celiac artery stenosis. Specificity, positive predictive value, and negative predictive value were 87, 57, and 100 %, respectively [23, 24]. A later retrospective analysis on children and adolescents further substantiated the suitability and value of the Doppler ultrasound in diagnosing MALS.

For the examination, patients should fast for a minimum of 8 h prior to the study. Given the vague clinical presentation, the entire mesenteric system should be evaluated. Lower frequency (in the range of 3–7.5 MHz) and harmonic imaging provide clearer images. All velocity measurements should be obtained with angle correction of less than 60° [25]. Wolfman et al. have demonstrated the importance of acquiring both supine and erect Doppler images, noting a tendency of pathological values to normalize when children are positioned erect. The stage of the respiratory cycle dramatically affects the results, with much higher peak velocities observed at peak expiration than peak inspiration due to the dorsal movement of the aorta upon inhalation. One study in adults suggested that 73 % of the patients with end-expiration celiac artery stenosis observed via ultrasound demonstrated at least partial resolution of the pathology at end-inspiration [26, 27]. Consensus for the proper moment in the respiratory cycle to examine the patient has not been established, with authors alternatively opting for either the best-case or worst-case ultrasonagraphic results. Examinations require fewer than 20 min for experienced ultrasongraphers to complete.

While normal blood flow velocities for adults and neonates are available, such data are not well-established for children, and no rigorously verified criteria for defining MALS in the pediatric population exist. For adults, prospective studies have shown that peak systolic velocities greater than 200 cm/s in the celiac artery (or no flow detected) correlate with at least 70 % stenosis of the vessel, with 75 % sensitivity and 89 % specificity [25]. Most subsequent publications have adopted these standards, even for children, and have demonstrated their reliability in diagnosing the MALS [24]. The largest series of children with MALS (n = 59) entertained more liberal criteria, including greater than twofold acceleration in flow between the aorta and celiac artery, but a lack of confirmatory data prevents us from endorsing this expanded definition. Figure 9.5 illustrates the findings in MALS.

When appropriate, surgical intervention can proceed via either open or laparoscopic means. For either approach, the use of intraoperative ultrasound can confirm the efficacy of the repair and the resolution of the stenosis by showing decreased peak velocities in the celiac artery [28]. Thus, for screening, diagnosis, and post-treatment verification, Doppler ultrasound is a highly effective, inexpensive modality well-suited for the pediatric population.

Superior Mesenteric Artery Syndrome (SMAS)

SMAS (also referred to as Wilkie's disease, cast syndrome, arterial mesenteric duodenal compression) occurs when the SMA and aorta entrap and compress the third portion of the duodenum. It was first noted by Rikitansky in 1842 and

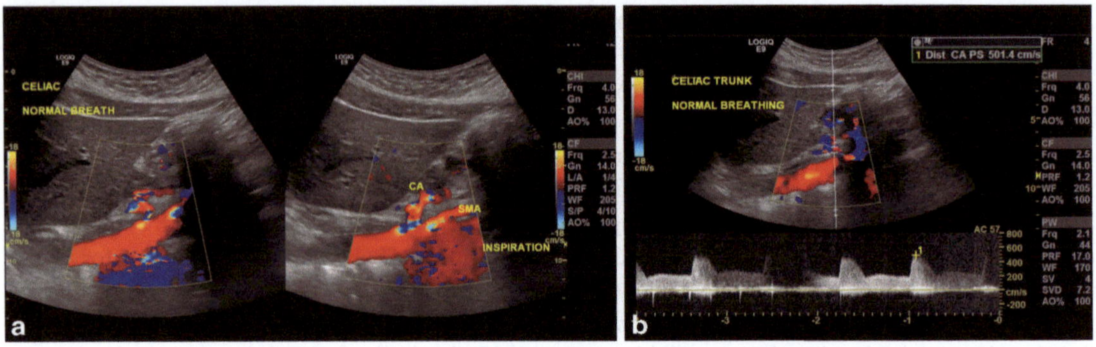

Fig. 9.5 Median arcuate ligament syndrome *(MALS)*. **a** the angle between the celiac axis and the *SMA* is seen and measured erect and supine as well as in deep inspiration. **b** The velocity measured is > 200 cm/s

more completely described by Wilkie in 1927 [29].

Ultrasound has now assumed an important role in screening for the condition. A 2005 controlled prospective study in adults clearly demonstrated the ability of ultrasound to match CT scans in accurately identifying the vascular features of this syndrome [30, 31]. Exams are performed after an overnight fast and during the expiratory phase of respiration. Low MHZ probes provide the best images. There was no significant difference between conducting the exam in the supine or standing positions, although the lateral position was less sensitive.

Ultrasound can help diagnose SMAS by assessing the angle between the aorta and the SMA (Fig. 9.6a and b) as well as the distance from the aorta to the SMA at the level of the duodenum [32]. In adults, these values have been well studied, and while measurements vary, the literature generally considers a normal angle to be between 25 and 60° and a normal distance to be between 10 and 28 mm. These values in children have recently been studied in 205 consecutive pediatric abdominal CT scans in patients presenting without suspicion for SMAS. This series showed the mean angle to be 45.6±19.6° [33]. The few published cases demonstrating the utility of ultrasound to diagnose SMAS in young patients with otherwise unexplainable abdominal pain have used adult measurements [34]. However, the study of 205 pediatric abdominal CT scans revealed

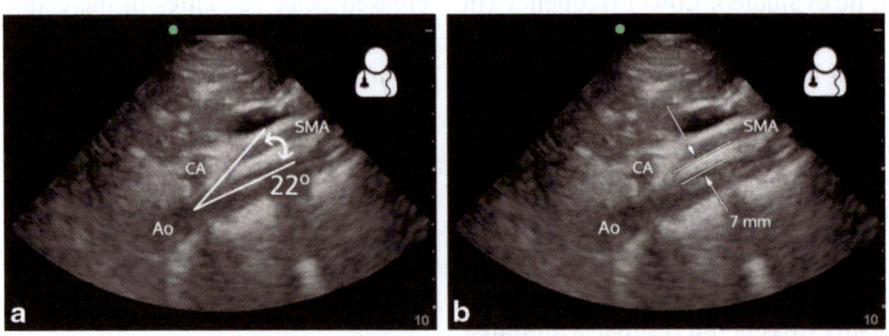

Fig. 9.6 Superior mesenteric artery syndrome *(SMAS)*. A normal aortomesenteric angle is approximately 45°, and an aortomesenteric angle of 6–25° confirms the diagnosis. This angle can be readily measured on ultrasound. **a** To measure the aortomesenteric angle, first obtain a sagittal view of the aorta and delineate landmarks: *Ao*, *CA*, and *SMA*. Measure the *SMA* angle as it takes off from the aorta. **b** A normal aortomesenteric distance is 10–28 mm. An aortomesenteric distance <8–10 mm suggests *SMA* syndrome in the appropriate clinical setting [32]

that over 20% of the cases demonstrated angles less than 8°—values that meet diagnostic criteria for SMAS, yet the patients denied any symptoms of the syndrome [33]. Moreover, other data show significant inter-operator variability with Doppler measurements of the SMA, challenging the reliability of test. Clearly, clinicians must have a high index of suspicion to evaluate for SMAS and use imaging to confirm clinical assessment rather than solely relying on angles and distances. At present, ultrasound serves well as a screening modality for SMAS, but CT scans ought to be obtained to confirm the diagnosis and clarify the anatomy, particularly if operative intervention is planned.

Nutcracker Syndrome

Nutcracker syndrome refers to an array of symptoms associated with the compression of the LRV. It is crucial to distinguish the syndrome from nutcracker phenomenon, which refers to anatomical and radiological evidence of such constriction without any corresponding symptoms. Anatomists have recognized compression of the LRV between the aorta and SMA since the 1930s [35, 36], but the condition of nutcracker syndrome was not elucidated until the 1970s [37]. Children suffering from the disease report flank and/or abdominal pain, gross hematuria, and varicoceles; some present with asymptomatic proteinuria or microhematuria [38]. Today, ultrasound has an important role in establishing the diagnosis.

Prior to ultrasound, renal venography with pressure gradients established the presence of the disease, with pressure differentials of greater than 3 mm Hg between the LRV and vena cava confirming the disease. This methodology remains the gold-standard, if rarely implemented. (Normal pressure differentials in children have not been established, forcing clinicians to rely on adult parameters). The invasiveness, radiation, and contrast load, not to mention cost, render this technique unappealing, especially in children. In 1986, Wolfish et al. proposed using ultrasound as an alternative [39]. Specifically, they suggested a 50% increase in the diameter of the LRV between the renal hilum and the aorta compared to the segment between the aorta and vena cava reflected compression. The first recorded case of the nutcracker syndrome diagnosed by ultrasound occurred in 1988 in Japan using Wolfish's criteria [40]. Further Japanese studies established clear guidelines for the diagnoses nutcracker phenomenon based on LRV dilation ratios [41, 42], but additional investigation revealed normal LRV diameter varied too much in children to rely on it for diagnostic purposes [43, 44].

The advent of Doppler technology offered a new option in measuring blood flow. However, the anatomy of pediatric patients complicated its initial deployment. With a very short LRV that runs almost perfectly horizontal, children challenged the acquisition of acceptable Doppler angles [45]. As such, early Doppler investigations relied on the identification of the collateral veins to diagnose nutcracker phenomenon, which had a relatively low sensitivity (78%) but 100% specificity when observed [46, 47]. Rarely found on CT scans, Doppler-identified collateral veins remain useful in confidently diagnosing nutcracker phenomenon.

More recently, Doppler-acquired flow velocities have demonstrated reliability and accuracy in identifying the nutcracker phenomenon. With the advent of new technology and the introduction of techniques like instructing patients to drink water prior to the exam (thus eliminating bowel gas and creating clearer windows), Doppler exams became more feasible. A 1996 South Korean study compared Doppler ultrasound directly to LRV pressure gradient measurements in adult patients with the nutcracker syndrome verses controls and found significant differences in the peak velocity of blood flowing in the LRV between the vena cava/aorta and aorta/hilum [48]. The ratio of velocity differences Kim elucidated has since become the foundation of Doppler-diagnosed nutcracker phenomenon. Subsequent investigators worked to apply these findings to children [49], and in 2001, the first child was diagnosed with the nutcracker syndrome based on this ratio [50].

Since Kim et al. established the ratio, other groups have worked to refine the value and apply it to children. Kim et al. established the cut off ratio for adults to be 5.0 [50]. Pediatric studies have suggested ratios ranging from 4.1 to 4.8, with sensitivities of 100 % and specificities ranging in the low 90s [51–53]. These ratios have proven accurate enough and are so widely accepted that physicians reporting continued use of other modalities like MRA and CT-A scans have been criticized in the literature [54]. Which exact number to use remains debatable, and the ethnic homogeneity of all subjects in these studies is less than ideal, but the repeatability of the results and the relatively narrow range of ratios strongly substantiate the methodology. More recent investigations have also looked to the measuring the aorta–SMA angle as an adjunct to help diagnose nutcracker phenomenon, but given (a) the high sensitivity and specificity of ratios; (b) the dependence of the angle on child positioning; and (c) the aforementioned wide variability of this angle in children, clinicians need not pursue this additional measurement.

Several well-controlled studies have clearly demonstrated the ability of Doppler ultrasound to diagnose nutcracker phenomenon in children by comparing the peak velocities of blood flow in different segments of the LRV. Ultrasound provides a welcome advance from the invasive, expensive, radioactive methods of the 1980s, and, based on the above investigations, can be used exclusively to diagnose the LRV compression characteristic of the nutcracker syndrome.

Stenosis, Aneurysm, Collaterals, and Thrombosis

Renal Artery Stenosis

Ultrasound can be used to evaluate the causes of renovascular hypertension, specifically renal artery stenosis, often induced by Takayasu's arteritis in children [55]. Typically, the patient is placed in a lateral decubitus position, with an angle of insonation of about 60°. A velocity in the renal artery >200 m/s is consistent with renal artery stenosis, and a difference in the resistive indices >0.05 between the two kidneys with the lower resitive index (RI) being on the side of the kidney with the elevated velocities is consistent with renal artery stenosis of >60 %.

Aneurysms

Abdominal aneurysms are uncommon in children and most often occur with Kawasaki's disease [56], pancreatitis [57], or after trauma to the liver and spleen [58]. Ultrasound can be used to evaluate for pseudoaneurysm or true aneurysm and is a useful technique to monitor success after intervention. Ultrasound can reliably measure the dimensions of the aneurysm and characterize the flow of blood in the lesion.

Collaterals and Portosystemic Shunts

Portal hypertension is caused by a number of conditions that create an increase in the PV pressure. These are generally classified as pre-hepatic, post-hepatic, or sinusoidal (intra-hepatic). There are a number of physiologic sequelae to prolonged portal hypertension. In pediatric surgery, pre-hepatic causes can be due to PV thrombosis after umbilical vein catheterization (although more often from unclear etiology). If portal hypertension progresses, appropriate flow can become hepatofugal in direction, and ultimately there is shunting of portal blood flow to the systemic veins that return blood to the heart via the inferior vena cava. Ultrasound can be used to document and follow shunts and collaterals that develop in patients with the chronic portal hypertension. Ultrasound can demonstrate changes in flow through portosystemic shunts [59], along with changes in the characteristics of flow (i.e.,

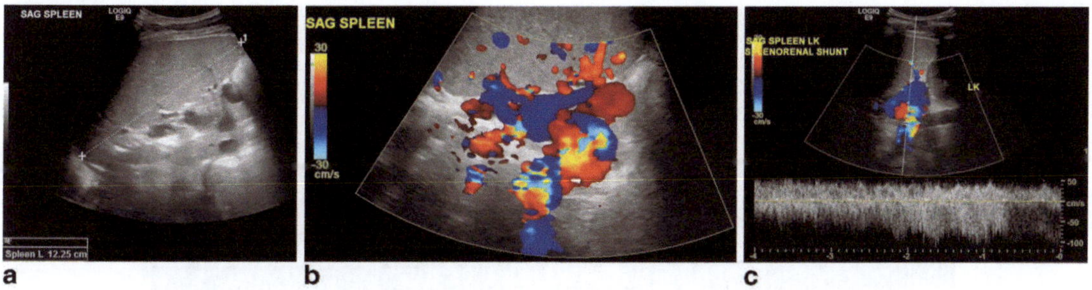

Fig. 9.7 Splenorenal shunt. **a** Ultrasound identifies the dilated vessels at the splenic hilum and documents the splenomegaly. **b** Hepatopetal flow identified in the splenic parenchyma. **c** Close proximity of flow between the liver and kidney, patent renal vein

reliably demonstrative of loss of variation with respiration or changes in Doppler waveform patterns).

As an example, Fig. 9.7 demonstrates a splenorenal shunt. In the top panel, the spleen is measured and noted to be enlarged with normal parenchyma. The tortuous splenic collaterals are seen at the hilum. In the middle panel, the central PV is not identified. However, hepatopedal (appropriate directional) portal venous flow is detected within the parenchyma. The hepatic veins demonstrate gross patency. In the bottom panel, the limited image of the left kidney demonstrates no abnormality. Flow is toward the kidney, compatible with a splenorenal shunt. This is patent and demonstrates flow above and below the baseline. Peak velocity ranges between 50 and 100 cm/s. The main renal vein is grossly patent.

Thrombosis

Duplex sonography is the main radiographic method for detecting and monitoring thrombosis of the larger veins. All major veins can be easily visualized and examined for flow characteristics except the superior vena cava (SVC) and the more distal SMV, which are often obscured by air from lungs or bowel. To evaluate the SVC, MRA, or venous phase CTA are needed for optimal evaluation. Clinically, thrombosis is common in the femoral, iliac, internal jugular, and subclavian veins, mostly secondary to central venous catheters [60] (Fig. 9.8). Extent and resolution after anticoagulation therapy is preferably monitored with the ultrasound, which can even be performed as a bedside study in the intensive care unit (Fig. 9.9). Ultrasound-guided placement of vena cava filters is standard of care in many centers for adolescents with increased risk of peripheral deep venous thrombosis to prevent a large pulmonary embolus [63]. The exact position for deployment just inferior to the confluence with the renal veins is paramount when placing these devices (Fig. 9.10).

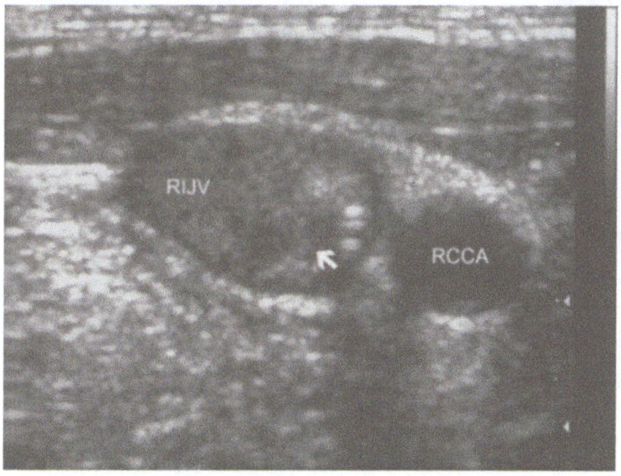

Fig. 9.8 Thrombus visualized within the right internal jugular vein *(RIJV) (arrow)*. The vessel could not be compressed. *RCCA* right common carotid artery [61]

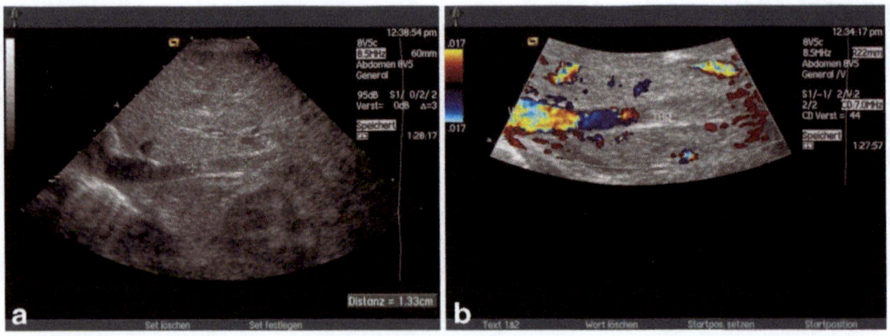

Fig. 9.9 Newborn 36th gestational week with massive swelling of abdomen and thorax. The extremities were only mildly edematous. **a** Depiction of an echogenic thrombus in the area of the middle inferior vena cava at about the level of the renal vein junction. The increased echogenicity of the thrombus indicates that the clot is at least 7 days old. **b** The color Doppler shows that the retrohepatic inferior vena cava above the level of the thrombus *(THR)* is patent without any clot burden [62]

Summary

Ultrasonography of abdominal vessels aids in the workup of many abdominal conditions in children. Simple to employ with no risks to the patient, ultrasound has become a very important implement in the physician's armamentarium for diagnostic workup and management decisions involving the major vessels. Every abdominal organ, their vascular supply, and the large central vessels are able to be imaged with ultrasound, making it a very versatile tool. Color Doppler can picture and quantify pathology within the vasculature itself. As ultrasound involves no contrast or radiation and is noninvasive and repeatable, it is a logical study to be included in the workup of the many diagnoses involving the abdominal vasculature.

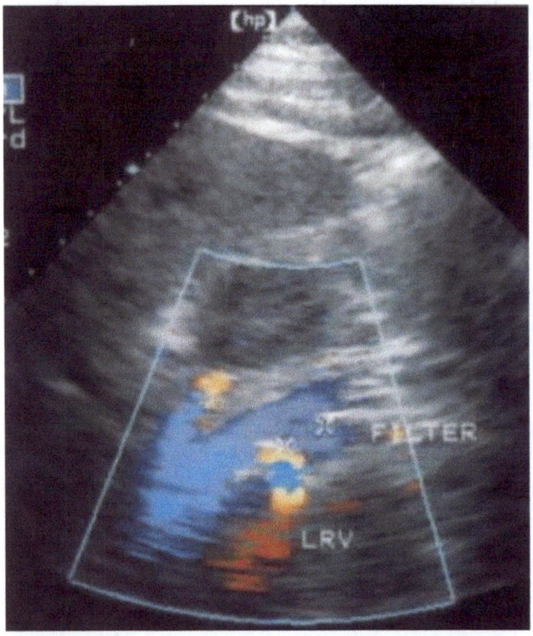

Fig. 9.10 Color-flow duplex ultrasound scan with patent *IVC* with tip of Greenfield filter seen just distal to the *LRV*. The patient is scanned from the right flank while in left decubitus position. The head of the patient is to the left [63]

References

1. Epelman M. The whirlpool sign. Radiology. 2006;240(3):910–1.
2. Applegate KE. Evidence-based diagnosis of malrotation and volvulus. Pediatr Radiol. 2009;39:161–3.
3. Stephens LR, Donoghue V, Gillick J. Radiological versus clinical evidence of malrotation, a tortuous tale–10-year review. Eur J Pediatr Surg. 2012;22(3):238–42.
4. Chao H-C, Kong M-S, Chen J-Y, Lin S-J, Lin J-N. Sonographic features related to volvulus in neonatal intestinal malrotation. J Ultrasound Med. 2000;19(6):371–6.
5. Gaines P, Saunders A, Drake D. Midgut malrotation diagnosed by ultrasound. Clin Radiol. 1987;38(1):51–3.
6. Loyer E, Eggli KD. Sonographic evaluation of superior mesenteric vascular relationship in malrotation. Pediatr Radiol. 1989;19(3):173–5.

7. Weinberger E, Winters W, Liddell R, Rosenbaum D, Krauter D. Sonographic diagnosis of intestinal malrotation in infants: importance of the relative positions of the superior mesenteric vein and artery. AJR Am J Roentgenol. 1992;159(4):825–8.
8. Zerin JM, DiPietro M. Superior mesenteric vascular anatomy at US in patients with surgically proved malrotation of the midgut. Radiology. 1992;183(3):693–4.
9. Dufour D, Delaet M, Dassonville M, Cadranel S, Perlmutter N. Midgut malrotation, the reliability of sonographic diagnosis. Pediatr Radiol. 1992;22(1):21–3.
10. Pracros J, Sann L, Genin G, Tran-Minh V, de Finfe CM, Foray P, et al. Ultrasound diagnosis of midgut volvulus: the "whirlpool" sign. Pediatr Radiol. 1992;22(1):18–20.
11. Shimanuki Y, Aihara T, Takano H, Moritani T, Oguma E, Kuroki H, et al. Clockwise whirlpool sign at color Doppler US: an objective and definite sign of midgut volvulus. Radiology. 1996;199(1): 261–4.
12. Patino MO, Munden MM. Utility of the sonographic whirlpool sign in diagnosing midgut volvulus in patients with atypical clinical presentations. J Ultrasound Med. 2004;23(3):397–401.
13. Yeh WC, Wang HP, Chen C, Wang HH, Wu MS, Lin JT. Preoperative sonographic diagnosis of midgut malrotation with volvulus in adults: the "whirlpool" sign. J Clin Ultrasound. 1999;27(5):279–83.
14. Van Winckel M, Voet D, Robberecht E. "Whirlpool sign": not always associated with volvulus in intestinal malrotation. J Clin Ultrasound. 1996;24(7): 367–70.
15. Marine MB, Karmazyn B. Imaging of malrotation in the neonate. Semin Ultrasound CT MR. 2014;35(6):555–70.
16. Applegate KE, Anderson JM, Klatte EC. Intestinal malrotation in children: a problem-solving approach to the upper gastrointestinal series. Radiographics. 2006;26(5):1485–500.
17. Yousefzadeh DK. The position of the duodenojejunal junction: the wrong horse to bet on in diagnosing or excluding malrotation. Pediatr Radiol. 2009;39(2):172–7.
18. Orzech N, Navarro OM, Langer JC. Is ultrasonography a good screening test for intestinal malrotation? J Pediatr Surg. 2006;41(5):1005–9.
19. Esposito F, Vitale V, Noviello D, Serafino MD, Vallone G, Salvatore M, et al. Ultrasonographic Diagnosis of midgut volvulus with malrotation in children. J Pediatr Gastroenterol Nutr. 2014;59(6):786–8.
20. Quail MA. Question 2 is Doppler ultrasound superior to upper gastrointestinal contrast study for the diagnosis of malrotation? Arch Dis Child. 2011;96(3):317–8.
21. Ashley LM, Allen S, Teele RL. A normal sonogram does not exclude malrotation. Pediatr Radiol. 2001;31(5):354–6.
22. Harjola PT. A rare obstruction of the coeliac artery. Report of a case. Ann Chir Gynaecol Fenn. 1963;52:547–50.
23. Aschenbach R, Basche S, Vogl TJ. Compression of the celiac trunk caused by median arcuate ligament in children and adolescent subjects: evaluation with contrast-enhanced MR angiography and comparison with Doppler US evaluation. J Vasc Interv Radiol. 2011;22(4):556–61.
24. Moneta GL, Yeager RA, Dalman R, Antonovic R, Hall LD, Porter JM. Duplex ultrasound criteria for diagnosis of splanchnic artery stenosis or occlusion. J Vasc Surg. 1991;14(4):511–20.
25. Lynch K. Celiac artery compression syndrome a literature review. J Diagn Med Sonogr. 2014;30(3): 143–8.
26. Wolfman D, Bluth EI, Sossaman J. Median arcuate ligament syndrome. J Ultrasound Med. 2003;22(12):1377–80.
27. Papacci P, Giannantonio C, Cota F, Latella C, Semeraro CM, Fioretti M, et al. Neonatal colour Doppler ultrasound study: normal values of abdominal blood flow velocities in the neonate during the first month of life. Pediatr Radiol. 2009;39(4):328–35.
28. Moneta GL, Lee RW, Yeager RA, Taylor LM, Porter JM. Mesenteric duplex scanning: a blinded prospective study. J Vasc Surg. 1993;17(1):79–86.
29. Roayaie S, Jossart G, Gitlitz D, Lamparello P, Hollier L, Gagner M. Laparoscopic release of celiac artery compression syndrome facilitated by laparoscopic ultrasound scanning to confirm restoration of flow. J Vasc Surg. 2000;32(4):814–7.
30. Kohn GP, Bitar RS, Farber MA, Marston WA, Overby DW, Farrell TM. Treatment options and outcomes for celiac artery compression syndrome. Surg Innov. 2001;18(4):338–43.
31. Wilkie D. Chronic duodenal ileus. Am J Med Sci. 1927;173(5):643–8.
32. Neri S, Signorelli S, Mondati E, Pulvirenti D, Campanile E, Di Pino L, et al. Ultrasound imaging in diagnosis of superior mesenteric artery syndrome. J Intern Med. 2005;257(4):346–51.
33. Unal B, Aktas A, Kemal G, Bilgili Y, Guliter S, Daphan C, et al. Superior mesenteric artery syndrome: CT and ultrasonography findings. Diagn Interv Radiol. 2005;11(2):90–5. http://www.ultrasoundoftheweek.com/uotw-21-answer/.
34. Arthurs O, Mehta U, Set P. Nutcracker and SMA syndromes: what is the normal SMA angle in children? Eur J Radiol. 2012;81(8):e854–e61.
35. Abu-Zidan F, Hefny A, Saadeldinn Y, El-Ashaal Y. Sonographic findings of superior mesenteric artery syndrome causing massive gastric dilatation in a young healthy girl. Singapore Med J. 2010;51(11):e184–6.
36. Chin L-W, Chou M-C, Wang H-P. Ultrasonography diagnosis of superior mesenteric artery syndrome in the ED. Am J Emerg Med. 2005;25:864.e5–.e6.

37. Fagarasanu I. Recherches anatomiques sur la veine renale gauche et ses collaterales; leurs rapports avec la pathogenie du varicocele essential et des varices du ligament large. (Demonstrations experimentales). Ann Anat Pathol. 1938;15:9–52.
38. Grant J. Method of anatomy. Baltimore: Williams and Wilkins; 1938. p. 1.
39. De Schepper A. " Nutcracker" phenomenon of the renal vein and venous pathology of the left kidney. J Belge Radiol. 1971;55(5):507–11.
40. Alaygut D, Bayram M, Soylu A, Cakmakcı H, Türkmen M, Kavukcu S. Clinical course of children with nutcracker syndrome. Urology. 2013;82(3): 686–90.
41. Wolfish N, McLaine P, Martin D. Renal vein entrapment syndrome: frequency and diagnosis. A lesson in conservatism. Clin Nephrol. 1986;26(2):96–100.
42. Arima M, Hosokawa S, Ogino T, Ihara H, Terakawa T, Ikoma F. Ultrasonographically demonstrated nutcracker phenomenon: alternative to angiography. Int Urol Nephrol. 1990;22(1):3–6.
43. Okada M, Tsuzuki K, Ito S. Diagnosis of the nutcracker phenomenon using two-dimensional ultrasonography. Clin Nephrol. 1998;49(1):35–40.
44. Takahashi Y, Sano A, Matsuo M. An ultrasonographic classification for diverse clinical symptoms of pediatric nutcracker phenomenon. Clin Nephrol. 2005;64(1):47–54.
45. Zerin J, Hernandez R, Sedman A, Kelsch R. "Dilatation" of the left renal vein on computed tomography in children: a normal variant. Pediatr Radiol. 1991;21(4):267–9.
46. Buschi AJ, Harrison RB, Norman A, Brenbridge A, Williamson B, Gentry R, et al. Distended left renal vein: CT/sonographic normal variant. Am J Roentgenol. 1980;135(2):339–42.
47. Park SJ, Shin JI. Renal Doppler ultrasonography in the diagnosis of nutcracker syndrome. Eur J Pediatr. 2013;172(1):135–6.
48. Stavros AT, Sickler KJ, Menter RR. Color duplex sonography of the nutcracker syndrome (aortomesenteric left renal vein compression). J Ultrasound Med. 1994;13(7):569–74.
49. Takebayashi S, Ueki T, Ikeda N, Fujikawa A. Diagnosis of the nutcracker syndrome with color Doppler sonography: correlation with flow patterns on retrograde left renal venography. Am J Roentgenol. 1999;172(1):39–43.
50. Kim SH, Cho SW, Kim HD, Chung JW, Park JH, Han MC. Nutcracker syndrome: diagnosis with Doppler US. Radiology. 1996;198(1):93–7.
51. Cho BS, Choi YM, Kang HH, Park SJ, Lim JW, Yoon TY. Diagnosis of nut-cracker phenomenon using renal Doppler ultrasound in orthostatic proteinuria. Nephrol Dial Transplant. 2001;16(8): 1620–5.
52. Kavukcu S, Kasap B, Göktay Y, Seçil M. Doppler sonographic indices in diagnosing the nutcracker phenomenon in a hematuric adolescent. J Clin Ultrasound. 2004;32(1):37–41.
53. Cheon J-E, Kim WS, Kim I-O, Kim SH, Yeon KM, Ha IS, et al. Nutcracker syndrome in children with gross haematuria: Doppler sonographic evaluation of the left renal vein. Pediatr Radiol. 2006;36(7):682–6.
54. Shin JI, Park JM, Lee JS, Kim MJ. Effect of renal Doppler ultrasound on the detection of nutcracker syndrome in children with hematuria. Eur J Pediatr. 2007;166(5):399–404.
55. Shin JI, Park JM, Lee JS, Kim MJ. Doppler ultrasonographic indices in diagnosing nutcracker syndrome in children. Pediatr Nephrol. 2007;22(3): 409–13.
56. Park SJ, Oh JY, Shin JI. Diagnostic value of renal Doppler ultrasonography for detecting nutcracker syndrome in children with recurrent gross hematuria. Clin Pediatr (Phila). 2012;51(10):1001-.
57. TA L, Gajjar P, McCulloch M, Scott C, Numanoglu A, Nourse P. Impact of revascularization on hypertension in children with Takayasu's arteritis-induced renal artery stenosis: a 21-year review. Pediatr Nephrol. 2015. Feb 4.
58. Hoshino S, Tsuda E, Yamada O. Characteristics and fate of systemic artery aneurysm after Kawasaki disease. J Pediatr. 2015;167:108–12.e2.
59. Puri A, Acharya H, Tyagi S, Curian S, Chadha R, Anand R, Choudhary SR. Pseudoaneurysm of the radial branch of the splenic artery with pancreatic pseudocyst in a child with recurrent acute pancreatitis: treatment with endovascular stent graft and cystogastrostomy. J Pediatr Surg. 2012;47(5):1012–5.
60. Safavi A, Beaudry P, Jamieson D, Murphy JJ. Traumatic pseudoaneurysms of the liver and spleen in children: is routine screening warranted? J Pediatr Surg. 2011;46(5):938–41.
61. Pinter SZ, Rubin JM, Kripfgans OD, Novelli PM, Vargas-Vila M, Hall AL, Fowlkes JB. Volumetric blood flow in transjugular intrahepatic portosystemic shunt revision using 3-dimensional Doppler sonography. J Ultrasound Med. 2015;34(2):257–66.
62. Shah SH, West AN, Sepanski RJ, Hannah D, May WN, Anand KJ. Clinical risk factors for central line-associated venous thrombosis in children. Front Pediatr. 2015;3:35.
63. Karakitsos D, Labropoulos N, De Groot E, Patrianakos AP, Kouraklis G, Poularas J, et al. Real-time ultrasound-guided catheterisation of the internal jugular vein: a prospective comparison with the landmark technique in critical care patients. Crit Care. 2006;10(6):R162. http://www.radiologyteacher.com/index.cgi?&nav=view&DatID=95.
64. Cahn MD, Rohrer MJ, Martella MB, Cutler BS. Long-term follow-up of Greenfield inferior vena cava filter placement in children. J Vasc Surg. 2001;34(5):820–5.

Gastrointestinal Tract

10

Christine M. Leeper, Sara K. Rasmussen
and Stefan Scholz

Introduction

Abdominal and gastrointestinal (GI) problems in children comprise a large part of routine daily practice of pediatricians and pediatric surgeons. In many cases, history and physical examination can be pathognomonic, but the correct diagnosis can often be confirmed by a general or focused ultrasound examination of the abdomen. For children, ultrasound plays a dominant role under imaging methods either for screening or for definite diagnosis. In many parts of the world, it is considered as the "stethoscope of the surgeon." As a dynamic real-time method, sonography can be performed at the bedside, has no ionizing radiation, and can be easily repeated. It succeeds as a child-friendly nonintimidating imaging technique and enjoys high acceptance with parents.

S. Scholz (✉)
Division of Pediatric General and Thoracic Surgery, Children's Hospital of Pittsburgh of UPMC, University of Pittsburgh School of Medicine, One Children's Hospital Drive, 4401 Penn Avenue, Pittsburgh, PA 15224, USA
e-mail: stefan.scholz@chp.edu

C. M. Leeper
Department of General Surgery, University of Pittsburgh Medical Center, 200 Lothrop Street, Pittsburgh, PA 15213, USA
e-mail: leepercm@upmc.edu

S. K. Rasmussen
Department of Surgery, University of Virginia, 1215 Lee Street, Charlottesville, VA 22908, USA
e-mail: Skr3f@virginia.edu

The ultrasound examination of the GI tract poses relatively high demands on the expertise of the examiner. Pathologies can only be recognized if one is familiar with the sonographic appearance of normal structure and function. The intestine offers a great variation of its normal anatomy. Further, structures can be very subtle and the scanning field can be confusing due to the lack of landmarks needed for orientation. However, the learning curve even for providers untrained in advanced sonographic techniques can be steep and the skill can be acquired with little practice [1, 2].

Routine clinical practice in pediatric centers is changing. Today, focused abdominal ultrasound is used to confirm the clinical suspicion of hypertrophic pyloric stenosis (HPS) and intussusception rather than clinical examination alone (the palpable "olive" or a sausage-like palpable mass, respectively), abdominal radiograph or upper GI contrast study under fluoroscopy. Sonographic screening abdominal examinations can be performed quickly and it can successfully discover many problems such as mesenteric, pancreatic, or choledochal cysts, localized fluid collections and general ascites, or hemorrhage.

One example for which abdominal ultrasound has largely replaced computed tomography (CT) scan as a first-line study in many pediatric centers is for the diagnosis of acute appendicitis. The goal is to visualize and measure the appendix directly, with success rates directly linked to the examiner's patience, skill, and experience. Peri-appendiceal fluid can be detected as

S. Scholz, M. D. Jarboe (eds.), *Diagnostic and Interventional Ultrasound in Pediatrics and Pediatric Surgery*, DOI 10.1007/978-3-319-21699-7_10

well as a fecalith and, once found, the appendix' compressibility is directly tested. A focal sonographic "Murphy's sign" directly over the appendix can confirm the clinical and sonographic suspicion (Murphy's sign is traditionally reserved for focal tenderness elicited over the gallbladder by the ultrasound probe in the setting of acute cholecystitis). Perforated appendicitis leading to a phlegmon or an abdominal or pelvic abscess can be detected. Alternative diagnoses such as kidney stones or ovarian pathology can be ruled out relatively easily.

In centers dedicated to the care of children, abdominal ultrasound has become a mainstay of the diagnostic algorithm for many common clinical questions. The expertise of examiners is growing and may open the door for more sophisticated sonographic applications.

Scanning Technique and Normal Anatomy

Ultrasound scanning of the abdomen should be performed with a linear probe capable of color-flow Doppler imaging since the wide area of contact allows painless compression of the abdominal wall. Individual anatomical variations require the operator to search for the best acoustic window in a dynamic, flexible fashion. Compression of the abdominal wall pushes intestinal gas sideways to allow scanning of the abdominal contents without artifacts. In addition, the distance between the probe and the target area is shortened resulting in a higher-quality picture since a higher-frequency probe can be used.

Fine abdominal structures require high-resolution imaging, ideally with a linear probe of 7 MHz or higher. This frequency allows differentiation of the intestinal wall up to a scanning depth of 4–5 cm, which is sufficient for infants and children up to 15 years of age. Older or adipose children require a 5-MHz-probe, which limits resolution and does not allow fine differentiation of the intestinal wall. Even with this relatively low-frequency probe a number of pathological problems can be identified such as a peri-appendiceal abscess or thickened intestinal wall in active Crohn's disease. A sector or curved array ultrasound probe is needed for the examination of the distal esophagus, the cardia, and the rectum. A 5-MHz-probe is sufficient since the exact differentiation of the intestinal wall is usually not needed.

There is a large variability in the sonomorphology of the intestinal tract and the abdomen. Anatomical knowledge is a prerequisite to recognize pathological findings.

The stomach cannot be evaluated without preparation due to severe gas artifacts. The patient has either to be fasting or to have taken only clear liquids. A fasting study may also be of advantage for examining the upper abdomen since the picture is not disturbed by air artifacts or increased peristalsis of the small bowel. Standard examination of the remainder of the intestinal tract does not require special preparation of the patient but examination about 1–2 h postprandially will yield the best results.

The examination is performed in a supine position. The arms should be positioned parallel to the body and not behind the head; this would place the abdominal wall under tension and interfere with abdominal compression with the probe. A shallow pillow under the head can help to relax the abdominal wall as can pulling the knees towards the chest. The ultrasound gel should be warmed before the examination, either in the microwave or in a bottle warmer. A small child can be distracted with a bottle, a pacifier, or by reading a book. School-age children and teenagers can be shown the live image of their scan as a feedback to let them actively participate in the process and assure their cooperation. The patient can be turned to move gas out of the scanning field and improve visualization.

A systematic screening examination of the abdomen should include all the four quadrants and also the parenchymatous organs to exclude alternate pathological findings. This should not take longer than 10 min during which the patient gains confidence.

The gastroesophageal junction can be visualized and measures about 18 mm in newborns and 34 mm in children. The esophagus is usually empty and decompressed unless a pathology such as a stricture or achalasia is suggested. A dynamic evaluation can be performed while pressing on the stomach to give a quantitative impression of the severity of gastroesophageal reflux disease (GERD).

The gastric wall has a hypoechoic muscularis propria, a hyperechoic submucosa, a hypoechoic muscularis, and an echogenic serosa. The thickness of the stomach wall varies depending on its amount of filling from 1 to 9 mm. When fasted, the antrum is always found empty and can be located between the left lobe of the liver and the pancreas. Postprandially, the antrum is filled with gas and food and hard to evaluate by ultrasound, especially in infants.

The pylorus, found between the antrum and duodenal bulb, opens to allow the passage of food. Once the transverse plane of the pylorus is identified and the thickness of its hypoechoic muscle wall is measured, the probe can be turned by 90° to find the longitudinal plane to measure its length.

To scan the intestine, ultrasound should be performed with slightly increasing pressure always moving sideways. The bowel should be characterized by the diameter of its lumen, intestinal contents, peristalsis, morphology, and thickness of the wall. The upper limit of the bowel wall thickness is 1.5 mm for ileum and 2.0 mm for colon [3].

Passing the pylorus, the duodenal bulb can be seen. Its wall has the typical three-layered structure with a thin muscle layer (1.0 mm), mostly filled with a small amount of air. The distal duodenum is usually contracted with an empty lumen. In the left mid abdomen, the jejunum can be found with a wall thickness around 1.0 mm and good peristalsis. There is a great variability depending on food content or gas. The probe is moved through the right mid and lower abdomen to examine the ileum and its variable morphology. It can be very hard to differentiate intestinal loops due to gas artifacts. The terminal ileum is often empty and contracted. It can be seen overlying the psoas muscle, has no high folds typical for jejunum and a similar wall thickness of 1.0 mm. If conditions are good, the ileocecal valve is visualized resembling lips protruding into the cecum. The valve is closed at baseline, but stool passage can be observed at times.

The cecum has a large lumen filled with gas and stool, and lacks peristalsis. Look for the appendix around the cecum and the ileocecal valve area as a short blind ending part of the intestine with its own lumen. The appendix can often be found more medially between the cecum and the ileum and is much easier to find when inflamed and enlarged. The normal appendiceal wall measures 3.0 mm in thickness with a total diameter up to 6.0 mm.

The ascending colon is up to 2.0 mm thick with very little peristalsis and has a more echogenic submucosa. Its taenia can be seen as a circumscript wall thickening in the axial plane. Axial planes are obtained for the evaluation of the colon. Moving upwards along the colon, turn the ultrasound probe 90° to evaluate the transverse colon below the liver edge which often appears contracted and narrow with little gas. Again, turn the probe 90° to evaluate the descending colon in left abdomen which is often filled with gas and also has little peristalsis. Use a sector or curved array probe to find the sigmoid colon and the rectum. Evaluate the wall morphology and thickness of the colon by ultrasound, it may be filled with fluid by enema.

In general, there is great variability within the intestine and pathologies can be difficult to detect by ultrasound. Abnormal wall thickening and atypical wall morphology, a pathological size of the lumen, unexpected intestinal contents (foreign bodies, magnets), or changes in normal peristalsis could indicate an underlying problem

Gastroesophageal Reflux

GER in infants and children is diagnosed through the use of multiple modalities; abdominal ultrasound is not recommended for use as an isolated diagnostic test [4–6]. However, ultrasound can be used in conjunction with other tests to aid in diagnosis and has a role in the anatomic and functional evaluation of the upper GI tract. Important anatomic criteria in the diagnosis of GER include shorter length of the abdominal esophagus and more obtuse angle of His, both of which are reliably measured by ultrasound [6, 7].

Ultrasound offers the clinician functional information as well. This is particularly valuable in the context of GER, where ultrasound permits direct visualization of reflux episodes with assessment of frequency, duration and characteristics, and correlation with patient symptoms. Further, nonacid reflux events and other upper GI issues that share symptoms with GER like intestinal obstruction, masses, malrotation, HPS, and hiatal hernia may be identified at the time of ultrasound [8].

Hiatal Hernia

A hiatal hernia occurs when a portion of the stomach traverses an abnormally widened esophageal hiatus of the diaphragm into the mediastinum. It is important to perform ultrasound under defined and consistent clinical conditions, as variables such as stomach volume can affect data acquisition [9]. In addition to shorter length of the abdominal esophagus and more obtuse angle of His previously discussed in relation to the diagnoses of GER, some diagnosticians also cite a "beak sign" or widening of the stomach end of the gastric triangle as an indicator of hiatal hernia [7]. Cakmakci and colleagues suggest that absence of the periesophageal fat pad sign is another indicator of hiatal hernia. Hiatal hernia is clinically relevant as its presence is associated with degree of reflux severity [10]. Ultrasound findings for hiatal hernia correlate well with CT [11].

Hypertrophic Pyloric Stenosis

HPS is relatively common (incidence: 1.5–3:1000) with an increased incidence in firstborns, males, and children with a family history of HPS [12]. The classic presentation is a 2–12 week old with projectile nonbilious emesis after enteral feeds, the physical examination finding of a "palpable olive" in the midepigastric region, and laboratory evidence of a hypokalemic hypochloremic metabolic alkalosis. For reasons thought to be related to abnormal innervation of the muscular layer of the intestine that remain incompletely explained, the pylorus becomes abnormally thickened, resulting in narrowing and elongation of the pyloric channel and producing a gastric outlet obstruction with compensatory gastric hyperperistalsis [13]. The treatment is fluid resuscitation followed by surgical pyloromyotomy.

Ultrasound is currently the imaging study of choice for diagnosis of HPS. Recommended probe selection includes 6–10 MHz linear array mid-high frequency or 6–8 MHz small foot print, high-frequency annular array, or curvilinear probes. Scanning should start medial to gallbladder with localization of the fluid-filled stomach. The stomach may be followed distally to the pylorus, which will be lateral and anterior to the aorta–superior mesenteric artery (SMA) junction.

Ideally, the patient has to fast for 4 h to minimize gas interference. A warm room and warm gel are essential for patient comfort; crying increases gas in the stomach making visualization much more difficult. The baby should then be fed (water is best for a good acoustic window), which will allow the stomach to be seen as hypoechoic with small hyperechoic air bubbles. Milk is suboptimal as it appears as echogenic heterogeneous material.

The thickness and the length of the hypoechoic pyloric muscle make the diagnosis of HPS. A pyloric muscle thickness of greater than 3 mm (100 % sensitive and 99 % specific), and pyloric canal length greater than 14 mm (100 % sensitive and 97 % specific) are considered abnormal (Fig. 10.1a—normal, b—HPS). The pyloric channel will also be filled with crowded and redundant mucosa in HPS. If the stomach is filled with gas, use of gravitational maneuvers during an ultrasound examination may be useful with placement of the patient in a right anterior oblique position or left posterior oblique position to reveal the hypertrophied pylorus [14]. During the ultrasound examination, the pyloric channel should be observed for the passage of any gastric contents and this should also be a part of the study report. Passage of large amounts of gastric contents during a 10–15 min-long examination contradicts the diagnosis of pyloric stenosis.

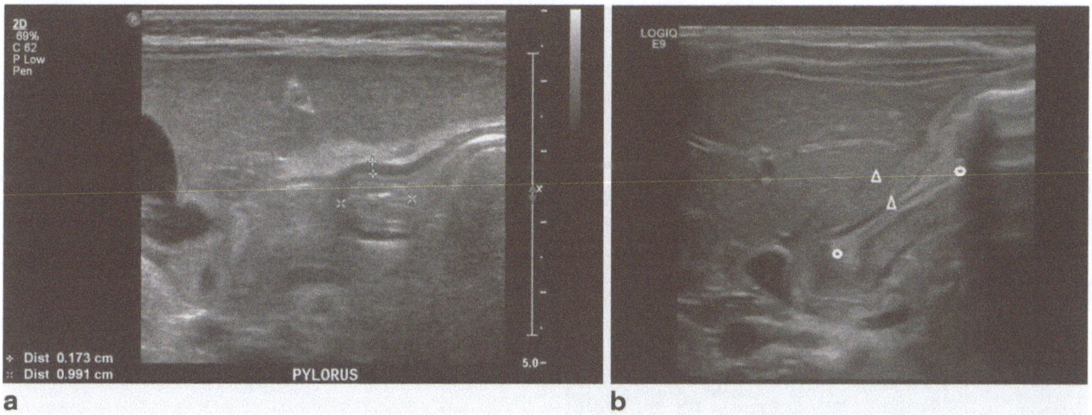

Fig. 10.1 **a** Normal *pylorus* **b** Hypertrophic pyloric stenosis—4-week-old male who presented with forceful nonbilious emesis. Pyloric muscle measured 4 mm *(triangles)*, pyloric channel measured 17 mm *(circles)*

Malrotation and Volvulus

Malrotation (incidence 1:6000) is caused by failure of the intestine to undergo the normal 270° counterclockwise rotation around the SMA during embryologic development. Midgut volvulus results from torsion of the bowel around an abnormally narrow mesentery that results from malrotation and improper fixation of the bowel. It can result in catastrophic necrosis and loss of a majority of the intestine if not recognized and treated promptly with surgical derotation. The typical patient is a previously healthy term infant in the first month of life who presents with sudden onset bilious emesis. Traditionally, the diagnosis is made with abdominal radiograph and upper GI studies [15].

Currently, ultrasound is utilized in some centers when the diagnosis of malrotation or acute midgut volvulus is equivocal. Color Doppler is employed to demonstrate the "whirlpool" sign, a swirling of the blood vessels caused by the twisting of the mesentery (Fig. 10.2), or an inversion of the location of the SMA and superior mesenteric vein [16]. Malrotation is often accompanied by dilation of the duodenum. There is a potential role for diagnosing malrotation based on the position of the duodenum relative to the SMA and aorta. Yousefzadeh and colleagues demonstrated the feasibility and validity of this technique in 33 neonates [17]. If normal anatomy is seen on abdominal ultrasound, additional studies and radiation exposure may be avoided.

Intussusception

Intussusception, or intestinal invagination is the process by which one segment of proximal bowel telescopes onto the adjacent distal segment. It can result in obstruction, abdominal pain, and ultimately ischemic bowel due to compromised blood flow. Abdominal ultrasound, first described for the evaluation of this entity in 1977, is the primary imaging modality for diagnosis of

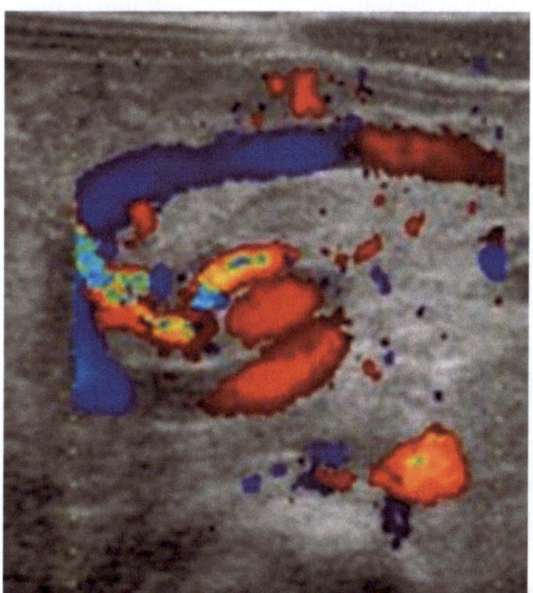

Fig. 10.2 Malrotation with volvulus—color Doppler ultrasound demonstrates "whirlpool" sign

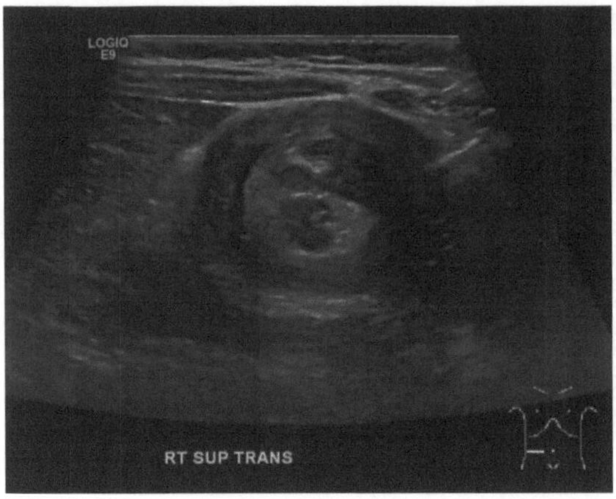

Fig. 10.3 Intussusception—5-month-old male who presented with fussiness, drawing legs up to chest, and blood per rectum. Ultrasound showed ileocolic intussusception, "target" sign

intussusception today. The hallmark sign is the "target" or "doughnut" sign (Fig. 10.3), an image seen in the transverse plain that demonstrates bowel wall and mesenteric fat within the intussusceptum forming rings of high and low echogenicity. Another characteristic finding is the "pseudokidney" sign (Fig. 10.4), an image seen in the longitudinal plain that demonstrates the edema in the walls of the intussusceptum trapped inside the intussuscipiens [18].

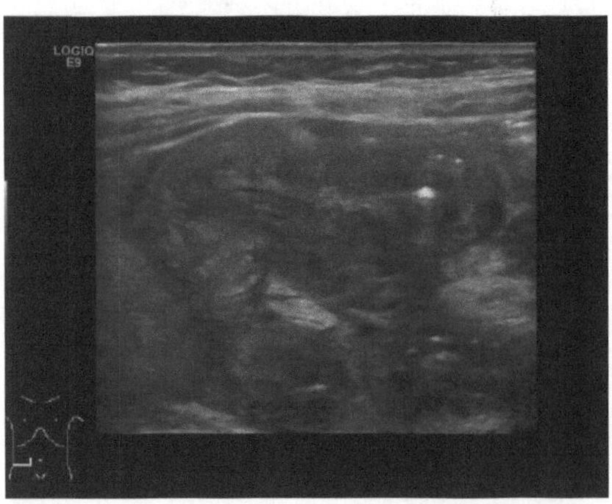

Fig. 10.4 Intussusception—5-month-old male who presented with fussiness, drawing legs up to chest, and blood per rectum. Ultrasound showed ileocolic intussusception, "pseudokidney" sign

Intussusception can be reduced with normal saline hydrostatic enema under ultrasound guidance. Many centers utilize air enema and fluoroscopy to confirm reduction. However, ultrasound can visualize the reduction of the ileo-ileocolic intussusception as well as the development of any pneumoperitoneum should perforation complicate the procedure [19]. Inability to complete the reduction under ultrasound guidance should prompt an attempt at conventional air/contrast enema reduction.

Intestinal Atresia

Intestinal atresias are congenital obstructions of the lumen of the duodenum, jejunum, or ileum thought to be due to vascular accidents in utero. They represent a relatively common etiology of neonatal bowel obstruction (incidence 1.3–2.8:10,000) and are frequently diagnosed on antenatal ultrasound. Duodenal atresia is reliably diagnosed prenatally through recognition of the classic "double bubble" sign, but identifying jejunal and ileal atresias can be more challenging with lower and more variable rates of prenatal diagnosis. Imaging characteristics including polyhydramnios and dilated bowel may not be present at the time of ultrasound [20].

For neonates who carry a diagnosis of suspected atresia, many centers utilize abdominal ultrasound as confirmatory testing and to evaluate for additional anomalies [21]. Characteristics of duodenal atresia include massive dilation of the stomach and normal pylorus with decompressed distal intestine (Fig. 10.5).

Characteristics of intestinal atresia on ultrasound may include dilated loops of proximal bowel and decompressed distal bowel segments; direct visualization of the atretic segment is also possible (Figs. 10.6 and 10.7). In previously healthy neonates who present with symptoms of bowel obstruction, a variety of imaging techniques are employed for evaluation including plain radiograph, upper GI series, contrast enema, and ultrasound, among others. Ultrasound

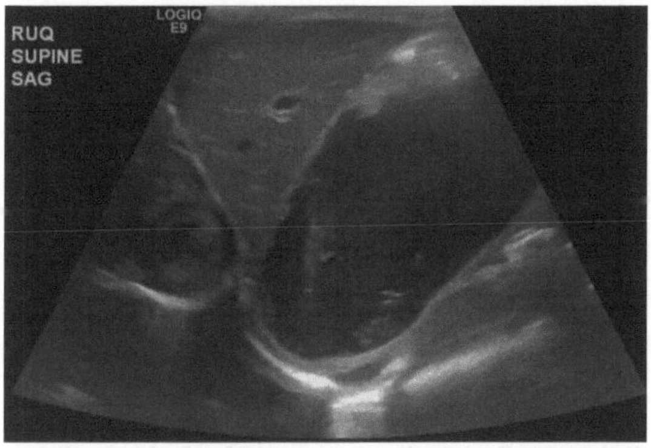

Fig. 10.5 Duodenal atresia—5-day-old male with emesis and no passage of stool. Ultrasound showed hugely distended stomach containing anechoic fluid, anatomically and functionally normal pylorus that opened well to allow passage of a small amount of gastric contents into the duodenum seen during the scanning process

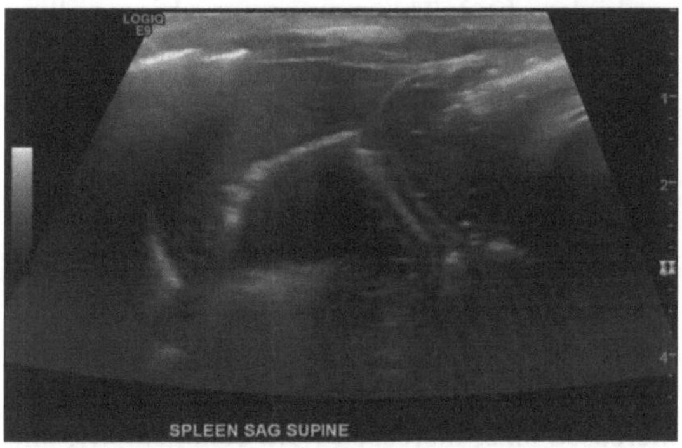

Fig. 10.6 Jejunal atresia: 2-day-old male with intestinal atresia type 4, total of 15 atretic segments. Ultrasound shows multiple dilated loops of bowel

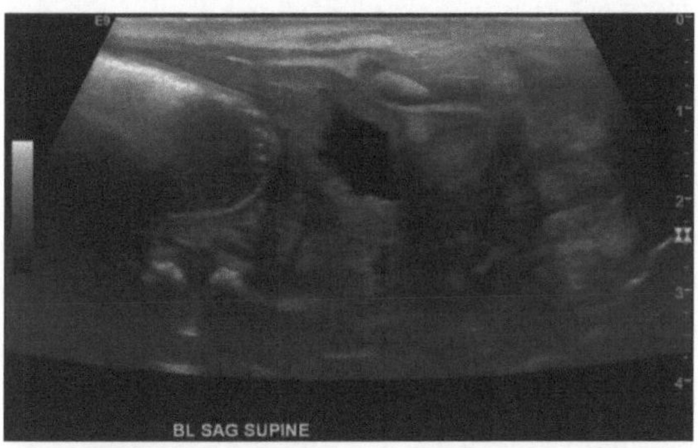

Fig. 10.7 Jejunal atresia: 2-day-old male with intestinal atresia type 4, total of 15 atretic segments. Ultrasound shows multiple dilated loops of bowel

has the advantage of not only demonstrating the intestinal atresia but also ruling out ascites, perforation, abdominal masses, or other etiology of obstruction.

Meckel Diverticulum

Meckel diverticulae represent the most common anomaly of the GI tract with prevalence in the general population from 1 to 4%. The clinical presentation can be variable and includes GI bleed, obstruction, diverticulitis, perforation, and volvulus [22]. An inflamed Meckel's diverticulum functions commonly as the lead point of a nonreducible intussusception, then diagnosed and resected in the operating room. Abdominal ultrasound is frequently obtained in the evaluation of pediatric abdominal pain, particularly when patients present with symptoms that are nonspecific. A Meckel's diverticulum appears on ultrasound as a long tubular structure and can mimic a duplication cyst. It can also be confused for an acutely inflamed appendix, as in the case of Meckel's diverticulitis (Fig. 10.8). If a diverticulum is the lead point causing intussusception, ultrasound will reveal a "double-target sign," a target-shaped mass of rings of high and low echogenicity with an additional central area of hyperechogenicity.

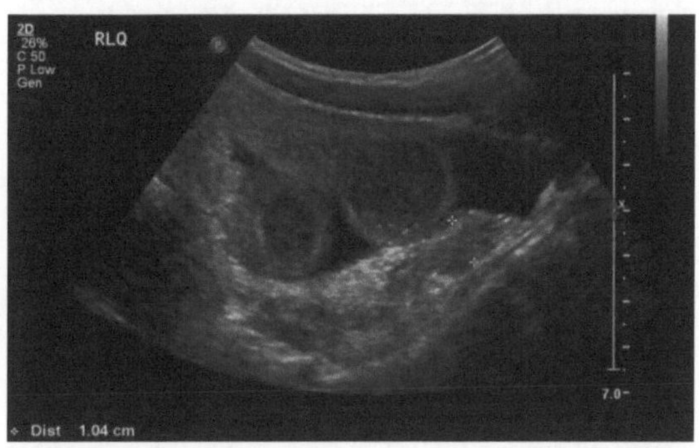

Fig. 10.8 9-year-old male with Meckel's diverticulitis—distended, blind-ending tubular structure in right lower quadrant consistent with the appendix which measures 1 cm in diameter. Several loops of dilated bowel with wall thickening are also seen. Additionally, free fluid is identified in the right lower quadrant and in Morison's pouch

Abdominal Cysts

Enteral Duplication Cyst

Intestinal duplication cysts are uncommon congenital anomalies (incidence 1–2:10,000) that can be seen throughout the GI tract (Figs. 10.9 and 10.10), but are most commonly found in the ileum. Most are diagnosed before age 2 after the patient presents with obstructive symptoms, vague pain or constipation, or rarely with GI bleeding or malignant degeneration. The treatment is surgical excision of the lesion. Ultrasound diagnosis is made by the "double wall" appearance (Fig. 10.11)—a hyperechoic edge surrounding the mucosal wall inside and a hypoechoic wall surrounding the smooth muscular layer outside, which are continuous with the corresponding structures of the adjacent bowel [23].

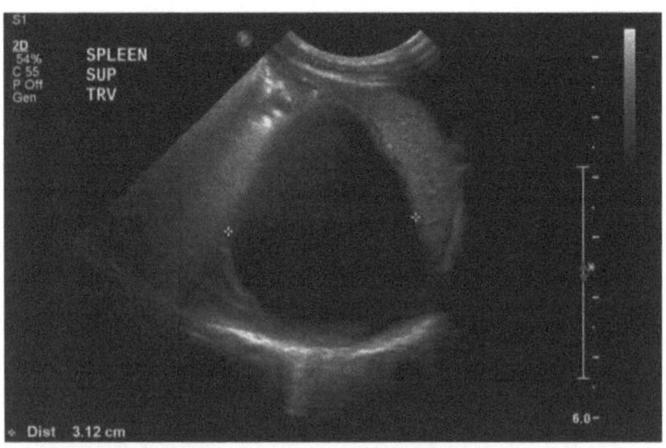

Fig. 10.9 Gastric duplication cyst at the level of the fundus, adjacent to the spleen—abdominal view

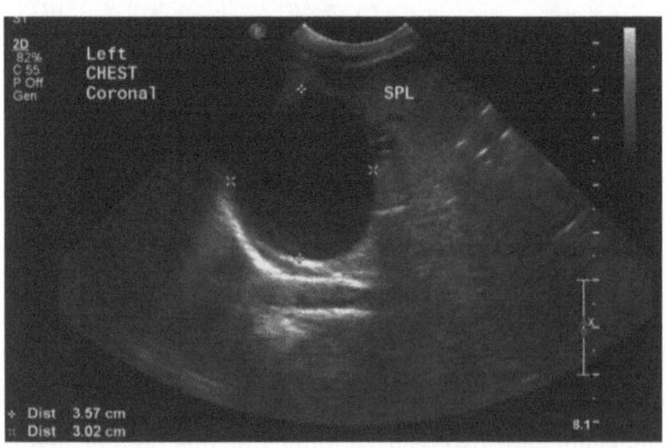

Fig. 10.10 Gastric duplication cyst at the level of the fundus, adjacent to the spleen—transthoracic view

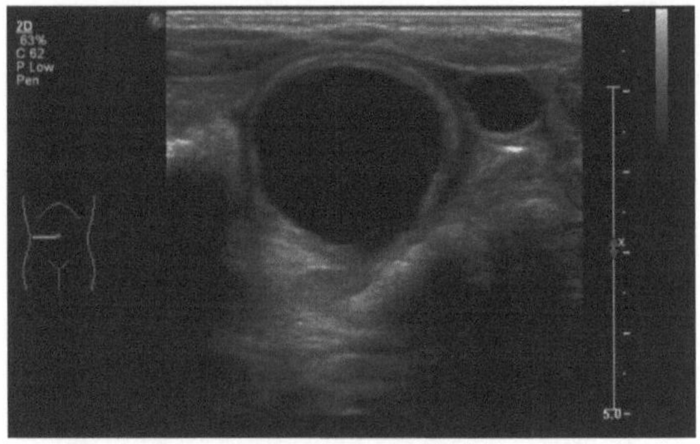

Fig. 10.11 Ileal duplication cyst with "double wall" appearance

Mesenteric Cysts

Mesenteric cysts are a rare anomaly (incidence 1:100,000) with only 25–30 % of these diagnosed in children [24]. They can be found in small or large bowel mesentery after patients present with abdominal pain and undergo imaging to rule out other presumed pathology like appendicitis. Ultrasound evaluation is sensitive and specific, and can be used for diagnosis as well as to follow lesions of uncertain etiology. Imaging characteristics include a multiloculated septated cystic mass and ascites may or may not be present (Fig. 10.12). Sequential images may show increased size, increased fluid echogenicity, and thickening or multiplication of septae [25]. Surgical excision is the treatment of choice; pathology

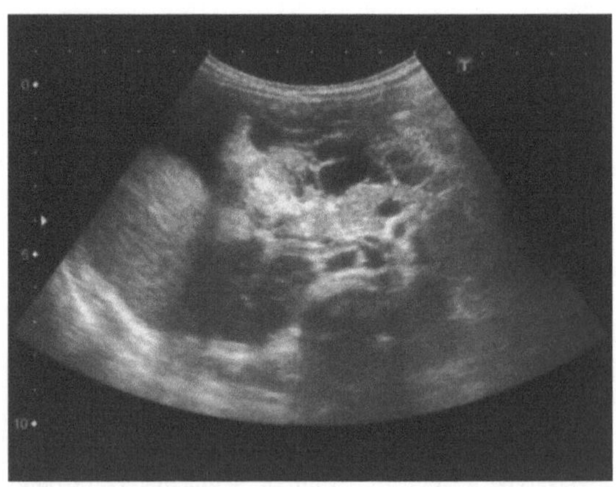

Fig. 10.12 Mesenteric cyst—multiloculated, septated cystic intra-abdominal mass

typically reveals benign tissue though complications may arise from cyst growth over time [26].

Necrotizing Enterocolitis

Necrotizing enterocolitis (NEC) is a multifactorial disease that leads to disruption of intestinal integrity followed ultimately by bowel necrosis and bacterial translocation. Birth weight is inversely associated with incidence (1:1000) and mortality (15–30 %). Younger gestational age is also a predictor of poor outcome. The clinical presentation of NEC includes feeding intolerance, abdominal distention, and often bloody stool [27].

Currently, abdominal radiograph remains the preferred modality of choice for diagnosis and classification of NEC. However, abdominal ultrasound is increasingly being applied in NEC diagnosis and management for the advantages it offers over standard radiographs. Ultrasound permits visualization of bowel wall thickness and echogenicity, peristalsis, free fluid, and bowel wall perfusion [28]; this may allow for earlier diagnosis of bowel compromise and expedition of needed surgical intervention when bowel is threatened, but before actual perforation or frank necrosis occurs.

Pneumatosis intestinalis (PI) has been used as a marker for the condition. Most often observed in the ileum and colon, the finding is almost pathognomonic for NEC, though its presence ranges between 13 and 100 % of cases, depending on the study examined. Ultrasound has proven superior in the early diagnosis of PI. In a study of 40 neonates with Bell stage I NEC, ultrasound located PI in all 40, despite the lack of such findings on abdominal radiographs, demonstrating the value of ultrasound in making an early, definitive diagnosis [29]. However, for patients in ≥Bell stage II NEC, abdominal radiographs have been shown, in some studies, to be superior in identifying pneumatosis. Given this variation, more studies are needed to clarify the role of ultrasound in diagnosing PI in neonates with NEC.

The protocol for ultrasound of the abdomen for NEC has been well described by Faingold et al. [30] and includes evaluation of the intestine for increased wall echogenicity, wall thickening (greater than 2.7 mm) suggestive of edema, wall thinning (less than 1.0 mm) suggestive of ischemia, intramural gas (PI; Fig. 10.13), bowel wall perfusion on color Doppler, and bowel peristalsis. The peritoneal cavity of the abdomen and pelvis is then evaluated for free-fluid or discrete-fluid collections, and the liver and portal venous system are evaluated for portal venous gas (Fig. 10.14). The splanchnic and hepatic circulation should then be assessed via Doppler for flow and perfusion. The sensitivity, specificity,

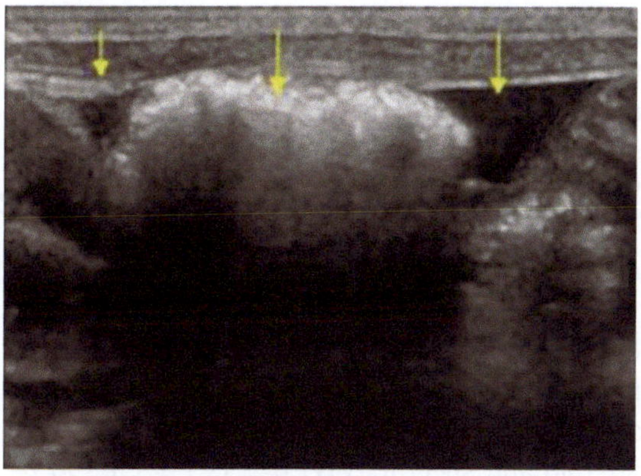

Fig. 10.13 Necrotizing enterocolitis—intramural gas

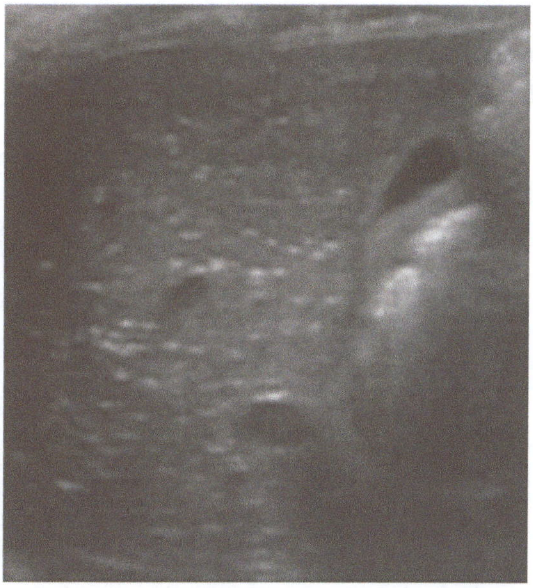

Fig. 10.14 Necrotizing enterocolitis—portal venous gas

positive predictive value, and negative predictive values of sonography for the detection of bowel necrosis were reported to be 100, 95, 80, and 100 %, respectively [31].

Appendicitis

Ultrasound is a reliable tool in the workup of pediatric abdominal pain and diagnosis of acute appendicitis (sensitivity 72.5 % (95 % CI = 58.8–86.3 %) and specificity 97.0 % (95 % CI = 96.2–97.9 %)) [32, 33]. It is now the standard of care in pediatric centers to obtain ultrasound imaging as the first-line modality with selective use of CT scan in some cases. This demonstrates a change in practice that has decreased the burden of ionizing radiation in pediatric patients without an increase in the negative appendectomy or missed appendectomy rates [34, 35].

The sonographic criteria to diagnose acute appendicitis in children include visualizing a blind-ending tubular structure that is noncompressible (Fig. 10.15) and lacks peristalsis, with an appendicular diameter greater than 6 mm and/or a wall thickness greater than 2.0 mm.

Other signs to support the diagnosis of appendicitis include the lack of air in the appendiceal lumen, periappendiceal fat stranding, presence of appendicolith, complex right lower quadrant mass, enlarged mesenteric lymph nodes, and presence of free fluid [36] (Fig. 10.16). Recent evidence suggests that using a cutoff point of 7.0 mm appendicular diameter and 1.7 mm wall thickness [37] may be more predictive of acute appendicitis in pediatric patients.

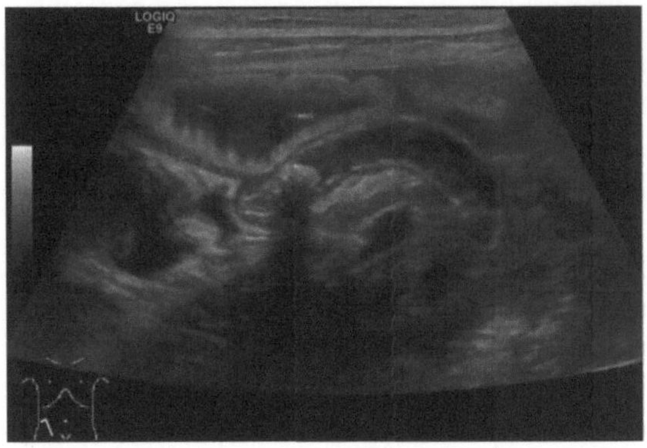

Fig. 10.16 Appendicitis—enlarged tubular blind-ending structure in right lower quadrant with fecalith visible at the base, longitudinal view

Ultrasound is operator dependent and is limited by the lie of the appendix. In up to one third of the cases, the appendix may be nonvisualized on ultrasound imaging with the patient in the traditional supine position. Some protocols recommend turning the patient to left posterior oblique position in an attempt to identify a potentially retrocecal appendix [38]. In the absence of a leukocytosis, patients with a nonvisualized appendix can be safely observed without the immediate need for additional imaging [39].

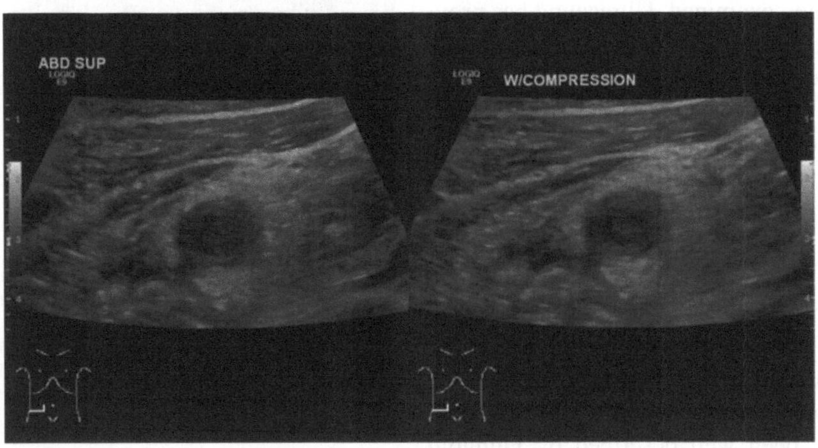

Fig. 10.15 Appendicitis—sagittal view of noncompressible enlarged appendix

Anorectal Malformations

Anorectal malformations are a complex group of congenital anomalies with an incidence of approximately 1:5000 births. The most common presentation in males is imperforate anus (anal atresia) with a rectourethral fistula, and in females imperforate anus with a rectovestibular fistula [39]. Some patients are diagnosed antenatally after visualizing dilated distal bowel or rectum on obstetric ultrasound [40, 41], though the technical difficulty in making that diagnosis means that most patients are identified by physical examination on the first day of life. Ultrasound plays many roles in the care of patients with anorectal malformations, including diagnosis and preoperative planning, intraoperative guidance, and postoperative assessment.

For children with imperforate anus, early diagnosis and clarification of the patient's anatomy is critical in planning the appropriate surgical intervention. The distance from bowel to skin is a determining factor in the type of procedure that is indicated: for a low defect (< 1 cm bowel-skin distance), an anoplasty typically can be done without a colostomy; but for an intermediate or high defect (> 1 cm bowel-skin distance), a decompressive colostomy may be created before posterior sagittal anorectoplasty described by Pena [42]. Both radiographs (invertogram and prone cross-table lateral views) and ultrasound can be utilized to obtain this information. Transperineal ultrasound is feasible and valid for determining bowel-skin distance with sensitivity 100 % and specificity 86 % with an error in distance measurement of 0.12 cm (±0.33) [43, 44] (Fig. 10.17).

Another important consideration in patients with imperforate anus is the location of fistulae to adjacent anatomic structures. Transperineal ultrasound can be utilized to identify the presence of multiple types of fistulae including rectourethral, rectovaginal, rectovestibular, rectovesical, and rectocloacal [45, 46]. Finally, preoperative evaluation is not complete without identification of any associated anomalies that frequently accompany imperforate anus—a thorough evaluation typically includes abdominal, pelvic, and spine ultrasound [46].

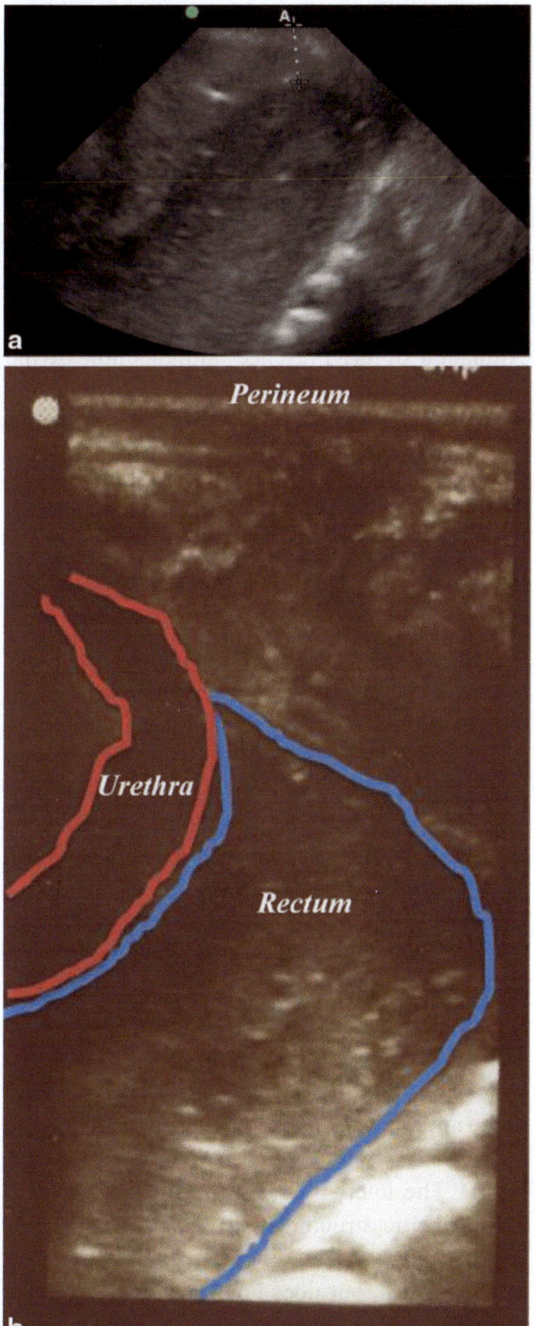

Fig. 10.17 **a** and **b** Imperforate anus—**a** Transperineal ultrasound shows blind-ending rectum of a low imperforate anus without fistula (note the *round shape* of the rectal tip), the ruler measures the bowel-skin distance (*A* = skin); **b** Transperineal ultrasound of a different patient: the position of the *rectum,* the rectourethral fistula and the *urethra* can be clearly differentiated. To aid identification of the *urethra,* placement of a Foley catheter is helpful

Laparoscopy-assisted sagittal anorectoplasty with intraoperative ultrasound is an alternative to the traditional open procedure in some centers. A transperineal ultrasound probe in addition to electrical stimulation of the anal sphincter complex is applied to aid in identification of anatomic structures and creation of the pull through canal [47, 48].

Endoanal ultrasound may also be useful following repair of anorectal malformations. An evaluation of the presence and function of the internal and external anal sphincters can guide therapy such as feedback training for symptoms like constipation or incontinence with the goal of improving quality of life [49].

Hirschsprung's Disease

Hirschsprung's disease (HD; incidence 1:5000) is the congenital absence of ganglion cells in the myenteric and submucosal plexuses of the intestine. In over 80% of the cases, the affected location is the rectum or rectosigmoid. The diagnostic pathway at present includes either a contrast enema or anorectal manometry followed by confirmation with tissue biopsy [50]. Abdominal ultrasound is not a first-line test in HD but, if utilized, will show massively dilated colon, possibly filled with meconium, and a contracted and empty rectum [51]. Orno and colleagues validated the use of ultrasound in visualizing the rectoanal inhibitory reflex, the reflex relaxation of the internal anal sphincter caused by distention of the normally innervated rectum that is absent in HD. The internal anal sphincter is viewed as a hypoechoic structure that decreases in diameter and allows passage of injected contents in a reactive test, but does not contract or result in movement of rectal contents in an inconclusive or nonreactive test [52].

Peritoneal Fluid

Ultrasound can detect as little as 5–10 mL of fluid within the abdominal cavity. The differential diagnosis for intraperitoneal fluid is vast;

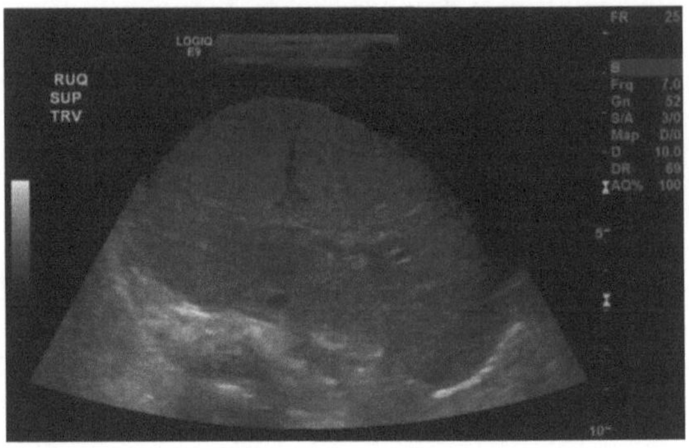

Fig. 10.18 Ascites—anechoic, mobile fluid overlying the liver

sonographic characteristics of the fluid, such as wall structure, contour, and echogenicity, can aid in determining the underlying etiology [53]. A fluid collection may be anechoic (acute hemorrhage, ascites; Fig. 10.18), hypoechoic (old hematoma, bile, and pus; Fig. 10.19), or hyperechoic (air). A collection may be fixed (mass) or mobile (fluid), well circumscribed or poorly defined [54] (Fig. 10.20). Abdominal ultrasound is capable of providing an accurate depiction of peritoneal fluid which can greatly impact the management of the pediatric patient.

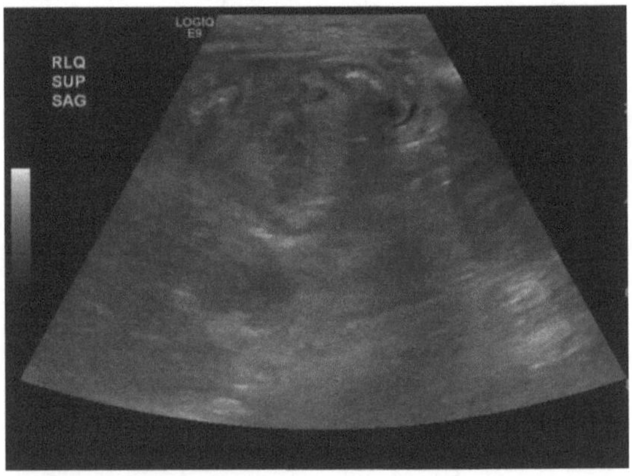

Fig. 10.19 Organized hematoma—large, irregular, complex fluid collection in the pelvis displacing loops of intestine

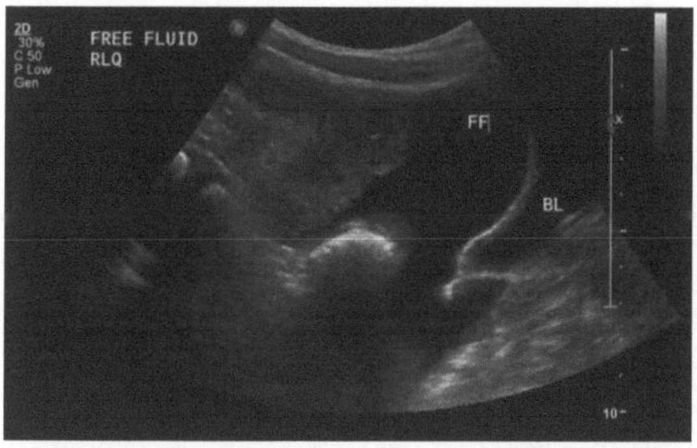

Fig. 10.20 Free fluid—anechoic, mobile, ill-defined pelvic fluid adjacent to bladder, associated with acute appendicitis

Abscess

Ultrasound is useful in both the diagnosis and management of abdominal and pelvic abscesses. The etiology is attributed to the introduction of enteric microorganisms into the peritoneal compartment. This may occur from perforated appendicitis, inflammatory bowel disease (IBD), and NEC, or ischemic enteritis; it may also occur after direct contamination from surgery or trauma. Mixed aerobic and anaerobic flora are typically found within the abscess [55].

Walled-off fluid collections can be localized by scanning the subhepatic, subdiaphragmatic, pelvic, and interloop locations. Diagnosis is made through the identification of a hypoechoic mass with irregular contour or an extraluminal air fluid level, with or without a localized ileus (Fig. 10.21). Ultrasound in the diagnosis of abscess is sensitive but not very specific, meaning that it is difficult to exclude abscess with ultrasound alone.

Traditional ultrasound can be used to guide transabdominal percutaneous drainage of these abscesses with published success rates of anywhere from 33 to 100% depending on abscess location and etiology [55]. Transrectal ultrasound can also be used for localization and drainage of deep pelvic abscesses. Transrectal aspiration and/or drain placement can be accomplished with high success rates and low incidence of complication [56].

Inflammatory Bowel Disease

Crohn's disease (annual incidence 1–8.5:100,000) and ulcerative colitis (annual incidence 1–4.3:100,000) are common GI pathologies in pediatric patients. Diagnosis can be delayed due to the nonspecific nature of patient complaints and often relies on a variety of imaging studies as well as endoscopy, tissue biopsy, and laboratory testing [57]. The low cost, lack of radiation, and high-negative predictive value make abdominal ultrasound an important initial imaging modality in the workup of suspected IBD. It can also be

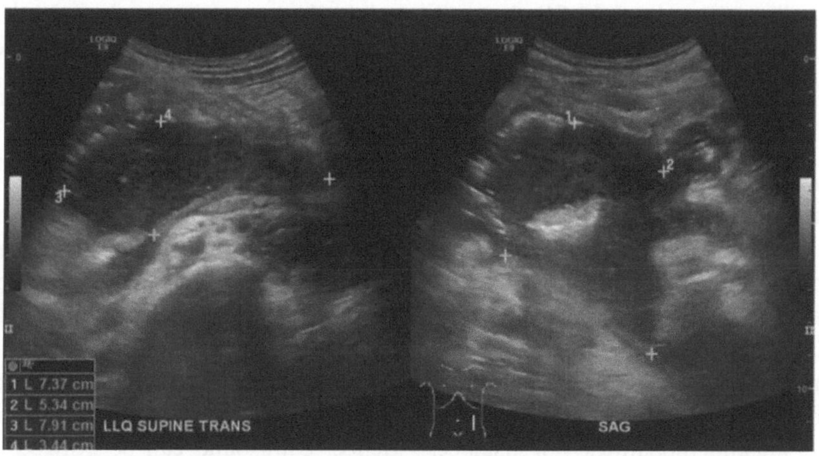

Fig. 10.21 Abscess—17-year-old female patient who presented with ruptured appendicitis, ultrasound demonstrated an irregular, localized, hypoechoic fluid collections in the pelvis and left lower quadrant (pictured)

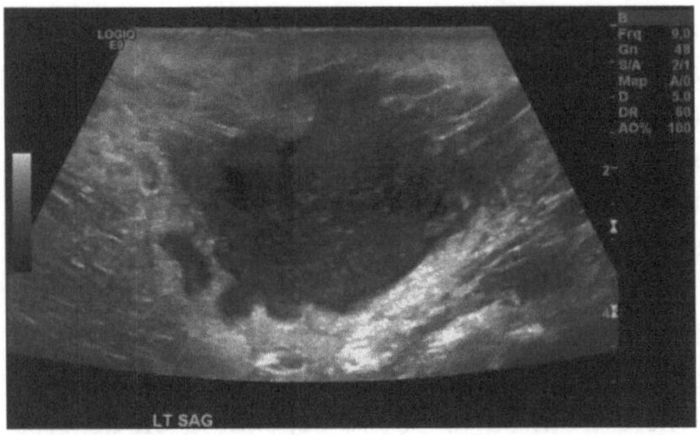

Fig. 10.22 Perianal abscess—Transrectal ultrasound demonstrates a perianal, heterogeneous, localized fluid collection measuring 6.3 × 3.3 × 5.9 cm that is surrounded by hyperemia

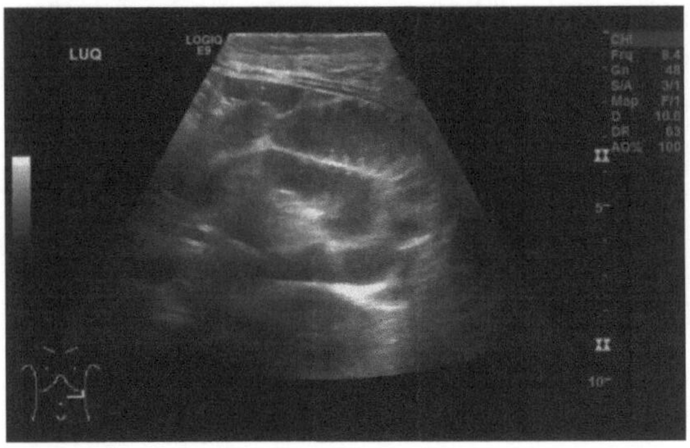

Fig. 10.23 Nonspecific finding of mildly dilated, thickened loops of small bowel

used to surveil patients who carry a diagnosis of IBD for active inflammation and complications like abscess or stricture [58] (Fig. 10.22). Accuracy for diagnosing the number and site of small bowel lesions is enhanced when oral contrast is given [59]. Importantly, limitations to the use of ultrasound in IBD include the fact that many findings are nonspecific, the intestine cannot be assessed over its entire length, and the quality of the images and interpretation are operator dependent [57].

Other Diseases

Ultrasound may also demonstrate nonspecific findings including dilated, fluid-filled loops of intestine, wall thickening or hyperemia (Fig. 10.23). These findings are seen across a range of pathology and may indicate infectious or inflammatory enteritis, partial obstruction, or other issue. Imaging in this case is not diagnostic but can help to guide the clinician in conjunction with the clinical history, laboratory testing, and physical examination.

Abdominal ultrasound is a common first-line test for pediatric patients presenting with general abdominal pain, and consequently may identify unusual pathology that is more commonly associated with other imaging modalities. For instance, a patient with Henoch–Schönlein purpura who presented with hematochezia was found to have severe bowel-wall thickening throughout the abdomen, consistent with intramural hemorrhage (Fig. 10.24a and b). A bezoar can be detected as an intraluminal mass with a hyperechoic curved surface and an acoustic shadow [60]. In developing regions where certain infectious etiologies are more common and in patients who offer a history of travel to such locations, the differential must include parasitic and tuberculin disease. Intestinal ascariasis may be diagnosed after visualizing echogenic structures within the lumen at multiple locations, arranged in a thin line or coil [61]. Intestinal tuberculosis may appear as bowel-wall thickening with intramural abscesses, with or without fistula; there may also be evidence of mesenteric thickening accompanied by enlarged mesenteric lymph nodes [62]. Hydatid cysts, commonly located in the abdomen or the liver, show a typical ultrasound appearance.

Summary

Abdominal ultrasound is a popular modality for the screening and diagnosis of GI pathology in pediatric patients. There is a steep learning curve for the operator given the challenges of imaging the dynamic and variable intestine; however, proficiency can be achieved with training and experience. Ultrasound can be utilized to identify a broad spectrum of pathology.

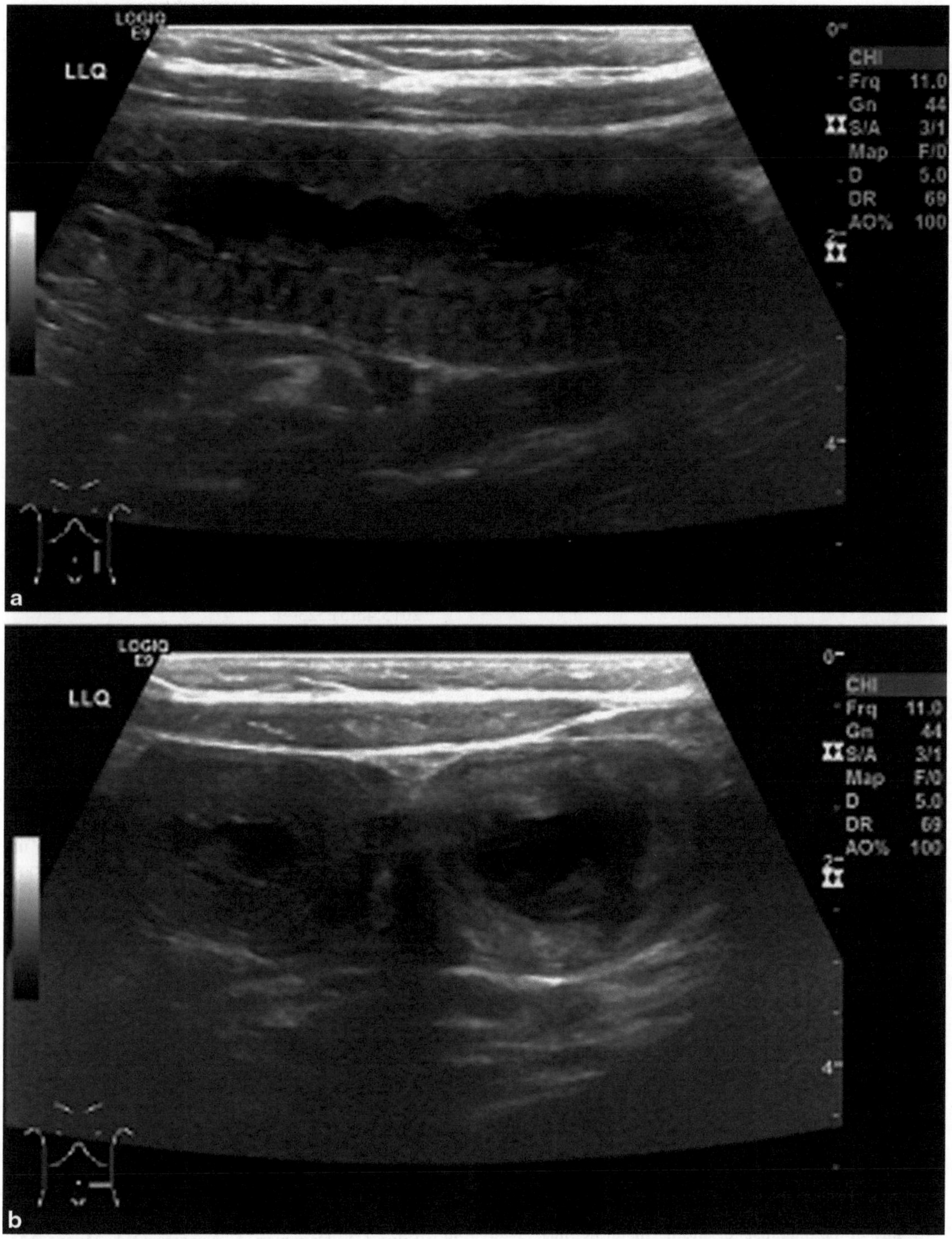

Fig. 10.24 **a** and **b** Henoch–Schoenlein purpura—extreme wall thickening consistent with intramural hemorrhage

References

1. Copeland DR, Cosper GH, McMahon LE, Boneti C, Little DC, Dassinger MS, et al. Return of the surgeon in the diagnosis of pyloric stenosis. J Pediatr Surg. 2009;44(6):1189–92. discussion 92.
2. McVay MR, Copeland DR, McMahon LE, Cosper GH, McCallie TG, Kokoska ER, et al. Surgeon-performed ultrasound for diagnosis of pyloric stenosis is accurate, reproducible, and clinically valuable. J Pediatr Surg. 2009;44(1):169–71. discussion 71–2.
3. Esposito F, Lombardi R, Grasso AC, Dolezalova H, Sodano A, Tarantino L, et al. Transabdominal sonography of the normal gastroesophageal junction in children. J Clin Ultrasound. 2001;29(6):326–31.
4. Milocco C, Salvatore CM, Torre G, Guastalla P, Ventura A. Sonography versus continuous 24 h oesophageal pH-monitoring in the diagnosis of infant gastroesophageal reflux. La Pediatr Med Chir Med Surg Pediatr. 1997;19(4):245–6.
5. Matrunola M, Grandin A, Mazza ML, Panetta A, Giardini V, Corrado G. Role of radiography and ultrasonography in the diagnosis of the pediatric gastro-esophageal reflux disease. Eur Rev Med Pharmacol Sci. 2003;7(5):147–9.
6. Vandenplas Y, Rudolph CD, Lorenzo C D, Hassall E, Liptak G, Mazur L, et al. Pediatric gastroesophageal reflux clinical practice guidelines: joint recommendations of the North American society for pediatric gastroenterology, hepatology, and nutrition (NASPGHAN) and the European society for pediatric gastroenterology, hepatology, and nutrition (ESPGHAN). J Pediatr Gastroenterol Nutr. 2009;49(4):498–547.
7. Westra SJ, Wolf BH, Staalman CR. Ultrasound diagnosis of gastroesophageal reflux and hiatal hernia in infants and young children. J Clin Ultrasound. 1990;18(6):477–85.
8. Savino A, Cecamore C, Matronola MF, Verrotti A, Mohn A, Chiarelli F, et al. US in the diagnosis of gastroesophageal reflux in children. Pediatr Radiol. 2012;42(5):515–24.
9. Gomes H, Lallemand A, Lallemand P. Ultrasound of the gastroesophageal junction. Pediatr Radiol. 1993;23(2):94–9.
10. Koumanidou C, Vakaki M, Pitsoulakis G, Anagnostara A, Mirilas P. Sonographic measurement of the abdominal esophagus length in infancy: a diagnostic tool for gastroesophageal reflux. AJR Am J Roentgenol. 2004;183(3):801–7.
11. Cakmakci E, Celebi I, Tahtabasi M, Tabakci ON, Ozkurt H, Basak M, et al. Accuracy of ultrasonography in the diagnosis of sliding hiatal hernias. Acad Radiol. 2013;20(4):453–6.
12. Krogh C, Fischer TK, Skotte L, Biggar RJ, Oyen N, Skytthe A, et al. Familial aggregation and heritability of pyloric stenosis. JAMA. 2010;303(23):2393–9.
13. Ranells JD, Carver JD, Kirby RS. Infantile hypertrophic pyloric stenosis: epidemiology, genetics, and clinical update. Adv Pediatr. 2011;58(1):195–206.
14. Hernanz-Schulman M. Infantile hypertrophic pyloric stenosis. Radiology. 2003;227(2):319–31.
15. Dassinger MS, Smith SD. Malrotation. In: Holcomb G, Murphy JP, Ostlie DJ, editors. Ashcraft's pediatric surgery. 6th ed. Philadelphia: Elsevier; 2014.
16. Patino MO, Munden MM. Utility of the sonographic whirlpool sign in diagnosing midgut volvulus in patients with atypical clinical presentations. J Ultrasound Med Off J Am Inst Ultrasound Med. 2004;23(3):397–401.
17. Yousefzadeh DK, Kang L, Tessicini L. Assessment of retromesenteric position of the third portion of the duodenum: an US feasibility study in 33 newborns. Pediatr Radiol. 2010;40(9):1476–84.
18. Intussusception MACFM. In: Holcomb G, Murphy JP, Ostlie DJ, editors. Ashcraft's pediatric surgery. Philadelphia: Elsevier; 2014. p. 531–8.
19. Wang GD, Liu SJ. Enema reduction of intussusception by hydrostatic pressure under ultrasound guidance: a report of 377 cases. J Pediatr Surg. 1988;23(9):814–8.
20. Virgone C, D'Antonio F, Khalil A, Jonh R, Manzoli L, Giuliani S. Accuracy of prenatal ultrasound in detecting jejunal and ileal atresia: systematic review and meta-analysis. Ultrasound Obstet Gynecol: Off J Int Soc Ultrasound Obstet Gynecol. 2015;45(5):523–9.
21. Aguayo P, Ostlie DJ. Duodenal and intestinal atresia and stenosis. In: Holcomb G, Murphy JP, Ostlie DJ, editors. Ashcraft's pediatric surgery. 6th ed. Philadelphia: Elsevier; 2014. p. 414–29.
22. Pepper VK, Stanfill AB, Pearl RH. Diagnosis and management of pediatric appendicitis, intussusception, and Meckel diverticulum. Surg Clin North Am. 2012;92(3):505–26. vii.
23. Gebesce A, Korkmaz M, Keles E, Korkmaz F, Mahmutyazicioglu K, Yazgan H. Importance of the ultrasonography in diagnosis of ileal duplication cyst. Gastroenterol Res Pract. 2013;2013:248625.
24. Pampal A, Yagmurlu A. Successful laparoscopic removal of mesenteric and omental cysts in toddlers: 3 cases with a literature review. J Pediatr Surg. 2012;47(8):e5–e8.
25. Konen O, Rathaus V, Dlugy E, Freud E, Kessler A, Shapiro M, et al. Childhood abdominal cystic lymphangioma. Pediatr Radiol. 2002;32(2):88–94.
26. Bliss DP Jr, Coffin CM, Bower RJ, Stockmann PT, Ternberg JL. Mesenteric cysts in children. Surgery. 1994;115(5):571–7.
27. Dominguez K, Moss RL. Necrotizing enterocolitis. In: Holcomb G, Murphy JP, Ostlie DJ, editors. Ashcraft's pediatric surgery. 6th ed. Philadelphia: Elsevier; 2014. p. 454–73.
28. Silva CT, Daneman A, Navarro OM, Moore AM, Moineddin R, Gerstle JT, et al. Correlation of sonographic findings and outcome in necrotizing enterocolitis. Pediatr Radiol. 2007;37(3):274–82.
29. Kim WY, Kim WS, Kim IO, Kwon TH, Chang W, Lee EK. Sonographic evaluation of neonates with early-stage necrotizing enterocolitis. Pediatr Radiol. 2005;35(11):1056–61.

30. Faingold R, Daneman A, Tomlinson G, Babyn PS, Manson DE, Mohanta A, et al. Necrotizing enterocolitis: assessment of bowel viability with color Doppler US. Radiology. 2005;235(2):587–94.
31. Yikilmaz A, Hall NJ, Daneman A, Gerstle JT, Navarro OM, Moineddin R, et al. Prospective evaluation of the impact of sonography on the management and surgical intervention of neonates with necrotizing enterocolitis. Pediatr Surg Int. 2014;30(12):1231–40.
32. Mittal MK, Dayan PS, Macias CG, Bachur RG, Bennett J, Dudley NC, et al. Performance of ultrasound in the diagnosis of appendicitis in children in a multicenter cohort. Acad Emerg Med. 2013;20(7):697–702.
33. Rubin SZ, Martin DJ. Ultrasonography in the management of possible appendicitis in childhood. J Pediatr Surg. 1990;25(7):737–40.
34. Russell WS, Schuh AM, Hill JG, Hebra A, Cina RA, Smith CD, et al. Clinical practice guidelines for pediatric appendicitis evaluation can decrease computed tomography utilization while maintaining diagnostic accuracy. Pediatr Emerg Care. 2013;29(5):568–73.
35. Thirumoorthi AS, Fefferman NR, Ginsburg HB, Kuenzler KA, Tomita SS. Managing radiation exposure in children–reexamining the role of ultrasound in the diagnosis of appendicitis. J Pediatr Surg. 2012;47(12):2268–72.
36. Prendergast PM, Poonai N, Lynch T, McKillop S, Lim R. Acute appendicitis: investigating an optimal outer appendiceal diameter cut-point in a pediatric population. J Emerg Med. 2014;46(2):157–64.
37. Goldin AB, Khanna P, Thapa M, McBroom JA, Garrison MM, Parisi MT. Revised ultrasound criteria for appendicitis in children improve diagnostic accuracy. Pediatr Radiol. 2011;41(8):993–9.
38. Chang ST, Jeffrey RB, Olcott EW. Three-step sequential positioning algorithm during sonographic evaluation for appendicitis increases appendiceal visualization rate and reduces CT use. AJR Am J Roentgenol. 2014;203(5):1006–12.
39. Cohen B, Bowling J, Midulla P, Shlasko E, Lester N, Rosenberg H, et al. The non-diagnostic ultrasound in appendicitis: is a non-visualized appendix the same as a negative study? J Pediatr Surg. 2015;50(6):923–7.
40. Vijayaraghavan SB, Prema AS, Suganyadevi P. Sonographic depiction of the fetal anus and its utility in the diagnosis of anorectal malformations. J Ultrasound Med Off J Am Inst Ultrasound Med. 2011;30(1):37–45.
41. Taipale P, Rovamo L, Hiilesmaa V. First-trimester diagnosis of imperforate anus. Ultrasound Obstet Gynecol. 2005;25(2):187–8.
42. Pena A. Management of anorectal malformations during the newborn period. World J Surg. 1993;17(3):385–92.
43. Niedzielski JK. Invertography versus ultrasonography and distal colostography for the determination of bowel-skin distance in children with anorectal malformations. Eur J Pediatr Surg: Off J Austrian Assoc Pediatr Surg. = Z Kinderchir. 2005;15(4):262–7.
44. Haber HP, Seitz G, Warmann SW, Fuchs J. Transperineal sonography for determination of the type of imperforate anus. AJR Am J Roentgenolog. 2007;189(6):1525–9.
45. Kim IO, Han TI, Kim WS, Yeon KM. Transperineal ultrasonography in imperforate anus: identification of the internal fistula. J Ultrasound Med: Off J Am Inst Ultrasound Med. 2000;19(3):211–6.
46. Levitt M, Peña A. Imperforate anus and cloacal malformations. In: Holcomb GWMJ, Ostlie DJ, editors. Ashcraft's pediatric surgery. 6th ed. Philadelphia: Elsevier; 2014. p. 492–514.
47. Kubota A, Kawahara H, Okuyama H, Oue T, Tazuke Y, Tanaka N, et al. Laparoscopically assisted anorectoplasty using perineal ultrasonographic guide: a preliminary report. J Pediatr Surg. 2005;40(10):1535–8.
48. Yamataka A, Yoshida R, Kobayashi H, Lane GJ, Kurosaki Y, Segawa O, et al. Intraoperative endosonography enhances laparoscopy-assisted colon pull-through for high imperforate anus. J Pediatr Surg. 2002;37(12):1657–60.
49. Caldaro T, Romeo E, De Angelis P, Gambitta RA, Rea F, Torroni F, et al. Three-dimensional endoanal ultrasound and anorectal manometry in children with anorectal malformations: new discoveries. J Pediatr Surg. 2012;47(5):956–63.
50. Langer JC. Hirschsprung disease. In: Holcomb G, Murphy JP, Ostlie DJ, editors. Ashcraft's pediatric surgery. 6th ed. Philadelphia: Elsevier; 2014. p. 474–91.
51. Chavhan GB, Babyn PS, Cohen RA, Langer JC. Multimodality imaging of the pediatric diaphragm: anatomy and pathologic conditions. Radiographics. 2010;30(7):1797–817.
52. Orno AK, Lovkvist H, Marsal K, von Steyern KV, Arnbjornsson E. Sonographic visualization of the rectoanal inhibitory reflex in children suspected of having Hirschsprung disease: a pilot study. J Ultrasound Med Off J Am Inst Ultrasound Med. 2008;27(8):1165–9.
53. Doust BD, Quiroz F, Stewart JM. Ultrasonic distinction of abscesses from other intra-abdominal fluid collections. Radiology. 1977;125(1):213–8.
54. Schmidt WOSG, Kurjak A. Differential diagnosis in ultrasound: a teaching atlas. Stuttgart Thieme; 2005.
55. Brook I. Intra-abdominal, retroperitoneal, and visceral abscesses in children. Eur J Pediatr Surg: Off J Austrian Assoc Pediatr Surg [et al] = Z Kinderchir. 2004;14(4):265–73.
56. Koral K, Derinkuyu B, Gargan L, Lagomarsino EM, Murphy JT. Transrectal ultrasound and fluoroscopy-guided drainage of deep pelvic collections in children. J Pediatr Surg. 2010;45(3):513–8.
57. Chiorean L, Schreiber-Dietrich D, Braden B, Cui XW, Buchhorn R, Chang JM, et al. Ultrasonographic imaging of inflammatory bowel disease in pediatric

patients. World J Gastroenterol. 2015;21(17):5231–41.

58. Nylund K, Hausken T, Gilja OH. Ultrasound and inflammatory bowel disease. Ultrasound Q. 2010;26(1):3–15.
59. Pallotta N, Civitelli F, Nardo G D, Vincoli G, Aloi M, Viola F, et al. Small intestine contrast ultrasonography in pediatric Crohn's disease. J Pediatr. 2013;163(3):778–84. e1.
60. Ripolles T, Garcia-Aguayo J, Martinez MJ, Gil P. Gastrointestinal bezoars: sonographic and CT characteristics. AJR Am J Roentgenol. 2001;177(1):65–9.
61. Ghonge NP. Gastric migration of intestinal ascariasis: B-mode sonographic depiction. J Ultrasound Med: Off J Am Inst Ultrasound Med. 2008;27(12):1799–801.
62. Barreiros AP, Braden B, Schieferstein-Knauer C, Ignee A, Dietrich CF. Characteristics of intestinal tuberculosis in ultrasonographic techniques. Scand J Gastroenterol. 2008;43(10):1224–31.

Intra-abdominal and Retroperitoneal Masses

11

Kevin M. Riggle and Kenneth W. Gow

Introduction

Abdominal and retroperitoneal masses in children and adolescents present the clinician with diagnostic and therapeutic challenges. Because of the number of different structures in the abdomen, the differential diagnosis is quite broad. Further, the management of these lesions may involve biopsy, drainage, or resection of the mass. For all of these reasons, ultrasound may serve as a valuable diagnostic and therapeutic tool for the surgeon.

Diagnosis

The most common entities in early childhood arise from the retroperitoneum. As children age, the lesions trend towards intra-abdominal. Ultrasound is often used as the initial study for pediatric abdominal masses and will, in most instances, at least narrow the differential diagnosis. Ultrasound is advantageous for this purpose as it is widely available, noninvasive, and provides information without the use of ionizing radiation. Important aspects of the ultrasound examination include identifying the location of the lesion—whether it is located in the abdomen, retroperitoneum, or the pelvis. This, along with the patient's age, will guide the focus to the most likely organ of origin. Echogenicity and vascularity of the mass can further differentiate between solid and cystic masses. Also, continuity with adjacent abdominal organs or mass effect on adjacent vasculature may aid in determining the origin of the abdominal mass. Further information can be gained by examining for vascular invasion, adjacent solid organ involvement, lymphadenopathy, or vessel thrombosis.

After examining the sonographic characteristics of the mass and adding that information to the sex, age, and location of the mass, a narrow list of differential diagnoses can be made. We will now examine the imaging characteristics of cystic and solid abdominal and retroperitoneal masses, subcategorized by organ or origin and age at diagnosis to aid in the creation of a diagnostic algorithm.

Cystic Masses

Retroperitoneal

Kidney

Up to two third of abdominal masses in the neonate are renal in origin, with hydronephrosis and

K. W. Gow (✉)
Department of General and Thoracic Surgery, Seattle Children's Hospital, 4800 Sand Point Way NE, Seattle, WA 98105, USA
e-mail: Kenneth.gow@seattlechildrens.org

K. M. Riggle
Department of Surgery, University of Washington, 1959 NE Pacific Street, Box 356410, Seattle, WA 98195, USA
e-mail: rigglk@uw.edu

S. Scholz, M. D. Jarboe (eds.), *Diagnostic and Interventional Ultrasound in Pediatrics and Pediatric Surgery,* DOI 10.1007/978-3-319-21699-7_11

simple cysts accounting for most of the benign masses [4]. Common causes of hydronephrosis in the neonate are ureteropelvic obstruction, vesicoureteral reflux, posterior urethral valves, or ureterovesicular junction obstruction. A detailed discussion of these is beyond the scope of this chapter, but should be accounted for when evaluating cystic renal masses. Cystic masses in the neonate can also be caused by multicystic dysplastic kidney (MCDK), autosomal recessive polycystic kidney disease (ARPKD), and congenital mesoblastic nephroma (CMN), which we will discuss further.

Multicystic Dysplastic Kidney

Most renal cysts detected in childhood are secondary to congenital cystic diseases of the kidney. MCDK is the most likely cystic disease to present as a palpable abdominal mass in childhood [20]. Sonographic examination will show multiple, noncommunicating anechoic structures of varying sizes. In general, no ureter or collecting system will be seen in the involved kidney. In fact, no discernible normal renal parenchyma is typically visualized. Further evaluation with renal scintigraphy would show a nonfunctioning kidney. Continued follow-up ultrasound will show eventual involution of the involved kidney.

Autosomal Recessive Polycystic Kidney Disease

ARPKD usually presents with bilateral enlarged kidneys, detected on prenatal ultrasound. Renal enlargement is secondary to hyperplasia of the remaining collecting tubules. Sonographic appearance is variable, but typically demonstrates bilaterally enlarged, echogenic kidneys with multiple anechoic spaces and poor corticomedullary differentiation caused by dilated collecting ducts [21]. This pathology, i.e., numerous tiny cysts that are smaller than the sonographic resolution, results in multiple acoustic interfaces of the ultrasound beam, and hence, hyperechogenicity.

Abdominal

Liver

Mesenchymal Hamartoma

Mesenchymal hamartomas are benign hepatic tumors that typically present as a palpable abdominal mass between birth and 10 years of age, most often occurring between 15 and 20 months [7]. These tumors arise from the mesenchyme of the periportal tracts, and thus have cystic and stromal architecture. Sonography demonstrates an anechoic, cystic structure with interspersed solid, echogenic septations representing the stromal component.

Biliary/Gallbladder

Choledocal Cyst

Choledocal cyst (CC) refers to dilation of the common bile duct (CBD), the intrahepatic bile ducts, or both. It is believed to be secondary to an abnormal junction of the pancreatic duct with the CBD, resulting in reflux of pancreatic enzymes into the CBD followed by chemical cholangitis and dilation of the ducts [5]. Congenital CCs are classified based on the location and type of dilation. Most patients with CC present in the first decade of life, and the “classic” triad of episodic abdominal pain, jaundice, and right upper quadrant mass is present in only one fourth of patients. Ultrasound evaluation will show dilation of either the extrahepatic ducts, intrahepatic ducts, or both, depending on type of CC [17]. The diagnosis is made by the presence of a cystic structure near the porta hepatis. Visualization of multiple planes on ultrasound is necessary to confirm that the CC is in continuity with the CBD, a requirement for the diagnosis [10]. Further evaluation with magnetic resonance cholangiopancreatography (MRCP) is usually performed prior to surgical therapy.

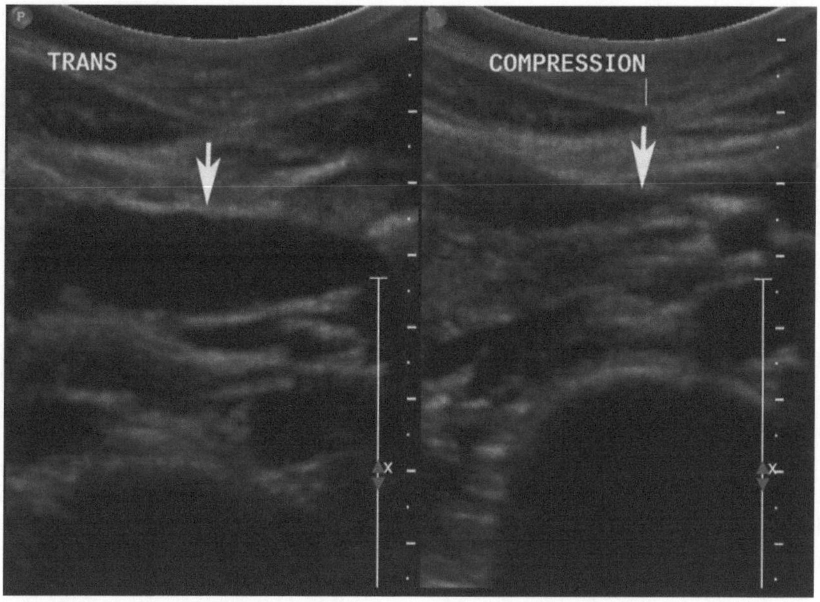

Fig. 11.1 Transabdominal ultrasound of cystic abdominal mass demonstrating an anechoic, irregularly shaped cystic lesion at midline located anterior to the SMA and SMV and inferior to the pancreas. Lesion measured 8 × 3 cm and was compressible (*arrows*). Surgery demonstrated this to be a mesenteric cyst. *SMA* superior mesenteric artery, *SMV* superior mesenteric vein

Bowel

Duplication Cyst

Enteric duplication cysts are rare congenital cysts that may occur anywhere along the gastrointestinal (GI) tract, but are most common in the small intestine. They arise from the mesenteric side of the intestine and range from a few centimeters in length up to the size of the entire bowel [2]. The most common presenting signs and symptoms include a palpable abdominal mass, intestinal obstruction, or hemorrhage. Additionally, they may serve as a lead point for intussusception. Ultrasound examination will show a hypoechoic to anechoic cystic structure. The wall of the cyst may show an echogenic inner mucosal layer and a hypoechoic outer mucosal layer. Layering of debris within the cyst can often be seen. [23]

Lymphangioma

Abdominal lymphangiomas are benign mesenteric (Fig. 11.1) or omental cysts that occur secondary to congenital malformations of the abdominal and/or retroperitoneal lymphatic tissue (Fig. 11.2). They are most commonly found in the mesentery, followed in frequency by the omentum, mesocolon, and retroperitoneum [11]. Ultrasound will demonstrate a thin-walled, hypo- to anechoic structure with posterior acoustic enhancement. They may also have

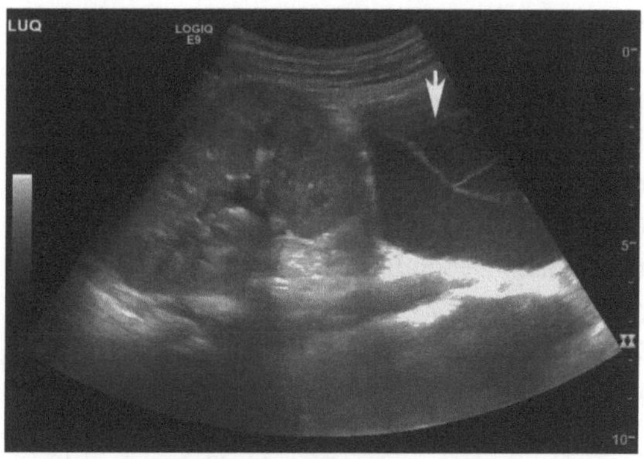

Fig. 11.2 Transabdominal ultrasound of cystic retroperitoneal mass (*arrows*) demonstrating multicompartmental collections filled with fluid adjacent to the kidney. Lesion was noted by CT scan to be consistent with retroperitoneal lymphatic malformation

some internal echoes from debris, hemorrhage, or infection [13]. Usually, a computed tomography (CT) or magnetic resonance imaging (MRI) is necessary to determine involvement of adjacent structures prior to surgical resection [19].

Pseudocyst

A meconium pseudocyst forms secondary to an intestinal perforation during fetal life. The inflammatory reaction from this chemical peritonitis causes the perforation to seal, and the meconium that was released into the peritoneal cavity is walled off into a pseudocyst. Ultrasound examination will demonstrate a cystic mass with heterogeneous echogenicity [3]. There may also be calcifications present, causing shadowing of the cyst, which can sometimes be seen on plain radiographs.

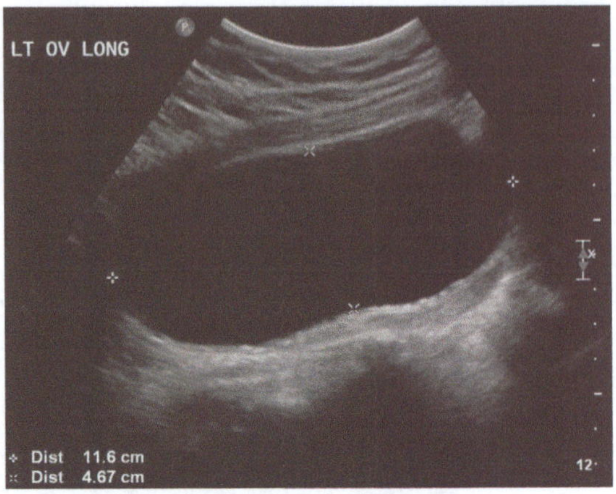

Fig. 11.3 Transabdominal ultrasound of the pelvis demonstrating an anechoic cyst near an ovary measuring 11.6 × 4.7 cm. Laparoscopic examination demonstrated this to be a paratubular cyst, which was excised

Urachal Cyst

Urachal cysts are most frequently seen in infants and young children. They arise when the urachus obliterates at the umbilicus and the bladder, but not in between. Most urachal cysts remain asymptomatic, but some may present as a palpable abdominal mass, an infection of the cyst, or as symptoms from compression of adjacent structures. Ultrasound demonstrates a hypoechoic, thick-walled cystic structure, often just superior to the bladder wall. [18]

Pelvis

Uterus/Ovaries

Ovarian Cysts

Ovarian cysts are common in the neonatal period, likely secondary to in utero hormone exposure [22]. They may be diagnosed on prenatal ultrasound, or present symptomatically with pain, abdominal distension, or fever—usually as a result of torsion or hemorrhage. Sonography of ovarian cysts (Fig. 11.3) usually demonstrates a simple cyst with no internal echoes, and a thin wall. If there has been torsion or hemorrhage, the inner part of the cyst will contain echogenic debris. Doppler ultrasound may differentiate a hemorrhagic cyst from other ovarian neoplasms, as the latter would demonstrate internal flow. Ovarian torsion may be demonstrated by the whirlpool sign, which represents the twisted pedicle of the ovary [14]. Doppler flow to the ovarian parenchyma may be absent (Fig. 11.4) but this absence should not be used to rule out torsion since some studies have demonstrated Doppler flow in up to 50 % of torsed ovaries. Simple cysts that are less than 4 cm and have no solid component may be monitored

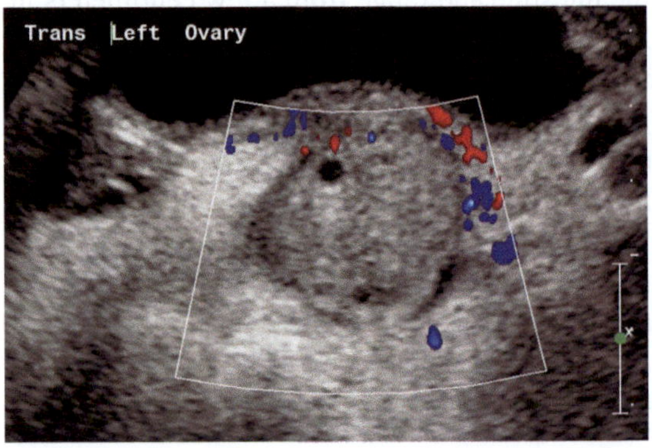

Fig. 11.4 Transabdominal ultrasound of the pelvis demonstrating an enlarged left ovary with small peripherally displaced follicles and heterogenous stromal echogenicity. Ovary measure 3 × 2 × 4 cm. Color and spectral Doppler demonstrated no arterial or venous flow. Laparoscopic detorsion was performed immediately thereafter

with serial ultrasound examinations [16]. Removal of cysts is generally reserved for large, symptomatic, or torsed cysts.

Solid Masses

Retroperitoneal

Kidney

Wilms' Tumor

Wilms' tumor is the most common renal malignancy in childhood. The majority of patients are between 1 and 5 years of age, and present with an asymptomatic abdominal mass. The diagnosis of Wilms' tumor is associated with various conditions, including Beckwith–Weidemann syndrome, sporadic aniridia, Drash syndrome, and hemihypertrophy [8]. In fact, it is recommended that patients with either Beckwith–Weidemann or hemihypertrophy should be screened with an abdominal ultrasound every few months due to their increased risk of Wilms' tumor. Ultrasound examination of Wilms' tumor will reveal an echogenic, solid mass within the kidney that may contain some cystic areas (Fig. 11.5). Increased tumor vascularity will be noted with Doppler sonography.

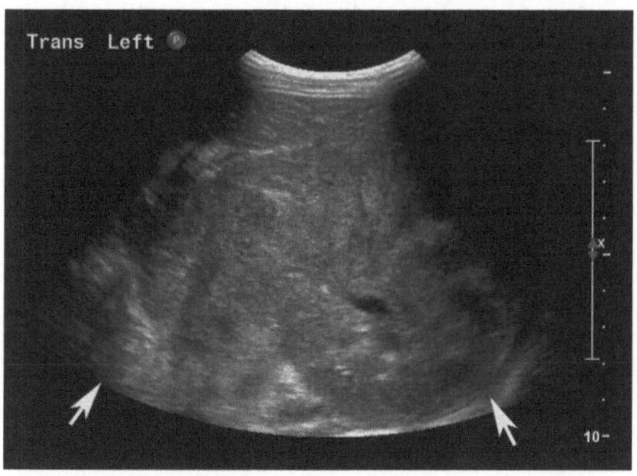

Fig. 11.5 Transabdominal ultrasound of a diffusely enlarged and heterogenous left kidney (*arrows*)

Careful attention should be paid to the extent of tumor involvement in regard to the perinephric space, inferior vena cava (IVC) (Fig. 11.6), and rarely, the right atrium. Peritoneal lymphadenopathy may also be seen. Further staging via a CT scan is recommended following the diagnosis of Wilms' tumor in order to determine tumor rupture, contralateral kidney involvement, and/or lung involvement.

Congenital Mesoblastic Nephroma

CMN is the most common renal neoplasm of infancy, with 85 % of CMNs diagnosed prior to 6 months of age [15]. Presentation is often with a palpable abdominal mass and, occasionally, with a paraneoplastic syndrome such as hypertension or hypercalcemia. Sonography demonstrates a large, solid renal mass with heterogeneous echogenicity. Color Doppler will demonstrate internal flow. Often, there is a central area of necrosis that is hypoechoic in nature. Though this tumor may extend beyond the renal capsule, involvement of the renal vein is uncommon. CMN may be similar in appearance to Wilms' tumor, but is differentiated based on age of presentation given that Wilms' tumor is rarely seen in neonates.

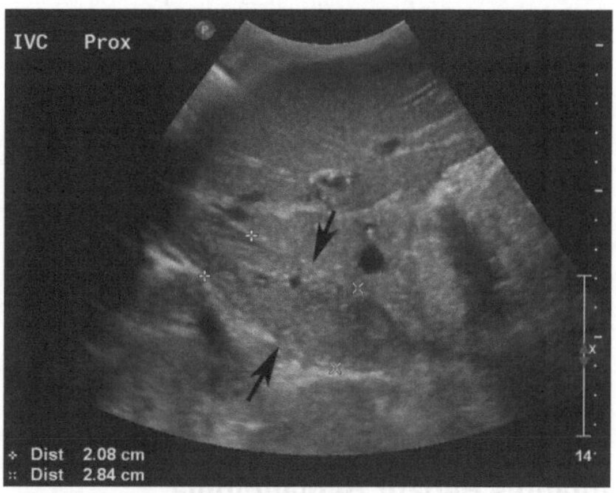

Fig. 11.6 Transabdominal ultrasound of patient with a renal tumor and associated large IVC tumor thrombus (*arrows*). Patient was treated with preoperative chemotherapy and subsequently underwent nephrectomy with tumor thrombectomy

Adrenal Gland

Neuroblastoma

Neuroblastomas are tumors derived from neural crest cells, and have an incidence of 1:10,000 live births in the USA. Advances in prenatal ultrasound have increased the prenatal detection of neuroblastoma. Furthermore, screening ultrasound in early neonates may also reveal adrenal masses, such that 30% of neuroblastomas may be diagnosed in the neonatal period [9]. It was unknown if some of the early detection of these lesions was merely a result of increased sensitivity of the screening ultrasound, and therefore not clinically significant. Indeed, ultrasound screening performed in Japan and Quebec has demonstrated that many of these small lesions will regress spontaneously [12]. Such screening has been discontinued as the lesions detected early were low-staged tumors and the program did not alter the overall survival in the entire cohort. Ultrasound findings of neuroblastoma tend to vary with the stage of the tumor. In lower-stage tumors, ultrasound reveals a homogeneous or slightly heterogeneous solid mass that replaces the adrenal gland. At more advanced stages, this mass tends to have a much more heterogeneous echotexture, increased vascularity, and multiple intralesional calcifications [1]. All patients with neuroblastoma should receive a staging CT and a metaiodobenzylguanidine (MIBG) scan to determine the extent of involvement. Treatment is based on tumor stage, and certain neuroblastomas (4S) may be followed with serial ultrasound or CT to determine regression and need for surgery.

Abdominal

Liver

Infantile Hepatic Hemangioma

Hemangioma is the most common benign liver mass in infants and children, with a peak presentation between 3 and 6 months of age [5]. Presenting signs and symptoms range from a palpable abdominal mass to congestive heart failure and thrombocytopenia as a result of Kasabach–Merritt syndrome. Sonography will demonstrate a complex, solid mass with heterogeneous echotexture (Fig. 11.7) and robust Doppler flow. Infantile hemangiomas typically increase in size until 9–10 months of age, and then slowly involute [6]. Medical therapies for those that do not involute spontaneously include the use of propranolol and corticosteroids. Embolization or surgical removal is reserved for those that do not involute with medical therapy, or for patients with severe complications.

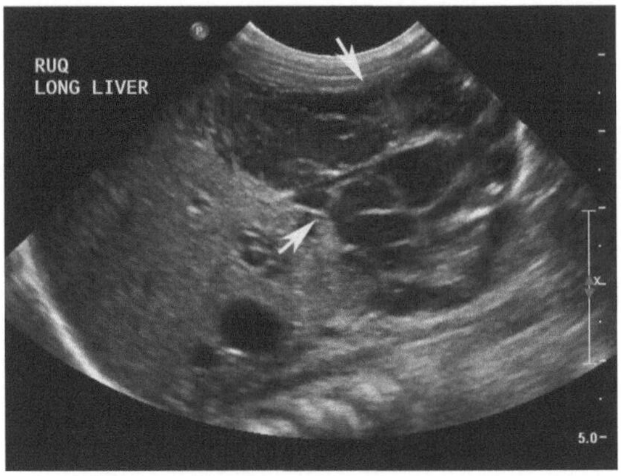

Fig. 11.7 Transabdominal ultrasound of infant with large right hepatic mass with cystic spaces and increased blood flow. Patient also had congestive heart failure. Image and presentation is typical of a large, symptomatic hepatic hemangioma. The child was started on oral propranolol and has had significant improvement in symptoms and resolution of the liver mass

Hepatoblastoma

Malignant tumors comprise the majority of hepatic masses in children, with the most common tumor being hepatoblastoma [5]. Hepatoblastoma typically presents in children between the ages of one and three as a palpable abdominal mass. Initial ultrasound evaluation typically shows a well-defined, heterogeneous tumor often with cystic areas caused by necrosis and calcifications. Use of a high-frequency (>7 MHz) linear transducer will aid in the evaluation of portal and hepatic venous involvement. The tumor may invade the venous system, or cause the formation of an echogenic tumor thrombus within the lumen of the vessels. The intraluminal material may be examined with Doppler sonography, and if there is arterial flow within the intraluminal material, venous invasion by the tumor is likely.

Hepatocellular Carcinoma

Hepatocellular Carcinoma (HCC) is the second most common type of childhood liver tumor, and is more often found in older children (median 10–12 years of age) compared to hepatoblastoma [5]. Ultrasound examination of HCC will demonstrate a hyperechoic, solid mass with a thin, hypoechoic capsule that resembles a halo around the mass. As with hepatoblastoma, evaluation of invasion into portal structures is paramount when evaluating HCC. Unfortunately, only 18–36% of HCCs in children are amenable to complete surgical resection. Often, chemotherapy, embolization, and/or radiofrequency ablation are used to shrink the tumor in hopes of subsequent resection, or as palliative therapy.

Bowel

Lymphoma

Non-Hodgkin's Lymphoma (NHL) often presents in extranodal sites in children. The bowel is the most common extranodal site involved in NHL, up to one third of the time [4]. The presentation may be of a palpable abdominal mass, or the lymphoma may serve as a lead point for intussusception. Because of this, any intussusception in a child older than 5 years must be evaluated for intestinal lymphoma. Sonography will demonstrate a lobular, solid mass within and extending from the bowel wall. There may be circumferential involvement, and often there is internal vascularity on Doppler ultrasound. If intestinal NHL is suspected via ultrasound, a CT must be performed for initial staging.

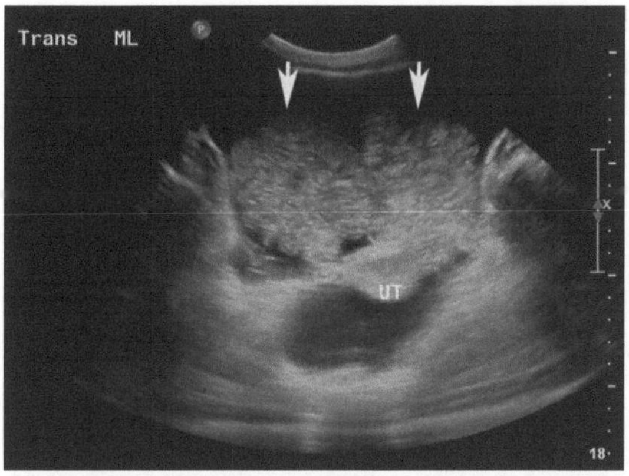

Fig. 11.8 Transabdominal ultrasound demonstrating large soft tissue peritoneal implants in close contiguity to the right ovary. There is a large amount of ascites noted with multiple other peritoneal implants. Resection of these masses followed with histological assessment revealed papillary serous cystadenoma

Rhabdomyosarcoma

Rhabdomyosarcoma is the fourth most common solid tumor of childhood, and the genitourinary (GU) tract is the second most common site for rhabdomyosarcomas, behind the head and neck [9]. Median age at presentation, which is usually that of a palpable abdominal mass, is approximately 7 years. Ultrasound examination can help to identify the tumor as well as to evaluate the other pelvic and abdominal organs to determine the origin of the tumor. The sonographic appearance of rhabdomyosarcomas is variable, but most often is a solid mass with heterogeneous echogenicity. There are frequently hypoechoic areas within the tumor, signifying previous hemorrhage and necrosis.

Pelvic

Ovary

Germ Cell Tumors

Ovarian germ cell tumors account for up to two third of all pediatric ovarian tumors (Figs. 11.8 and 11.9). Similar to simple cysts, they may

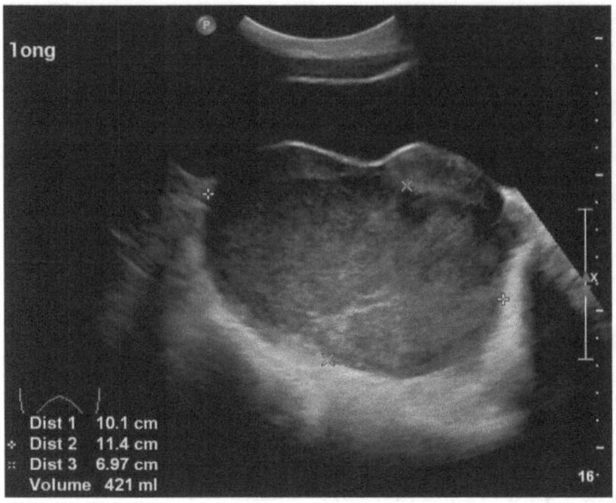

Fig. 11.9 Transabdominal ultrasound demonstrating a large, solid, heterogenous, hypervascular midline pelvic mass posterior to the uterus measuring 10.1 × 11.4 × 7.0 cm. There are multiple echogenic foci within the mass, and the tumor caused anterior displacement of the uterus and posterior wall of the bladder. Mass was resected and histologically determined to be a dysgerminoma of the ovary

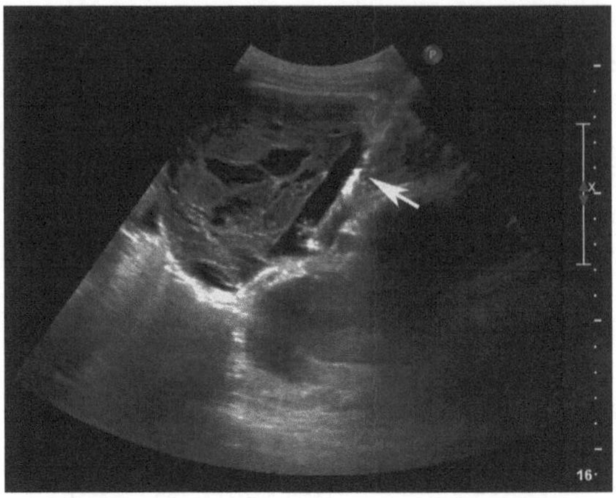

Fig. 11.10 Ultrasound-guided insertion of needle into a retroperitoneal lymphatic malformation. Ultrasound allowed for positioning of the needle, wire, and drain into the largest fluid pocket to provide access for sclerotherapy with doxycycline

present as a palpable abdominal mass, or with signs of ovarian torsion [16]. Ultrasound findings will vary based on the type of germ cell tumor. Teratomas are formed from all three embryonic germ layers, and as such may have complex internal components, i.e., hair, mucus, or calcium deposits. Most commonly, there will be a cystic structure with echogenic foci and variable internal acoustic shadowing. Often, the dermoid mesh sign can be seen, which shows areas of linear hyperechogenicity. Doppler flow is used to determine the location of the involved ovary. Surgical removal is recommended for ovarian germ cell tumors based on the increased risk for ovarian torsion.

Therapeutic

Masses that are either cystic or solid may require ultrasound to help perform drainage, sclerotherapy, or biopsy. Care must be taken to consider the whole picture and involve all interested care providers. Further, ultrasound may be used intraoperatively to help identify vascular structures to aid dissection and resection.

Percutaneous Drainage

Selected lesions, i.e., those that are either difficult to resect or infected and need drainage, will benefit from percutaneous ultrasound-guided drainage. The most common example of this would be perforated appendicitis with associated abscess, where drainage will allow at least partial treatment of the infectious process, and either obviate or alter an urgent need for an elective operation. Also, percutaneous drainage may be considered therapy for lymphatic malformation when used in conjunction with a sclerosant agent (Figs. 11.10 and 11.11).

Biopsy

In situations where it is deemed unwarranted for initial resection of a mass (due to large size, adjacent or involving other structures, or metastasis), a biopsy is often undertaken to obtain tissue for diagnostic purposes. In these scenarios, ultrasound guidance is often helpful whether it be by transabdominal, open, or laparoscopic means. Biopsy may be performed with a Tru-cut (core) biopsy needle, whereby the ultrasound is

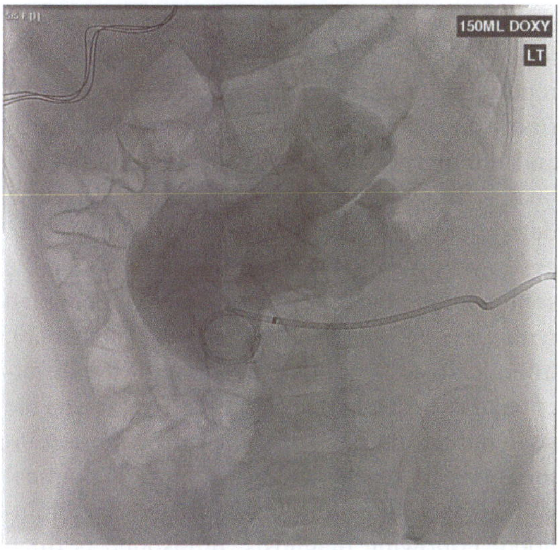

Fig. 11.11 Fluoroscopic image of the pigtail retroperitoneal drainage with contrast within the retroperitoneal lymphatic malforamation

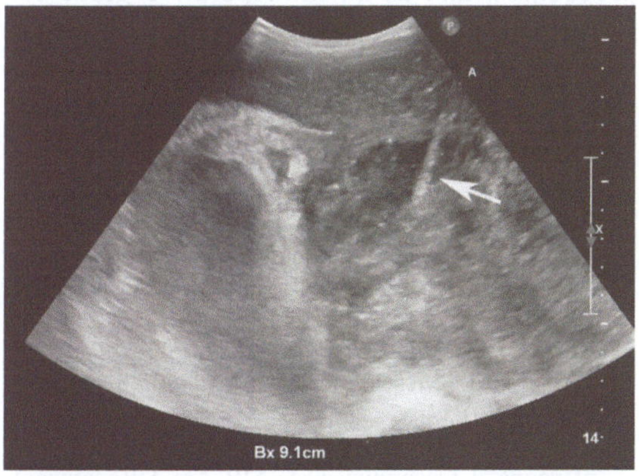

Fig. 11.12 Transabdominal ultrasound-guided liver biopsy with Tru-cut core needle (*arrow*)

used to identify and then follow the passage of the needle (Fig. 11.12). Doppler may be useful in order to identify and avoid vascular structures to minimize bleeding from the biopsy procedure. Prior to biopsy, the clinical team must always consider a working diagnosis, as a biopsy is not recommended in all clinical situations and may result in an upstaging of the tumor (e.g., Wilms' tumor).

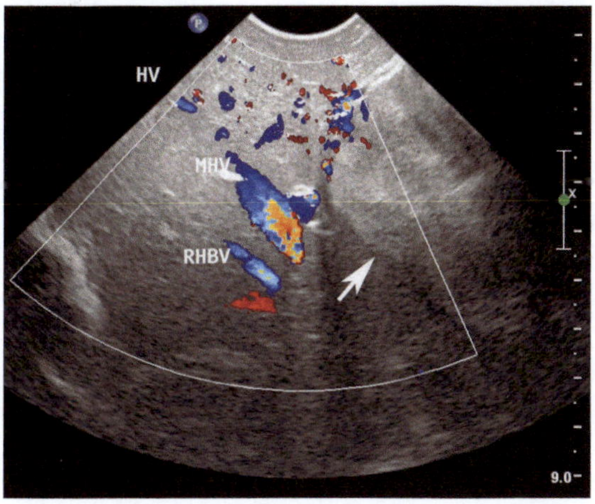

Fig. 11.13 Intraoperative cavitary ultrasound demonstrating hepatic mass adjacent to the hepatic veins. Mass is identified by the *arrow*. *MHV* middle hepatic vein, *RHV* right hepatic vein

Intraoperative Guide

Surgical resection requires the operator to be able to identify what should and should not be resected. While preoperative imaging is extremely helpful in most instances, the operator sometimes requires real-time imaging to guide the surgical resection. The added benefit of using ultrasound as a real-time imaging modality is clear: tools are commonplace, radiation is avoided, Doppler ultrasound can identify vessels, and the study can be easily repeated if needed. Examples of clinical scenarios in which ultrasound may be beneficial include:

- Identification of vascular anatomy in liver resections—in situations in which the tumor is adjacent to hepatic or portal veins (Figs. 11.13 and 11.14), the use of ultrasound has been key to determining the extent of resection, often leading to the conversion of what might otherwise be an extensive resection into a smaller one. Alternatively, ultrasound may identify situations where a resection is not possible, and therefore hasten the conclusion of surgery.
- Identification of vascular and collecting system anatomy in partial renal resections—there are well-established clinical scenarios in which a partial nephrectomy is warranted (e.g., bilateral renal tumors to preserve neph-

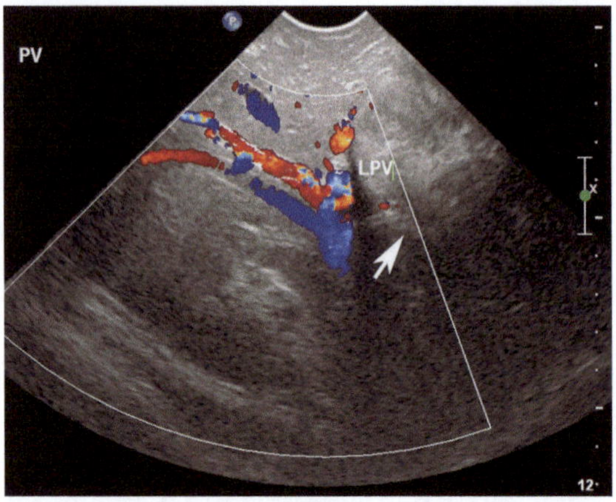

Fig. 11.14 Intraoperative cavitary ultrasound demonstrating hepatic mass adjacent to the left portal vein *(LPV)*. Mass is identified by the *arrow*

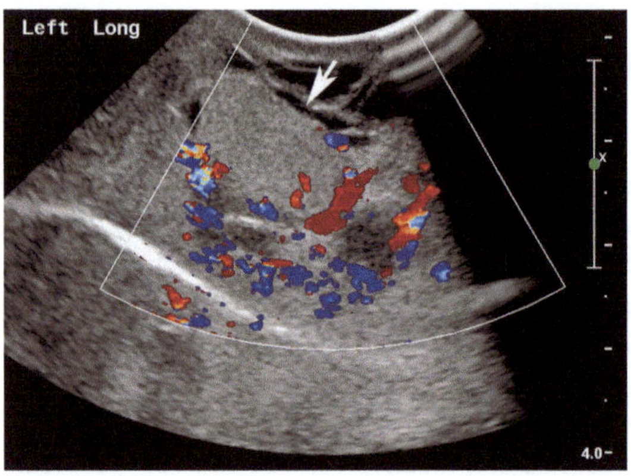

Fig. 11.15 Intraoperative cavitary ultrasound demonstrating renal mass *(arrow)* adjacent to renal artery. A partial nephrectomy was performed using ultrasound guidance

rons; syndromic patients where future resections are likely; horseshoe kidney; renal cell carcinoma). In these situations, intraoperative ultrasound may provide valuable real-time assessment of whether a partial nephrectomy is feasible (Fig. 11.15).

Summary

Abdominal and retroperitoneal masses in children and adolescents present the clinician with diagnostic and therapeutic challenges. Ultrasound is a valuable diagnostic and therapeutic tool that should become part of the surgeon's repertoire. Ultrasound can often be used as the first diagnostic test for many intra-abdominal and retroperitoneal masses in children and neonates. Importantly, ultrasound can be used to determine the size, location, vascularity, and cystic versus solid nature of the mass. Using the sonographic characteristics of a mass, coupled with the age, sex, and history of the patient, often leads to a precise narrowing of the differential diagnosis. In this chapter, we reviewed the sonographic findings of some of the most commonly seen cystic and solid intra-abdominal and retroperitoneal masses of infancy and childhood. Following diagnosis, ultrasound is often an important adjunct for bedside procedures as well as in the operating room. The chapter also discussed descriptions on how ultrasound is useful when performing biopsies, guided drainage procedures, and as an intraoperative guide for tumor resection.

References

1. Berdon WE, Ruzal-Shapiro C, Abramson SJ, Garvin J. The diagnosis of abdominal neuroblastoma: relative roles of ultrasonography, CT, and MRI. Urol Radiol. 1992;14(4):252–62.
2. Bliss DP, Coffin CM, Bower RJ, Stockmann PT, Ternberg JL. Mesenteric cysts in children. Surgery. 1994;115(5):571–7.
3. Carroll BA, Moskowitz PS. Sonographic diagnosis of neonatal meconium cyst. AJR Am J Roentgenol. 1981;137(6):1262–4. doi:10.2214/ajr.137.6.1262.
4. Crane GL, Hernanz-Schulman M. Current imaging assessment of congenital abdominal masses in pediatric patients. Semin Roentgenol. 2012;47(1):32–44. doi:10.1053/j.ro.2011.07.004.
5. Dezsöfi A, McLin V, Hadzic N. Hepatic neoplasms in children: a focus on differential diagnosis. Clin Res Hepatol Gastroenterol. 2014;38(4):399–402. doi:10.1016/j.clinre.2014.05.001.
6. Friedman AP, Slovis TL, Haller JO, Lebensart DP. The role of sonography in evaluating right upper quadrant disease in children. Clin Pediatr (Phila). 1980;19(9):591–6.
7. Haddad MC, Birjawi GA, Hemadeh MS, Melhem RE, Al-Kutoubi AM. The gamut of abdominal and pelvic cystic masses in children. Eur Radiol. 2001;11(1):148–66. doi:10.1007/s003300000487.

8. Kim S, Chung DH. Pediatric solid malignancies: neuroblastoma and Wilms' tumor. Surg Clin North Am. 2006;86(2):469–87, xi. doi:10.1016/j.suc.2005.12.008.
9. Ladd AP, Grosfeld JL. Gastrointestinal tumors in children and adolescents. Semin Pediatr Surg. 2006;15(1):37–47. doi:10.1053/j.sempedsurg.2005.11.007.
10. Lee HC, Yeung CY, Chang PY, Sheu JC, Wang NL. Dilatation of the biliary tree in children: sonographic diagnosis and its clinical significance. J Ultrasound Med. 2000;19(3):177–82; quiz 183–4.
11. Luo CC, Huang CS, Chao HC, Chu SM, Hsueh C. Intra-abdominal cystic lymphangiomas in infancy and childhood. Chang Gung Med J. 2004;27(7):509–14.
12. Nuchtern JG. Perinatal neuroblastoma. Semin Pediatr Surg. 2006;15(1):10–6. doi:10.1053/j.sempedsurg.2005.11.003.
13. Okur H, Küçükaydin M, Ozokutan BH, Durak AC, Kazez A, Köse O. Mesenteric, omental, and retroperitoneal cysts in children. Eur J Surg. 1997;163(9):673–7.
14. Onur MR, Bakal U, Kocakoc E, Tartar T, Kazez A. Cystic abdominal masses in children: a pictorial essay. Clin Imaging. 2013;37(1):18–27. doi:10.1016/j.clinimag.2012.03.010.
15. Riccabona M. Imaging of renal tumours in infancy and childhood. Eur Radiol. 2003;13(Suppl 4):L116–29. doi:10.1007/s00330-003-2001-x.
16. Milla SS, Lee EY, Buonomo C, Bramson RT. Ultrasound evaluation of pediatric abdominal masses. Ultrasound Clin. 2007;2(3):541–59.
17. Sato M, Ishida H, Konno K, Naganuma H, Hamashima Y, Komatsuda T, Watanabe S. Liver tumors in children and young patients: sonographic and color Doppler findings. Abdom Imaging. 2000;25(6):596–601.
18. Ueno T, Hashimoto H, Yokoyama H, Ito M, Kouda K, Kanamaru H. Urachal anomalies: ultrasonography and management. J Pediatr Surg. 2003;38(8):1203–7.
19. Vargas-Serrano B, Alegre-Bernal N, Cortina-Moreno B, Rodriguez-Romero R, Sanchez-Ortega F. Abdominal cystic lymphangiomas: US and CT findings. Eur J Radiol. 1995;19(3):183–7.
20. White KS. Imaging of abdominal masses in children. Semin Pediatr Surg. 1992;1(4):269–76.
21. Wicks JD, Silver TM, Bree RL. Giant cystic abdominal masses in children and adolescents: ultrasonic differential diagnosis. AJR Am J Roentgenol. 1978;130(5):853–7. doi:10.2214/ajr.130.5.853.
22. Wootton-Gorges SL, Thomas KB, Harned RK, Wu SR, Stein-Wexler R, Strain JD. Giant cystic abdominal masses in children. Pediatr Radiol. 2005;35(12):1277–88. doi:10.1007/s00247-005-1559-7.
23. Yamaguchi M, Takeuchi S, Akiyama H, Sawaguchi S. Ultrasonic evaluation of abdominal masses in the pediatric patient. Tohoku J Exp Med. 1980;130(1):25–39.

Emergency Ultrasound in the Evaluation of Pediatric Blunt Abdominal Trauma

12

Seth Goldstein and F. Dylan Stewart

Ultrasound (USN) has been an integral, but poorly understood, adjunct in the care of the acutely injured patient for decades. Use of ultrasound in the evaluation of blunt abdominal trauma is very well accepted, such that it has even become an extension of the physical exam. Although USN was used as early as the 1970s in Europe, it did not achieve widespread use in North America until the introduction of the American College of Surgeons Focused Abdominal Sonography for Trauma (FAST) exam, which has been an integrated part of Advanced Trauma Life Support (ATLS) since the early 1990s. USN is prized for its noninvasive, rapid, reproducible, safe, and inexpensive qualities. With the recent increased attention and awareness of the potential risks of malignancy in children with the use of ionizing radiation, USN has become an even more attractive modality in the evaluation of the pediatric trauma patient with suspected intra-abdominal injury (IAI). However, whereas the accuracy and utility of the FAST exam in adults is well documented, its usefulness and sensitivity in children has remained less clear, and therefore widespread usage of this potentially important technology is lacking. A survey published in 2009 showed use of FAST in 96 % of adult trauma centers, but only in 15 % of freestanding children's hospitals [1]. This is paradoxical, as the pediatric surgical and emergency medicine communities have historically been on the forefront of the effort to minimize ionizing radiation exposure in children, and USN may be a key to achieving this goal. Part of the reluctance to embrace a new diagnostic modality may be due to the fact that pediatric surgeons have also been leaders in development of nonoperative management of IAIs, making the diagnosis of these injuries less likely to change the clinical course of the child. It is also well described that one third of children with solid organ injury after blunt trauma have no intra-abdominal free fluid, which is the diagnostic hallmark of a positive FAST exam. Furthermore, well-designed studies that are likely to demonstrate accuracy of USN in children are unlikely to show a statistically significant change in the clinical course of injured children.

Despite these challenges, we suspect USN will play an ever-expanding role in the evaluation of children with blunt abdominal trauma, especially as more and more surgeons become comfortable with the performance of the FAST exam. In this chapter, we will demonstrate the proper technique in detail, briefly review the existing literature in regards to the academic evaluation of the use of USN in injured children, and detail the authors' proposed algorithm

F. D. Stewart (✉)
Department of Pediatric Surgery, Johns Hopkins Hospital, 1800 Orleans St, Bloomberg Building, 7335, Baltimore, MD 21287, USA
e-mail: dstewart@jhmi.edu

S. Goldstein
Department of Surgery, Johns Hopkins Hospital, 1800 Orleans St, Tower 110, Baltimore, MD 21287, USA
e-mail: sgoldstein@jhmi.edu

S. Scholz, M. D. Jarboe (eds.), *Diagnostic and Interventional Ultrasound in Pediatrics and Pediatric Surgery,* DOI 10.1007/978-3-319-21699-7_12

for including USN into the pediatric blunt torso trauma evaluation.

Technique

The FAST exam is typically performed with the patient in the supine position and the sonographer on the right side of the patient with a curvilinear transducer in his or her right hand. The ultrasound machine should be set to B-mode imaging on a preconfigured abdominal setting, if available. The sequence principally comprises four views: hepatorenal, splenorenal, suprapubic, and pericardial. An extended version of the FAST (eFAST) also includes bilateral views of the chest for hemo- and pneumothorax, but this technique is not well studied in children and will not be discussed here.

The hepatorenal recess of the subhepatic space, also known as Morison's pouch, is the most dependent area of the supramesocolic peritoneum and is thus the most sensitive for upper abdominal trauma. For this view, the probe is placed in the right posterior axillary line at the most inferior intercostal spaces and positioned to provide a coronal view of the interface between the liver and the right kidney (Fig. 12.1). The probe marker should point cephalad, and the probe adjusted to the intercostal space in which both organs can be clearly seen. In a normal examination the renal, or Gerota's, fascia will directly abut the liver and may appear as a bright stripe. In the presence of free abdominal fluid, the classic finding is an anechoic band between kidney and liver.

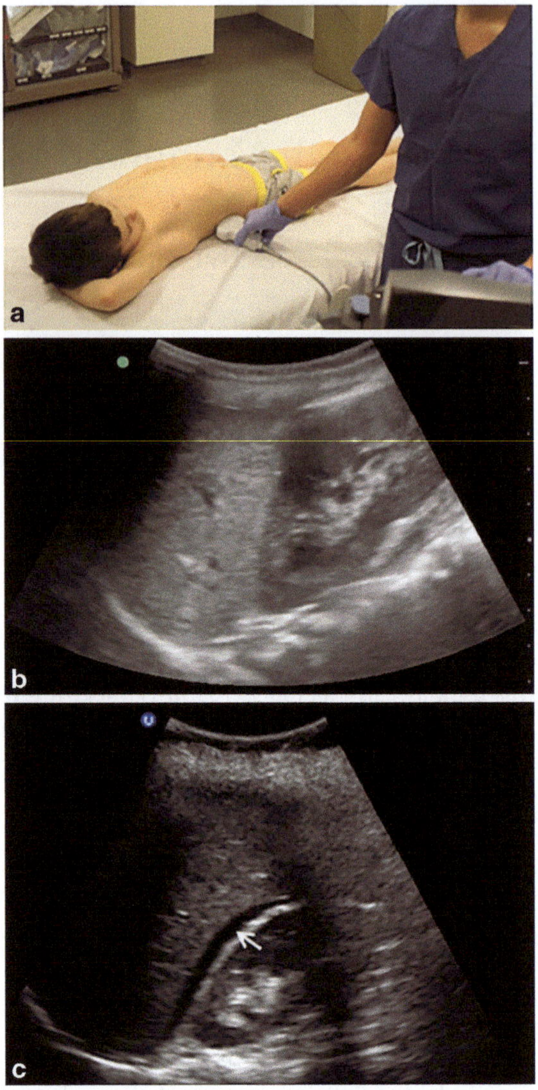

Fig. 12.1 Transducer positioning for the hepatorenal area (**a**), normal view of Morison's pouch (**b**), and an abnormal exam with free fluid between liver and kidney denoted by *white arrow* (**c**). Panel **c** courtesy of Geoffrey E. Hayden, MD, RDMS

The splenorenal fossa is in an analogous position on the left side of the abdomen and is often relevant in the setting of suspected splenic trauma. The probe is placed in the left posterior axillary line at the inferior intercostal spaces and positioned to provide a coronal view of the interface between spleen and left kidney (Fig. 12.2). The entirety of the spleen can be seen with slight translation and rotation of the probe in this fashion. Positive findings again entail anechoic areas representing free intraperitoneal fluid in either the splenorenal or splenodiaphragmatic spaces. If difficulties are encountered visualizing either the hepatorenal or splenorenal views, asking the patient to hold full inspiration, if possible, can slide the area of interest more inferiorly and into better view. More posterior positioning of the probe to the extent that the bed or gurney allows is also often helpful in avoiding bowel gas.

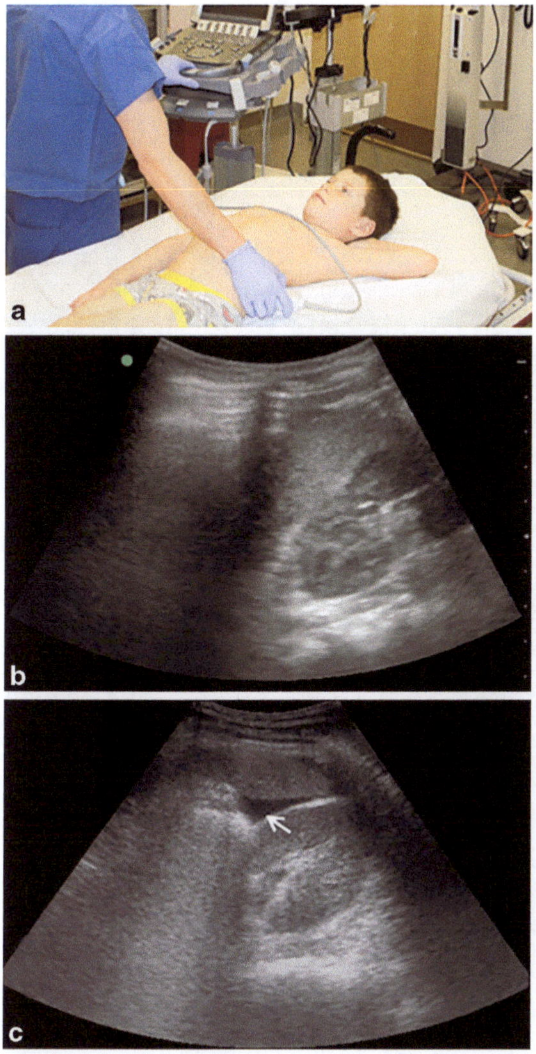

Fig. 12.2 Transducer positioning for the splenorenal area (**a**), normal view of the recess (**b**), and an abnormal exam with free fluid between spleen and kidney denoted by *white arrow* (**c**). Panel **c** courtesy of Geoffrey E. Hayden, MD, RDMS

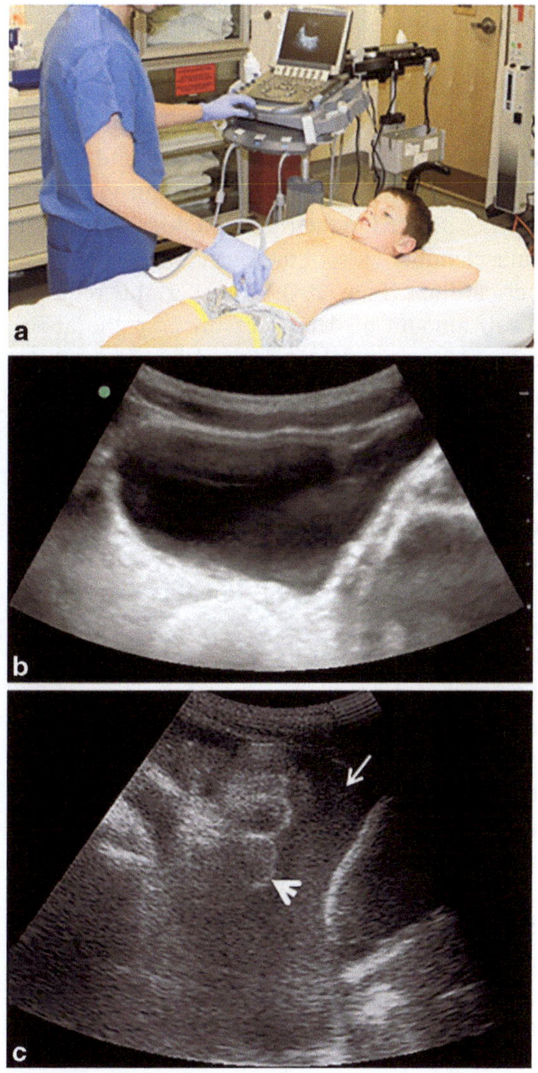

Fig. 12.3 Transducer positioning for the suprapubic area (**a**), normal view of the bladder (**b**), and an abnormal exam with free fluid around bladder and freely floating bowel loops, denoted by *white arrow* and *arrowhead*, respectively (**c**). Panel **c** courtesy of Geoffrey E. Hayden, MD, RDMS

Suprapubic positioning of the probe allows assessment of the dependent areas of the inframesocolic peritoneum, which are the rectovesicular pouch in males and the rectouterine pouch (of Douglas) in females. The transducer is placed immediately cephalad to the pubic bone and the array angled inferiorly into the pelvis (Fig. 12.3), where the bladder is generally easily seen. Longitudinal and transverse images are both typically obtained, with particular attention paid to the posterior border of the bladder, where fluid can be seen as an anechoic stripe.

Finally, interrogation of the pericardial space is a useful benefit of the FAST exam in blunt trauma. Hemopericardium and the resultant tamponade can be a consequence of either direct sternal impact or a deceleration injury that coincides with subxiphoid abdominal impact. There are two acceptable ways in which cardiac views can be obtained by ultrasound. A subxiphoid approach entails placing a transducer just inferior to the xiphisternum and directing it towards the left shoulder with the probe marker pointed to the right shoulder to aquire a four-chamber view of the heart and surrounding pericardium (Fig. 12.4). However, this requires a fair amount of deep pressure into the abdomen and may not be tolerated by all patients. Alternatively, a parasternal long-axis view can be achieved by orienting the probe in a parasagittal axis just to the left of the sternum and locating an interspace that permits identification of the heart. In either view, finding more than trace fluid in the dependent posterior pericardial space is abnormal and should be considered a positive finding.

The FAST can easily be employed as a routine part of the secondary trauma survey, and is often performed in parallel to other therapeutic and resuscitative care. By giving immediate realtime images of the most commonly injured solid abdominal organs as well as the dependent areas in which fluid accumulates, ultrasound is a valuable adjunct to trauma diagnostic algorithms. Serial examinations may be appropriate in many instances, as hemoperitoneum can take time to acculULate. We particularly recommend FAST in time-sensitive situations in which the decision must be made to manage critical illness following trauma in either an intensive care unit or in an operating room.

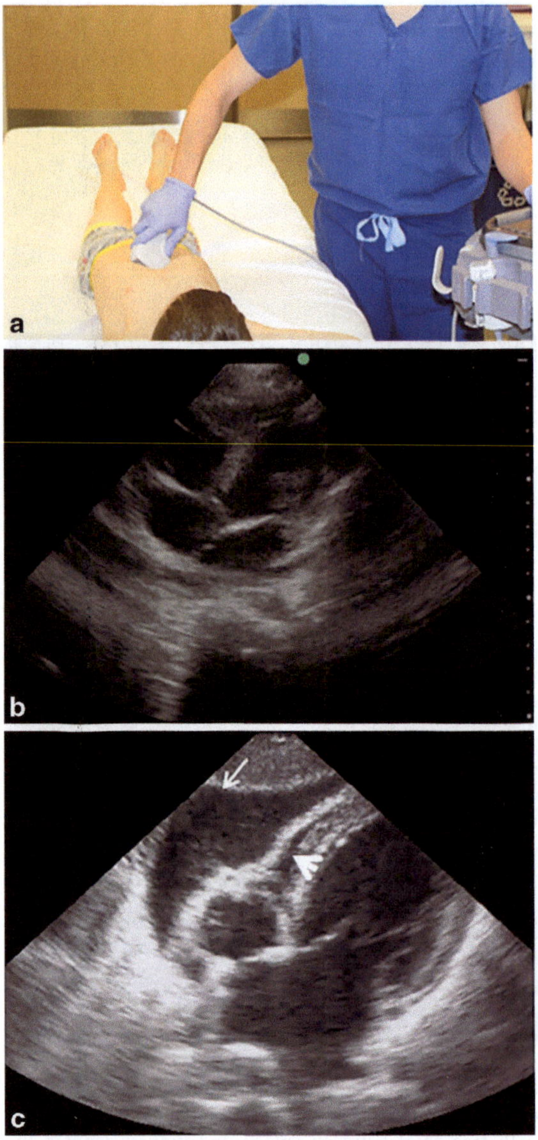

Fig. 12.4 Transducer positioning for subxiphoid view of pericardium (**a**), normal four-chamber view of the heart (**b**), and pericardial tamponade with pericardial fluid and right ventricular collapse denoted by *white arrow* and *arrowhead*, respectively (**c**). Panel **c** courtesy of Geoffrey E. Hayden, MD, RDMS

Review of Literature

Many authors have attempted to evaluate the usefulness of the FAST exam in the clinical practice of pediatric trauma. Scaife et al. reported a well-designed study where surgeons received intensive ultrasound training, and then compared the FAST findings to CT scans that were subsequently obtained [1]. The overall sensitivity of FAST was only 36 % when all four views were taken into account, and of the eight patients in the study with significant intra-abdominal injury, four had a negative FAST exam. Of note, at the conclusion of the study, the usage of FAST by the pediatric surgeons quickly dropped from 70 to 30 % of patient of trauma evaluations. The authors concluded that reliable

Table 12.1 Predictors of clinically significant blunt intraabdominal injury

Age-adjusted hypotension
Abnormal abdominal physical examination
Presence of femur fracture
Elevated hepatic transaminases (AST > 200 U/L or ALT > 125 U/L)
Microscopic hematuria (> 5 RBCs/HPF)
Hematocrit on presentation less than 30 %

FAST exam required a significant commitment to surgeon training, and the benefit gained from that expenditure remained unclear.

Holmes et al. [2] performed a large meta-analysis on all studies of pediatric ultrasound to evaluate the test performance of FAST. They reported that the exam has only a modest sensitivity (80 %) for the detection of hemoperitoneum in children, but that when only the most methodologically rigorous studies were included, that sensitivity dropped to 66 %. Of interest, the authors discuss several studies where an attempt was made to add imaging of solid organs to the performance of the standard FAST exam, but with only a modest increase in sensitivity for IAI, and no data was obtained as to how well non-radiologists could be trained to interpret solid organ imaging. The authors concluded that the FAST exam has a highly questionable role as the only diagnostic test when IAI was suspected.

Few would argue that FAST should be (or will become) the sole diagnostic test for blunt traumatic injuries. Sola et al. in 2009 published a study on the addition of elevated liver transaminases to the FAST exam as a screening tool for blunt abdominal trauma. They retrospectively reviewed 400 patients who had all received FAST, abdominal CT, and transaminases. They found that FAST had a sensitivity of only 50 % on its own for identifying IAI confirmed by CT scan. This increased to 88 % when the addition of an AST or ALT value over 100 U/L was included in the analysis with the positive FAST scans. They concluded that children with a negative FAST and liver transaminases under 100 U/L should not undergo CT scanning given the low risk of missed injuries.

Menaker and the authors of the Pediatric Emergency Care Applied Research Network (PECARN) [3] evaluated the usage of FAST and its effect on Abdominal CT scanning in a retrospective study of 20 PECARN pediatric trauma centers. They found high levels of variation in the usage of FAST, but definite decrease in the use of Abdominal CT in patients considered low risk for IAI when the FAST exam was normal. The results of the FAST did not influence physician behavior, however, when the clinical suspicion for injury was higher.

One of the clinical challenges in treating children with IAI is that the majority of injuries are not of clinical significance. Most children are managed with nonoperative therapy, so the importance of correctly diagnosing IAI is unclear. Several authors have responded to this challenge by proposing a clinical predication model to identify children who will have a higher likelihood of a significant injury. The six high-risk variables from the study by Holmes et al. are listed in Table 12.1.

Abdominal CT scanning presents a significant risk of malignancy. The risk of a fatal cancer is estimated to be as high as 1 per 1000 pediatric CT scans, or a 0.18 % lifetime risk for a 1-year-old child [4]. Therefore, it is clear that the usage of this modality must decrease in the standard clinical practice of pediatric trauma, and that CT scanning must be reserved for children where the management will change based on the results of the scan, and not simply to satisfy physician curiosity nor to practice defensive medicine. We believe that FAST scanning, despite its limitations, will play a key role in this practice management change. Below, we propose an algorithm developed using the concept that FAST is valuable, but will only increase in value the more it is utilized and perfected (Fig. 12.5). Pediatric Emergency providers, trained in the American College of Surgeon's Ultrasound course, should be expected to perform FAST on all pediatric trauma evaluations. The results of the FAST should then be considered in light of the previously described clinical predic-

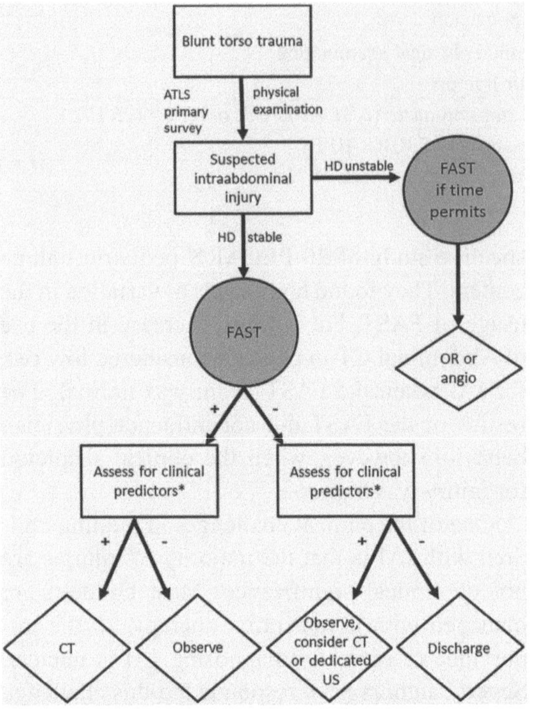

Fig. 12.5 Proposed algorithm for incorporation of ultrasound into trauma bay management. *clinical predictors listed in Table 1. *ATLS*=advanced trauma life support; *HD*=hemodynamically; *FAST*=focused abdominal sonography for trauma. *CT*=computed tomography; *US*=ultrasound; *OR*=operating room; angio=angiography suite

tion model. Patients with both a positive FAST and positive clinical predictors would be the most appropriate for CT scanning. Patients with negative FAST and no concerning factors would be most likely discharged to home. A combination of the two results will result in patients undergoing observation, possibly a dedicated USN exam by an ultrasonographer, or CT scanning. We also believe that parents should be involved in the decision-making, so they are aware of the risks of malignancy with CT scanning, and understand that their child may need a longer period of observation, hospital admission, NPO status, etc., in an attempt to rule out clinically significant injury without ionizing radiation. Continued studies of such decision-making algorithms are crucial to prove the safety of these new clinical pathways, and to produce a culture change in pediatric emergency rooms that have for too long practiced over-reliance on CT imaging.

Summary

In conclusion, FAST scanning is likely to play a larger role in the evaluation of the pediatric blunt abdominal trauma patient as the risks of CT scanning become better understood. Encouragement of consistent and routine FAST scanning in academic centers should be the standard, as the FAST exam will likely become more valuable when it is performed by more experienced providers. Incorporation of the FAST results into clinical decision pathways using validated predictors can achieve the goal of discovery of injuries without the overuse of harmful radiation.

References

1. Scaife ER, Fenton SJ, Hansen KW, et al. Use of focused abdominal sonography for trauma at pediatric and adult trauma centers: a survey. J Pediatr Surg. 2009;44:1746–9.
2. Holmes JF, Gladman A, Chang CH. Performance of abdominal ultrasonography in pediatric blunt trauma patients: a meta-analysis. J Pediatr Surg. 2007 Sep;42(9):1588–94.
3. Menaker J, Blumberg S, Wisner DH, Dayan PS, Tunik M, Garcia M, Mahajan P, Page K, Monroe D, Borgialli D, Kuppermann N, Holmes JF, Intra-abdominal Injury Study Group of the Pediatric Emergency Care Applied Research Network (PECARN). Use of the focused assessment with sonography for trauma (FAST) examination and its impact on abdominal computed tomography use in hemodynamically stable children with blunt torso trauma. J Trauma Acute Care Surg. 2014;77:427–32.
4. Brenner D, Elliston C, Hall E, et al. Estimated risks of radiation-induced fatal cancer from pediatric CT. AJR Am J Roentgenol. 2001;176:289–96.

The Kidney

13

Oliver L. Sanchez, Raimondo M. Cervellione
and Kimberly M. Lumpkins

Introduction

Ultrasonography (US) is the most fundamental tool in the armamentarium of the pediatric urologist. US allows excellent visualization of the kidney and bladder and is a well-tolerated modality with few adverse effects on the patient. As ultrasound is highly dependent on the experience of the technician, experience with the pediatric population improves the quality and utility of the imaging.

Scanning Technique and Normal Sonographic Findings

Pediatric patients are generally thin with more superficial positioning of the kidneys and therefore require a higher frequency probe (7 MHz) for quality imaging. Warmed ultrasound gel can be useful in avoiding distress in young patients. All patients should be well hydrated prior to the study. Examination of the bladder is a critical part of the ultrasound and should be performed with the bladder distended. All children past the age of toilet training should have pre- and post-micturition imaging. Hydronephrosis may partially improve with micturition depending on the underlying pathology. In younger children, the bladder should be examined first, as pressure, cold ultrasound gel, and stimulation often lead to reflex micturition. If the bladder is empty, then the scan can proceed, hoping for refilling of the bladder during this period. Abnormalities of the bladder wall may be clearer when viewed with and without bladder distention. Normal bladder thickness is less than 3 mm in the well-distended bladder, and increased bladder thickness suggests the possibility of a bladder outlet obstruction or acute urinary tract infection (UTI). Documentation of the post-void residual volume is of importance in the assessment of lower urinary tract symptoms. Bladder volume pre- and post-micturition can be estimated by the formula: volume (ml) $=0.9\times$ depth $\times$ height $\times$ width in centimeters, however this formula is not reliable in very irregular bladders [1]. This can be compared to the expected bladder capacity by age using the formula: capacity $=30\times$ (age in years $+1$) in milliliters [2]. An extensive discussion of bladder imaging and lower urinary tract dysfunction is beyond the scope of this chapter. Care should be taken to search for dilated ureters behind the bladder. The normal, nondilated ureter should not be visible on US.

The renal ultrasound scan requires imaging of both kidneys in the coronal and transverse planes, usually imaged from the midaxillary line.

K. M. Lumpkins (✉)
Department of Surgery, University of Maryland School of Medicine, 29 S Greene St Suite 110, Baltimore, MD, USA
e-mail: klumpkins@smail.umaryland.edu

O. L. Sanchez
Department of Pediatric Surgery, Children's Hospital Geneva, Rue Willy-Donzé 6, Geneve, Switzerland
e-mail: oliversanchez@lopecito.net

R. M. Cervellione
Royal Manchester Children's Hospital, Oxford Road, Manchester, M13 9WL England, UK

S. Scholz, M. D. Jarboe (eds.), *Diagnostic and Interventional Ultrasound in Pediatrics and Pediatric Surgery,* DOI 10.1007/978-3-319-21699-7_13

However, actual transducer positioning is determined by the unique requirements of each individual patient. Younger patients are often unable or unwilling to cooperate with the instructions to hold breath, requiring flexibility on the part of the operator. The kidneys lie in the retroperitoneum in close proximity to the liver and duodenum on the right and the spleen, pancreas, and colon on the left. Kidney dimension should be measured in the longitudinal view. The normal kidney in an adult measures 9–11 cm. Nomograms have been published establishing the reference ranges for kidney size in the pediatric population, including preterm infants [3, 4].A small kidney falling below the expected size for age may suggest renal scarring or other pathologic process and warrant further inquiry [5]. Solitary kidneys are expected to display significant compensatory growth and can be expected to fall more than two standard deviations above the expected renal length for age. This can be estimated using the equation: length (cm) $=0.4\times$ age (years) $+7$ [6]. Kidney growth should be monitored serially over time to ensure proper growth velocity in selected patients. Measurement of the anteroposterior diameter (APD) of the renal pelvis, an important measure of hydronephrosis, is facilitated by a clear coronal image of the kidney, showing the point where the renal pelvis exits the parenchyma.

Anatomically, the renal cortex is clearly visualized at the periphery of the kidney. The renal medulla is arranged in columns (the columns of Bertin) with the base of the pyramids adjacent to the cortex and the apex projecting into the center of the kidney (Fig. 13.1). The renal pyramids are hypoechoic in comparison to the renal cortex, and renal fat located in the sinus is brightly echogenic (although not visible in the very young due to a relative paucity of renal fat) [7]. The difference in echogenicity between the cortex and medulla is the cause for the corticomedullary differentiation seen on a normal renal ultrasound. Although the kidney is typically hypoechoic to the liver and spleen, it is normal for the newborn kidney to be isoechoic or hyperechoic [8]. This is believed to be due to an increased density of glomeruli in the cortex. The density decreases to its typical hypoechoic appearance within the first several months after birth. The spleen may serve as a useful reference for density in patients who may have altered liver density due to intrinsic liver disease. Hyperechoic renal parenchyma is often reflective of underlying medical renal disease, even in newborns, but may be present in normal kidneys (Fig. 13.2). Fetal lobation may be seen as a multiple, smooth, rounded contours outlining the lobes of the kidney in neonates [7]. This may be confused for scarring, but the boundary of the lobes lies between the medullary pyramids instead of overlying them.

Doppler US can be a useful adjunct in the assessment of vascular problems of the kidney (see below) and is an essential part of the evaluation for renal transplants. Doppler US relies on the frequency shift of blood or other fluid in motion to determine the speed and direction of flow. Flow altering conditions in vessels, such as renal

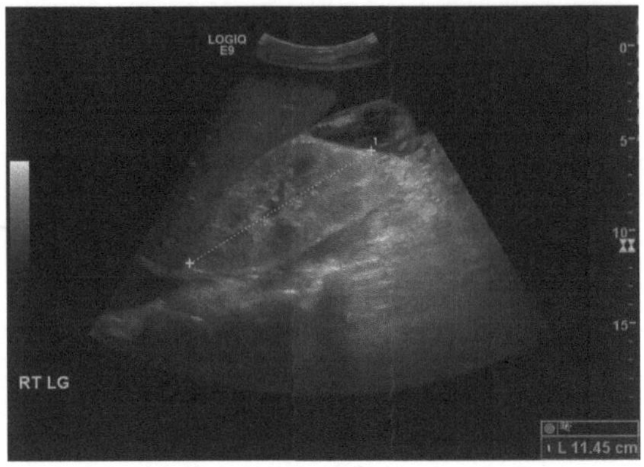

Fig. 13.2 Hyperechoic kidney in congenital nephrotic syndrome. Compare the echogenicity to the adjacent liver

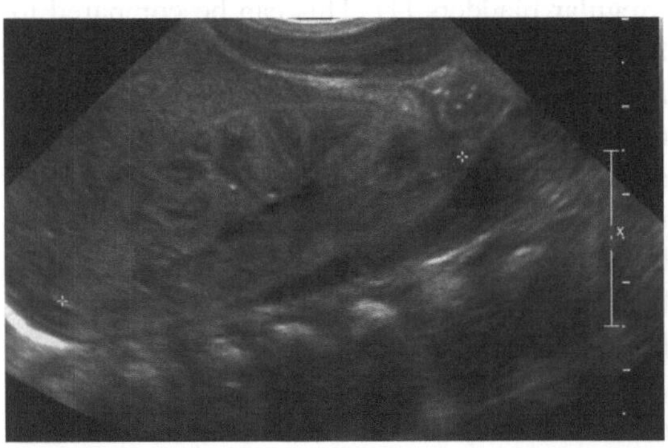

Fig. 13.1 Normal neonatal kidney

artery stenosis, may be suspected based on alterations in velocity pre- and post-stenosis. Imaging of the native renal vessels may be complicated by overlying bowel gas, and thus fasting beforehand can be helpful [9].

Renal Agenesis and Cystic Dysplasia

Congenital absence of one kidney occurs in approximately 1 in 1000 patients [7]. It is due to agenesis of the Wolffian duct or lack of induction of the metanephros during development. When agenesis is suspected on ultrasound, a careful search for ectopic renal tissue should be made. In females, unilateral renal agenesis may be associated with gynecologic abnormalities such as unicornuate uterus, obstructed hemivagina and ipsilateral renal agenesis (OHVIRA) syndrome, and Mayer–Rokitansky syndrome [10, 11]. Magnetic resonance imaging (MRI) may be indicated if there is a clinical suspicion of other gynecological abnormalities. Forty percent of the patients with a solitary kidney have other urinary tract anomalies such as vesicoureteral reflux (VUR), and a voiding cystourethrogram (VCUG) should be considered [12].

Regardless of whether a solitary kidney is the result of unilateral agenesis, dysplasia, or nephrectomy, long-term follow-up is indicated. The lower limits of acceptable glomerular filtration rate (GFR) in pediatric patients with a solitary kidney, representing two standard deviations below the norm, have been reported to be 78 ml/min/1.73 m^2 in children under 2 years, 73 ml/min/1.73 m^2 in girls older than 2 and boys 2–13 years old, and 70 ml/min/1.73 m^2 in boys older than 13 [13]. Patients falling below these levels should have more in-depth evaluation. Experimental data suggest that decreased nephron mass leads over time to possible hyperfiltration injury and ongoing kidney damage [14]. Patients with a solitary kidney may demonstrate higher blood pressure and increased proteinuria or microalbuminuria [15]. On the other hand, some studies have not found this association [16]. Higher renal vascular resistive indices have also been reported in young children with a solitary kidney, of unclear significance [17]. Thus, although the overall prognosis of patients with a solitary kidney is excellent, they should receive long-term follow-up of blood pressure, proteinuria, and kidney function.

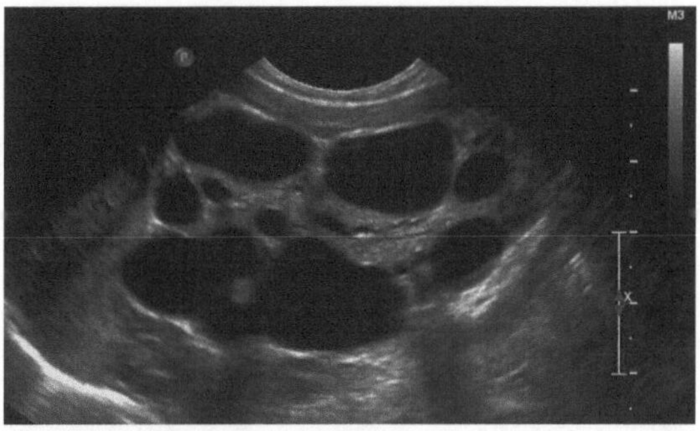

Fig. 13.3 Multicystic dysplastic kidney

Multicystic dysplastic kidney (MCDK) represents an anomaly of ureteral formation during early development and is the most common neonatal abdominal mass (Fig. 13.3). MCDK is often associated with an atretic or absent ureter [18]. It is characterized by multiple cysts of varying size that do not communicate [19]. There may or may not be visible renal parenchyma. Involution is common and may lead to confusion with renal agenesis if not detected until after involution is complete. Involution appears to occur most rapidly soon after birth. Serial US is an excellent modality for long-term monitoring. The need for nephrectomy in patients whose MCDK does not completely involute is a matter of debate [20]. Increased risk of hypertension has traditionally been used as an argument in favor of nephrectomy, but recent data suggest that this risk is only 5 in 1000, similar to the general population [21].

Other cystic disorders may be diagnosed by US. Simple renal cysts, which are quite common in adults, are unusual in children. Simple cysts are anechoic without evidence of septae or debris. Cystic changes in the setting of end stage renal disease (ESRD) are common and appear to relate to the duration of dialysis [22]. Annual ultrasound surveillance of pediatric patients on dialysis is prudent due to long-term risk of malignant degeneration. Genetic cystic renal diseases are rare but often suggested by the ultrasound

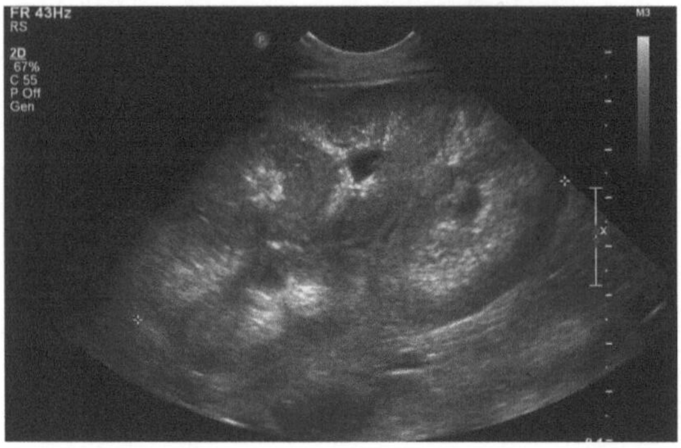

Fig. 13.4 Autosomal recessive polycystic kidney disease (ARPKD) in a neonate. The kidney measures 9 cm (normal for this age is 4.5 cm)

appearance of the kidneys. Identification of multiple cysts in the kidneys should lead to an ultrasonographic survey of other abdominal solid organs, as many cystic renal diseases involve other organs.

Autosomal dominant polycystic kidney disease (ADPKD), the most common genetic cystic disease, generally does not manifest itself until adulthood, but changes may be visible even prenatally. Recently, a fetal pattern of a hyperechoic cortex and hypoechoic medulla has been described with this condition, but the significance of this remains unclear [23]. A few scattered cysts may be evident early in childhood. In a child with a known family history, two or more cysts on ultrasound are diagnostic. Although liver cysts commonly develop, significant hepatic dysfunction is rare. The natural history of this disorder is progression of the cystic disease and development of renal insufficiency in young adulthood [24].

Autosomal recessive polycystic kidney disease (ARPKD) is generally symptomatic early in childhood and may lead to in utero or neonatal death due to pulmonary hypoplasia and Potter sequence. The kidneys are massively enlarged, and the cysts are often small enough that the kidneys appear solid on ultrasound, with loss of corticomedullary differentiation (Fig. 13.4). This condition is associated with hepatic fibrosis and portal hypertension. Perinatal mortality is 30 %, but some patients with a milder phenotype may maintain renal function into adulthood [25]. A variety of rarer pediatric cystic renal diseases exists; a combination of clinical suspicion and genetic analysis may be necessary to diagnose these in the correct clinical setting [26].

Anomalies of Renal Fusion and Rotation

Anomalies of renal fusion and rotation are relatively common. The kidneys form in the pelvis and rise by differential growth, and failure of ascent leads to ectopic positioning of the kidney. This is commonly in the pelvis below the level of the aortic bifurcation, but may occur at any point along the line of ascent of the kidney. In rare cases, the kidney can be located in the thoracic cavity. This frequently but not exclusively occurs in association with a congenital diaphragmatic hernia [27, 28]. Fusion of the lower pole of the developing kidneys across the midline can lead to horseshoe kidney, which occurs in 1 in 400–500 patients [29]. The ascent of a horseshoe kidney is typically arrested below the inferior mesenteric artery, leading to a low position. It is also possible for both kidneys to ascend ipsilaterally, known as crossed ectopia, and these kidneys may be fused or unfused. In both horseshoe kidney and crossed ectopia, the ureters of each renal moiety drain to their respective sides of the bladder (the ureters originate from the trigone in the normal positions). Malrotation of the pelvis is a common accompanying finding in all forms of renal ectopia, and this may predispose to ureteropelvic junction (UPJ) obstruction [30].

Ultrasound is easily able to identify the location and orientation of ectopic and fused kidneys. The blood supply of these kidneys may be very unusual, with feeding vessels originating at a variety of levels. Doppler US can evaluate the vasculature of the kidneys; however, magnetic resonance angiogram (MRA) or computed tomography angiography (CTA) may be indicated to more precisely delineate the vascular anatomy prior to an operative intervention. Ectopic kidneys have a relatively high incidence of associated urologic abnormalities, including vesicoureteral reflux (VUR) (20–30 % or more), and a VCUG should be considered [31]. Isolated renal ectopia itself is asymptomatic and has no long-term impact on kidney function or hypertension [32].

Duplex Kidney

A duplex kidney is composed of two separate pelvicalyceal systems, with either complete or partial ureteral duplication. This is a common finding, occurring in 1:125 patients. It is a variant of normal anatomy, and patients are often entirely asymptomatic. However, duplex kidneys carry an increased risk for VUR or obstruction. They may be difficult to identify if not associated with dysplasia or hydronephrosis. Suggestive findings on ultrasound include dilated ureter, the presence of a ureterocele in the bladder, or significant hydronephrosis of one pole (Fig. 13.5). Presence of more than one of these features increases the likelihood of a duplex kidney. According to the Weigert–Meyer law, in which the upper pole ureter inserts into the bladder caudally and more medially than the laterally placed lower pole ureter, upper pole moieties are associated with ureterocele and obstruction while lower pole moieties are associated with VUR. A full discussion on the management of duplex kidney is beyond the scope of this chapter.

Hydronephrosis

Hydronephrosis represents the lion's share of renal pathology presenting to a pediatric urologist. Antenatal hydronephrosis is very common, and the majority of patients never requires surgical intervention [33]. Evaluation of hydronephrosis is complicated by the fact that the severity can vary according to the patient's hydration status, and description of hydronephrosis is often subjective and vague. Terms such as "mild," "moderate," or "severe" may have very different meanings depending on the observer. The Society of Fetal Urology has established a classification system for the description of hydronephrosis in the neonatal population [34]. This is designed to be used only after the exclusion of VUR, but in practice is commonly used to describe the ultrasound findings without regard to diagnostic status. Grade 0 represents no hydronephrosis, grade 1 only the renal pelvis is seen, grade 2 a few calyces are visualized, and in grade 3 virtually all calyces are dilated. Grade 4 additionally demonstrates cortical thinning. Whenever possible, the Society of Fetal Urology (SFU) criteria or objective measurements such as the APD [35] and should be used to minimize the subjective nature of descriptive terminology.

The pattern of dilation seen on the ultrasound often suggests the underlying etiology. Massive dilation of the renal pelvis with a normal ureter is very suspicious for UPJ obstruction (Fig. 13.6). Follow-up with a diuretic renogram is generally indicated in moderate to severe hydronephrosis in order to confirm the diagnosis, assess the degree of obstruction, and determine differential renal function [36]. Congenital hydronephrosis can often be managed conservatively, but increasing hydronephrosis (particularly with an

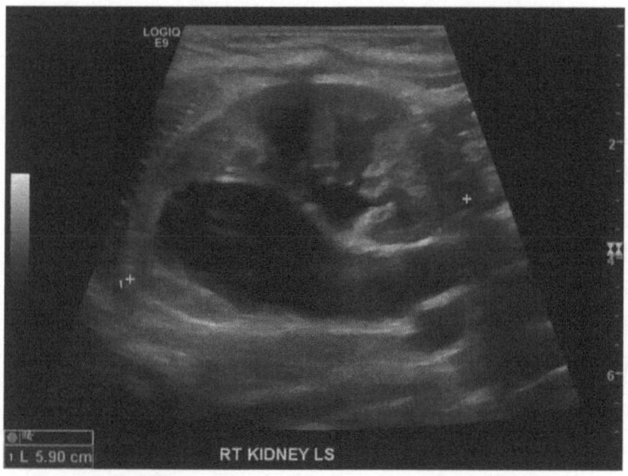

Fig. 13.5 Duplex kidney with upper pole hydroureteronephrosis

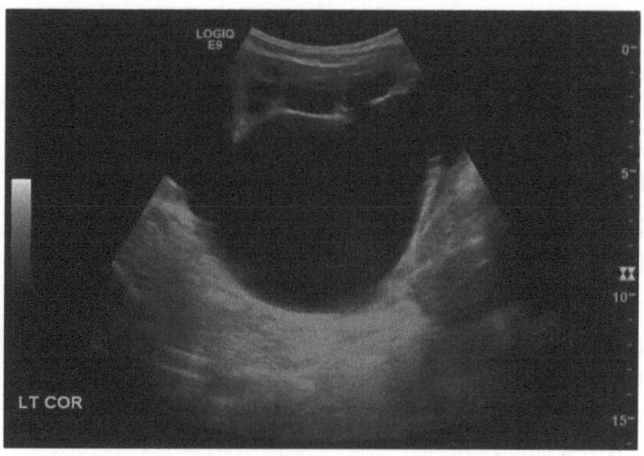

Fig. 13.6 Ureteropelvic junction obstruction with massive hydronephrosis

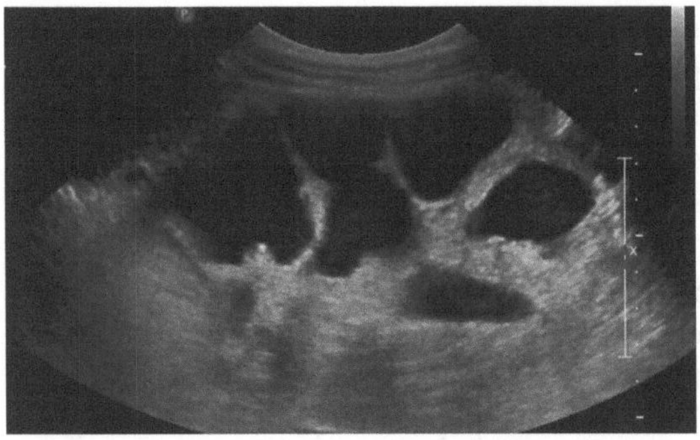
Fig. 13.7 Severe hydronephrosis due to grade V vesicoureteral reflux

APD >3 cm) and deteriorating differential renal function on mercaptoacetyltriglycine (MAG3) renogram indicate UPJ obstruction which requires operative intervention [37].

Hydronephrosis with concomitant hydroureter is suggestive of a congenital megaureter which can be either obstructive or refluxing (Fig. 13.7). Lower grades of VUR that are not associated with dilation are easily missed on US. Formal diagnosis of VUR is typically made with a voiding cystourethrogram (VCUG) or radionuclide voiding cystography (RVC). Both these methods involve exposure to radiation and placement of a urethral catheter. In toilet-trained children, VUR can be diagnosed via indirect radioisotope cystogram using intravenous injection of MAG3.

Although several groups have attempted to identify US methods of diagnosis that might allow avoidance of both radiation and urethral catheterization, at this date none has been found to be sufficiently sensitive to replace VCUG or RVC [38]. Contrast-enhanced ultrasound has been advocated as a diagnostic tool to avoid radiation exposure. In this technique, a complete renal and bladder ultrasound is performed prior to the instillation of microbubble ultrasound contrast into the bladder via urethral catheter. The US is repeated several times before and after voiding. The presence of microbubbles in the ureter supports the diagnosis of VUR. A grading system has been established corresponding to the traditional VCUG classification of VUR. Microbubbles in the ureter alone represents grade I reflux, while microbubbles in the renal pelvis with hydronephrosis and tortuous ureters represents grade V reflux [39]. VUS is highly operator dependent, does not image the urethra, and the study time is prolonged. Additionally, the cost of ultrasound contrast is much greater than that of fluoroscopic contrast. These factors have limited its widespread adoption, and at this point VCUG remains the gold standard imaging test [40].

Bilateral hydroureteronephrosis in a male infant should raise suspicion of posterior urethral valves (PUV) [41]. The partial urethral obstruction caused by the congenital valves leads to a thick-walled, "keyhole" bladder that can be seen on ultrasound, and careful scanning from the perineal approach may demonstrate the dilated posterior urethra proximal to the valves. Catheter decompression followed by VCUG is the first line of management and should be performed prior to hospital discharge for any infant with suspected valves.

Infection

UTI is very common and represents a significant health care burden; 6.6% of girls and 1.8% of boys develop a UTI by age 6 [42]. Despite the frequency of this problem, the indication for imaging and timing of imaging remain a matter of considerable debate in the pediatric urology community, particularly with regard to the use of VCUG after UTI. Although a complete discussion of this topic is beyond the scope of this chapter, a brief discussion of the application of renal sonography to UTI is warranted. UTI can be divided into lower tract infection (cystitis) and upper tract infection (pyelonephritis). In the setting of lower UTI, US may demonstrate thickening of the bladder wall or debris within the bladder. This generally does not add much information to the history and physical exam, urinalysis, and urine culture, and routine use of US to diagnose cystitis cannot be recommended. However, US has the utility in identifying anatomic abnormalities such as hydronephrosis or ureterocele that may require intervention. Recommendations vary as to the indication for and timing of ultrasound after UTI. American Academy of Pediatrics guidelines currently recommend that all infants 2–24 months old with febrile UTI have a screening renal ultrasound performed at some point following treatment [43]. The National Institute for Health and Care Excellence (NICE) guidelines in the UK recommend a renal ultrasound within 6 weeks for infants less than 6 months old with an uncomplicated UTI and imaging during the acute episode for infants with a recurrent UTI or severe illness. For children older than 6 months, US is recommended in the acute setting for seriously ill children and within 6 weeks for a recurrent UTI. No ultrasound is recommended for simple UTI in children older than 6 months [44].

Diagnosis of pyelonephritis as opposed to cystitis may be made based on clinical and radiologic criteria. Pyelonephritis is typically associated with fever and flank pain, with or without symptoms of cystitis [45]. US is often normal in the setting of acute pyelonephritis, but there are several suggestive findings. Inflammation of the renal pelvis and ureter may be seen, and edema of the kidney parenchyma can lead to increased renal volume. Corticomedullary differentiation may be focally lost in the acute setting [46]. If clear documentation of acute pyelonephritis is clinically warranted, a dimercaptosuccinic acid (DMSA) scan to detect renal cortical perfusion abnormalities is indicated [47]. CT may also reveal wedge-shaped hypodensities in contrast uptake due to acute infection. Several investigators have explored the use of Doppler US in the diagnosis of acute pyelonephritis [48, 49]. Doppler US had good ability to detect renal cortical involvement, with 87–89 % sensitivity and 53–92 % specificity but was not as accurate as DMSA overall.

US may reveal layering echoes in the dependent portions of the infected collecting system, which may represent clot, sediment, or pus. These echoes shift with changes in patient position. With clinical evidence of significant infection and echogenic urine on ultrasound, urgent decompression of the pyonephrosis should be considered by nephrostomy tube or internal stenting.

The long-term sequelae of pyelonephritis can include renal scarring, and this risk is increased in the presence of VUR [50]. Although the gold standard investigation for renal scarring is a DMSA scan, several findings on US may suggest the presence of scar. A globally small kidney may represent diffuse renal scarring or alternatively hypoplasia (Fig. 13.8). Focal renal scars may be evident by locally thinned cortical parenchyma, irregular outline, and calyceal dilatation [51]. If clinically indicated, a DMSA scan at 6–12 months post infection can be used to confirm the presence of scarring [47].

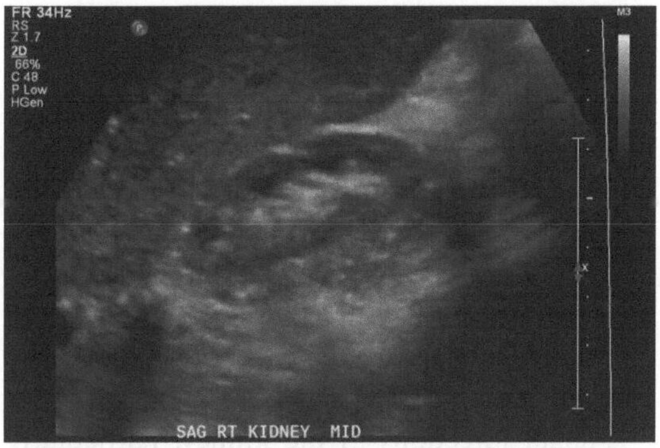

Fig. 13.8 Small globally scarred right kidney in 5-year-old boy with unilateral grade IV vesicoureteral reflux and multiple urinary tract infections

Xanthogranulomatous pyelonephritis (XPN) is a severe chronic renal inflammatory disorder of uncertain origin that is associated with kidney stones, urinary obstruction, and infection [52]. The end result of XPN is a burnt out, nonfunctional kidney characterized by granulomatous inflammatory infiltrate with xanthomatous histiocytes [53]. It is unknown why urinary obstruction due to a stone leads to XPN in some circumstances and not others. Staghorn calculi are common [54]. Although this is usually a process involving the entire kidney, it may occur in a focal form (unassociated with urinary obstruction). Ultrasound may show an enlarged, heterogenous kidney suspicious for a mass. Evidence of urinary obstruction and renal or ureteral stones are often present. Presence of local calcifications may suggest the true diagnosis, but XPN may be mistaken for a neoplastic process. CT scan is generally obtained for better characterization of the process and demonstrates abscess, pyonephrosis, renal atrophy, and inflammatory changes of the perinephric fat or accumulation of perinephric fat. Treatment is generally nephrectomy, although there have been case reports of successful treatment of the focal form of XPN in the pediatric population with long-term intravenous antibiotics [55]. Laparoscopic nephrectomy is being increasingly attempted but the conversion rate to open nephrectomy remains high due to the severe inflammation [56].

Fungal infections of the kidney, particularly candidiasis, are rare but potentially devastating. Preterm infants and immunosuppressed patients are most at risk for fungal involvement of the urinary tract [57]. The classic finding of fungus balls within the collecting system is rare but highly suspicious for candidiasis. These appear as hyperechoic round densities in the collecting system which do not have an acoustic shadow, differentiating them from stones. This finding should prompt an evaluation for systemic fungemia including blood cultures and ophthalmologic exam. In severe cases, bilateral fungal balls or unilateral fungal balls in a solitary kidney may lead to acute renal failure [58]. Fungal obstruction of the bladder outlet has also been described [59]. The mainstay of treatment is systemic antifungal therapy with fluconazole or amphotericin B, but surgical removal of fungal balls may be required in severe or refractory cases [60].

Renal Vascular Disorders

The early onset of severe hypertension in a pediatric patient should raise suspicion of renal artery stenosis (RAS). RAS is usually due to fibromuscular dysplasia in children and as a result commonly involves segmental renal arteries. It is bilateral in 30 % of cases [61]. Other pathologies leading to renal or aortic stenosis include Takayasu's arteritis and mid-aortic syndrome (stenosis of the abdominal aorta) in neurofibromatosis type I. Angiography remains the gold standard for diagnosis [62], but duplex ultrasound is commonly used as an initial screening test. Doppler interrogation of the renal waveforms suggests stenosis by an elevated peak systolic velocity above 2 m/s or the presence of a tardus et parvus waveform, where the peak systolic velocity is low and slow to reach its maximum. Branch vessel stenoses may be missed if they are distal to the point where the systolic velocities are measured. As branch vessel involvement is common in pediatric RAS, this represents a serious cause of false negative studies. Chhadia and colleagues compared duplex ultrasound in the pediatric population to renal artery angiogram. The sensitivity of US was only 64 %. The majority of patients with missed RAS had branch vessel involvement and severe hypertension, leading the authors to recommend that in the clinical setting of severe hypertension, consideration should be made to proceeding with a diagnostic angiogram despite a negative US study [63]. Endovascular techniques are being increasingly applied to RAS. Angioplasty has been widely used. Stenting has traditionally been avoided in fibromuscular dysplasia as well as in the pediatric population in general, but has been used with some reported success [64]. In the event of unsuitable anatomy or stenosis refractory to endovascular therapy, open repair may be required. Ex vivo repair may be necessary in the case of complex branch vessel stenosis [62].

Renal and Adrenal Neoplasms

US often represents the first-line imaging modality in the diagnosis of abdominal masses. Cystic masses of the kidney are commonly MCDK (discussed above), although cystic nephroma is a rare tumor of the kidney. More commonly, a solid renal tumor may contain cystic components. Antenatal or neonatal detection of a solid renal mass by physical exam or ultrasound should raise the suspicion of a congenital mesoblastic nephroma (CMN). These masses are generally large and often associated with polyhydramnios. The tumor exhibits low echogenicity and often has concentric hyper- and hypoechoic rings. CMN is characterized by infiltration of surrounding renal parenchyma without infiltration of the renal vein. Further imaging with CT or MR is indicated prior to definitive surgical excision, but clear differentiation from a Wilms' tumor may not be possible preoperatively. These tumors have low malignant potential, except in the case of the cellular form of CMN. Cellular CMN has cytogenetic similarity to congenital fibrosarcoma and may exhibit more aggressive behavior [65].

Wilms' tumor (WT) appears as a large heterogenous lesion arising from the kidney, without calcifications (although calcifications may be present in 5–10 % of WT). Unlike in CMN, there tends to be a well-defined pseudocapsule [66]. Anechoic components represent necrosis, hemorrhage, or cysts within the tumor. Doppler US is very helpful in the assessment of venous extension of tumor into the renal vein and inferior vena cava. Vessel patency must be interrogated to the level of the hepatic veins. Nephrogenic rests may sometimes be observed; however, on ultrasound these have similar echogenicity to the renal parenchyma and may be missed. Once the diagnosis of tumor is made by US, current Children's Oncology Group (COG) and Society of Paediatric Oncology (SIOP) protocols mandate appropriate cross sectional imaging (MRI or CT) for further characterization of the tumor and operative planning.

Other rarer renal tumors include clear cell sarcoma of the kidney, rhabdoid tumor, and juvenile renal cell carcinoma. Renal medullary carcinoma is a highly lethal tumor associated with sickle cell trait [65]. US cannot reliably distinguish between these renal tumors. Further imaging and biopsy are generally necessary. Angiomyolipoma is a hamartomatous tumor associated with tuberous sclerosis. The classic defining feature is the presence of fat, which lends a very hyperechoic appearance to the tumor on US. Approximately 33 % of small angiolipomas demonstrate some degree of posterior acoustic shadowing [67].

Renal US is indicated for screening purposes in genetic syndromes associated with WT, such as Beckwith–Wiedemann syndrome and Simpson–Golabi–Behmel syndrome. Screening is generally performed every 3 months for the first several years of life, typically at least until the age of 8 [68].

Renal Transplantation in the Pediatric Population

Ultrasound has an excellent track record in the evaluation of renal allograft function and assessment of complications after transplantation. Transplant kidneys are typically placed in the retroperitoneum, generally in the right iliac fossa, with vascular anastomoses to the external iliac arteries. Small pediatric patients do not have adequate space in the retroperitoneum for an adult kidney, and in this situation the kidney is placed intraperitoneally with vascular anastomoses to the aorta and inferior vena cava [69]. Most transplant surgeons obtain an initial baseline ultrasound within 1–2 days postoperatively.

Vascular complications are the most feared in the early postoperative period. Renal artery thrombosis is rare (<1 %) but devastating. It typically occurs within 1 week and is visualized as absence of flow distal to the renal artery in a hypoechoic kidney. Segmental thrombosis can occur with wedge-shaped areas of the kidney that lack flow on Doppler [70]. Absence of renal vein flow with reversal of arterial flow during diastole is a sign of renal vein thrombosis. Significant vascular compromise in the immediate postoperative period generally requires urgent operative revision. RAS of the transplant artery usually develops within a year of transplant and shows the same signs as in the native kidney, with increased systolic velocity and tardus et parvus waveforms [71].

Ultrasound is very sensitive in the detection of perinephric fluid collections, but cannot reliably distinguish between hematoma, urinoma, and lymphocele. Generally, hematomas appear in the immediate postoperative period, while urine leaks often present after several days and lymphoceles after several weeks [72]. Hematoma tends to have a very heterogenous appearance on ultrasound as opposed to the simple anechoic fluid of lymphocele or urinoma. In the case of ongoing diagnostic uncertainty, aspiration of the fluid may be helpful in determining the etiology as a urine leak demonstrates a very high creatinine level in the aspirated fluid, while a lymphocele has a composition similar to serum.

Urine leak from an intraperitoneal kidney leads to ascites. Treatment of a urine leak may include percutaneous nephrostomy or stenting to divert the urine flow and allow for healing of the ureteral anastomosis, but open surgical revision is necessary in large leaks or where ureteral necrosis is suspected. [73] Lymphoceles are frequently septated on US and benefit from image-guided drainage with or without concomitant sclerosis, but operative marsupialization may be necessary if persistent [74].

Measurement of the vascular resistive index (RI) is an essential part of the transplant assessment. It is measured at the arcuate or interlobar arteries and is calculated by the formula (peak systolic velocity—end diastolic velocity)/peak systolic velocity [70]. Less than 0.7 represents a normal value. Elevated RI may be found in acute tubular necrosis, rejection, renal vein thrombosis, and renal dysfunction due to immunosuppressive toxicity from calcineurin inhibitors. Unfortunately, rejection, calcineurin toxicity, and acute tubular necrosis all have nonspecific imaging findings and elevated RI, and renal biopsy is often needed in the case of graft dysfunction without clear vascular abnormalities [9, 75].

Ultrasound Guidance in Renal Biopsy

Ultrasound represents an ideal modality for image-guided biopsy of native or transplant kidneys. Ultrasound guidance allows selection of a safe track for core needle biopsy of kidney parenchyma, avoiding injury to vessels via use of Doppler imaging. Spring-loaded biopsy guns allow easy acquisition of cores of tissue for histologic analysis. The patient is placed in the prone or lateral position (for native kidneys) or supine position (for transplant kidneys), and an initial ultrasound survey with Doppler examines the orientation of the kidney and vessels. The lower pole is the preferable target in the native kidney. After appropriate skin preparation, a small puncture incision is made to allow easy passage of the biopsy gun, passed through a needle guide on the ultrasound probe. The needle should be directed with the tip away from the renal hilum, towards the corticomedullary junction. A tangential approach, with the needle aimed 45–60° from the renal capsule, has been advocated [76]. Several passes may be taken to maximize the specimen available for pathologic analysis.

The reported complication rate of renal biopsy varies widely from 2–32 % [77]. Most complications are evident within several hours of the procedure. Hematuria represents the most frequent complication of biopsy (5–7 %) and is usually self-limited. It typically presents with the first void. Arteriovenous fistula is a more serious complication and may require embolization to correct. Perirenal hematoma is another possible outcome of biopsy and can require blood transfusion. A postprocedure ultrasound is very accurate at identifying arteriovenous (AV)fistulae and hematoma and determining which patients may require embolization. Despite these risks, renal biopsy is generally quite safe and performed as an outpatient procedure [78].

Renal Trauma

The kidney is frequently injured in pediatric trauma, but the vast majority of even severe kidney injuries can be managed nonoperatively [79, 80]. The focused assessment with sonography in trauma (FAST) scan is a widely used screening tool in the urgent evaluation of the pediatric trauma patient. Images are taken in four windows (pericardial, pelvic, perihepatic, perisplenic) to identify the presence of free fluid [81]. The FAST scan is designed to evaluate for intraperitoneal blood, but by definition it is not sensitive for retroperitoneal injuries and cannot be used to rule out renal injury [82, 83]. The finding of gross or microscopic hematuria (>50 red blood cells per high-powered field) in a pediatric trauma patient requires additional investigation with a definitive study. The gold standard evaluation for renal trauma is CT with intravenous contrast, which clearly delineates renal vasculature, parenchymal lacerations, and perirenal fluid collections [84]. Delayed imaging during the excretory phase improves detection of urine leaks. Ultrasound is not as sensitive as CT in the diagnosis of renal injury. While perinephric collections can be seen, it is difficult to distinguish between hematoma and urinoma by US. Parenchymal contusions are often missed on ultrasound. However, the desire to avoid unnecessary radiation exposure—the "as low as reasonably achievable" principle [85]—has motivated further investigation into the use of ultrasound as a primary modality in the investigation of blunt pediatric trauma patients. The rationale for this is that although ultrasound is overall less sensitive than CT, clinically significant injuries are likely to be apparent [86]. Doppler interrogation of the vessels is critical as part of this evaluation to ensure that the kidney has not been devascularized. Amerdorfer recommends the use of primary US with Doppler imaging in patients with minor or moderate trauma who are stable. Patients with a normal examination or minor pathology undergo a follow-up US within 24 h, while patients with inconclusive or severely abnormal scans receive a CT [87]. Recent recommendations of the European Society of Radiology recommend the use of US with Doppler as a first-line modality in minor to moderate trauma and in severe trauma isolated to the flank in a stable patient [88]. CT may be used where additional information is expected to alter the treatment plan. Application of these protocols in clinical practice is dependent on the quality of pediatric US available at a given institution.

Although its use as a primary imaging modality remains debatable, US is recommended for serial examinations of documented renal injury

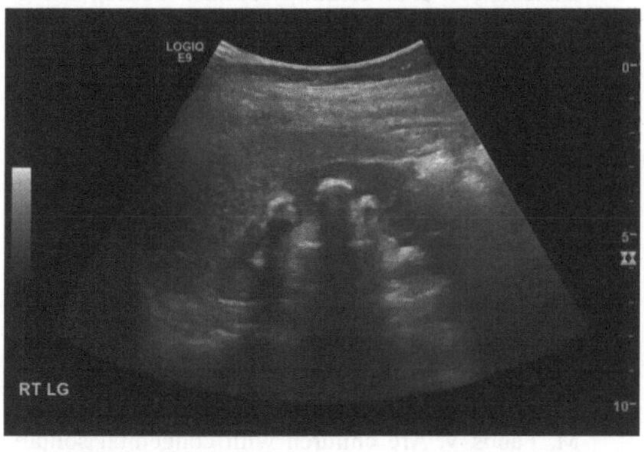

Fig. 13.9 Staghorn renal calculus with posterior acoustic shadowing

to avoid further radiation exposure caused by routine repeat CT scan [88]. Ultrasound is sensitive in the detection of perinephric fluid collections and hence the detection of an expanding urinoma or hematoma requiring treatment. Eeg presented a series of 73 patients with CT-documented renal injury who underwent reevaluation with ultrasound 36–48 h after injury. No missed complications were identified in this cohort [89]. Other authors have also published favorable experiences with the use of US for reevaluation of documented renal injury [90].

Urolithiasis

Stone disease represents an increasing problem in the pediatric population. Seven percent of all stones are found in patients younger than 16 (Coran), and emergency department visits for pediatric renal colic have doubled between 1999 and 2008 [91]. The main etiologies for stone formation are metabolic disease, drug-induced calculi, anatomic anomalies causing obstruction or stasis, foreign bodies (stents), and infections, but around 12% are idiopathic. Nearly 70% of pediatric patients suffer a recurrence of stone disease over a 5-year period [92], and this presents concern for radiation exposure in the setting of repeated CT scans. Many authors consider US to be the primary investigation for suspected urinary tract calculi in the pediatric population [93–95] Clinical presentation depends on age with abdominal or loin pain, hematuria, and infection being the typical presenting symptoms.

The diagnosis of a urinary tract stone requires the presence of a hyperechoic focus with an acoustic shadow (Fig. 13.9). Specificity of stone detection is greater in the ureter than in the kidney due to surrounding tissues in the kidney which can be mistaken for stones, while sensitivity is greater in the kidney due to bowel gas and other intervening tissues obstructing the visualization of the ureter [94]. The mid ureter is the most difficult location to visualize stones, but is also the least likely site of stone impaction in a pediatric patient [96]. Stones are most common in the distal ureter and renal pelvis. Following the hydroureter to the point of obstruction may help find an otherwise obscure calculus [97]. The anatomical localization of a stone inside the kidney may be difficult to assess in the absence of pelvicalyceal dilation [98]. The measurement of stone size is essential to help decide on the therapeutic approach, and this is based on the maximum recorded length. Stone size can be overestimated when using only US [94].

US has a broad reported sensitivity from 44–90% in all age groups, as compared to 94–99% in CT [95]. There are several associated findings that can improve the effectiveness of the initial sonographic investigation [94, 99]. Obstruction of the upper urinary tract induces changes in the intrarenal blood flow which can be evaluated by measuring the RI. An RI >0.70 or a difference, when comparing both sides, of >0.06 is suggestive of obstruction and increases specificity and sensitivity when investigating for a suspected stone [100]. This is less valid if the patient is taking nonsteroidal anti-inflammatory drugs, in the setting of acute obstruction (<6 h), or in partial obstruction. Documentation of frequency, peak velocity, and duration of the ureteral jets has been described to have a very high sensitivity and good specificity when looking for obstruction, and confounding effect of poor hydration can be overcome by comparing jets from both sides [101]. Comparison of a plain abdominal film to the initial US helps improve sensitivity and specificity of the radiological workup, more so in the presence of ureteral stones where US detection rate is around 38% [102] , with results of the combined modalities approaching what is expected from CT investigations [99]. In the clinical setting where a stone is strongly suspected but not observed on US, CT should be considered as it remains the gold standard evaluation and has better sensitivity for small stones and ureteral stones [103].

Summary

Renal US is a fundamental tool in the armamentarium of the pediatric surgeon and urologist. Renal ultrasound should routinely include evaluation of the kidneys, ureters, and bladder, both pre- and post-micturition. Doppler imaging adds valuable information about vasculature. US defines unusual renal anatomy and has a critical role in the evaluation of hydronephrosis and hydroureter. It is the initial imaging study in the evaluation of abdominal masses. It serves a valuable role in postinjury evaluation of the renal trauma patient and is a cornerstone of evaluation of the renal transplant patient. US contributes functional information to the evaluation of urolithiasis.

References

1. Bis K, Slovis T. Accuracy of ultrasonic bladder volume measurement in children. Pediatr Radiol. 1990;20:457–60.
2. Austin PF, et al. The standardization of terminology of lower urinary tract function in children and adolescents: update report from the standardization committee of the international children's continence society. J Urol. 2014;191:1863–5.
3. Erdemir A, et al. Reference ranges for sonographic renal dimensions in preterm infants. Pediatr Radiol. 2013;43:1475–84.
4. Han BK, Babcock DS. Sonographic measurements and appearance of normal kidneys in children. AJR Am J Roentgenol. 1985;145:611–6.
5. Peratoner L, et al. Kidney length and scarring in children with urinary tract infection: importance of ultrasound scans. Abdom Imaging. 2005;30:780–5.
6. Krill A, et al. Evaluating compensatory hypertrophy: a growth curve specific for solitary functioning kidneys. J Urol. 2012;188:1613–7.
7. Williams H. Renal revision: from lobulation to duplication--what is normal? Arch Dis Child Educ Pract Ed. 2007;92:ep152–8.
8. Daneman A, et al. Renal pyramids: focused sonography of normal and pathologic processes. Radiographics. 2010;30:1287–307.
9. Lockhart ME, Robbin ML. Renal vascular imaging: ultrasound and other modalities. Ultrasound Q. 2007;23:279–92.
10. Schantz-Dunn J, Laufer MR. Obstructed hemivagina and ipsilateral renal anomaly. (OHVIRA) syndrome with a single septate uterus: first case report. Fertil Steril. 2007;88:192.
11. Rousset P, et al. Ultrasonography and MRI features of the Mayer-Rokitansky-Kuster-Hauser syndrome. Clin Radiol. 2013;68:945–52.
12. Zaffanello M, Brugnara M, Zuffante M, Franchini M, Fanos V. Are children with congenital solitary kidney at risk for lifelong complications? A lack of prediction demands caution. Int Urol Nephrol. 2009;41:127–35.

13. Hellerstein S, Chambers L. Solitary kidney. Clin Pediatr (Phila). 2008;47:652–8.
14. Brenner BM, Lawler EV, Mackenzie HS. The hyperfiltration theory: a paradigm shift in nephrology. Kidney Int. 1996;49:1774–7.
15. Shirzai A, et al. Is microalbuminuria a risk factor for hypertension in children with solitary kidney? Pediatr Nephrol. 2014;29:283–8.
16. Hegde S, Coulthard MG. Renal agenesis and unilateral nephrectomy: what are the risks of living with a single kidney? Pediatr Nephrol. 2009;24:439–46.
17. Siomou E, et al. Growth and function in childhood of a normal solitary kidney from birth or from early infancy. Pediatr Nephrol. 2014;29:249–56.
18. Vester U, Kranz B, Hoyer PF. The diagnostic value of ultrasound in cystic kidney diseases. Pediatr Nephrol. 2010;25:231–40.
19. Fufezan O, Asavoaie C, Blag C, Popa G. The role of ultrasonography for diagnosis the renal masses in children. Pictorial essay. Med Ultrason. 2011;13:59–71.
20. Hains DS, Bates CM, Ingraham S, Schwaderer AL. Management and etiology of the unilateral multicystic dysplastic kidney: a review. Pediatr Nephrol. 2009;24:233–41.
21. Narchi H. Risk of hypertension with multicystic kidney disease: a systematic review. Arch Dis Child. 2005;90:921–4.
22. Mattoo TK, Greifer I, Geva P, Spitzer A. Acquired renal cystic disease in children and young adults on maintenance dialysis. Pediatr Nephrol. 1997;11:447–50.
23. Avni FE, et al. Perinatal assessment of hereditary cystic renal diseases: the contribution of sonography. Pediatr Radiol. 2006;36:405–14.
24. Rizk D, Chapman A. Treatment of autosomal dominant polycystic kidney disease (ADPKD): the new horizon for children with ADPKD. Pediatr Nephrol. 2008;23:1029–36.
25. Hartung Ea, Guay-Woodford LM. Autosomal recessive polycystic kidney disease: a hepatorenal fibrocystic disorder with pleiotropic effects. Pediatrics. 2014;134:e833–45.
26. Avni FE, Hall M. Renal cystic diseases in children: new concepts. Pediatr Radiol. 2010;40:939–46.
27. Hampton LJ, Borden TA. Ureteropelvic junction obstruction in a thoracic kidney treated by dismembered pyeloplasty. Urology. 2002;60:164.
28. Jefferson KP, Persad RA. Thoracic kidney: a rare form of renal ectopia. J Urol. 2001;165:504.
29. Weizer AZ, et al. Determining the incidence of horseshoe kidney from radiographic data at a single institution. J Urol. 2003;170:1722–6.
30. Daneman A, Alton D. Radiographic manifestations of renal anomalies. Radiol Clin North Am. 1991;29:351–63.
31. Guarino N, et al. The incidence of associated urological abnormalities in children with renal ectopia. J. Urol. 2004;172:1757–59 (discussion 1759).
32. Van den Bosch CM, et al. Urological and nephrological findings of renal ectopia. J Urol. 2010;183:1574–8.
33. Gökaslan F, Yalçınkaya F, Fitöz S, Özçakar ZB. Evaluation and outcome of antenatal hydronephrosis: a prospective study. Ren Fail. 2012;34:718–21.
34. Fernbach SK, Maizels M, Conway JJ. Ultrasound grading of hydronephrosis: introduction to the system used by the society for fetal urology. Pediatr Radiol. 1993;23:478–80.
35. Pereira AK, et al. Antenatal ultrasonographic anteroposterior renal pelvis diameter measurement: is it a reliable way of defining fetal hydronephrosis? Obstet Gynecol Int. 2011;2011:861865.
36. Burgu B, et al. When is it necessary to perform nuclear renogram in patients with a unilateral neonatal hydronephrosis? World J Urol. 2012;30:347–52.
37. Subramaniam R. European society for pediatric urology web book. 2013;8–24. https://www.espu.org/educational-committee/espu-web-book.
38. Kljucevšek D, Kljucevšek T, Levart TK, Novljan G, Kenda RB. Catheter-free methods for vesicoureteric reflux detection: our experience and a critical appraisal of existing data. Pediatr Nephrol. 2010;25:1201–6.
39. Snow BW, Taylor MB. Non-invasive vesicoureteral reflux imaging. J Pediatr Urol. 2010;6:543–9.
40. Darge K. Voiding urosonography with US contrast agents for the diagnosis of vesicoureteric reflux in children: II. Comparison with radiological examinations. Pediatr Radiol. 2008;38:54–63.
41. Williams CR, Pérez LM, Joseph DB. Accuracy of renal-bladder ultrasonography as a screening method to suggest posterior urethral valves. J Urol. 2001;165:2245–7.
42. Mårild S, Jodal U. Incidence rate of first-time symptomatic urinary tract infection in children under 6 years of age. Acta Paediatr. 1998;87:549–52.
43. Guideline CP. Urinary tract infection: clinical practice guideline for the diagnosis and management of the initial UTI in febrile infants and children 2 to 24 months. Pediatrics. 2011;128:595–610.
44. National collaborating centre for women's and children's health (UK). Urinary tract infection in children: diagnosis, treatment and long-term management (NICE Clin. Guidel.). London: RCOG Press; 2007 (54).
45. Shortliffe L. Campbell Walsh urology. 10. Edn. vol. 4. 2012. pp. 3085–3122. https://www.nice.org.uk/guidance/cg54.
46. Craig WD, Wagner BJ, Travis MD. Pyelonephritis: radiologic-pathologic review. Radiographics. 2008;28:255–77 (quiz 327–328).
47. Ghasemi K, Montazeri S, Pashazadeh AM, Javadi H, Assadi M. Correlation of 99mTc-DMSA scan with radiological and laboratory examinations in childhood acute pyelonephritis: a time-series study. Int Urol Nephrol. 2013;45:925–32.
48. Halevy R, et al. Power doppler ultrasonography in the diagnosis of acute childhood pyelonephritis. Pediatr Nephrol. 2004;19:987–91.
49. Basiratnia M, Noohi AH, Lotfi M, Alavi MS. Power doppler sonographic evaluation of acute childhood pyelonephritis. Pediatr Nephrol. 2006;21:1854–7.

50. Lee YJ, Lee JH, Park YS. Risk factors for renal scar formation in infants with first episode of acute pyelonephritis: a prospective clinical study. J Urol. 2012;187:1032–6.
51. Barry BP, et al. Improved ultrasound detection of renal scarring in children following urinary tract infection. Clin Radiol. 1998;53:747–51.
52. Smith EA, Styn N, Wan J, McHugh J, Dillman JR. Xanthogranulomatous pyelonephritis: an uncommon pediatric renal mass. Pediatr Radiol. 2010;40:1421–5.
53. Li L, Parwani AV. Xanthogranulomatous pyelonephritis. Arch Pathol Lab Med. 2011;135:671–4.
54. Loffroy R, et al. Xanthogranulomatous pyelonephritis in adults: clinical and radiological findings in diffuse and focal forms. Clin Radiol. 2007;62:884–90.
55. Gupta S, Araya CE, Dharnidharka VR. Xanthogranulomatous pyelonephritis in pediatric patients: case report and review of literature. J Pediatr Urol. 2010;6:355–8.
56. Korkes F, et al. Xanthogranulomatous pyelonephritis: clinical experience with 41 Cases. Urology. 2008;71:178–80.
57. Sobel JD, Fisher JF, Kauffman CA, Newman CA. Candida urinary tract infections—Epidemiology. Clin Infect Dis. 2011;52:433–6.
58. Aysel K, et al. Acute renal failure caused by fungus balls in renal pelvises. Pediatr Int. 2009;51:836–8.
59. Baetz-Greenwalt B, Debaz B, Kumar ML. Bladder fungus ball: a reversible cause of neonatal obstructive uropathy. Pediatrics. 1988;81:826–9.
60. Vázquez-Tsuji O, Campos-Rivera T, Ahumada-Mendoza H, Rondán-Zárate A, Martínez-Barbabosa I. Renal ultrasonography and detection of pseudomycelium in urine as means of diagnosis of renal fungus balls in neonates. Mycopathologia. 2005;159:331–7.
61. Srinivasan A, et al. Spectrum of renal findings in pediatric fibromuscular dysplasia and neurofibromatosis type 1. Pediatr Radiol. 2011;41:308–16.
62. Tullus K. Renal artery stenosis: Is angiography still the gold standard in 2011? Pediatr Nephrol. 2011;26:833–7.
63. Chhadia S, Cohn RA, Vural G, Donaldson JS. Renal doppler evaluation in the child with hypertension: a reasonable screening discriminator? Pediatr Radiol. 2013;43:1549–56.
64. Colyer JH, Ratnayaka K, Slack MC, Kanter JP. Renal artery stenosis in children: therapeutic percutaneous balloon and stent angioplasty. Pediatr Nephrol. 2014;29:1067–74.
65. Ahmed H, et al. Part II: treatment of primary malignant non-Wilms' renal tumours in children. Lancet Oncol. 2007;8:842–8.
66. Riccabona M. Imaging of renal tumours in infancy and childhood. Eur Radiol. 2003;13:116–29.
67. Jinzaki M, et al. Renal angiomyolipoma: a radiological classification and update on recent developments in diagnosis and management. Abdom Imaging. 2014;39:588–604.
68. Tan TY, Amor DJ. Tumour surveillance in Beckwith-Wiedemann syndrome and hemihyperplasia: a critical review of the evidence and suggested guidelines for local practice. J Paediatr Child Health. 2006;42:486–90.
69. Van Heurn E, De Vries EE. Kidney transplantation and donation in children. Pediatr Surg Int. 2009;25:385–93.
70. Sharfuddin A. Renal relevant radiology: imaging in kidney transplantation. Clin J Am Soc Nephrol. 2014;9:416–29.
71. Friedewald SM, Molmenti EP, Friedewald JJ, DeJong MR, Hamper UM. Vascular and nonvascular complications of renal transplants: sonographic evaluation and correlation with other imaging modalities, surgery, and pathology. J Clin Ultrasound. 2005;33:127–39.
72. Irshad A, Ackerman SJ, Campbell AS, Anis M. An overview of renal transplantation: current practice and use of ultrasound. Semin Ultrasound CT MRI. 2009;30:298–314.
73. Castagnetti M, et al. Ureteral complications after renal transplant in children: timing of presentation, and their open and endoscopic management. Pediatr Transplant. 2014;18:150–4.
74. Lee HS, et al. Laparoscopic fenestration versus percutaneous catheter drainage for lymphocele treatment after kidney transplantation. Transplant Proc. 2013;45:1667–70.
75. Surratt JT, Siegel MJ, Middleton WD. Sonography of complications in pediatric renal. Radiographics. 1990;10:687–99.
76. Cakmakci E, et al. A modified technique for real time ultrasound guided pediatric percutaneous renal biopsy: the angled tangential approach. Quant Imaging Med Surg. 2014;4:190–4.
77. Franke M, et al. Ultrasound-guided percutaneous renal biopsy in 295 children and adolescents: role of ultrasound and analysis of complications. Plos One. 2014;9:e114737.
78. Al Makdama A, Al-Akash S. Safety of percutaneous renal biopsy as an outpatient procedure in pediatric patients. Ann Saudi Med. 2006;26:303–5.
79. Rogers CG, et al. High-grade renal injuries in children—Is conservative management possible? Urology. 2004;64:574–9.
80. Umbreit EC, Routh JC, Husmann DA. Nonoperative management of nonvascular grade IV blunt renal trauma in children: meta-analysis and systematic review. Urology. 2009;74:579–82.
81. Scalea TM, et al. Focused assessment with sonography for trauma (FAST): results from an international consensus conference. J Trauma. 1999;46:466–72.
82. Coley BD. Pediatric applications of abdominal vascular doppler imaging: part I. Pediatr Radiol. 2004;34:757–71.
83. Emery KH, et al. Absent peritoneal fluid on screening trauma ultrasonography in children: a prospective comparison with computed tomography. J Pediatr Surg. 2001;36:565–9.

84. Stanescu AL, Gross JA, Bittle M, Mann FA. Imaging of blunt abdominal trauma. Semin Roentgenol. 2006;41:196–208.
85. Slovis TL, Berdon WE. Perfect is the enemy of the very good. Pediatr Radiol. 2002;32:217–8.
86. McGahan JP, Richards JR, Jones CD, Gerscovich EO. Use of ultrasonography in the patient with acute renal trauma. J. Ultrasound Med. 1999;18:207–213 (quiz 215–216).
87. Amerstorfer EE, Haberlik A, Riccabona M. Imaging assessment of renal injuries in children and adolescents: CT or ultrasound? J Pediatr Surg. 2014;50:448–55.
88. Riccabona M, et al. ESPR uroradiology task force and ESUR paediatric working group: imaging recommendations in paediatric uroradiology, part IV: minutes of the ESPR uroradiology task force minisymposium on imaging in childhood renal hypertension and imaging of renal trauma. Pediatr Radiol. 2011;41:939–44.
89. Eeg KR, et al. Single center experience with application of the ALARA concept to serial imaging studies after blunt renal trauma in children-is ultrasound enough? J Urol. 2009;181:1834–40.
90. Canon S, et al. The utility of initial and follow-up ultrasound reevaluation for blunt renal trauma in children and adolescents. J Pediatr Urol. 2014;10:815–8.
91. Ng C, Tsung JW. Avoiding computed tomography scans by using point-of-care ultrasound when evaluating suspected pediatric renal colic. J Emerg Med. 2015:1–7. doi:10.1016/j.jemermed.2015.01.017.
92. Milliner DS, Murphy ME. Urolithiasis in pediatric patients. Mayo Clin Proc. 1993;68:241–8.
93. Smith SL, Somers JM, Broderick N, Halliday K. The role of the plain radiograph and renal tract ultrasound in the management of children with renal tract calculi. Clin Radiol. 2000;55:708–10.
94. Ray AA, Ghiculete D, Pace KT, Honey RJD. Limitations to ultrasound in the detection and measurement of urinary tract calculi. Urology. 2010;76:295–300.
95. Passerotti C, et al. Ultrasound versus computerized tomography for evaluating urolithiasis. J Urol. 2009;182:1829–34.
96. Abhishek, et al. Pediatric urolithiasis: experience from a tertiary referral center. J Pediatr Urol. 2013;9:825–30.
97. Ripollés T, et al. Suspected ureteral colic: plain film and sonography vs unenhanced helical CT. A prospective study in 66 patients. Eur Radiol. 2004;14:129–36.
98. Sandhu C, Anson KM, Patel U. Urinary tract stones—Part I: role of radiological imaging in diagnosis and treatment planning. Clin Radiol. 2003;58:415–21.
99. Catalano O, Nunziata A, Altei F, Siani A. Suspected ureteral colic: primary helical CT versus selective helical CT after unenhanced radiography and sonography. Am J Roentgenol. 2002;178:379–87.
100. Geavlete P, Georgescu D, Cauni V, Nita G. Value of duplex doppler ultrasonography in renal colic. Eur Urol. 2002;41:71–8.
101. Jandaghi AB, et al. Assessment of ureterovesical jet dynamics in obstructed ureter by urinary stone with color Doppler and duplex Doppler examinations. Urol Res. 2013;41:159–63.
102. Palmer JS, Donaher ER, O'Riordan MA, Dell KM. Diagnosis of pediatric urolithiasis: role of ultrasound and computerized tomography. J Urol. 2005;174:1413–6.
103. Copelovitch L. Urolithiasis in children. Medical approach. Pediatr Clin North Am. 2012;59:885–96.

Adrenal Gland

14

Nathalie Kremer and Judy H. Squires

Introduction

Ultrasound (US) performed with high-frequency (5.0 or 7.5 MHz) transducers provides high-resolution images of the normal adrenal glands in neonates and young infants due to the relatively large size of the glands in relation to the kidney size and the small amount of retroperitoneal fat. It can identify lesions as small as 1 cm in size in all age groups and allows assessment of the nature of the lesions. US imaging in children is a safe, effective, and inexpensive diagnostic imaging tool and is used as a first-line modality. Computed tomography (CT) can often be less useful to diagnose adrenal abnormalities due to the small amount of retroperitoneal fat in infants and the limited ability of CT to distinguish between different soft tissue densities. Magnetic resonance imaging (MRI) has excellent soft tissue differentiation and is the modality of choice for adrenal tumor characterization and staging [1].

N. Kremer (✉)
Department of Pediatric Surgery,
Cincinnati Children's Hospital Medical Center,
3333 Burnet Ave, MLC#5031,
Cincinnati, OH 45229-3026, USA
e-mail: nathalie.kremer@cchmc.org

J. H. Squires
Department of Pediatric Radiology,
Children's Hospital of Pittsburgh,
4401 Penn Avenue 2nd Floor Radiology,
Pittsburgh, PA 15224, USA

Development, Function, and Anatomy

Fetal Development of the Adrenal Glands

The adrenal glands are endocrine organs composed of two entities: the steroid hormone-producing cortex (aldosterone, cortisol, and androgens) and the catecholamine-synthesizing medulla, which have a dual embryological origin. Around the 5th week of gestation, the cortex develops from the mesoderm of the urogenital ridge that later develops into the pro-, meso-, and metanephros. The medulla arises from the neural crest. In the fetus, the cortex is further divided into a wide inner fetal cortex and an outer zone that later becomes the adult cortex. This occurs via hemorrhagic and then necrotic involution of the fetal cortex and proliferation of the adult cortex towards the center of the gland which causes a 30–50 % reduction in the gland weight (Fig. 14.1) [2, 3]. Prior to this, the adrenal glands are 10–20 times larger than adult glands in relation to the total body weight and approximately one third the size of the neonatal kidney [4]. After involution of the fetal cortex, the infant adrenal glands measure between 1 and 3.6 cm (mean 1.5 cm) in length and between 2 and 5 mm (mean 3 mm) in thickness [5, 6]. The adult cortex continues to develop until 3 years of age into three zones: zona glomerulosa, fasciculata, and reticularis.

S. Scholz, M. D. Jarboe (eds.), *Diagnostic and Interventional Ultrasound in Pediatrics and Pediatric Surgery,* DOI 10.1007/978-3-319-21699-7_14

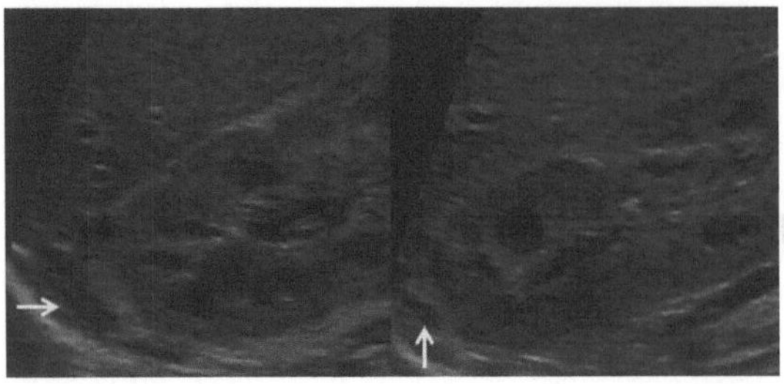

Fig. 14.1 Ultrasound performed on an 11-day-old male with a possible renal cyst seen on prenatal ultrasound screening demonstrates the normal appearance of the right adrenal gland with prominence of the cortex *(left image)*. Follow-up ultrasound at 8 weeks of life demonstrates interval decrease in size of the adrenal gland *(right image)*

Anatomy

The adrenal glands are located within the fascia of Gerota, superior and medial to the upper pole of the kidneys; however, their exact location can be quite variable, making them more challenging to locate with decreasing relative size [7]. Typically, the left gland is located slightly lower and more anteriorly while the right gland is posterior to the inferior vena cava and slightly higher [1]. Heterotopic adrenal glands, horseshoe adrenal glands, and unilateral adrenal gland agenesis have been described, but are rare [8].

The arterial blood supply is provided by the inferior phrenic artery, the aorta, and the renal artery. These arteries further subdivide into small channels that span over the capsule of the gland and form a rich plexus within the gland. There is a single draining vein, but smaller accessory veins are usually found following the anatomic course of the smaller arteries [6].

Ultrasound Appearance of the Normal Adrenal Glands

The glands have a pyramidal or triangular shape and lie just above the upper pole of the kidneys. During infancy, the shape of the adrenal limbs is more bulbous or convex, while in older children the contour tends to have straight or even concave margins. The surface of the glands is usually smooth or mildly undulated. With ipsilateral renal agenesis, the adrenal gland retains a flat or discoid appearance and can be easily confused with renal tissue [9, 10]. Corticomedullary differentiation can be identified on US imaging but varies greatly with age [1, 11]. The cortex has lower echogenicity than the medulla and is prominent in normal newborns because of the thick transient fetal cortical zone. This zone shows a narrow hyperechoic central stripe which represents the congested sinusoids, the central vein, and the small medulla [12]. The adult cortex at this age can be seen with high-resolution US as an echogenic line along the peripheral gland [10, 13]. In the weeks after birth, as the fetal cortex atrophies and is replaced by fibrous tissue, the hyperechoic central stripe becomes broader, while the hypoechoic fetal cortex thins [12].

Solid Tumors of the Adrenal Gland

Primary adrenal neoplasms can be categorized by their origin and function. They arise from either the medulla or cortex, and they are usually nonfunctioning or hyperfunctioning. Medullary neoplasms originate from the neural crest cells and therefore can occur anywhere along the sympathetic neural chain. These neoplasms include neuroblastoma, ganglioneuroblastoma, ganglioneuroma, and pheochromocytoma. Neoplasms arising from the adrenal cortex include adrenocortical carcinoma and adenoma and are very uncommon in children. The rarer adrenal neoplasms of childhood include teratoid rhabdoid tumor and smooth muscle tumors in patients with AIDS. In addition to masses of adrenal origin, extra-adrenal masses in the suprarenal fossa may be difficult to differentiate from primary masses of the adrenal glands. The most common examples are retroperitoneal lymphatic malformations and intra-abdominal extralobar pulmonary sequestrations [7].

Medullary Neoplasms

Neuroblastoma

Neuroblastoma is the second most common intra-abdominal neoplasm after Wilms' tumor and the third most common pediatric tumor after leukemia and tumors of the central nervous system (CNS), accounting for 10% of all pediatric neoplasms [14]. The majority (75%) of neuroblastomas arise in the abdomen, with one third of these in the adrenal glands. The remainder of the neuroblastomas can occur anywhere along the sympathetic nerve chain, from the neck to the pelvis [15]. Over 90% of the patients present between 1 and 5 years (median 2 years). Prenatal diagnosis occurs more frequently due to a rising number of fetal imaging, and currently 20% of all neuroblastomas are diagnosed prenatally or within the first 3 months of life [16].

Clinically, neuroblastoma most commonly presents as a palpable mass, but can be an incidental finding on US or sequential imaging. If symptomatic, children can present with signs of increased adrenal medullary hormone production or symptoms from direct tumor growth or metastatic disease.

Local invasion can occur into the liver, kidneys, and through the neural foramina into the spinal canal, causing cord compression symptoms. Neuroblastomas typically show encasement or displacement of the vascular structures and only rarely invade the vasculature or ureter, which can be helpful to distinguish them from Wilms' tumor. Distant metastases are present in half the cases at the time of diagnosis and are most commonly found in lymph nodes, bone marrow, liver, and skin [7].

US is often the first diagnostic imaging tool applied and can also be helpful in the diagnosis of metastatic disease, especially in liver involvement. On US, the neuroblastoma usually appears as a heterogeneous mass, with hyperechoic areas caused by calcifications, with or without posterior acoustic shadowing. Hypoechoic and anechoic areas in neuroblastoma correspond to cystic, hemorrhagic, or necrotic changes and are less common than in Wilms' tumor. Larger cystic areas are more often present in newborns, in whom bilateral cystic neuroblastoma with intracystic hemorrhage may occur (Fig. 14.2) [17].

Diagnosis of neonatal neuroblastoma is often more challenging for several reasons. Sonographic findings may resemble neonatal adrenal hemorrhage, and, in addition, tests specific to neuroblastoma such as metaiodobenzylguanidine (MIBG) scintigraphy and sampling of urine catecholamines are not reliable in this age group. Urinary catecholamines are increased in 90% of the cases beyond infancy, but only in half of the cases in the first year of life. However, neuroblastoma in neonates usually shows a 4-year survival of greater than 95% and is associated with a high rate of spontaneous regression, so that an expectant approach with serial short-term follow-up US with Doppler is often the only recommended testing [18]. If the mass does not decrease in size or enlarges, and/or shows increasing echogenicity, a more aggressive form of neuroblastoma should be considered [19].

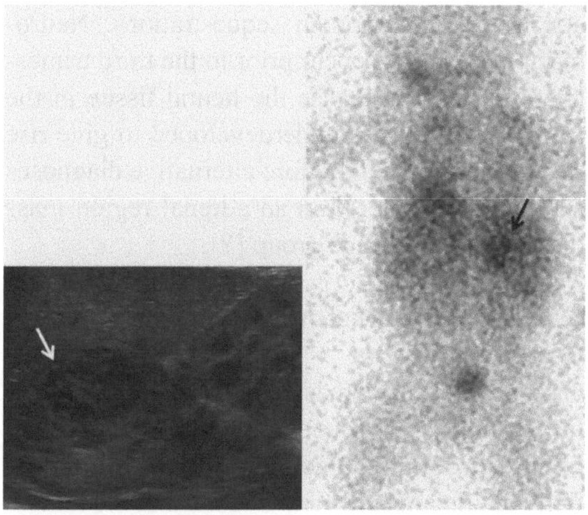

Fig. 14.2 Longitudinal ultrasound in a 29-day-old with a suprarenal mass noted on prenatal ultrasound demonstrates a heterogeneous cystic- and solid-appearing mass in the right adrenal gland. A posterior whole-body image from nuclear medicine I-123-MIBG study demonstrates intense uptake within the mass, consistent with neuroblastoma. No metastatic foci were seen

Other differential diagnoses in the neonatal period include intra-abdominal extralobar pulmonary sequestrations. Helpful hints are the location and morphology, with sequestrations being more commonly located in the left suprarenal region, while neonatal neuroblastoma is more commonly located on the right side and is more heterogeneous in morphology. Calcifications occur in neuroblastoma and have not been reported in sequestrations. Additionally, feeding arteries are common in sequestrations. Neuroblastoma does not occur prior to the third trimester of gestation because the neural tissue in the adrenal gland is too underdeveloped to give rise to neuroblastoma, therefore alternative diagnoses should be considered in an adrenal region mass discovered in this age group [7].

Ganglioneuroblastoma and Ganglioneuroma

Ganglioneuroblastomas arise from both, the mature ganglion cells and immature cells resembling neuroblastoma cells, resulting in a potentially malignant behavior. One third of the tumors arise in the adrenal gland, one third in the retroperitoneum, and the remaining one third in the posterior mediastinum, with only rare manifestations in the neck or pelvis [12].

Ganglioneuromas are the most mature neural crest tumors and are histologically benign. One third of the cases are located in the retroperitoneum, and only rarely do they arise in the adrenal gland. Ganglioneuromas occur in older children, can be completely asymptomatic, and are often incidental findings on US or chest radiographs. When they invade the spine, neurologic symptoms can occur related to cord compression. Ganglioneuroblastomas and Ganglioneuromas cannot be distinguished from neuroblastoma with imaging alone, and therefore there is no standard imaging protocol for follow-up [12].

Pheochromocytoma

Pheochromocytoma is an uncommon pediatric neoplasm. It accounts for less than 1 % of all tumors seen in pediatric centers and is rarely diagnosed in infancy with the mean age at diagnosis being 11 years in children [20]. In the pediatric age group, 80 % of pheochromocytomas occur in the adrenal gland with bilateral involvement in 25 % [20, 21]. In the 20 % of extra-adrenal cases, the most frequent site is the upper abdomen [22]. Less common extra-adrenal sites include the sympathetic chain in a cervical, thoracic, or pelvic location, and, in rare cases, they may occur in the urinary bladder, spinal cord, and vagina. When occurring outside the adrenal gland, the tumors are usually referred to as paragangliomas. Multiple tumors are present in 30–70 % of the patients, especially in those with a positive family history for pheochromocytoma and in association with multiple endocrine neoplasia (MEN) type II, neurofibromatosis 1, or von Hippel–Lindau disease. In addition to age at presentation, the clinical presentation also differs from neuroblastoma, as pheochromocytoma arises from the chromaffin cells of the medulla that are actively producing epinephrine and norepinephrine and occasionally vasoactive intestinal peptide (VIP). The first-line imaging modality is US, on which pheochromocytoma may present as a homogeneous soft tissue mass measuring 2–5 cm on average, but it may also contain heterogeneous areas, caused by hemorrhage, necrosis, or calcifications (Fig. 14.3) [7]. The tumor is often well encapsulated and color Doppler examination reveals hypervascularization [23]. MIBG scanning is more sensitive than US and can be positive, even when US shows no abnormalities [17].

Cortical Neoplasms

Primary tumors of the adrenal cortex are extremely rare in children, and their clinical presentation and outcome can differ greatly from the adult-onset disease. Adrenocortical carcinoma is rarely reported, and there are no reports of Conn's

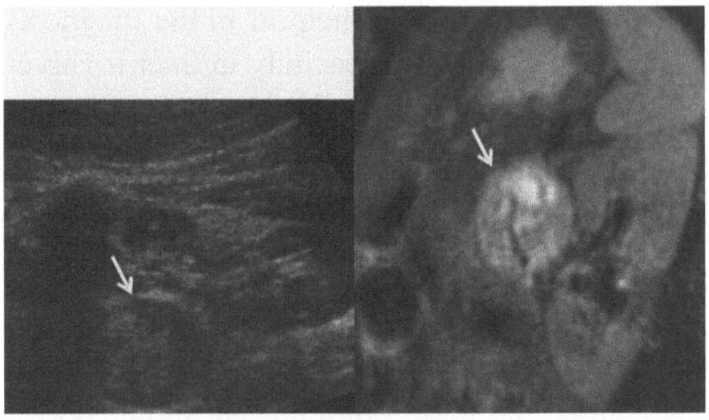

Fig. 14.3 A 14-year-old female with hypertension and elevated urine metanephrines. Longitudinal ultrasound demonstrates a heterogeneously hypoechoic mass in the left adrenal gland. Sagittal T2-weighted fast spin-echo magnetic resonance image demonstrates a heterogeneously hyperintense T2 mass. Pheochromocytoma was confirmed at surgical resection

syndrome resulting from aldosterone-producing adenomas in a pediatric patient.

Adrenocortical carcinoma has an overall incidence of 1–1.5/million/year, peaking in childhood and in the fifth decade of life. The outcome tends to be more favorable when the diagnosis is made under the age of 4; however, the overall 5-year survival of less than 30% is poor [1, 24]. As opposed to adults, where adrenocortical neoplasms are usually nonfunctioning, most pediatric patients present with hormonally active tumors, displaying endocrinologic abnormalities. These include virilization in girls or precocious puberty and Cushing's syndrome in both sexes. Physical exam often will not reveal a palpable tumor; if they are large enough to be found on clinical exam, they are often carcinomas rather than benign neoplasms. US is the first-line imaging method and can be helpful in determining local invasion of the vena cava (Fig. 14.4) [7].

Other Tumors

Other tumors of the adrenal gland are often incidental findings with no further clinical intervention needed. These include myelolipomas and angiomyolipomas that are extremely rare in children [5]. Angiomyolipomas arise from the perivascular epithelioid cells and are typically found in the kidneys. They can be associated with tuberous sclerosis and appear as multiple masses of varying echogenicity depending on the fat content [25]. Myelolipomas contain fatty as well as hematopoietic elements and appear rather homogenous and hyperechoic with no substantial vascularity. They can look impressive on imaging as they can reach sizes reported as large as 10 cm; however, they are benign in nature (Fig. 14.5) [26].

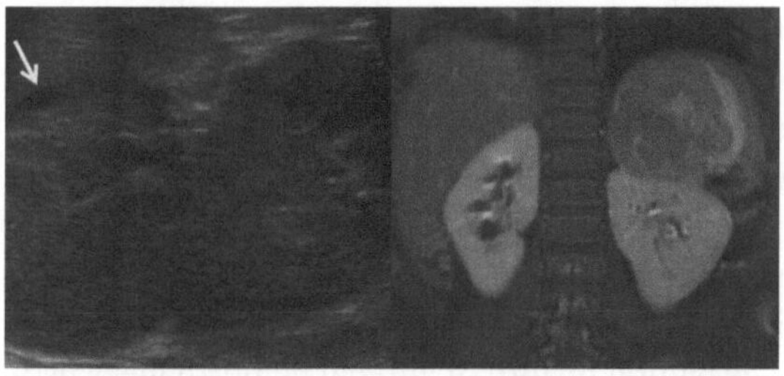

Fig. 14.4 A 2-year-old with abdominal distention and weight gain. Longitudinal ultrasound demonstrates a large heterogeneous mass in the left adrenal gland *(arrow)*. Coronal post-contrast T1 with fat saturation demonstrates heterogeneous enhancement of the mass. Pathologic evaluation at surgical resection confirmed adrenal cortical carcinoma

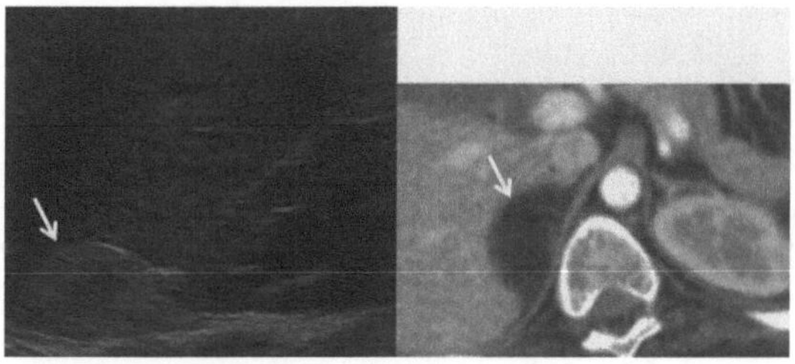

Fig. 14.5 Longitudinal ultrasound in a 25-year-old female with a urinary tract infection shows a relatively hyperechoic circumscribed mass in the right adrenal gland. The fat-attenuation mass did not enhance following contrast administration on computed tomotgraphy (CT), consistent with adrenal myelolipoma

Other adrenal masses that are nonneoplastic in nature include hemorrhage, cysts, and abscesses. They are generally rare and often incidental findings [7].

Hemorrhage

Neonatal Adrenal Hemorrhage

Neonatal adrenal hemorrhage is a rare event commonly presenting within the first week of life with unexplained hyperbilirubinemia. Clinical findings can be subtle and vary. Reports include newborns with hypovolemia, anemia, abdominal mass, or even scrotal or inguinal ecchymosis [27]. Infants at risk are usually macrosomic newborns who underwent stressful delivery, with a higher incidence in vaginal deliveries. In addition, single reports mention an association with anoxia, sepsis, bleeding disorders, and maternal diabetes [28]. Hemorrhage more commonly occurs in the right adrenal gland than left. In the acute phase, US will reveal a heterogeneously hypoechoic mass with a hyperechoic rim [5].

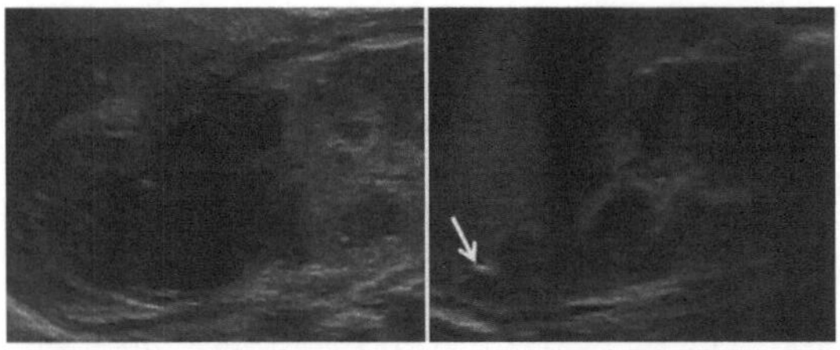

Fig. 14.6 A 7-day-old infant with polycythemia and hypertension. Longitudinal ultrasound demonstrates a heterogeneous, predominantly hypoechoic mass in the left adrenal gland. Follow-up imaging at 1.5 months of life demonstrates decreased size of the mass and a small focus of possible calcification *(arrow)*, compatible with hemorrhage evolution

However, infants often have a delayed presentation, and the sonographic appearance varies depending on the age of the hemorrhage. Typically, as it resolves, the hematoma will increase in size and become more hypoechoic, although there are reports of increased echogenicity [29]. Serial US exams are mandatory to distinguish hemorrhage from a tumor, most importantly, neuroblastoma (Fig. 14.6) [5]. Color Doppler interrogation usually shows no vascular flow within the hemorrhage in contrast to a tumor mass. Also, hemorrhage will gradually decrease in size over time with complete resolution within 3 weeks to 6 months of life. Calcifications can be a late finding after neonatal hemorrhage on long-term follow-up, but the adrenal gland should maintain an adreniform rather than a lobular shape (Fig. 14.7) [29]. Calcification does not occur in the neonatal period. Calcification, mass-like calcification, or Doppler flow in an adrenal mass in a patient of any age should raise suspicion for a solid tumor [30].

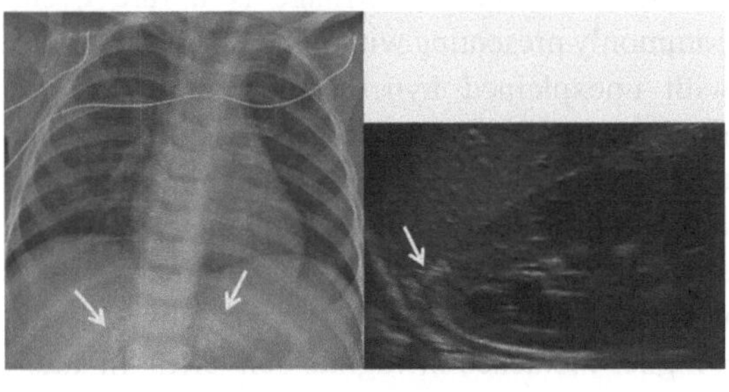

Fig. 14.7 A 2-year-old male with lethargy and incidentally noted calcifications in the region of the adrenal glands on screening chest radiograph *(arrows)*. Longitudinal abdominal ultrasound demonstrates mild non-mass-like enlargement of the right adrenal gland with multiple calcifications *(arrow)*. The left adrenal gland (not shown) had a similar appearance. No etiology was identified

Adrenal Hemorrhage in the Older Child

Adrenal hemorrhage may be seen in association with sepsis and shock due to infection with bacteria such as *Neisseria meningitides, Haemophilus influenzae,* and *Streptococcus pneumoniae* (Waterhouse–Friderichsen syndrome). It has also been reported as a result of anticoagulation therapy and in the setting of heparin-induced thrombocytopenia and in patients with antiphospholipid syndrome or other coagulopathies [31–34]. Most commonly, adrenal hemorrhage in these cases is an incidental finding upon sequential imaging for other causes in a usually severely ill patient. US will demonstrate a heterogeneous mass with areas of hypoechoic necrosis, usually in the cortex, that ultimately heals by the process of fibrosis [31].

Traumatic Adrenal Hemorrhage

Similar to adrenal hemorrhage in the setting of acute illness, adrenal trauma in children is often an incidental finding. However, to the increasing numbers of CT imaging for evaluation of blunt abdominal trauma, the diagnosis of traumatic adrenal hemorrhage is on the rise. In cases where US is obtained, adrenal hemorrhage presents as a well-circumscribed hypoechoic mass superior to the kidney, surrounded by an ill-defined hyperechoic material [1, 35, 36].

As with neonatal hemorrhage, the right adrenal gland is more commonly involved. The liver is the most common associated organ injured. The natural history of adrenal hemorrhage is usually self-limited and of little clinical importance with only single reports of adrenal insufficiency in the setting of massive hemorrhage [35]. If persistent extravasation is documented, only very few cases will require intervention. Angiographic embolization of adrenal hemorrhage as well as surgical exploration has been reported [37].

Adrenal Cysts

Cystic lesions of the adrenal gland are in general rare, usually found in older children, and often asymptomatic. Most adrenal cystic lesions are lymphatic malformations or hemorrhagic pseudocysts (39%) [38]. Simple cysts are round anechoic lesions with an imperceptible wall and have increased through-transmission. Lymphatic malformations may be hypoechoic or anechoic, and there may be internal septae. US in the longitudinal plane and MRI in the coronal plane have been found to be most useful to distinguish cystic lesions of the adrenal gland from renal or hepatic cysts [38]. Management depends on age and is usually conservative [7].

Nonneoplastic Changes of the Adrenal Glands

Congenital Adrenal Hyperplasia

The syndromes of congenital adrenal hyperplasia (CAH) result from a series of autosomal recessive enzymatic defects in the synthesis of adrenal steroids with different presentations depending on the affected enzyme and the severity of the enzyme deficiency. Adrenal hyperplasia in these syndromes results from insufficient production of mineralo- and glucocorticoids, leading to the buildup of precursors and subsequent pituitary adrenocorticotropic hormone (ACTH) overstimulation of the cortex. The most common deficiency affects the enzyme 21-hydroxylase and is responsible for approximately 95% of all cases of CAH [39]. Affected individuals have varying symptoms of cortisol deficiency, including aldosterone deficiency with salt wasting, and excess androgen production with signs of virilization, presenting as ambiguous genitalia in females. Deficiency of 11b-hydroxylase accounts for approximately 5% of all cases of CAH and is associated with increased production of androgens and deoxycorticosterone, leading to virilization and hypertension [31, 40, 41].

While the diagnosis of CAH is mainly made by clinical presentation and hormonal testing, it can be supported by sonographic assessment of the glands. Few infants with CAH will have completely normal-appearing adrenal glands on US, but the findings may be subtle. At the same time, normal-sized adrenal glands do not exclude the diagnosis of CAH. Sequential studies and thorough assessment of all planes in search for these characteristics can be helpful especially in newborns due to the variable size of the normal adrenal glands. In these studies, the width of the gland is often reported a more reliable measurement, and a width greater than 0.5 cm is suspicious for CAH [5]. A wrinkled or cerebriform-appearing cortex has been described in infants with CAH with or without enlargement of the adrenal glands. Due to the high variation in size measurement, some centers find the alteration of echogenicity to be more specific with the most common pattern reported being replacement of the central hyperechoic stripe by diffusely stippled echoes involving the entire adrenal gland (Fig. 14.8). Characteristics of size,

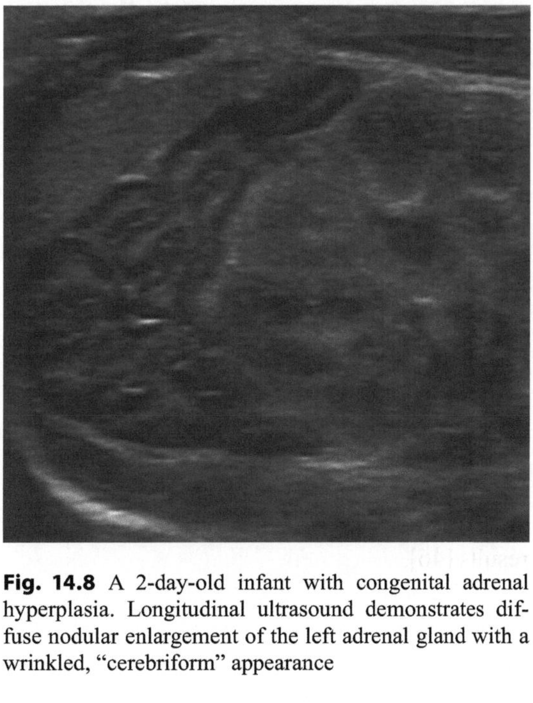

Fig. 14.8 A 2-day-old infant with congenital adrenal hyperplasia. Longitudinal ultrasound demonstrates diffuse nodular enlargement of the left adrenal gland with a wrinkled, "cerebriform" appearance

shape, and echogenicity are considered sufficiently sensitive and specific to make the diagnosis of CAH if two out of three characteristic criteria are met.

Generally, US changes appear to be completely reversible with introduction of steroid replacement therapy, and fetuses who receive intrauterine therapy can have sonographically normal-appearing adrenal glands at birth [12].

In rare untreated cases of CAH in an older child, adrenal enlargement manifests as diffuse hyperplasia or with nodular cortical hyperplasia related to adenoma development resulting from chronic ACTH stimulation [1, 42].

Storage Diseases

Wolman's disease (primary familial xanthomatosis) is a rare lipid storage disorder caused by an autosomal recessive deficiency of lysosomal acid lipase [31, 41, 43]. Patients develop bilateral adrenal enlargement with small calcifications, hepatosplenomegaly, diarrhea, severe failure to thrive due to malabsorption, and death within 6 months of life [44]. Adrenoleukodystrophy (Addison–Schilder's disease) is a rare, X-linked recessive disorder characterized by progressive demyelination of the central and peripheral nervous systems and by adrenal cortical insufficiency [31]. The role of adrenal imaging studies in adrenocortical insufficiency is limited.

Interventional Ultrasound

Abscess formation in the adrenal gland is uncommon in young infants and neonates [45]. Bacterial colonization of an adrenal hematoma is presumably the most likely cause, and timely diagnosis and adequate treatment are of key importance. Surgical exploration is still considered standard treatment; however, reports exist of US- or CT-guided percutaneous drainage with good results [46].

Summary

US imaging of the infant adrenal gland is a very helpful diagnostic tool in the initial assessment of a suspected adrenal pathology. With increasing age, the importance of US decreases as the adrenal glands are harder to visualize; however, US remains the preferred imaging modality in childhood for the initial assessment of the parenchymal organs of the abdomen and retroperitoneum. In the neonate with a suspected adrenal mass, US performed serially over time is often the only imaging necessary to distinguish between a benign, self-limited adrenal hemorrhage and neuroblastoma that may require further investigation and treatment. In experienced hands, US may be used as imaging guidance of percutaneous adrenal procedures.

References

1. Westra SJ, Zaninovic AC, Hall TR, Kangarloo H, Boechat MI. Imaging of the adrenal gland in children. Radiographics. 1994;14(6):1323–40.
2. Sadler TW, Langman J. Langman's medical embryology. 10th ed. Philadelphia: Lippincott Williams & Wilkins; 2006. pp. 314–5.
3. Beck K, Tygstrup I, Nerup J. The involution of the fetal adrenal cortex: a light microscopic study. Acta Pathol Microbiol Scand. 1969;76:391–400.
4. Blake MA, Cronin CG, Boland GW. Adrenal imaging. Am J Roentgenol. 2010;194(6):1450–60. (Erratum in: Am J Roentgenol 2012 May;198(5):1232.
5. Rumack C, Wilson S, Charboneau W, Levine D. Diagnostic Ultrasound. 3rd ed. Vol. 2. Philadelphia: Mosby; 2005.
6. Stephen AE, Haynes AB, Hodin RA. Adrenal surgery. In: Blake MA, Cronin CG, Boland GW, editors. Adrenal imaging. Totowa: Humana Press; 2009. pp. 77–89.
7. Balassy C, Navarro OM, Daneman A. Adrenal masses in children. Radiol Clin North Am. 2011;49(4):711–27.
8. Paterson A. Adrenal pathology in childhood: a spectrum of disease. Eur Radiol. 2002;12(10):2491–508.
9. Kenney PJ, Robbins GL, Effis DA, Spin BA. Adrenal glands in patients with congenital renal anomalies: CT appearance. Radiology. 1985;155:181–2.
10. Kangarloo H, Diament MJ, Gold RH, Barrett C, Lippe B, Geffner M, et al. Sonography of adrenal glands in neonates and children: changes in appearance with age. J Clin Ultrasound. 1986;14:43–7.
11. Mahboubi S, Patel K, O'Neill JA. Computed tomography in the evaluation of adrenal glands in infants

and children. J Comput Tomogr. 1988;12:240–4.
12. Al-Alwan I, Navarro O, Daneman D, Daneman A. Clinical utility of adrenal ultrasonography in the diagnosis of congenital adrenal hyperplasia. J Pediatr. 1999;135(1):71–5.
13. Scott EM, Thomas A, McGarrigle HHG, Lachelin GCL. Serial adrenal ultrasonography in normal neonates. J Ultrasound Med. 1990;9:279–83.
14. Hiorns MP, Owens CM. Radiology of neuroblastoma in children. Eur Radiol. 2001;11:2071–81.
15. Rha SE, Byun JY, Jung SE, et al. Neurogenic tumors in the abdomen: tumor types and imaging characteristics. Radiographics. 2003;23:29–43.
16. Nuchtern JG. Perinatal neuroblastoma. Semin Pediatr Surg. 2006;15:10–6.
17. McHugh K. Renal and adrenal tumours in children. Cancer Imaging. 2007;7:41–51.
18. Stevens MC. Neonatal tumours. Arch Dis Child. 1988;63:1122–5.
19. Deeg KH, Bettendorf U, Hofmann V. Differential diagnosis of neonatal adrenal haemorrhage and congenital neuroblastoma by colour coded Doppler sonography and power Doppler sonography. Eur J Pediatr. 1998;157:294–7.
20. Ross JH. Pheochromocytoma. Special considerations in children. Urol Clin North Am. 2000;27:393–402.
21. Lenders JW, Eisenhofer G, Mannelli M, Pacak K. Phaeochromocytoma. Lancet. 2005;366:665–75.
22. Daneman A, Navarro O, Haller JO. The adrenal and retroperitoneum. Caffey's pediatric diagnostic imaging. 11th ed. Philadelphia: Mosby, Elsevier; 2008. pp. 2214–33.
23. Fan J, Tang J, Fang J, Li Q, He E, Li J, Wang Y. Ultrasound imaging in the diagnosis of benign and suspicious adrenal lesions. Med Sci Monit. 2014;20:2132–41.
24. Mihai R. Rare adrenal tumors in children. Semin Pediatr Surg. 2014;23(2):71–5.
25. Goswami A, Sharma A, Khullar R, Soni V, Baijal M, Chowbey P. Adrenal angiomyolipoma: a case report and review of literature. J Minim Access Surg. 2014;10(4):213–5.
26. Cobanoglu U, Yaris N, Cay A. Adrenal myelolipoma in a child. Pediatr Surg Int. 2005;21(6):500–2.
27. Portnov I, Reznik I. Neonatal adrenal hemorrhage presenting as Bryant's and Stabler's signs. Isr Med Assoc J. 2014;16(6):395.
28. Gyurkovits Z, Maróti A, Rénes L, Németh G, Pál A, Orvos H. Adrenal haemorrhage in term neonates: a retrospective study from the period 2001–2013. J Matern Fetal Neonatal Med. 2014;7:1–4.
29. Postek G, Streich H, Narębski K. Assessment of diagnostic methods in adrenal gland hemorrhage in neonates on the basis of own material from the years 2007–2011. Pol J Radiol. 2011;76(3):62–4.
30. Hl E, Kim JH, Jang KM, Yoo SY, Lim GY, Kim MJ, et al. Comparison of clinico-radiological features between congenital cystic neuroblastoma and neonatal adrenal hemorrhagic pseudocyst. Korean J Radiol. 2011;12(1):52–8.
31. Mangray S, DeLellis RA. Adrenal embryology and pathology. In: Blake MA, Cronin CG, Boland GW, editors. Adrenal imaging. Totowa: Humana Press; 2009. pp. 1–33.
32. Warkentin TE, Safyan EL, Linkins LA. Heparin-induced thrombocytopenia presenting as bilateral adrenal hemorrhages. N Engl J Med. 2015;372(5):492–4.
33. Michon A, Darnige L, Pouchot J, Arlet JB. Catastrophic antiphospholipid syndrome presenting with bilateral massive adrenal haemorrhage. A case report. Joint Bone Spine. 2014. pii: S1297-319X(14)00263-2.
34. Sandal G, Arıkan E, Kuybulu AE, Ormecı AR. Unilateral Renal Vein Thrombosis and Adrenal Hemorrhage in A Newborn with Homozygous Factor V Leiden and Heterozygous Of MTHFR-677T, MTHFR-1298C Gene Mutations. Indian J Hematol Blood Transfus. 2014;30(Suppl 1):294–8.
35. Soundappan SV, Lam AH, Cass DT. Traumatic adrenal haemorrhage in children. ANZ J Surg. 2006;76(8):729–31.
36. Knorr M, Evans D. Bedside ultrasound of acute adrenal hemorrhage. Am J Emerg Med. 2012;30(9):2088. e1–2.
37. Liao CH, Lin KJ, Fu CY, Wang SY, Yang SJ, Ouyang CH. Adrenal Gland Trauma: Is Extravasation an Absolute Indication for Intervention? World J Surg. 2015;39(5):1312–9.
38. Broadley P, Daneman A, Wesson D, et al. Large adrenal cysts in teenage girls: diagnosis and management. Pediatr Radiol. 1997;27:550–2.
39. White PC, New MI, Dupont D. Congenital adrenal hyperplasia. N Engl J Med. 1987;316:1519–1524, 1580–1586.
40. DeLellis RA, Mangray S. The adrenal glands. Mills SE. Sternberg's diagnostic surgical pathology. Philadelphia: Lippincott Williams & Wilkins; 2004. pp. 621–67.
41. Hughes I. Congenital adrenal hyperplasia: phenotype and genotypes. J Pediatr Endocrinol Metab. 2002;15 (Suppl 15):1529–1340.
42. Lack EE. Pathology of the adrenal glands. New York: Churchill Livingstone; 1990.
43. Lloyd RV, Douglas BR, Young WF. Atlas of non-tumor pathology: endocrine diseases. Washington, D.C.: American Registry of Pathology & Armed Forces Institute of Pathology (AFIP); 2002. pp. 171–257.
44. Burch C. Cushing's disease: a review. Arch Intern Med. 1985;145:1106–11.
45. Kawashima A, Sandler CM, Ernst RD, Takahashi N, Roubidoux MA, Goldman SM, et al. Imaging of non-traumatic hemorrhage of the adrenal gland. Radiographics. 1999;19:949–63.
46. Diepstraten SC, Zwaveling S, Beek FJ. Diagnosis and subsequent US-guided percutaneous drainage of an adrenal abscess in a 5-week-old infant. Pediatr Radiol. 2012;42(9):1126–9.

The Pediatric Pelvis

15

Vincent Lee, Stacey Langford and Sameh Tadros

Introduction

Diagnosis of genital pathologies in the female pediatric population is largely dependent on imaging. Ultrasound (US) is considered the key screening modality for the diagnosis of ambiguous genitalia, pelvic masses, pelvic pain, and disorders of puberty. Sonography is also the initial modality in the investigation of the urinary bladder. The purpose of this chapter is to review the sonographic features of the normal and abnormal female pelvis and the urinary bladder in children and adolescents.

Female Pelvis—Uterus

Scanning Techniques

Ultrasonography is a key tool in the evaluation of the pediatric pelvis. With its low cost, lack of radiation, and no need for sedation, US is a great screening tool and may also be the only modality needed to confirm a diagnosis. For female pelvis US imaging, a full urinary bladder acts as an acoustic window. The distended bladder displaces air-filled loops of bowel allowing for improved transmission of the sound waves and easier identification of the uterus and ovaries [1–3]. In most children, oral hydration prior to the examination is sufficient to distend the bladder. When the oral route is not possible, catheterization for bladder filling is an option [1–3]. Overfilling of the urinary bladder should be avoided as it can distort the appearance of the uterus and can also displace or obscure the ovaries.

Particularly in neonates, the examination typically utilizes a small foot print high-frequency transducer [1–3]. With larger children, lower-frequency curvilinear transducers with better penetration are usually needed, sacrificing some near-field resolution [1–3]. Transvaginal scanning is not usually performed and is only done in older girls who are sexually active [3].

Longitudinal and transverse images should be obtained through the regions of the genital organs in relationship to the axis of the organs [4]. The uterus is located posterior to the urinary bladder and is measured in three dimensions [4]. Anteroposterior measurement is obtained on the longitudinal view at both, the fundus and the cervix. The thickness of the endometrium is measured, if visible. Images of the bilateral kidneys are also obtained to confirm their presence [4].

The vagina and the vaginal cuff are not typically evaluated on a routine pelvic evaluation.

S. Tadros (✉) · V. Lee · S. Langford
Department of Pediatric Radiology, Children's Hospital of Pittsburgh of UPMC, 4401 Penn Avenue, Pittsburgh, PA 15224, USA
e-mail: sameh.tadros@chp.edu

V. Lee
e-mail: dr.vincent.m.lee@gmail.com

S. Langford
e-mail: stace1212@gmail.com

S. Scholz, M. D. Jarboe (eds.), *Diagnostic and Interventional Ultrasound in Pediatrics and Pediatric Surgery,* DOI 10.1007/978-3-319-21699-7_15

Targeted evaluation can be performed when there is a clinical need. The vagina is generally not well visualized on a routine US and filling of the vagina with a saline infusion may be necessary [1, 7].

As there continues to be technological advances in the field of ultrasonography, additional techniques, such as 3-D and 4-D sonography, can be applied to help problem solve.

Normal Anatomy

The uterus changes in size and morphology as a child ages. In neonates, the fundus is more prominent in size compared to the cervix, due to the presence of maternal and placental hormones (Fig. 15.1a) and measures between 2.3 and 4.6 cm (mean 3.4 cm) in length [4]. The maximum anteroposterior diameter is between 0.8 and 2.2 cm [2]. The endometrium is also more prominent and visible [1, 3, 5]. The uterus then decreases in size with loss of the maternal and placental hormones with the fundus becoming smaller than the cervix and also loses the endometrial differentiation (Fig. 15.1b) [1, 3, 5]. The uterus then begins to grow and assumes a tubular morphology with the fundus now similar in size to the cervix (Fig. 15.1c). The prepubertal uterus measures between 2.5 and 3.3 cm in length and about 0.4–1.0 cm in maximum anteroposterior diameter [2]. With the onset of puberty, the uterus again grows and obtains the typical shape of an adult uterus with the fundus larger than the cervix with a prominent endometrium (Fig. 15.1d) [1, 3, 5]. The uterus also descends in the pelvis and loses its neutral position to become anteverted or retroverted [3]. The postpubertal uterus length ranges between 5 and 8 cm and has a maximum anteroposterior dimension of about 1.6–3 cm [2].

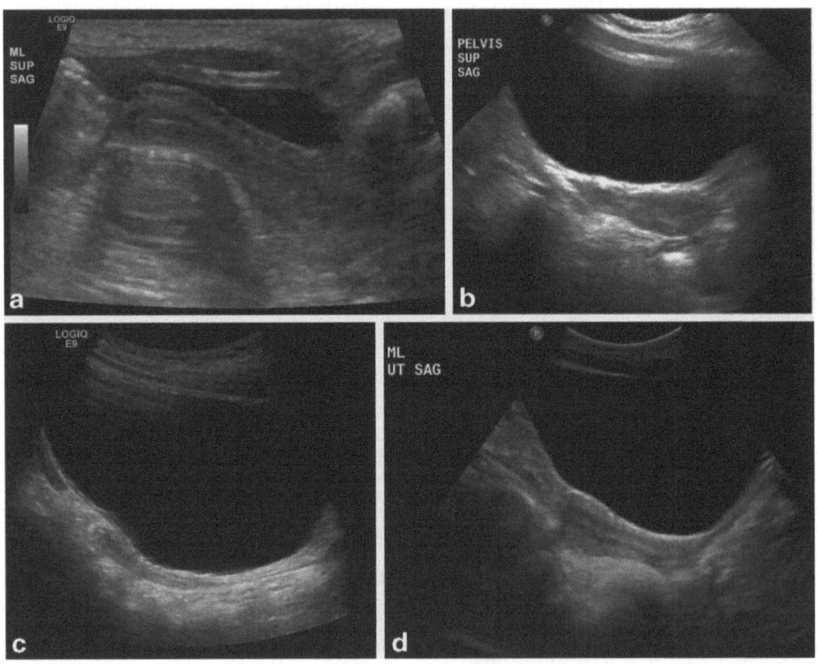

Fig. 15.1 **a** Ultrasound of a newborn demonstrates a more prominent fundus of the uterus in comparison to the cervix. The endometrium is also more prominent and visible. **b** Ultrasound of a 6-month-old shows a uterine fundus smaller than the cervix. **c** Ultrasound of an 8-year-old demonstrates a tubular appearance of the uterus with the fundus and cervix similar in size. **d** Ultrasound in a 15-year-old shows a typical postpubertal appearance of the uterus with a prominent fundus in relationship to the cervix as well as a prominent endometrium

Clinical Problems

Ambiguous Genitalia Ambiguous genitalia requires a complicated diagnostic evaluation. However, the role of sonography is straightforward to prove or disprove the presence of the uterus and to describe the degree of hypoplasia or agenesis, if applicable. Müllerian duct abnormalities affect the proximal two thirds of the vagina, cervix, and uterus [6]. The distal third of the vagina develops from the urogenital sinus [7]. US should also look for and describe the gonadal structures, if visible. Evaluation of the adrenal glands and kidneys is also necessary, as abnormalities of those organs can be linked.

Uterine Malformations Uterine malformations result from the disruption of the fusion of the Müllerian ducts during development [6]. Currently, magnetic resonance imaging (MRI) is the preferred means of evaluation. Ultrasonography, however, can provide a rapid, inexpensive, and relatively risk-free assessment. The US can evaluate the uterine contour, the shape of the endometrial cavity, and if there is duplication of the cervix and/or vagina. An arcuate uterus is demonstrated by a mild indentation of the endometrium at the fundus with a normal fundal contour [6]. If the endometrial cavity is further divided while maintaining the fundal contour, the uterus is considered septated [6]. Both didelphys and bicornuate uterus are characterized with a duplicated endometrial cavity as well as a fundal cleft [6]. Uterus didelphys also duplicates the cervix and proximal vaginas (Fig. 15.2a and b) [6]. In bicornuate uterus, the cervix may be duplicated (bicornuate bicollis) or without duplication (bicornuate unicollis) [6]. A unicornuate uterus is more easily characterized due to the presence of a single uterine horn with agenesis or hypoplasia of the contralateral horn [6].

Pelvic Mass Sonography is the initial examination of choice for evaluating a patient with a suspected pelvic mass. Primary tumors of the uterus and vagina are unusual in the pediatric population and are commonly malignant [3]. Rhabdomyosarcoma can arise from the uterus or vagina and has a nonspecific US appearance; the diagnosis is usually suggested by the location rather than a specific appearance. It typically exhibits as a well-circumscribed hypoechoic inhomogeneous mass and also has vascularity on color Doppler imaging [1]. Clear cell adenocarcinoma can arise from the vagina in children younger than 2 years of age who have a history of exposure to diethylstilbestrol in utero [2]. It has a similar appearance to rhabdomyosarcoma [2].

More commonly, genital tract obstruction presents as a pelvic mass in the pediatric population. The vagina (hydrocolpos) or the vagina and uterus (hydrometrocolpos) can become distended

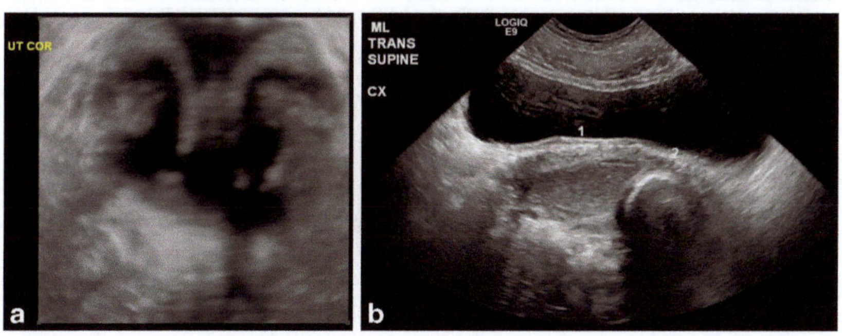

Fig. 15.2 **a** 3-D ultrasound demonstrates a uterus with two separate endometrial cavities and two cervixes. **b** A didelphys uterus is confirmed with the presence of duplication of the vagina. The first vagina is distended with complex fluid consistent with blood products. A tampon demonstrating acoustic shadowing is present in the second vagina

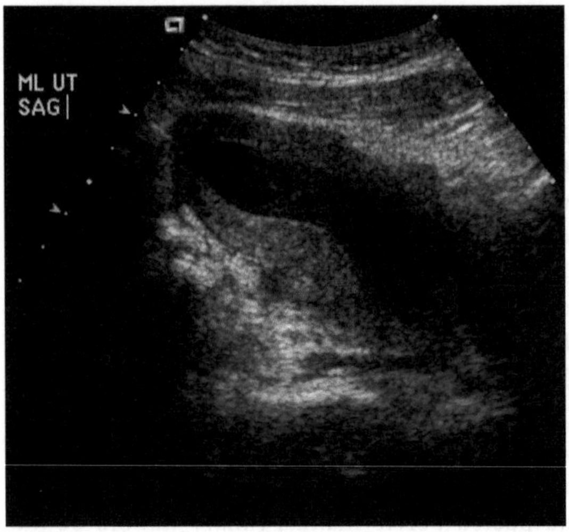

Fig. 15.3 Ultrasound shows a distended uterus and vagina with complex fluid representing blood products consistent with hematometrocolpos

with fluid and appear as a tubular cystic midline mass (Fig. 15.3) [2, 3, 5]. The uterus can be identified because of the thickness of its wall [3]. The obstruction is typically due to an imperforate hymen, but can also be secondary to cloacal or urogenital sinus malformations [2, 3, 5]. If the uterus is obstructed alone (hydrometra), this is usually due to cervical agenesis or obstruction of one horn of a bicornuate uterus [3]. If distended with blood, then the term is hematocolpos, hematometrocolpos, or hematometra.

Syndromes Pelvic anomalies are not always isolated findings. Congenital malformations may involve a part or all of the Müllerian or Wolffian duct, which can lead to associated anomalies. In Mayer–Rokitansky–Küster syndrome there is complete agenesis of the uterus and the upper two thirds of the vagina. Patients can have associated malformations including unilateral renal aplasia, ectopic locations of the kidney, horseshoe kidney, double ureter, and vertebral malformations [7].

Herlyn–Werner–Wunderlich syndrome is another constellation of anomalies affecting the Müllerian and Wolffian duct. The syndrome is characterized by uterine didelphys (Fig. 15.4a and b), obstructed hemivagina (Fig. 15.4b and c), and ipsilateral renal agenesis (Fig. 15.4e) [8].

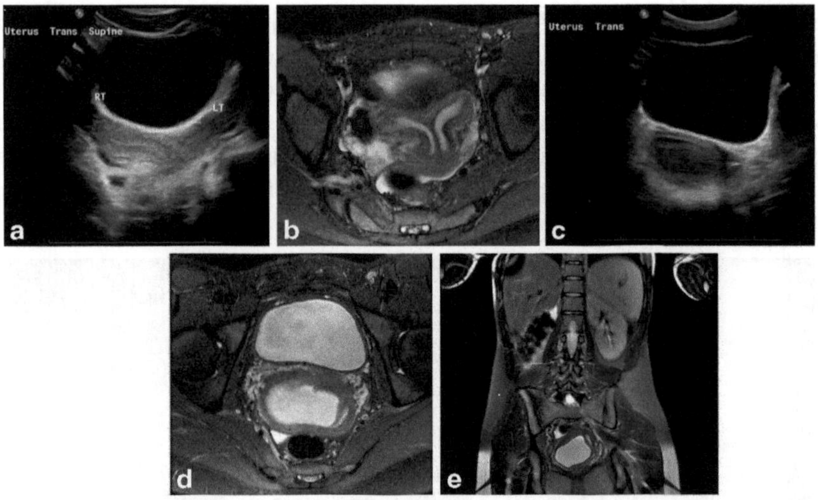

Fig. 15.4 **a** Transverse ultrasound view of the pelvis demonstrates a uterus with duplicated uterine bodies. **b** MRI coronal STIR sequence shows duplication of the uterine body and cervix consistent with uterine didelphys. **c** Traverse ultrasound view shows duplication of the vagina with distension of the right hemivagina with echogenic fluid consistent with right-sided hematocolpos. **d** MRI axial STIR sequence shows a duplicated vagina with distension of the right hemivagina with blood products consistent with right-sided hematocolpos. **e** MRI coronal T2 with fat saturation shows right-sided renal agenesis. *STIR* short tau inversion recovery

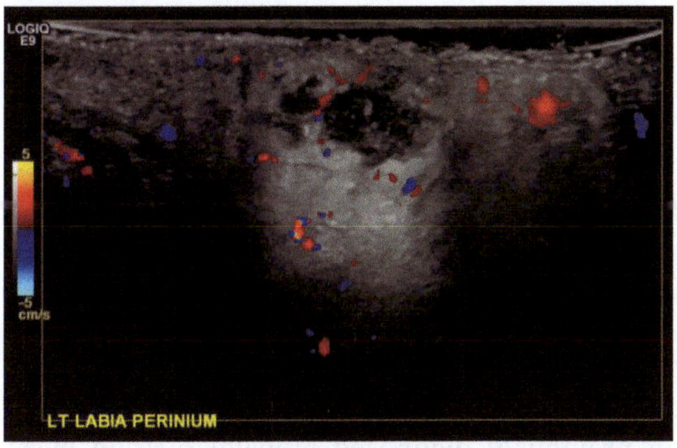

Fig. 15.5 Ultrasound of the left labia shows a complex fluid collection consistent with an abscess. There is also surrounding inflammatory changes and hyperemia

Disorders of Puberty With precocious puberty, pubertal delay, or amenorrhea, US is commonly used to evaluate the uterus and ovaries. The developmental morphology of the uterus can be identified with US and compared to the patient's level of sexual development. Uterine and ovarian volume can be measured and compared to a reference of normal volumes at a given age. The number and size of ovarian follicles can also be assessed.

Others Occasionally, targeted sonographic assessment is performed to evaluate the vaginal cuff. In the pediatric population, the common clinical indication is a site of inflammation and/or a palpable abnormality. With cellulitis of the labia, US can determine if there is an underlying fluid collection to suggest an abscess (Fig. 15.5). Vaginal cysts can also be identified, which can have superimposed infection. If US detects a cystic structure at the anterolateral wall of the vagina, above the inferior border of the pubic symphysis, this represents a Gartner duct cyst, which results from incomplete regression of the Wolffian ducts [9]. A cystic structure seen at or below the level of the pubic symphysis corresponds to a Bartholin gland cyst, which develops from obstruction of the gland's duct [9]. If the cystic structure is identified in the periurethral area, then this represents a Skene gland cyst, which is also secondary to obstruction of the gland [9].

Female Pelvis—Ovaries

Normal Appearance

The size of the ovary is traditionally reported in length, width, and depth, with an approximate ovarian volume calculated by multiplying the product of these numbers by 0.523 [2]. Ovarian size varies with age, and neonatal ovarian volume correlates with birth weight and length [10]. Neonatal ovaries, like the uterus, are larger due to maternal estrogen stimulation and can contain multiple follicles. Ovarian volume can reach up to 3 cm^3 during the first 3 months of life, decreasing in size over the first 2 years of life to a mean volume of approximately 0.67 cm^3. Ovaries remain small until about 6 years of age, at which time they begin to grow again, continuing their enlargement through the prepubertal and premenarchal stages. Postmenarchal ovarian volume averages 8 cm^3 with a wide range of normal volumes [11, 12]. Cystic spaces within ovaries are extremely common at all ages, usually representing follicles or functional cysts, and nearly all resolve spontaneously [11, 12]. The size and number of follicles generally increase throughout childhood.

The paired ovaries are best seen transabdominally through a fully distended bladder (Fig. 15.6). Longitudinal images can be obtained by scanning through the full bladder angled out toward the iliac vessels, and transverse images can be obtained through the bladder at around the level of the uterine fundus. In the neonate, the ovaries may be in an unsuspected higher and more ventral location within the abdomen [1, 2].

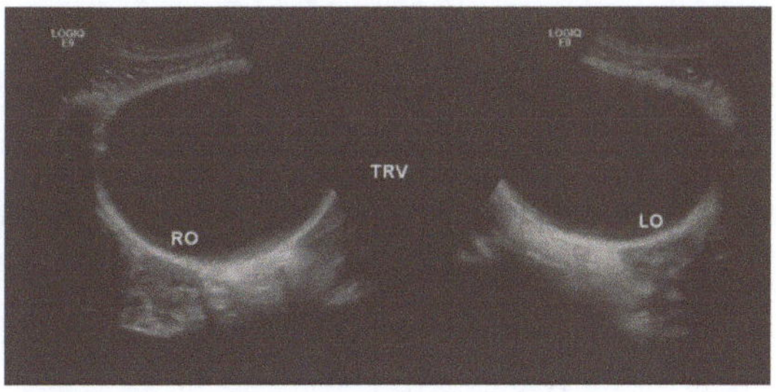

Fig. 15.6 Normal ovaries in an 18-year-old female seen through the fluid distended bladder

Ovarian detail is best seen transvaginally in adult patients, but endovaginal US is not used in routine pediatric practice [5].

Ovarian Torsion

Ovarian torsion may present with acute or subacute lower quadrant or pelvic pain, pelvic US is the imaging test of choice to evaluate for the presence of torsion. Torsion is common in pediatric patients due to the relative mobility of the ovary during childhood, and even more common in patients with predisposing lesions, such as cysts or neoplasms [12]. The ovarian salvage rate is overall low, largely due to delayed diagnosis and intervention.

US findings of ovarian torsion include marked enlargement, increased or decreased echogenicity, and decreased vascularity when compared to the unaffected side [1, 12]. The absence of flow on color Doppler US is not a reliable diagnostic criterion, and this phenomenon may be explained by the dual ovarian blood supply [12]. Multiple follicles at the periphery of the ovary may also indicate torsion (Fig. 15.7) [1, 12]. The ovary may be displaced superiorly and/or ventrally, and ascites may be present [1]. The presence of a predisposing lesion, such as a cyst or neoplasm, may complicate evaluation for torsion [1, 5]. In utero, ovarian torsion may be suggested by the presence of fluid-debris levels or septations seen in previously diagnosed prenatal ovarian cysts (Fig. 15.8) [2]. When torsion is suspected and the sonographic appearance of the ovary is equivocal or not definitely normal and symmetric, emergent diagnostic laparoscopy may be required [1].

Ovarian Cysts

Functional or follicular ovarian cysts are commonly seen at all ages, accounting for 60% of the pediatric ovarian masses, and nearly all invo-

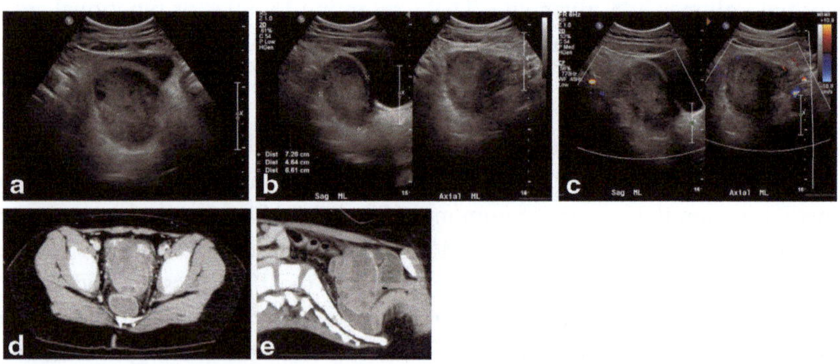

Fig. 15.7 **a**–**e** An 8-year-old female with pelvic pain initially thought to have pelvic mass, found to have enlarged left ovary with peripheral follicles, lacking internal Doppler flow, suggestion of central hypodense region found to have *ovarian torsion* with infarcted and gangrenous left ovary and fallopian tube intraoperatively

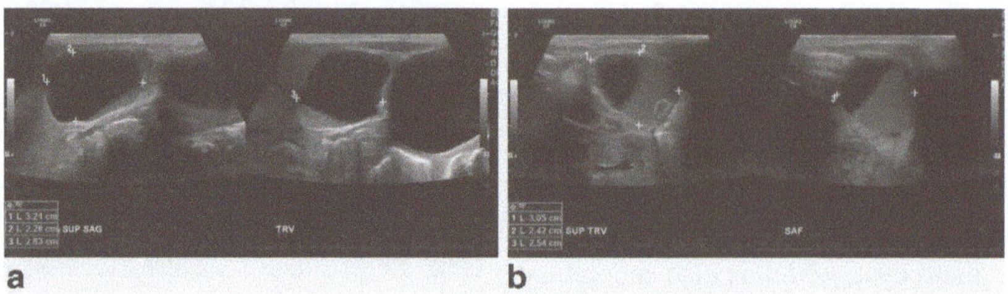

Fig. 15.8 **a** and **b** An 8-day-old female with bilateral ovarian cysts with fluid-debris levels and history of prenatal ovarian cysts, found to have *bilateral in utero ovarian torsion* on laparoscopy

lute spontaneously [12]. These appear as uncomplicated anechoic ovarian lesions with posterior acoustic enhancement that lack internal flow on color Doppler imaging, and these may be bilateral [2, 5]. Follicular size varies, but is often greater than 1 cm in neonates, less than 5 mm in infants, and up to 4 cm after puberty, depending on the phase of the menstrual cycle [1]. Management is typically conservative with or without serial US, and cystectomy or cyst aspiration is reserved for large or symptomatic cysts, typically greater than 5 cm [5], which may predispose to torsion. Autonomous ovarian follicular cysts may secrete estradiol and result in precocious puberty, but these are also often treated conservatively with symptoms regressing spontaneously along with the ovarian cyst on serial US [5, 12].

A hemorrhagic cyst consists of hemorrhage within a functional ovarian cyst. The presence of a hemorrhagic cyst may be suggested by severe acute pelvic pain at the midpoint of the menstrual cycle. On US, the hemorrhagic cyst appears as a complex or complicated adnexal or ovarian mass with increased through-transmission and absence of internal flow on color Doppler imaging [12], which can simulate torsion (Fig. 15.9). Hemorrhagic cysts may be homogenous and mimic a solid lesion, such as an ovarian tumor, may have a fluid-debris level, or may have a "retracting" angulated internal clot [5]. Differentiation from an ovarian tumor may be difficult, as a hemorrhagic cyst may appear solid [5], and follow-up US examinations may be necessary to differentiate the two [2]. Free fluid is often observed and may be complex. Treatment is often conservative, and serial US may demonstrate the cyst becoming anechoic as it regresses in size, unlike the ovarian tumors that do not change or decrease in size (Fig. 15.10) [2]. Occasionally, the presence of active bleeding resulting in acute abdomen and/or shock may warrant surgical intervention (Fig. 15.11).

Ovarian Neoplasms

The clinical manifestations of ovarian neoplasms include abdominal pain, palpable abdominal or pelvic mass, nausea, vomiting, anorexia, weight loss, constipation, and urinary frequency, although lesions are also often detected incidentally in an asymptomatic patient [13]. Depending on the age of the patient, evidence of endocrine abnormality may be the presenting feature in hormone-producing tumors, including precocious puberty, menstrual irregularity, and virilization [13]. Characterization of a pediatric ovarian neoplasm is crucial to the planning of surgical resection with potential ovarian salvage and fertility preservation [13], but US alone is often inadequate in reliably differentiating benign and malignant lesions and is complimented by computed tomography (CT) or MRI [5].

Ovarian neoplasms account for 40% of the pediatric ovarian masses, and most are benign. Up to two thirds are benign mature teratomas

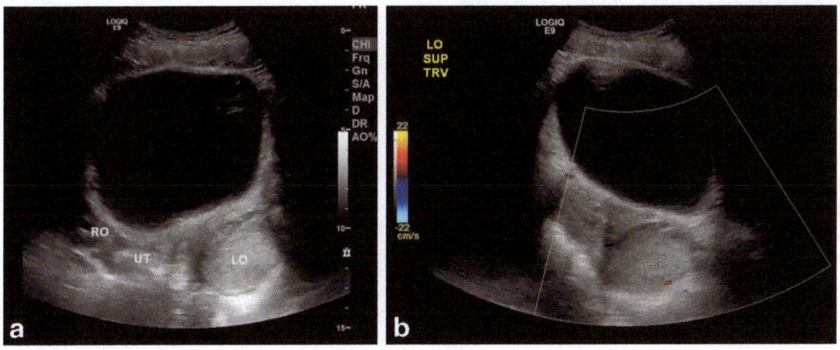

Fig. 15.9 **a** and **b** An 11-year-old female with midcycle left lower quadrant pain found to have enlarged, echogenic left ovary lacking internal Doppler flow. Initially thought to be torsion, but was *unruptured hemorrhagic cyst* on laparoscopy without torsion

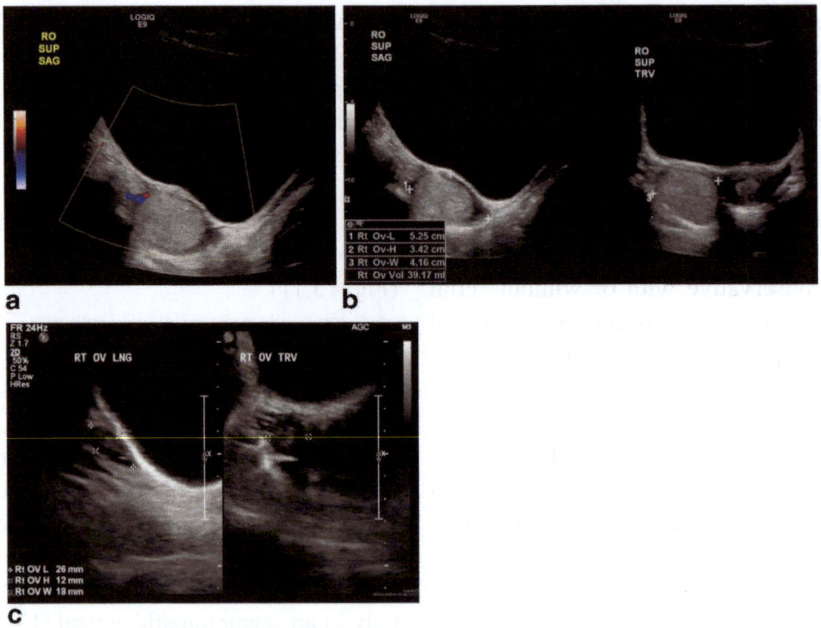

Fig. 15.10 **a–c** A 14-year-old female with acute midcycle right lower quadrant pain found to have an echogenic lesion in the right ovary that lacked internal Doppler flow, but flow was found in normal surrounding ovarian tissue. *Hemorrhagic cyst* was suspected, and this completely resolved on follow-up 4 weeks later (**c**)

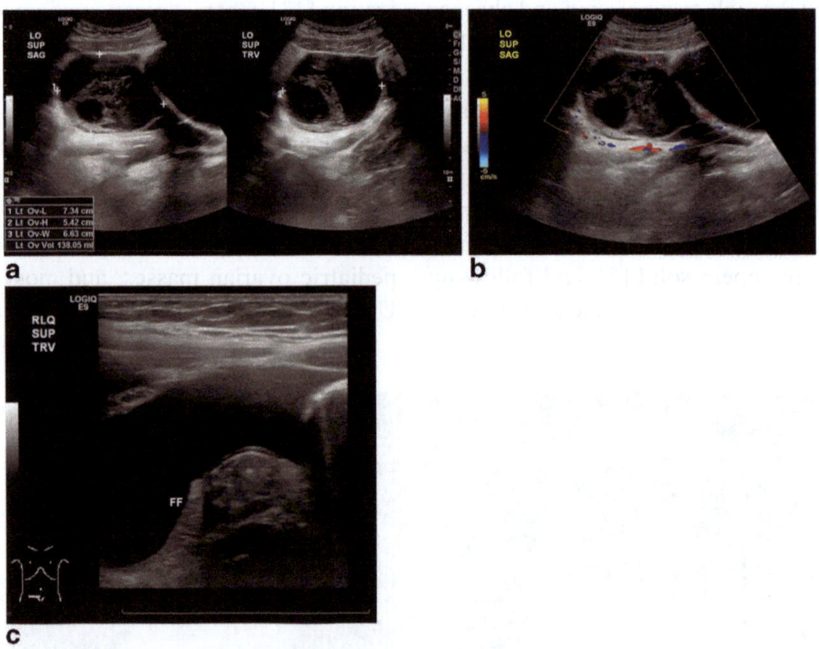

Fig. 15.11 **a–c** A 16-year-old female with acute midcycle left lower quadrant pain found to have free fluid and large left ovarian cyst lacking internal Doppler flow. Initially thought to have ovarian cyst with torsion, was found to have *ruptured hemorrhagic cyst* with hemoperitoneum without torsion on laparoscopy

[5, 12]. Approximately 10 % of the benign mature teratomas are bilateral, and up to 30 % ultimately result in ovarian torsion [12, 13]. Malignant transformation occurs in only 1–2 % [13]. The appearance of benign mature teratomas on US is highly variable depending on the histologic composition and ranges from cystic to solid and from homogenous to heterogeneous (Fig. 15.12). Common findings include unilocular (88 %) or multilocular cysts, mural nodules (55 % of cases), and shadowing echogenic foci (44 % of cases) relating to internal calcification, hair, or adipose elements [12, 13]. Additional US features that may support the diagnosis of benign mature teratoma include echogenic mass relating to internal sebaceous elements, thin echogenic bands attributable to hair, fat–fluid levels, and floating debris [13].

Benign serous and mucinous cystadenomas are the second most common benign pediatric ovarian mass, and these occur almost exclusively in postmenarchal patients [13]. US findings include unilocular or multilocular cystic lesions with thin wall or septa and no intracystic solid portion. Solid portions, large size (greater than 10 cm), thick wall or septa, and papillary projections are more indicative of a borderline or malignant cystadenoma (Fig. 15.13) [2, 13].

Up to 30 % of the ovarian neoplasms are malignant with 60–75 % representing germ cell tumors (including immature teratomas), 10–20 % representing epithelial tumors, and 10 % representing stromal tumors [5, 12], although histologically mixed lesions are not uncommon [13]. US features that may favor malignancy include a predominantly solid or heterogeneous mass as well as large size (Fig. 15.14). Additional US findings that may indicate malignancy include ascites, peritoneal implants, lymphadenopathy, pleural effusion, and hepatic metastases [12]. Careful scrutiny of the unaffected ovarian tissue is crucial, as coexisting ipsilateral and contralateral ovarian lesions can occur and may affect surgical planning [13]. Tumor markers including alpha-fetoprotein (AFP), beta human chorionic gonadotropin (β-HCG), and cancer antigen

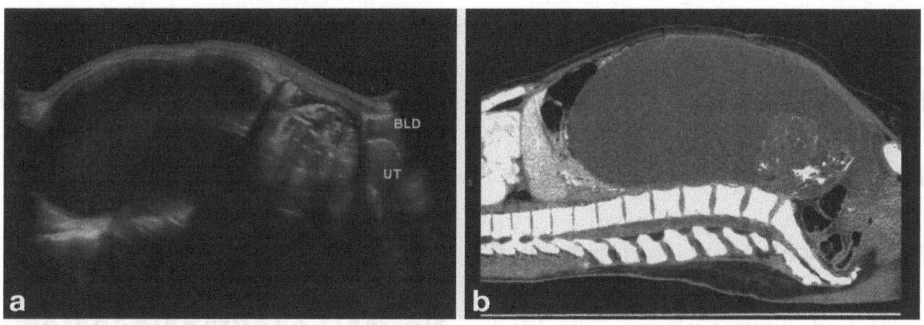

Fig. 15.12 **a** and **b** A 13-year-old female with 31 cm *mature cystic teratoma* arising from left ovary. Resected specimen contained elements of skin, hair, rudimentary teeth, fat, and bone

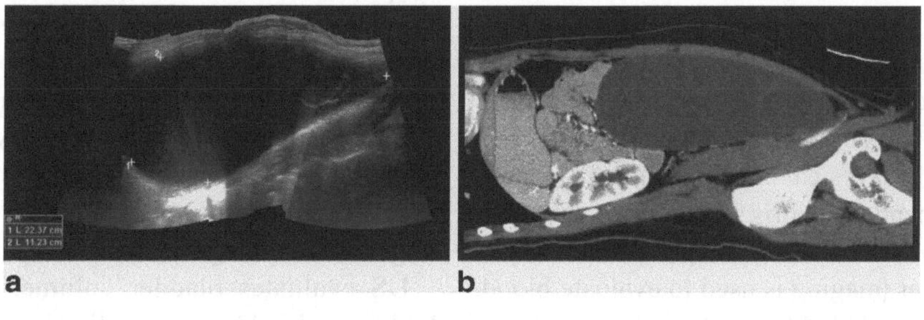

Fig. 15.13 **a** and **b** A 14-year-old female with abdominal and pelvic swelling and palpable mass found to have large left cystic ovarian mass that represented an *ovarian borderline mucinous* tumor upon surgical resection

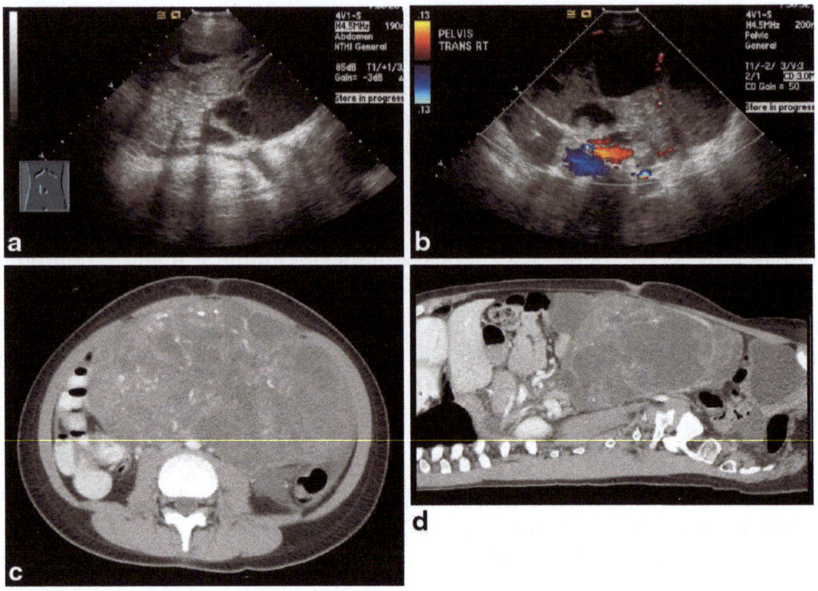

Fig. 15.14 **a–d** A 9-year-old female with history of constipation and abdominal pain found to have palpable mass on exam with positive α-FP and β-HCG. Found to have large, complex, solid abdominopelvic mass arising from the right ovary that was consistent with a *malignant mixed germ cell tumor* on surgical pathology, containing both yolk sac tumor and immature teratoma components

125 (CA-125) are elevated in only 54 % of the cases of pediatric ovarian malignancy [13].

Pediatric Urinary Bladder

Scanning Techniques

Imaging of the urinary bladder is performed with a high-frequency curvilinear or linear transducer in the transverse and sagittal planes. The bladder is examined when moderately distended. Bladder filling is accomplished by having the patient drink and not to void in the hour prior to the examination. In non-toilet trained infants, the bladder should be imaged before the kidneys and ureters, because the child may urinate as the transducer is moved over the abdomen. The patient is examined in the supine position. Mobility of intravesical contents such as stones, clots, or dependent debris is documented using cine capture while rolling the patient sideways. Color Doppler imaging is used to evaluate blood flow in thickened bladder wall and focal lesions, twinkle artifact in bladder or vesicoureteric junction calculi, and to demonstrate the ureteric jets. New techniques can further enhance sonographic potential such as echo-enhanced US for detection of vesicoureteral reflux after instillation of contrast material into the urinary bladder, or 3-D US can be used to assess the bladder luminal surface ("virtual cystoscopy") [14].

Normal Sonographic Anatomy

The urinary bladder is an ovoid pelvic organ that stores and evacuates urine. The smooth muscle component of the bladder is termed the *detrusor* and consists of interlacing muscle bundles [15]. Detrusor fibers continue into the bladder neck forming the "internal sphincter" which is under voluntary control and is the primary continence mechanism. The external striated sphincter surrounds the urethra, where it passes through the urogenital diaphragm.

US evaluates bladder volume, shape, wall thickness, bladder neck, distal ureters, retrovesical space/internal genitalia, ascites, and any perivesical pathologic process [16]. The normal bladder wall is smooth and uniform in thickness. The sonographic thickness of the bladder wall should not be more than 3 mm when distended and 5 mm when empty [17]. The bladder volume can be calculated from the transverse and sagittal views using the prolate ellipsoid method based on the following formula: volume (ml) = length × width × height × correction factor. The correction factor depends on bladder shape: 0.52 for spherical/elliptical configuration and 1.0 for rectangular shape [1]. Predictive bladder capacity can be estimated using the following linear equations—children less than 2 years old: capacity in ounces = 2 × age (years) + 2; children 2 years old or older: capacity in ounces = age (years)/2 + 6 (number of ounces × 30 = number in ml) [18]. A volume of 400 ml is used as the expected volume for children 11 years old or older. Pre- and post-void bladder volumes are always obtained; residual volumes can be considered clinically significant or pathologic when they represent, on repeated occasions, volume of ≥20 ml, or volumes of > 10 % of the bladder capacity [19]. Physiologically residual urine is noted in neonates due to immature bladder function [1].

Congenital Anomalies

Urachal Anomalies The urachus is an allantoic fibromuscular tube that extends upward from the anterior dome of the bladder toward the umbilicus. It lies in the space of Retzius behind the transversalis fascia and anterior to the peritoneum. The lumen is obliterated during fetal life extending from the umbilicus toward the bladder, and becomes the median umbilical ligament. A small, elliptical, hypoechoic structure is observed in 62 % of the pediatric bladder sonograms on the middle of the anterosuperior surface of the urinary bladder and represents a normal urachal remnant (Fig. 15.15) [20]. This normal remnant should not be mistaken for a pathologic process [21].

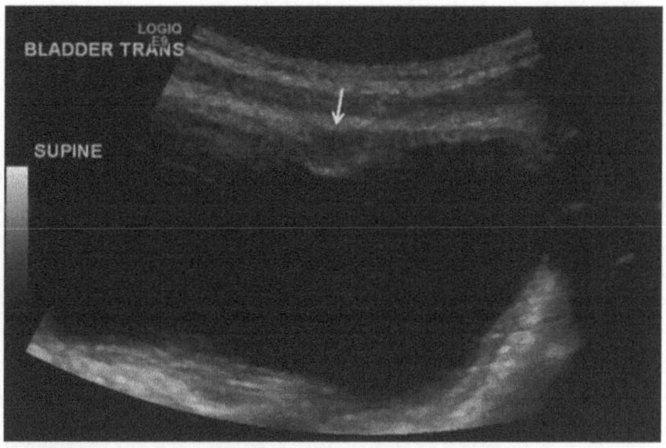

Fig. 15.15 Normal or physiological urachal remnant. Transverse bladder scan shows the urachal remnant (*arrow*) in the midline of the anterosuperior bladder surface; not to be mistaken for tumor

Failure of normal urachal regression can result in four types of congenital urachal anomalies: a patent urachus or vesico-umbilical fistula (50 % of cases), umbilical-urachal sinus (15 %), vesico-urachal diverticulum (3–5 %), or urachal cyst (30 %) [22]. Congenital urachal anomalies are twice as common in males as in females. Sonography is the initial study of choice to evaluate suspected urachal anomaly. *Patent urachus* appears as patent channel between the bladder and umbilicus on sagittal US and manifests clinically as neonatal urinary leakage from the umbilicus (Fig. 15.16a). *Umbilical-urachal sinus* consists of blind dilatation of the urachus at the umbilical end, and may result in periodic discharge. In *vesico-urachal diverticulum*, the urachus communicates only with the bladder dome and collapses when the bladder is empty (Fig. 15.16b). Patent urachus and urachal diverticula are frequent in infants with prune-belly syndrome. Urachal diverticulum may be complicated by urinary tract infection (UTI), intraurachal stone formation, and an increased prevalence of carcinoma after puberty. A *urachal cyst* develops if the urachus closes at both the umbilicus and bladder but remains patent between the two endpoints, more frequently in the lower one third of the urachus. Urachal cysts are usually small and infection is the most common complication. The spectrum of urachal remnant anomalies has recently expanded to include the newly recognized *intravesical urachal cysts*, which are characterized on US by

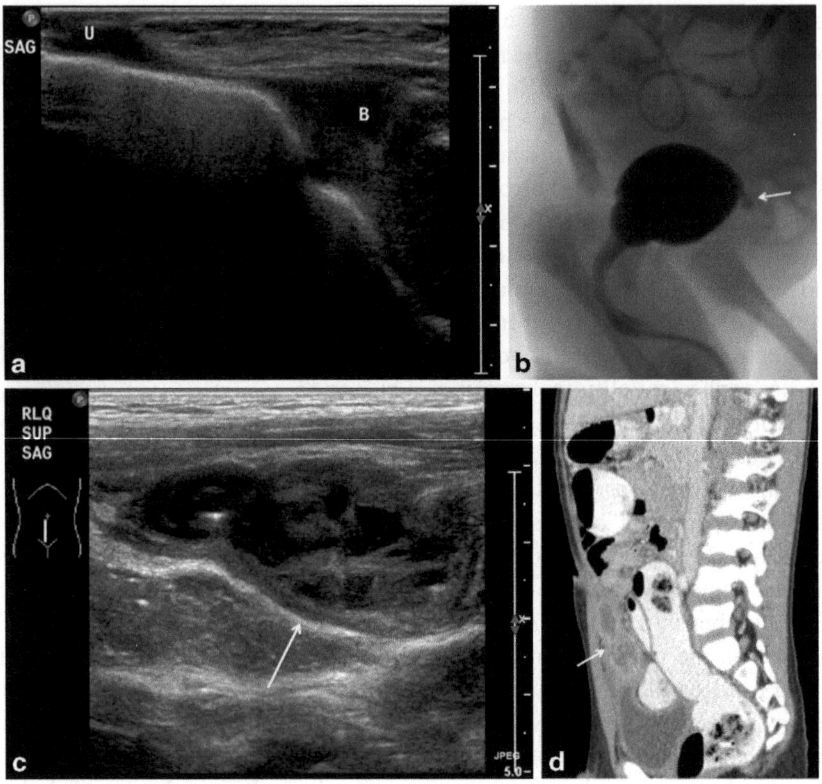

Fig. 15.16 Urachal anomalies. **a** Patent urachus. Longitudinal sonogram shows a fluid-filled channel extending from the bladder (*B*) to the umbilicus (*U*). **b** Urachal diverticulum. Lateral view during a voiding cystourethrography shows a small urachal diverticulum connected to the bladder dome (*arrow*). **c**, **d** Infected urachal cyst. Sagittal sonogram **(c)** shows a complex lesion (*arrow*) with thickened wall and containing internal debris. Sagittal reformatted contrast-enhanced CT image **(d)** demonstrates a heterogeneous hypoattenuating lesion with rim enhancement (*arrow*) and stranding of surrounding fat, extending between bladder dome and umbilicus

the presence of a thin-walled cyst along the midline anterosuperior aspect of the urinary bladder [23].

The majority of patients with urachal abnormalities (except those with a patent urachus) are asymptomatic. However, they may become symptomatic if these abnormalities are associated with infection and, rarely, urachal adenocarcinoma. Infected remnants, termed "pyourachus" [24], are frequently confused with a wide spectrum of midline intra-abdominal or pelvic inflammatory disorders at clinical examination and with malignant tumors at imaging (Fig. 15.16c and d) [22]. Ninety percent of the urachal carcinomas arise in the juxtavesical portion of the urachus and extend superiorly toward the umbilicus and inferiorly through the bladder wall. A primary bladder carcinoma arising in the mucosa of the bladder apex will usually manifest with less of an extravesical component than is seen in urachal cancer. Calcifications in a midline supravesical mass are considered nearly diagnostic for urachal carcinoma (calcification occurs in 50–70 % of the cases).

Bladder Exstrophy Exstrophy of the bladder is the result of failure of midline closure of the infraumbilical abdominal wall and anterior wall of the bladder. It occurs at a rate of 1 in 10,000–50,000 live births with male to female ratio ranging 1.5–5 to 1 [25]. The kidneys are usually normal at birth and produce urine that flows to the

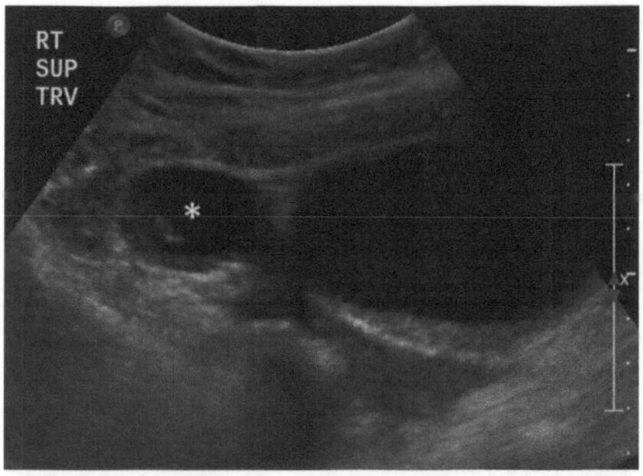

Fig. 15.17 Diverticulum in a neurogenic bladder. Transverse scan demonstrates a diverticulum *(*)* containing debris

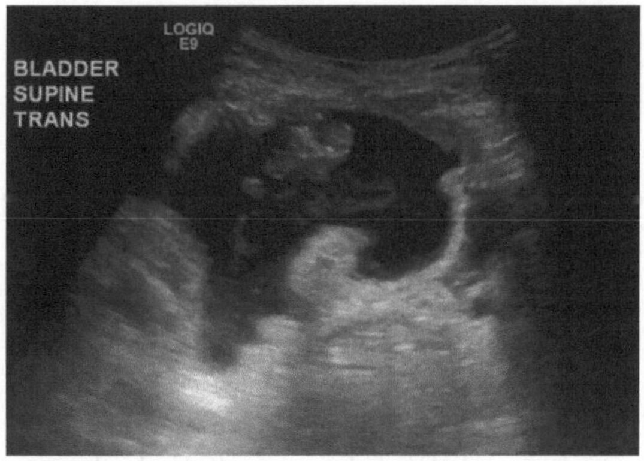

Fig. 15.18 Augmented neurogenic bladder. Transverse scan shows irregular bladder wall and intravesical debris consistent with mucus

open bladder and then along the abdominal wall. The diagnosis is obvious on physical examination at birth and a postnatal baseline renal US is obtained. Initial closure is often carried out within 72 h of life. Imaging is done soon after surgery to assess the condition of the anastomosis and evaluate bladder capacity and morphology [21]. Periodic renal US is obtained to detect hydronephrosis or renal scarring [26].

Bladder Diverticula Most bladder diverticula are *primary* developmental anomalies and result when the bladder mucosa protrudes through a congenital defect or point of weakness in the muscle wall [27]. Diverticula *secondary* to obstruction or neurogenic dysfunction are not as common as was once thought. They are really intravesical protrusions of mucosa between the hypertrophied muscle bundles and are better termed cellules or saccules, although chronically increased intravesical pressure can lead to protrusion of vesical mucosa through preexisting defects in the muscle (Fig. 15.17). The majority of diverticula are asymptomatic but they can cause vesico-ureteral reflux, obstruction, or residual urine. Diverticula can also be iatrogenic and occur after bladder surgery. Multiple diverticula have been described in children with Menkes syndrome, Williams syndrome, prune-belly syndrome, Ehlers–Danlos syndrome, and cutis laxa [21].

Neurogenic Bladder

In children, neurogenic bladder is most often congenital and occurs in 80–90% of the patients who suffer from myelodysplasia. Myelomeningocele is the most common defect. Children with neurogenic bladder dysfunction may be unable to retain urine normally, to evacuate normally, or both. A functional classification for neurogenic bladder includes contractile detrusor (detrusor hyperreflexia), acontractile detrusor (detrusor areflexia), which can be roughly linked to upper motor neuron lesion and lower motor neuron lesion, respectively, and intermediate detrusor (mixed type) [15]. Sonography readily demonstrates the trabeculated, small, thick-walled detrusor hyperreflexia bladder, and the smooth, large-capacity, thin-walled detrusor areflexia bladder [24]. US can also identify distal ureteral dilatation, incomplete bladder emptying by assessing post-void residual urine volume, and stone formation. Bladder augmentation is an operation designed to increase the volume of the small, high-pressure neurogenic bladder to prevent damage to the kidneys. Sonographically, the augmented bladder is irregular in shape, has an echogenic bowel mucosa, and may exhibit peristalsis. Mucus produced by the bowel lining appears as intraluminal debris (Fig. 15.18).

Inflammation (Cystitis)

Bacterial cystitis is frequently present in combination with pyelonephritis, although it may occur alone. Cystitis is usually bacterial or viral in origin; other causes include fungal infection and drug therapy (particularly cyclophosphamide). US may show diffuse wall thickening (more than 3 mm in a full bladder), focal wall thickening, or a polypoid mass (inflammatory pseudotumor) that mimics a tumor, and biopsy may be needed for diagnosis [24]. If there is extensive hemorrhage associated with cystitis, blood clots may appear as echogenic debris within the bladder (Fig. 15.19) [26]. *Eosinophilic cystitis* is an inflammatory condition of the bladder that has been linked to food allergies, infectious agents, medications, and other genitourinary conditions. It is characterized by an intense eosinophilic infiltrate in the acute phase and fibrosis in the chronic phase. On US, it appears as a focal mass simulating a rhabdomyosarcoma (Fig. 15.20), or as diffuse or localized bladder wall thickening.

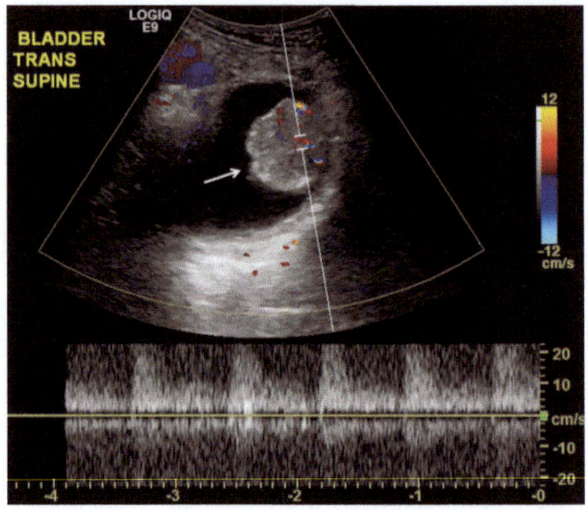

Fig. 15.20 Eosinophilic cystitis. Transverse sonogram shows a focal mass (*arrow*) arising from the bladder wall with evidence of internal vascularity on color Doppler. Biopsy confirmed the diagnosis

Bladder Stones

Bladder stones can either originate from the upper urinary tract or develop within the bladder. Predisposing factors associated with the formation of bladder stones include foreign body, infection with the urea-splitting organism *Proteus mirabilis*, bladder augmentation using intestinal mucosa, hypercalciuria, urinary stasis, bladder diverticulum, and urachal remnant. Bladder stones are echogenic and produce posterior acoustic shadowing (Fig. 15.21). They shift to the dependent portion of the bladder with changes in patient position. The endoscopic, submucosal injection of a small amount of Tef-

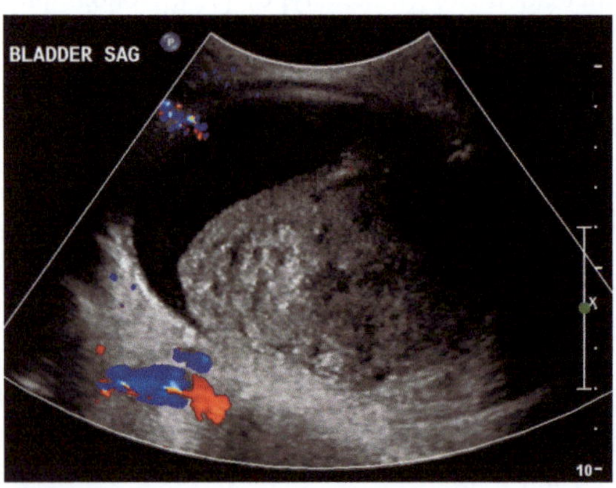

Fig. 15.19 Hemorrhagic cystitis with clot formation. Sagittal scan shows a large dependent bladder clot with absence of flow on color Doppler; it eventually resolved on follow-up scan

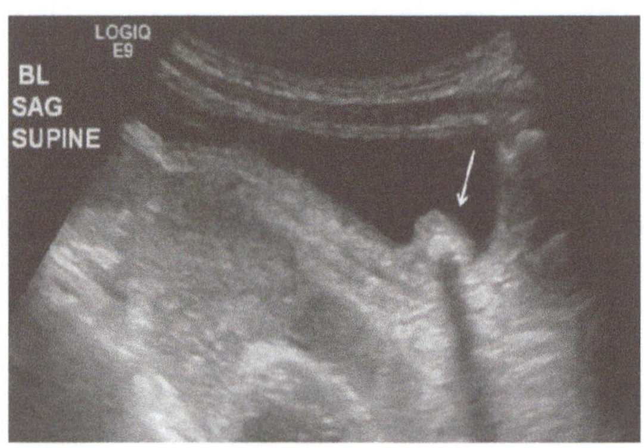

Fig. 15.21 Urinary bladder stone. Sagittal scan demonstrates a stone (*arrow*) with a sharp posterior acoustic shadowing. Three other mobile stones were noted within the bladder (not shown)

lon paste or dextranomer/hyaluronic acid (Deflux) immediately inferior to the ureterovesical junction in treatment of reflux can cause a hyperechoic focus with posterior shadowing that mimics bladder stones, but the injected material does not shift position [24].

Rhabdomyosarcoma

Bladder tumors in children are rare and more often malignant than benign. The most frequently encountered tumor is rhabdomyosarcoma, which may arise in the bladder wall itself or from adjacent structures, and secondarily involve the bladder. In males, more than 50 % of the cases arise from the prostate (Fig. 15.22). In females, rhabdomyosarcomas arise from the vagina and the uterine cervix [28]. Pathologic analysis of the tissue cannot always distinguish the site of origin. Rare tumors involving the child's bladder include pheochromocytoma, transitional cell carcinoma, hemangioma, and neurofibroma [21].

Boys and girls are equally affected by rhabdomyosarcoma. There are two peak age incidences: the first between 2 and 6 years and the second between 14 and 18 years. Tumors of the bladder and vagina occur primarily in infants. Tumors usually involve the submucosal region of the trigone, less often they arise in the bladder dome. The child presents with hematuria, dysuria, or urinary retention. Tumors appear either as a pedunculated soft-tissue mass projecting into the bladder lumen, referred to as *sarcoma botryoides* or "bunch of grapes" appearance (Fig. 15.23) or as focal or diffuse wall thickening. The embryonal botryoid subtype accounts for one fourth of the rhabdomyosarcoma cases and has the most favorable prognosis compared with all other histologies [28]. Tumor echogenicity is equal to or less than that of the bladder wall. Calcification and areas of necrosis or hemorrhage may be seen. The mass is hypervascular on color Doppler imaging. Hydronephrosis, invasion of perivesical structures, and metastases to pelvic lymph nodes can be noted. Diffuse bladder wall thickening by rhabdomyosarcoma can be confused with cystitis, although the thickening usually is uniform in cystitis, whereas it is irregular in tumor infiltration. The solitary polypoid form of bladder rhabdomyosarcoma is indistinguishable from an inflammatory polyp, collapsed ureterocele, or nehprogenic adenoma which may occur in association with bladder inflammation.

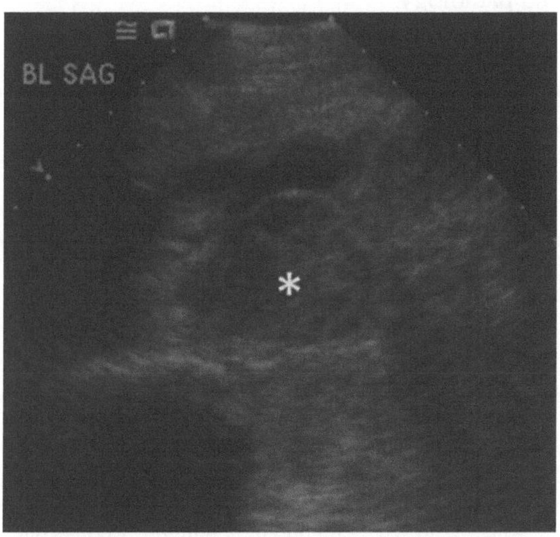

Fig. 15.22 Prostatic rhabdomyosarcoma. Sagittal scan of the pelvis shows a focal prostatic mass *(*)* extending into the base of the underfilled bladder

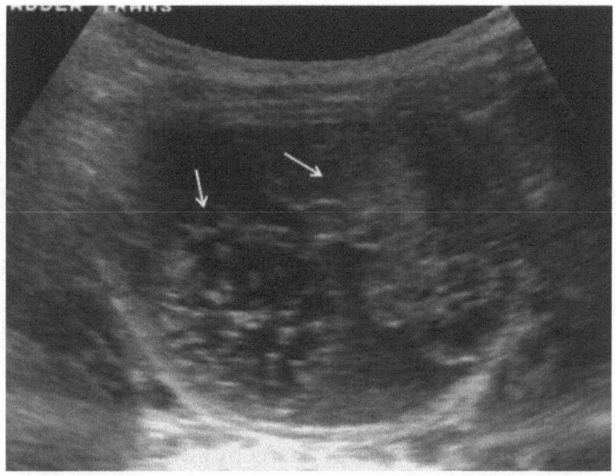

Fig. 15.23 Bladder rhabdomyosarcoma. Transverse sonogram of the bladder in an infant demonstrates a heterogeneous lobulated mass (*arrows*) arising from the bladder base. Biopsy confirmed the sarcoma botryoides subtype of rhabdomyosarcoma. (Courtesy of Kamaldine Oudjhane, MD, Toronto, Canada)

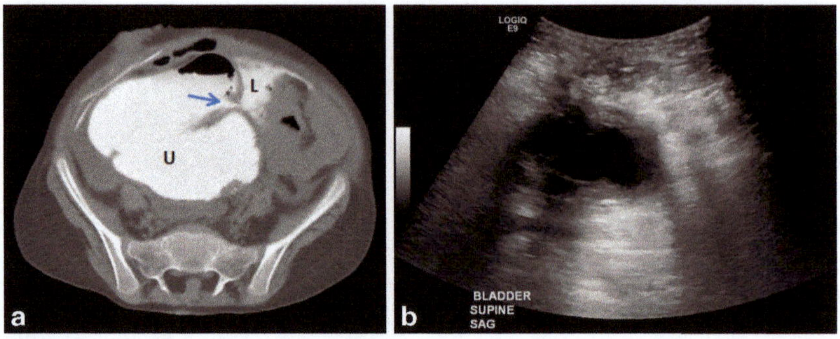

Fig. 15.24 Intraperitoneal rupture in a patient with augmented bladder status post cystoscopy and bladder irrigation. **a** Axial CT cystogram image shows contrast within the augmented bladder (*U*) and intraperitoneal leak of contrast (*L*) through a bladder wall perforation (*arrow*). **b** Immediate post-repair transverse sonogram of the bladder shows no appreciable residual perivesical fluid

Trauma

Injury of the bladder in childhood typically results from a blow to the lower abdomen when the bladder is distended or when the pelvis is fractured. The incidence of lower urinary tract injury in children is quite low, estimated at 0.2 % of the pediatric trauma admissions. Although 50 % of the children with bladder tears have a pelvic fracture, only 0.5–3.7 % of the children with pelvic fractures have associated bladder injuries [29]. Bladder injury can also be a complication of surgery or penetration by a foreign body. Bladder injuries are classified as intraperitoneal rupture (Fig. 15.24), extraperitoneal rupture, and combined type. In children, intraperitoneal rupture accounts for up to 60 % of all the bladder tears, and results from a direct blow tearing the bladder dome. Extraperitoneal rupture is less common in children than in adults, accounting for 40 % of all the cases. They are often associated with pelvic fractures that distort and shear the bladder base, below the peritoneal reflection.

CT cystogram is the study of choice in evaluating suspected bladder trauma, but US may be of value in follow-up evaluation. Sonographic findings of bladder trauma include diffuse wall thickening, intraluminal clot, and free pelvic and/or abdominal fluid [24].

Summary

US remains the modality of choice for imaging the genital organs of pediatric females because of its availability and reliability. US can assess the anatomy and hormonal status of children with sexual ambiguity and pubertal disorders. It is also the initial imaging technique to perform in children with pelvic pain or mass. In addition, sonography is very useful in the evaluation of the urinary bladder and its different disorders. Overall, the modality is well suited for the pelvis and is widely used in evaluation of pelvic anatomy and pathology.

References

1. Riccabona M. Ultrasound of the urogenital tract. In: Riccabona M, editor. Pediatric ultrasound: requisites and applications. Berlin: Springer; 2014. p. 321–95.
2. Siegel MJ, Surratt JT. Pediatric gynecologic imaging. Obstet Gynecol Clin North Am. 1992;19:103–27.
3. Cohen HL, Bober SE, Bow SN. Imaging the pediatric pelvis: the normal and abnormal genital tract and simulators of its diseases. Urol Radiol. 1992;14:273–83.
4. Teele RL, Share JC. Ultrasonography of the female pelvis in childhood and adolescence. Radiol Clin North Am. 1992;30:743–58.
5. De Bruyn R. The female reproductive system. In: De Bruyn R, editor. Pediatric ultrasound: how, why and when. 2nd ed. Edinburgh: Churchill Livingstone; 2010. p. 207–33.

6. Behr SC, Courtier JL, Qayyum A. Imaging of müllerian duct anomalies. Radiographics. 2012;32:E233–50.
7. Rousset P, Raudrant D, Peyron N, Buy JN, Valette PJ, Hoeffel C. Ultrasonography and MRI features of the Mayer–Rokitansky–Küster–Hauser syndrome. Clin Radiol. 2013;68:945–52.
8. Del Vescovo R, Battisti S, Paola V D, Piccolo CL, Cazzato RL, Sansoni I, Grasso RF, Zobel BB. Herlyn–Werner–Wunderlich syndrome: MRI findings, radiological guide (two cases and literature review), and differential diagnosis. BMC Med Imaging. 2012;12:4.
9. Walker DK, Salibian RA, Salibian AD, Belen KM, Palmer SL. Overlooked diseases of the vagina: a directed anatomic-pathologic approach for imaging assessment. Radiographics. 2011;31:1583–98.
10. Orbak Z, Kantarci M, Yildirim ZK, Karaca L, Doneray H. Ovarian volume and uterine length in neonatal girls. J Pediatr Endocrinol Metab. 2007;20:397–403.
11. Cohen HL, Shapiro MA, Mandel FS, Shapiro ML. Normal ovaries in neonates and infants: a sonographic study of 77 patients 1 day to 24 months old. AJR Am J Roentgenol. 1993;160:583–6.
12. Garel L, Dubois J, Grignon A, Filiatrault D, Van Vliet G. US of the pediatric female pelvis: a clinical perspective. Radiographics. 2001;21:1393–407.
13. Heo SH, Kim JW, Shin SS, Jeong SI, Lim HS, Choi YD, Lee KH, Kang WD, Jeong YY, Kang HK. Review of ovarian tumors in children and adolescents: radiologic–pathologic correlation. Radiographics. 2014;34:2039–55.
14. Riccabona M. Imaging of the neonatal genito-urinary tract. Eur J Radiol. 2006;60:187–98.
15. Fotter R. Neurogenic bladder in infants and children—a new challenge for the radiologist. Abdom Imaging. 1996;21:534–40.
16. Riccabona M, Avni FE, Blickman JG, Dacher J-N, Darge K, Lobo ML, Willi U. Imaging recommendations in paediatric uroradiology: minutes of the ESPR workgroup session on urinary tract infection, fetal hydronephrosis, urinary tract ultrasonography and voiding cystourethrography, Barcelona, Spain, June 2007. Pediatr Radiol. 2008;38:138–45.
17. Jequier S, Rousseau O. Sonographic measurements of the normal bladder wall in children. AJR Am J Roentgenol. 1987;149:563–6.
18. Kaefer M, Zurakowski D, Bauer SB, Retik AB, Peters CA, Atala A, Treves ST. Estimating normal bladder capacity in children. J Urol. 1997;158:2261–4.
19. Nørgaard JP, Van Gool JD, Hjälmås K, Djurhuus JC, Hellström A-L. Standardization and definitions in lower urinary tract dysfunction in children. Br J Urol. 1998;81(Suppl 3):1–16.
20. Cacciarelli AA, Kass EJ, Yang SS. Urachal remnants: sonographic demonstration in children. Radiology. 1990;174:473–5.
21. Fernbach SK, Feinstein KA. Abnormalities of the bladder in children: imaging findings. AJR Am J Roentgenol. 1994;162:1143–50.
22. Yu JS, Kim KW, Lee HJ, Lee YJ, Yoon CS, Kim MJ. Urachal remnant diseases: spectrum of CT and US findings. Radiographics. 2001;21:451–61.
23. Metwalli ZA, Guillerman RP, Mehollin-Ray AR, Schlesinger AE. Imaging features of intravesical urachal cysts in children. Pediatr Radiol. 2013;43:978–82.
24. Siegel MJ. Urinary tract. In: Siegel MJ, editor. Pediatric sonography. 4th ed. Philadelphia: Lippincott Williams & Wilkins; 2011. p. 384–460.
25. Ben-Chaim J, Docimo SG, Jeffs RD, Gearhart JP. Bladder exstrophy from childhood into adult life. J R Soc Med. 1996;89:39P–46P.
26. Barnewolt CE, Paltiel HJ, Lebowitz RL, Kirks DR. Genitourinary tract. In: Kirks DR, editor. Practical pediatric imaging. 3rd ed. Philadelphia: Lippincott Williams & Wilkins; 1998. p. 1009–170.
27. Boechat MI, Lebowitz RL. Diverticula of the bladder in children. Pediatr Radiol. 1978;7:22–8.
28. Bates DG. Bladder and urethra. In: Coley BD, editor. Caffey's pediatric diagnostic imaging. 12th ed. Philadelphia: Saunders; 2013. p. 1262–73.
29. Taylor GA. Genitourinary trauma. In: Coley BD, editor. Caffey's pediatric diagnostic imaging. 12th ed. Philadelphia: Saunders; 2013. p. 1285–9.

Groin and Testicle

16

Salmai Turial

Anatomy and Scanning Technique

Anatomy

Each of the two scrotal halves, divided longitudinally by the raphe, contains a testicle, epididymis, vas deferens, and spermatic cord. The testes are surrounded by the tunica albuginea, which is covered by the tunica vaginalis. The tunica vaginalis has two layers, an outer parietal layer and an inner visceral layer that are separated by a small volume of fluid.

The testis is ovoid in shape and the epididymis (consists of a head, body, and tail) lies along the posterolateral aspect of the testis. The largest portion of the epididymis is the head and is usually round or triangular in shape.

Structurally, the testes are divided into lobules by septa radiating from the tunica albuginea. Within the testicular parenchyma, seminiferous tubules converge at the mediastinum testis, an incomplete septum formed through invagination of the tunica albuginea (Fig. 16.1).

The appendix testis is a remnant of the Müllerian duct, which is attached to the upper pole of the testis and the appendix epididymis is a remnant of the mesonephron, which is found on the epididymal head [1, 2].

S. Turial (✉)
Department of Pediatric Surgery, University Medicine of the Johannes Gutenberg University Mainz, Langenbeckstraße 1, 55131 Mainz, Germany
e-mail: salmai.turial@unimedizin-mainz.de

Scanning Techniques

Position of the Patient

The patient is positioned in the supine position with the legs slightly spread apart. To improve

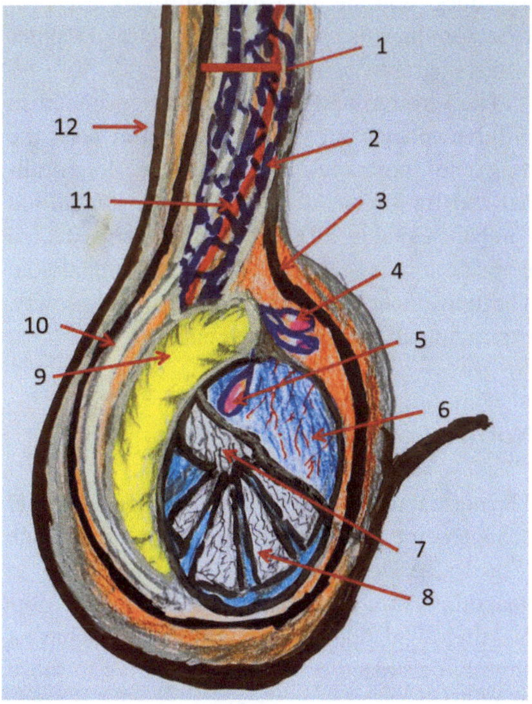

Fig. 16.1 Schematic illustration of the scrotal anatomy: *1* spermatic cord; *2* pampiniform plexus; *3* tunica vaginalis *(outer, parietal layer)*; *4* epididymal appendix; *5* testicular appendix; *6* testicle covered by tunica albuginea; *7* testicular mediastinum; *8* seminiferous tubules; *9* epididymis *(head)*; *10* ductus deferens; *11* testicular artery; *12* scrotal skin

S. Scholz, M. D. Jarboe (eds.), *Diagnostic and Interventional Ultrasound in Pediatrics and Pediatric Surgery,* DOI 10.1007/978-3-319-21699-7_16

exposure and to immobilize the testes, the scrotum is supported and slightly elevated by placing a towel beneath the scrotal sac. Ideally, it is placed in a towel sling. Prior to beginning with the ultrasound examination copious ultrasound jelly is applied to the scrotal area to provide sufficient surface interface of the linear transducer to the curvy scrotal surface and to avoid pressure on the testicle during the examination. It is very important for the child's comfort that the applied ultrasound gel is warmed close to body temperature. Utilizing cold gel may cause contraction of the scrotal skin or may elucidate the cremaster reflex with subsequent ascent of the testicles. Both effects may compromise the ultrasound examination.

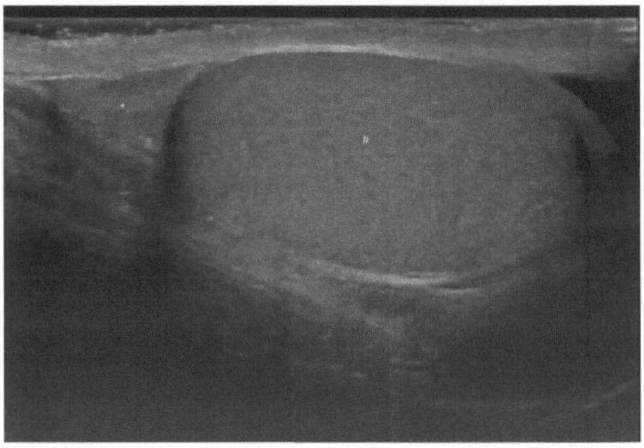

Fig. 16.2 Longitudinal scan of a pubertal testicle demonstrates granular homogenous echogenicity *(# testes; * head of epididymis)*

Scanning Techniques

The position of the scrotal and inguinal contents close to the surface requires use of a high-spatial resolution linear transducer dedicated to the study of soft tissues (9–15 MHz). Preferably, the transducer and the ultrasound software can provide simultaneous power and spectral Doppler ultrasonography as well.

The scrotum and its contents are scanned in different planes and documented in at least the long and short axes of the testicle (longitudinal and transverse scans). If one of the scrotal compartments is affected only, the unaffected hemiscrotum is scanned initially for comparison. The transducer is moved smoothly and slowly, examining all aspects of the anatomy.

Normal Sonographic Findings

The normal testis shows a granular medium-level echogenicity and is homogenous in appearance (Fig. 16.2). The testicular tissue echogenicity, in general, is similar to that of the liver or the normal thyroid gland [1, 2]. Prepubertal testes have a slightly decreased echogenicity relative to those in adults.

The tunica vaginalis appears as an echogenic outline of the testicle and a fold of it invaginates to the mediastinum of the testis. The mediastinum of the testis is visualized by ultrasound as a hyperechoic linear band running in craniocaudal direction.

The tubular rete testis appears as multiple small spherical or tubular hypoechoic regions close to the mediastinum testis.

The epididymis has an echogenicity slightly increased relative to the testicle. The epididymal head is round or ovoid in shape.

The appendix testis and the appendix epididymis are both embryological remnants of small ovoid hyperechoic protuberances found at the superior pole of the testis, normally hidden by the epididymal head. Unless torsed and swollen or outlined by fluid from a hydrocele, they are difficult to visualize on ultrasound.

In spectral Doppler sonography, the testis demonstrates a low-resistance arterial waveform. Color and spectral Doppler parameters should be set for low-flow power.

Some authors suggest that both, a short axis grayscale and a color Doppler image should be obtained of both testicles at the same time ("buddy shot" or "sunglasses view"), to compare relative echogenicity and blood flow. Most of the time, however, the transducer will not face both testicles at identical levels at the same time.

Size of the Testicle

The size of the testicle varies with age, increasing in size from birth to puberty. In a period of prepuberty, the testis contains a volume of about 2 cm^3 while it may develop a volume of up to 12–14 cm^3 during puberty [1].

In a population study of 769 boys (mean age=9.0 years; range: 0.6–19.0 years), Goede et al. [3] found no significant volume differences between the left and right testicle. Boys who had been born prematurely or who had an ethnic background other than Caucasian showed testicular volumes comparable to boys who had been born at term or who had Caucasian ethnicity. The mean testicular volume at 1 year of age was 0.48 ml. At 10 years of age it was 0.97 ml in their cohort [3].

Others also found no significant volume differences between the left and right testicle, and between the different ethnical groups. There were also no significant effects found correlating with birthweight and current body weight [4].

Volume Measurement Equations

The methodology for assessing testicular volume is not standardized. In the literature, the volumes obtained by ultrasound have been calculated by different equations for the ellipsoid.

The commonly used formula to measure the volume of a prolate ellipsoid, such as the testicle [4], has been described as:

$$\text{Testicularvolume}\left(\text{cm}^3\right) = \text{length}\left(\text{L}\right) \times \text{width}\left(\text{W}\right) \times \text{height}\left(\text{H}\right) \times \left(\pi/6\left(=0.5235\right)\right).$$

Further used equations are:

- The Hansen formula, in which W is squared, where:

$$V = L \times W^2 \times 0.52.$$

- The Lambert formula [4], where:

$$V = L \times W \times H \times 0.71.$$

However, there is no agreement which formula is the most accurate and the use of these mathematical equations is currently debated. Authors from Taiwan [5] state that larger errors result when applying the Lambert equation to estimate the volume of smaller testes. The authors conducted an interesting study to evaluate the accuracy of different equations for assessing testicular volume of smaller testes. The equations used usually for the testicular volume calculations were compared with the gold standard volume measurement obtained by water displacement (Archimedes principle). In their results, testicular volume estimates obtained from ultrasound measurements (Hansen and Lambert equations) correlated better with those obtained by water displacement measurement.

The authors suggest in their conclusion a new constant (0.59) for use in the Hansen equation to assess the volumes of smaller testes most accurately ($V=L \times W^2 \times 0.59$ [5]).

Undescended Testicle

Undescended testicles, located in the groin, or retractile testes are usually diagnosed by physical examination. There is no "true" indication for ultrasound examination routinely except for preoperative volume assessment and postoperative follow-up.

If the testicle is not found either in the scrotum or in the groin by physical examination (impalpable testicle; ectopic-, vanishing-, abdominal testes; testicular agenesis; true hermaphroditism), ultrasound is the first imaging modality performed. Twenty percent of the maldescended testes are non-palpable. Of the non-palpable testes, 50 % are abdominal, 45 % are atrophic, and 5 % are in the inguinal canal [6].

Imaging modalities including the MRI usually fail to detect non-palpable testis unless possibly located in the vicinity of the internal ring. The value of ultrasound for evaluation of non-palpable testes as discussed in the literature is controversial.

While Kanemoto et al. [7] and Wolverson et al. [8] showed that ultrasound had a sensitivity of 76–88 %, a specificity of 100 %, and an accuracy of 84–91 % for the diagnosis of non-palpable testis, others demonstrated limited diagnostic accuracy of imaging studies in non-palpable testes. Trasian et al. [9] conducted a meta-analysis including 12 studies of subjects younger than 18 years who had preoperative ultrasound evaluation for non-palpable testes and whose testes position was subsequently determined by surgery. They found that ultrasound had a sensitivity of 45 % and a specificity of 78 %, and concluded that ultrasound does not reliably localize non-palpable testes and does not rule out intra-abdominal testes.

Adesanya et al. [10] estimated the diagnostic accuracy of ultrasound evaluation for preoperative localization of undescended testes in children around 86.5 %.

Ultrasound is limited particularly in the evaluation of abdominal and retroperitoneal ectopic testes. For detection and evaluation of an atrophic testis, ultrasound may be inconclusive as it is difficult to differentiate the atrophic testicle from lymph nodes or parts of the infravaginal gubernaculum. Both structures can be mistaken for testicular tissue.

In our own experiences, diagnostic laparoscopy is the method of choice for suspected abdominal and non-palpable testes.

Shah and Shah [11] noted an overall diagnostic agreement between ultrasonography and laparoscopy in only 19 % of cases.

The undescended testicle might be smaller in volume and slightly hypoechoic in structure by ultrasound imaging compared to the normal testicle. The presence of a mediastinum testis (a longitudinal echogenic band) is diagnostic for the maldescended testis.

Hydrocele Testis, Spermatic Cord Hydrocele, Hydrocele of the Canal of Nuck

Hydrocele testis, spermatic cord hydrocele (funicolocele), and the hydrocele of the canal of Nuck (in girls only) are seen as anechogenic homogeneous fluid collections by ultrasound imaging (Fig. 16.3), occasionally containing septations and loculations (Fig. 16.4), calcifications and cholesterol.

Nuck's cyst presents as a cystic mass lying superficially and medially to the pubic bone at the level of the superficial inguinal ring enlarging toward the major labia. By clinical examination, Nuck's cysts may mimic an ovarial prolapse in female infants and a funicolocele (hydrocele of the cord) may mimic an irreducible inguinal hernia in boys. In those cases, a quick ultrasound

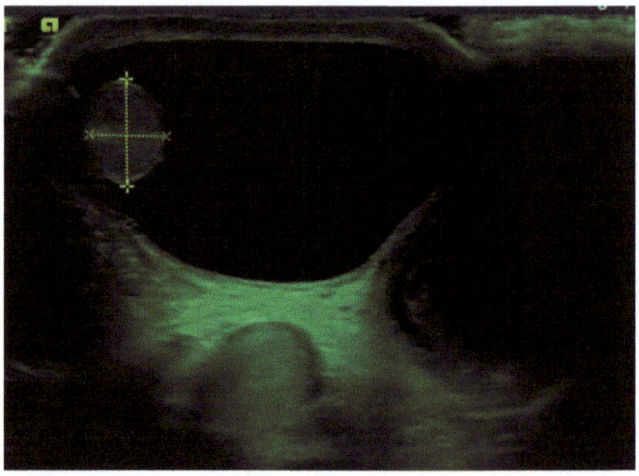

Fig. 16.3 Transverse sonogram shows the testis within a large, anechoic hydrocele *(clear fluid collection)*

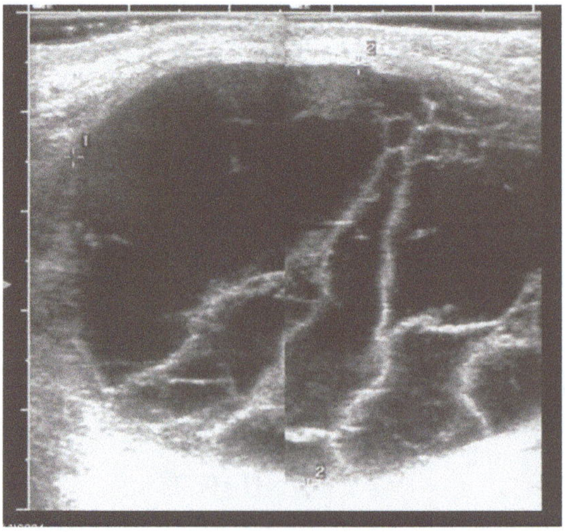

Fig. 16.4 Ultrasound image of a very large hydrocele containing multiple septations and loculations

evaluation brings clarity to the diagnosis very easily and can avoid repeated attempts of unsuccessful reduction by a physician, who is unfamiliar or inexperienced with these conditions.

Acquired or reactive hydroceles are seen in conjunction with infection, tumors, trauma, torsion, and incarcerated inguinal hernia.

The abdominoscrotal or communicating hydrocele represents a rare condition in children where a large scrotal hydrocele is connected with the abdominal cavity. The abdominal extension of the fluid collection may be preperitoneal or retroperitoneal, and the processus vaginalis may be patent or obliterated. The disorder has been associated with a variety of pathological entities (Fig. 16.4).

Varicocele

A varicocele is defined as a collection of abnormal enlarged tortuous veins of the pampiniform plexus of the spermatic cord. Dilatation of the pampiniform plexus larger than 1.5–2 cm in total diameter in adults (in resting state and in supine position) is considered as a varicocele. Correspondingly, in children, a diameter larger than 0.5 cm in prepuberty and larger than 0.8 cm in puberty is described as varicocele, respectively [1]. The veins of the pampiniform plexus normally range from 0.5 to 1.5 mm in diameter, and a dilatation greater than 2 mm in diameter is characteristic for varicocele.

The vast majority of the varicoceles are primary due to defective incompetent valves in the testicular vein. In contrast, the less common secondary varicoceles result from an increased pressure in the testicular veins caused by compression by an extrinsic mass, or obstruction.

Varicoceles are commonly located on the left side (85 %). This clear difference in predominance may be due to the shorter course of right testicular vein and its oblique insertion directly into the inferior vena cava, in contrast to the left testicular vein, which has a longer course and a right angle entry into the left renal vein.

Varicocele can be reliably diagnosed with ultrasound, which should be performed in both supine and standing positions including the Valsalva maneuvers (Figs. 16.5, 16.6, 16.7, 16.8 and 16.9). Power Doppler mode should be used to confirm flow in the varicocele, and there may even be flow reversal with the Valsalva maneuver, which is useful to grade the degree of reflux.

In the literature, several grading systems for varicocele severity have been proposed.

The most used ultrasound grading system was proposed by Sarteschi [12, 13], grading the varicocele into five grades according to its length, the characteristics of the reflux, and changes during the Valsalva's maneuver by CDU:

Grade 1 is characterized by non-dilated intrascrotal veins by grey-scale study, and prolonged reflux in the vessels in the inguinal canal during the Valsalva's maneuver.

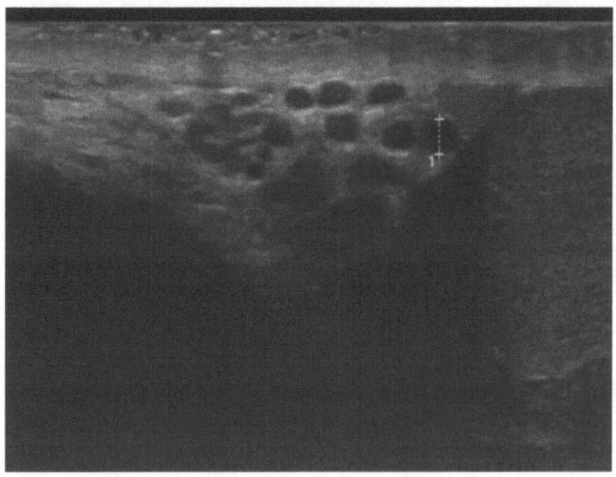

Fig. 16.5 Longitudinal scan of the pampiniform plexus in a 15-year-old boy with varicocele measuring the vein diameter in supine position of the patient

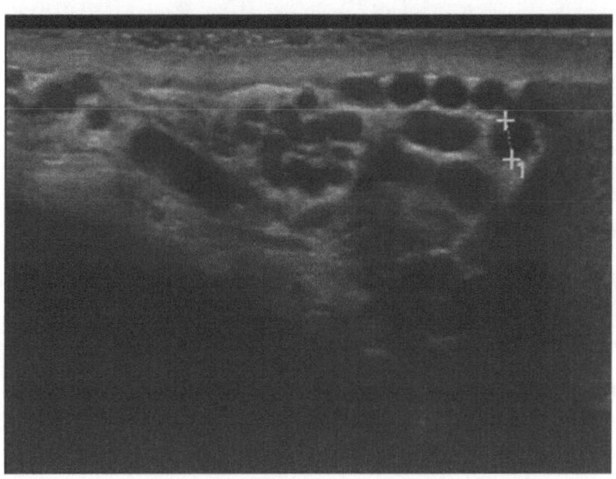

Fig. 16.6 Same patient as in Fig. 16.5 during the Valsalva maneuver resulting in moderate dilatation of the vessels

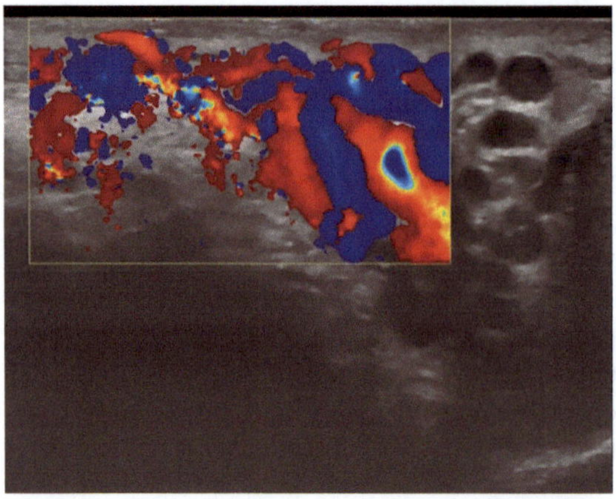

Fig. 16.7 CDU image of the same patient as in Fig. 16.6

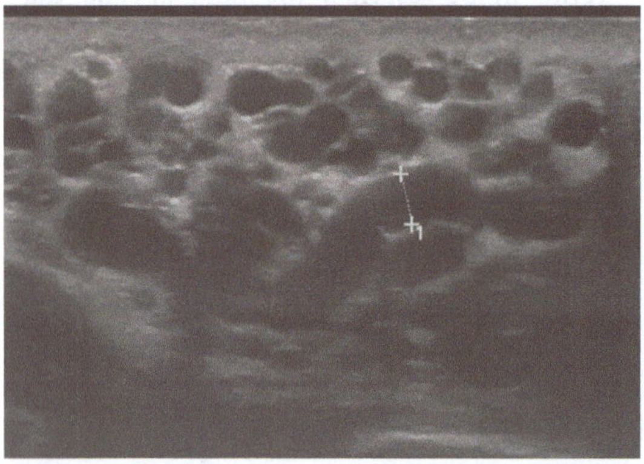

Fig. 16.8 The same patient as in Fig. 16.5: longitudinal scan after 2 min in standing position demonstrates impressive dilatation of the complete pampiniform plexus compared to the findings during the Valsalva maneuver in supine position (see Fig. 16.7 for comparison)

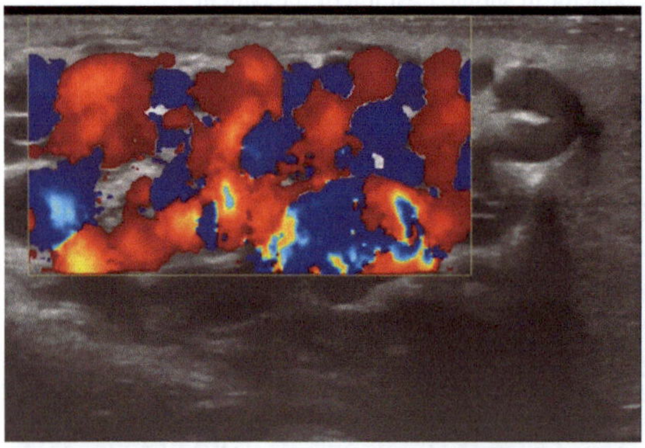

Fig. 16.9 Same patient as in Fig. 16.8 color Doppler ultrasound (CDU) image showed no further increase of the vein dilatation after 1 min of the Valsalva maneuver in standing position

Grade 2 shows a prominent posterior varicosity at the upper pole of the testis and reflux into the supratesticular region during the CDU evaluation.

Grade 3 is characterized by major dilatation of the venous vessels in the supine position, and to the inferior pole of the testis in standing position only. CDU demonstrates reflux at the lower pole veins only during the Valsalva maneuver.

Grade 4 has dilated veins in an supine position. This enlargement of the veins increases in the standing position over time and during Valsalva's maneuver. There is clear increase of the venous reflux after the Valsalva's maneuver. Hypotrophy of the testis is common at this stage.

Grade 5 shows venous dilatation even in a supine position. CDU demonstrates the presence of a baseline basal venous reflux without the Valsalva maneuver that does not further increase after the Valsalva maneuver (Table 16.1).

A total score of 4 or more determines the presence of a varicocele by CDU.

Iosa and Lazzarini in 2013 [15], proposed a new hemodynamic classification of the varicocele that could improve the accuracy of staging and the quality of the examination:

Table 16.1 Scoring system for CDU diagnosis of the varicocele [14]

	Score
Maximum vein diameter (mm)	
<2.5 0	0
2.5–2.9	1
3.0–3.9	2
>/=4.0	3
Plexus/sum of diameter of veins	
No plexus identified	0
Plexus (+) with sum diameter <3 mm	1
Plexus (+) with sum diameter 3–5.9 mm	2
Plexus (+) with sum diameter >/=6 mm	3
Change of flow velocity on the Valsalva maneuver	
<2 cm/s or duration <1 s	0
2–4.9	1
5–9.9	2
>/=10	3
Total score	0–9

Grade 1: Venous reflux lasting >1 s only during the Valsalva maneuver.

Grade 2: Spontaneous, discontinuous venous reflux that is not increased by the Valsalva maneuver.

Grade 3: Spontaneous, discontinuous venous reflux that is increased by the Valsalva maneuver.

Grade 4:

Level A: Spontaneous, continuous venous reflux that is not increased by the Valsalva maneuver.

Level B: Spontaneous, continuous venous reflux that is increased by the Valsalva maneuver.

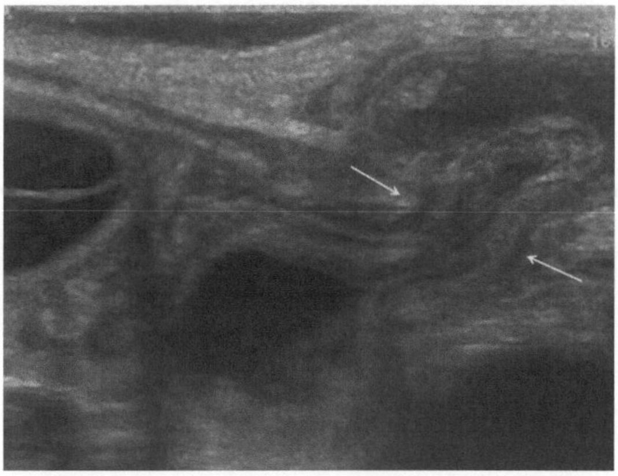

Fig. 16.10 Longitudinal sonogram of the inguinal region shows a bowel loop entering the inguinal canal traversing the internal inguinal ring *(arrows)*

Intestinal Hernia

In children and particularly in infants, the presence of an inguinal hernia by ultrasound is unreliable if the hernial sac is completely empty. The hernial sac most commonly contains bowel, followed by omentum. In female newborns and infants, visible and palpable swelling in the groin area is indicative of a hernia. The hernia sack frequently contains an ovary, the so called "ovarial prolapse" into a patent processus vaginalis [1, 16].

Ultrasound findings can include a fluid- or air-filled loop of bowel (Fig. 16.10). Omentum is visible as hyperechoic mass in the groin consistent with omental fat. The presence of real-time peristalsis in the inguinal canal is diagnostic for bowel in the hernia sac, and dilated bowel loops in the canal with complete absence of peristalsis is worrisome for incarceration. After an attempted reposition of an incarcerated hernia, ultrasound examination may be helpful to verify the complete reposition of the hernial sac contents into to the abdominal cavity.

The Acute Scrotum—Epididymitis, Orchitis, Torsion of Testis and Appendages, Trauma

Acute scrotal pain can have multiple causes. Up to 70% of young boys with acute scrotal symptoms have conditions other than testicular torsion, most commonly epididymitis. Ultrasound is helpful to rule in or rule out testicular torsion as it is a real urologic emergency with subsequent need for immediate surgical intervention or potential loss of the testicle.

Testicular Torsion Ultrasound is the modality of choice for evaluating both complete and incomplete testicular torsion. It is able to reliably assess the echogenicity of the testis, as well as the vascular perfusion. Testicular torsion can be classified as extravaginal or intravaginal and mesorchial (variance in mesenteric attachment (mesorchium)) [17]. Extra- or supravaginal torsion occurs in newborns and infants before the testis is fixed. Intravaginal torsion is much more common (65–80% [18]) with an age peak around puberty [1]. It is associated with a preexisting fixation anomaly of the testis, termed "bell clapper testis." The degree of torsion of the testis can range from 180 to 720°, but complete occlusion of blood flow typically does not occur before 450° of torsion. Transient or intermittent torsion (a torsion–detorsion sequence) with spontaneous resolution may sometimes occur.

During torsion, the spermatic cord twists upon itself resulting initially in venous congestion as the veins pose low-intravascular pressure and collapsible vessel walls. Venous obstruction is followed by a decrease in arterial inflow, which progresses to complete occlusion, testicular ischemia, and infarction [19].

Preferably, the ultrasound examination is started with the unaffected testicle to optimize the lower settings for flow, resistance, and velocity for CDU.

The testis is usually elevated and fixed in position as a result of the torsion, a so called high-riding testicle [18]. The Praen test can support the clinical suspicion.

Ultrasound findings can be variable, depending on the duration and of the torsion and the extent of vascular compromise. In the early period, 4–6 h after occurrence of the spermatic cord torsion, the testicle may appear slightly enlarged with normal or decreased echogenicity and the parenchyma of the testicle will become less homogenous. Reactive hydrocele and hyperechoic regions within the testicular tissue representing the initial hemorrhage may be present.

Later findings after 24 h are dominated by hypoechoic necrosis, heterogeneous structure (Figs. 16.11 and 16.12), enlargement of the epididymal head, scrotal wall thickening, and hyperemia of the surrounding tissue and the scrotal skin. Reactive hydroceles are common. Spiral twisting of the spermatic cord may be seen with color Doppler imaging. Downward movement of transducer along the cord may show a "whirlpool sign" [20] . A color Doppler study must be performed to confirm or rule out both, arterial and venous flow in the testicle. Color Doppler settings should be optimized to demonstrate low-velocity flow with a low-pulse repetition frequency and a low wall filter.

Unilateral diminished or absent central testicular blood flow is diagnostic for testicular torsion. In experienced hands, ultrasound evaluation of the testicle should read a very high sensitivity and specificity for torsion reaching close to 100%.

Power Doppler flow may be difficult to demonstrate in very young children, even within the normal testis due to its small size [21, 22].

More recently, imaging studies such as contrast-enhanced ultrasound, dynamic contrast magnetic resonance study, and near-infrared imaging are promising modalities for additional evaluation of testicular blood supply. At this time, availability is limited and the tidies are not used routinely for emergency cases.

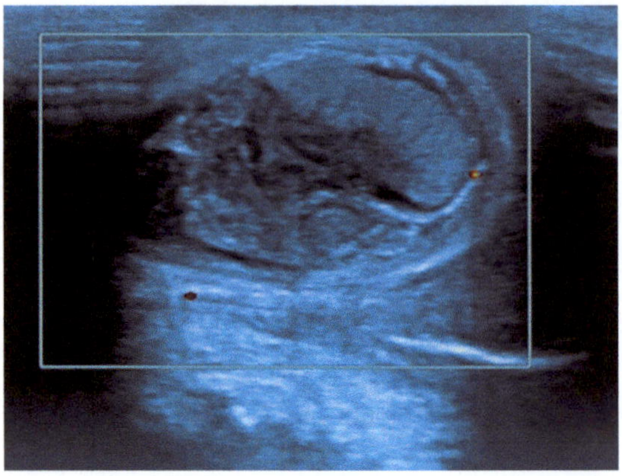

Fig. 16.11 Later ultrasound finding of a testicular torsion in a newborn: the transverse scan demonstrates hypoechoic necrosis and the heterogeneous structure of the testicle surrounded by a reactive hydrocele

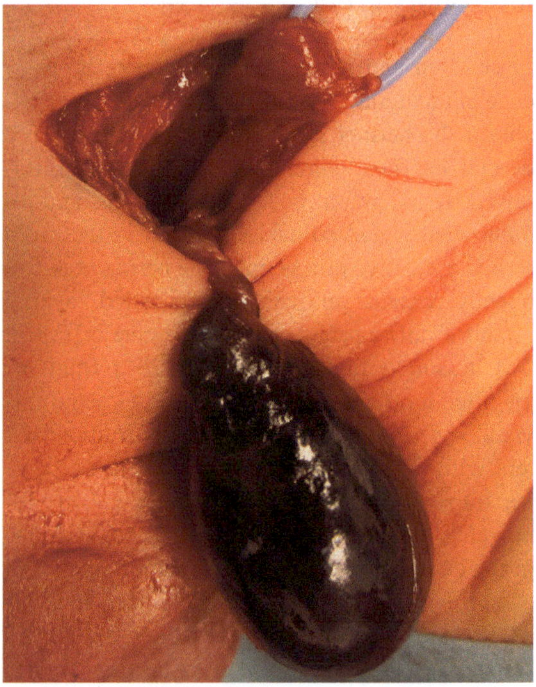

Fig. 16.12 Intraoperative finding of a prolonged extravaginal testicular torsion (same patient as in Fig. 16.11)

Torsion of Intrascrotal Appendices The most common cause of acute scrotum in prepubertal boys is torsion of the testicular or epididymal appendices. Most appendages are adjacent or in close proximity to the upper pole of the testis. A number of different localization of intrascrotal appendices exist, more frequently affected is the appendix testis compared to the epididiymal appendix. A testicular appendix may be seen between the testis and epididymis, and an epididymal appendix is attached to the head of the epididymis. Usually, unaffected intrascrotal appendices are difficult to pick up on gray scale ultrasound and CDU [23, 24].

Torsion of the testicular or epididymal appendix appears as a small pedunculated nodule. The tender and avascular lesion typically has low echogenicity with central hypoechogenic areas. Increased periappendiceal blood flow and hyperemia, hydrocele , and scrotal wall thickening are also suggestive of a torsed intrascrotal appendix (Figs. 16.13 and 16.14).

Epididymitis, Orchitis Infections generally originate in the lower urinary tract and spread retrograde to the epididymis, with its head most commonly involved. Orchitis is an acute infection of the testicle, usually following epididymitis.

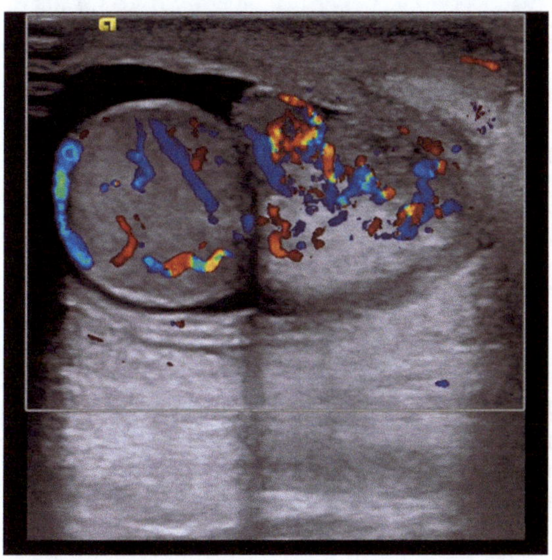

Fig. 16.13 Doppler image of a torsed intrascrotal appendix demonstrating increased periappendiceal blood flow, reactive inflammation of the epididiymis and of the testicle, as well as a reactive hydrocele

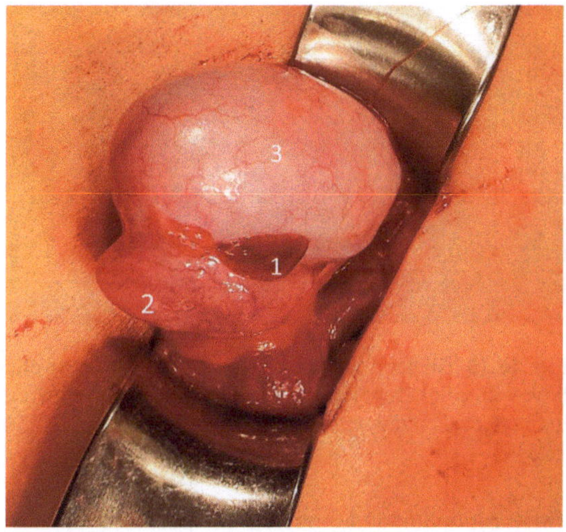

Fig. 16.14 Intraoperative picture of a torsed testicular appendix (*1* Torsed testicular appendix; *2* Epididymal head; *3* Testicle)

Ultrasound findings of acute epididymitis include an enlarged epididymis with decreased, heterogeneous echogenicity. Orchitis typically presents as an enlarged testicle with heterogeneous echogenicity and focal, peripheral, hypoechoic testicular lesions. Reactive hydroceles, hyperemia of epididymis and testicle, as well as scrotal wall thickening are frequently associated with both conditions.

This appearance is nonspecific and can be seen in many other conditions such as tumors, metastasis, infarction, and torsion [19].

With color Doppler, there is an increased blood flow in the affected epididymis and testicle noted (Fig. 16.15), whereas a normal epididymis has only limited color flow. The presence of normal or increased blood flow in CDU clearly differentiates epididymitis and orchitis from testicular torsion.

Color Doppler cannot differentiate malignant hypervascularity from inflammatory hypervascularity.

Acute Idiopathic Scrotal Edema Idiopathic scrotal edema is seen in 4–6 years aged boys. The pathophysiology is unclear with both infection

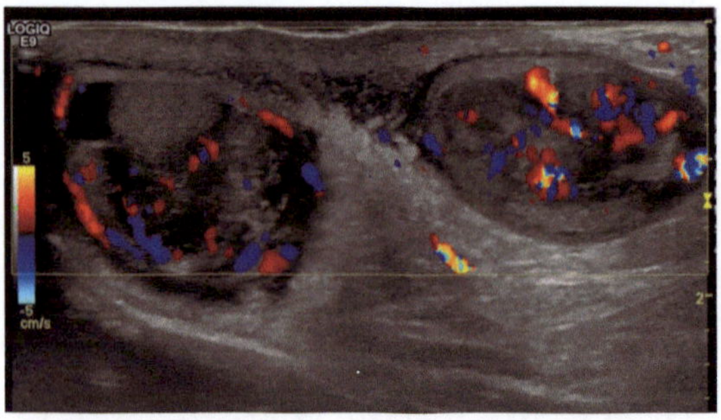

Fig. 16.15 Bilateral chronic epididymitis in a 1-year-old boy: with color Doppler, there is increased blood flow in both affected epididymises noted

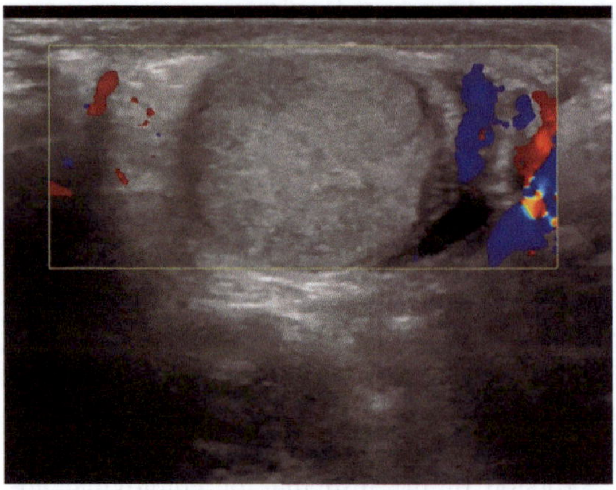

Fig. 16.16 Transverse CDU scan a few hours after blunt trauma to the testicle of a 9-year-old boy demonstrates hyperechogenic hemorrhage and fracture of the testicle

and angioedema suggested as possible causes [1]. The condition is self-limiting, with resolution usually within 3 days. Unilateral or bilateral scrotal wall thickening, edema, and erythema are characteristic. A "fountain sign" can be found on CDU [25]). Ultrasound demonstrates increased scrotal wall thickness and hypoechoic areas in the scrotal wall representing edema, with increased blood flow on color Doppler evaluation [25]. The condition is self-limiting, with resolution usually within 3 days.

Trauma

Injuries to the scrotum include blunt, penetrating, and degloving trauma. Blunt force trauma to the scrotum and the testicles is characterized by a hematocele or testicular hematoma, or testicular fracture. Patients can present with various degrees of pain, ecchymosis, and swelling.

Testicular rupture occurs when the testicle receives a direct blow or is squeezed against the hard bones of the pelvis. By ultrasound, testicular rupture appears as focal alterations of testicular echogenicity and irregularity of the testicular margins.

In the acute phase, the fresh hematoma and hemorrhage is echogenic (Fig. 16.16), but later appears more hypoechoic (Fig. 16.17). The collection may develop loculations and septations. Hematoceles are avascular on color Doppler imaging [26].

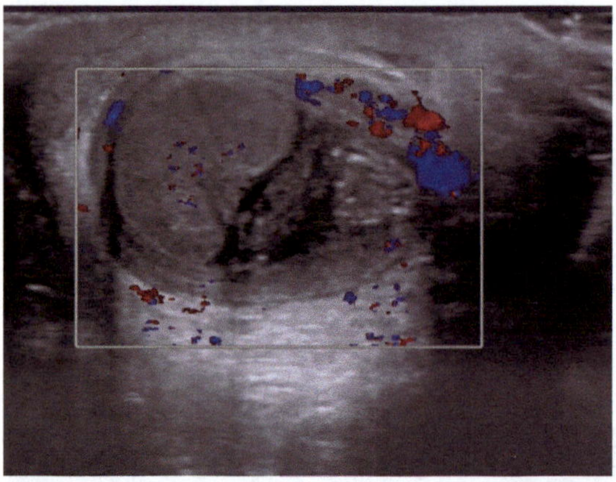

Fig. 16.17 Doppler imaging of the same patient as in Fig. 16.16 10 days after the initial trauma shows hypoechoic necrosis and loculations, as well as septations within the testicle

Tumor

Testicular tumors are very rare in the pediatric population (1 % of the entire malignancy in this population) with an average age of 3.8 years at time of diagnosis [1] with the mean age at diagnosis being 18 months [2].

Yolk sac tumors (endodermal sinus tumors) are the most commonly reported malignant testicular neoplasms (62 %) in prepubescent boys [2, 21, 27] and usually occur before the age of 2 years [27].

According to the Prepubertal Testis Tumor Registry of the Urologic Section of the American Academy of Pediatrics, the teratoma is the second most frequent primary testicular tumor (26 %) [28]. The seminoma is not seen in the pediatric population, and other malignant germ-cell tumors, including embryonal cell carcinoma and teratocarcinoma, typically occur only after puberty. Neoplasms from either Leydig or Sertoli cells of the testicular interstitium account for 10–30 %, and leukemia or lymphoma for less than 10 % of testicular masses in pediatric patients [2, 28].

The initial ultrasound images are useful for localizing palpable abnormalities in the scrotum in order to differentiate between solid or mixed cystic, extra- or intratesticular masses (Figs. 16.18 and 16.19).

The ultrasound characteristics of the intrascrotal tumors are not conclusive enough for reliable differentiation of tumor tissue types and histology remains the only certain diagnostic tool.

Yolk sac tumor may sonographically appear as a heterogeneous solid mass replacing the entire testis, or as a diffusely enlarged heterogeneous testis.

In a series of seven children with a pathologic diagnosis of mature teratoma of the testis reported by Epifanio et al. [29], the ultrasound findings were very variable. It can simulate other lesions, be single, multiseptated, small, or large. The testicle can contain diffuse or localized calcifications and may have an increased or normal volume [29]. Echogenic fat or calcifications may also be seen in teratomas [1, 22]. Immature teratomas tend to be more solid, but still heterogeneous with areas of hemorrhage and necrosis.

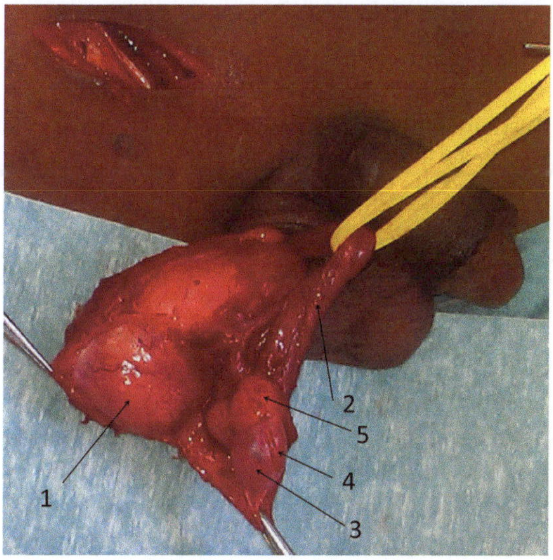

Fig. 16.19 The intraoperative finding (same patient as in Fig. 16.18) shows a mass (*rhabdomyosarcoma*) *(1)* at the *left aspect* of the photograph and a visually unaffected spermatic cord *(2)*, testicle *(3)* with an appendix testis *(4)* and the epididymal head *(5)* at the *right aspect* of the photograph

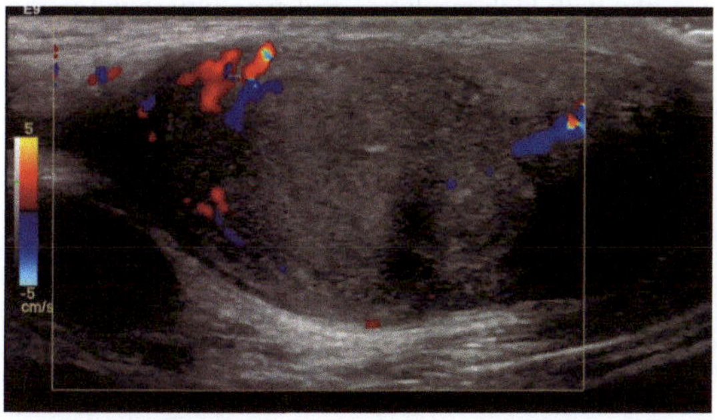

Fig. 16.18 Indifferent ultrasound findings at the initial evaluation of a paratesticular mixed rhabdomyosarcoma, which was initially misinterpreted as a chronic testicular torsion (please compare Fig. 16.19)

Lymphoma and leukemia are the most common metastases to the testes. Sonography may show a diffusely enlarged hypoechoic testicle or multifocal hypoechoic nodules [22].

Other benign cysts or tumors may include epidermoid, intratesticular, or tunica albuginea cysts, as well as adrenal rests and may appear cystic or heterogeneous on sonography.

The characteristic sonographic appearance of an epidermoid cyst presents as a heterogeneous mass, possibly as either a rounded hypoechoic lesion with a hyperechoic rim, or as the more classic lamellated "onion ring" or "onion skin" appearance. The epidermoid is often avascular on CDU [14, 30].

The sonographic appearance of adrenal rests is variable, with some series describing predominantly hypoechoic masses and others reporting heterogeneously hyperechoic masses with shadowing. Lesions are typically multiple, bilateral, and eccentrically located, usually within the testicular mediastinum.

Testicular Microlithiasis Testicular microlithiasis is a condition in which microcalcifications, composed of hydroxyapatite, are located within seminiferous tubules (≥5 microcalcifications within a testicle). With ultrasonography, the microcalcifications picture as punctuate, nonshadowing, echogenic foci [1, 31]. The condition is of clinical interest primarily due to its association with testicular malignancy.

In a recent study, Cooper et al. [31] reported that testicular microlithiasis has a prevalence of 2 % in boys who undergo scrotal ultrasound (out of a total of 3370 boys), and it was most commonly bilateral (75 %). Although they found a significant association of testicular microlithiasis and other testicular tumors, Volokhina et al. [32] reported no significant association between testicular microlithiasis and testicular germ-cell tumors.

In their study, the incidence of testicular germ-cell tumors was calculated in a group of patients with testicular microlithiasis and in a control group without testicular microlithiasis. The incidence of testicular microlithiasis was 3.8 % (out of 2266 boys). Incidence of testicular germ-cell tumors in testicular microlithiasis patients was 1.2 and 0.38 % in non-testicular microlithiasis patients (out of 2179 children).

Summary

Ultrasound examination is the modality of choice for imaging most of the conditions of the groin and scrotal area in the pediatric population. Sonography of the groin, but especially the scrotum demonstrates high levels of specificity, sensitivity, and overall diagnostic accuracy.

The value of ultrasound for evaluation of non-palpable testes as discussed in the literature is controversial. Diagnostic laparoscopy is the method of choice for suspected abdominal and non-palpable testes. A varicocele can be reliably diagnosed with ultrasound, which should be performed in both, supine and standing positions including a Valsalva maneuver. Ultrasound is the modality of choice to confirm or rule out a testicular torsion, and can clearly differentiate epididymitis and orchitis from testicular torsion, a urological emergency.

The sonographic imaging characteristics of variable intrascrotal tumors are not conclusive enough for differentiation of tumor tissue and reliable diagnosis, and a biopsy must be obtained.

References

1. Hofmann V, Deeg K-H, Hoyer PF. Ultraschalldiagnostik in Pädiatrie und Kinderchirurgie: Lehrbuch und Atlas. 3rd Ed. Thieme; 2005. ISBN-13:978-3131009531.
2. Carkaci S, Ozkan E, Lane D, Yang WT. Scrotal sonography revisited. J Clin Ultrasound. 2010 Jan;38(1):21–37.
3. Goede J, van der Voort-Doedens LM, Sijstermans K, Hack WW. The volume of retractile testes. J Urol. 2011 Nov;186(5):2050–4.
4. Kuijper EA, van Kooten J, Verbeke JI, van Rooijen M, Lambalk CB. Ultrasonographically measured testicular volumes in 0- to 6-year-old boys. Hum Reprod. 2008 Apr;23(4):792–6.
5. Lin CC, Huang WJ, Chen KK. Measurement of testicular volume in smaller testes: how accurate is the conventional orchidometer? J Androl. 2009 Nov–Dec;30(6):685–9.
6. Pradhan MR, Ansari MS. Imaging studies for non-palpable testis: are they at all required? Indian J Urol. 2012 Apr–Jun;28(2):227–9.
7. Kanemoto K, Hayashi Y, Kojima Y, Maruyama T, Ito M, Kohri K. Accuracy of ultrasonography and magnetic resonance imaging in the diagnosis of nonpalpable testis. Int J Urol. 2005;12:668–72.
8. Wolverson MK, Houttuin E, Heiberg E, Sundaram M, Shields JB. Comparison of computed tomography with high-resolution real-time ultrasound in the localisation of the impalpable undescended testis. Radiology. 1983;146:133–6.
9. Tasian GE, Copp HL. Diagnostic performance of ultrasound in nonpalpable cryptorchidism: a systematic review and meta-analysis. Pediatrics. 2011;127:119–28.
10. Adesanya OA, Ademuyiwa AO, Evbuomwan O,et al. Preoperative localization of undescended testes in children: comparison of clinical examination and ultrasonography. J Pediatr Urol. 2014;10(2):237–40.
11. Shah A, Shah A. Impalpable testes—is imaging really helpful? Indian Pediatr. 2006;43:720–3.
12. Liguori G, Trombetta C, Garaffa G, Bucci S, Gattuccio I, Salamè L, Belgrano E. Color Doppler ultrasound investigation of varicocele. World J Urol. 2004 Nov;22(5):378–81.

13. Pauroso S, Leo ND, Fulle I, Segni MD, Alessi S, Maggini E. Varicocele: ultrasonographic assessment in daily clinical practice. J Ultrasound. 2011 Dec;14(4):199–204.
14. Chiou RK, Anderson JC, Wobig RK, Rosinsky DE, Matamoros A Jr, Chen WS, Taylor RJ. Color Doppler ultrasound criteria to diagnose varicoceles: correlation of a new scoring system with physical examination. Urology. 1997 Dec;50(6):953–6.
15. Iosa G, Lazzarini D. Hemodynamic classification of varicoceles in men: our experience. J Ultrasound. 2013 Apr 30;16(2):57–63.
16. Agrawal AM, Tripathi PS, Shankhwar A, Naveen C. Role of ultrasound with color Doppler in acute scrotum management. J Family Med Prim Care. 2014 Oct-Dec;3(4):409–12.
17. Chan JL, Knoll JM, Depowski PL, Williams RA, Schober JM. Mesorchial testicular torsion: case report and a review of the literature. Urology. 2009 Jan;73(1):83–6.
18. Lin EP, Bhatt S, Rubens DJ, Dogra VS. Testicular torsion: twists and turns. Semin Ultrasound CT MR. 2007 Aug;28(4):317–28.
19. Yusuf GT, Sidhu PS. A review of ultrasound imaging in scrotal emergencies. J Ultrasound. 2013 Sep 4;16(4):171–8.
20. Vijayaraghavan SB. Sonographic differential diagnosis of acute scrotum: real-time whirlpool sign, a key sign of torsion. J Ultrasound Med. 2006 May;25(5):563–74.
21. Sharp VJ, Kieran K, Arlen AM. Testicular torsion: diagnosis, evaluation, and management. Am Fam Physician. 2013 Dec 15;88(12):835–40.
22. Sung EK, Setty BN, Castro-Aragon I. Sonography of the pediatric scrotum: emphasis on the Ts–torsion, trauma, and tumors. AJR Am J Roentgenol. 2012 May;198(5):996–1003.
23. Lev M, Ramon J, Mor Y, Jacobson JM, Soudack M. Sonographic appearances of torsion of the appendix testis and appendix epididymis in children. J Clin Ultrasound. 2015 Feb 20.
24. Osman S, Zaidi SF, Lehnert BE, Linnau KF. Core curriculum illustration: testicular torsion. Emerg Radiol. 2014 Jun;21(3):321–3.
25. Geiger J, Epelman M, Darge K. The fountain sign: a novel color Doppler sonographic finding for the diagnosis of acute idiopathic scrotal edema. J Ultrasound Med. 2010 Aug;29(8):1233–7.
26. Dalton DM, Davis NF, O'Neill DC, Brady CM, Kiely EA, O'Brien MF. Aetiology, epidemiology and management strategies for blunt scrotal trauma. Surgeon. 2014 Aug 20. pii: S1479-666X(14)00076-6.
27. Wei Y, Wu S, Lin T, He D, Li X, Liu J, Liu X, Hua Y, Lu P, Wei G. Testicular yolk sac tumors in children: a review of 61 patients over 19 years. World J Surg Oncol. 2014 Dec 29;12:400.
28. Renzo DD, Persico A, Sindici G, Lelli Chiesa P. Testicular teratoma, mimicking a simple testicular cyst, in an infant. Urology. 2013 Sep;82(3):701–3.
29. Epifanio M, Baldissera M, Esteban FG, Baldisserotto M. Mature testicular teratoma in children: multifaceted tumors on ultrasound. Urology. 2014 Jan;83(1):195–7.
30. Slawin J, Slawin K. Intratesticular epidermoid cyst masquerading as testicular torsion. Rev Urol. 2014;16(4):198–201.
31. Cooper ML, Kaefer M, Fan R, Rink RC, Jennings SG, Karmazyn B. Testicular microlithiasis in children and associated testicular cancer. Radiology. 2014 Mar;270(3):857–63.
32. Volokhina YV, Oyoyo UE, Miller JH. Ultrasound demonstration of testicular microlithiasis in pediatric patients: is there an association with testicular germ cell tumors? Pediatr Radiol. 2014 Jan;44(1):50–5.

Contrast-Enhanced Ultrasound (CEUS) for Children

17

Stefan Scholz

Introduction

Dynamic contrast-enhanced ultrasound (CEUS) uses microbubble contrast agents filled with different types of gases stabilized by a shell, which can be seen as echogenic dots on the ultrasound picture. Administered intravenously, the microbubbles enhance large and small vascular structures to easier identify larger vessels, demonstrate microperfusion, and discover potential tissue ischemia. Significant developments in ultrasound technology such as color overlay and background subtraction options can greatly enhance visualization of the microbubbles [1]. CEUS represents the most sensitive cross-sectional real-time method for measuring parenchymal perfusion and enhancement dynamics, which can be utilized to differentiate between benign and malignant tumors. It accurately predicts tumor response to chemotherapy within a very short time [2].

Routine and validated adult applications of CEUS include echocardiography as well as hepatic and a growing body of non-hepatic indications. Several second-generation microbubble contrast agents are approved in various parts of the world for intravenous or intracavitary use. However, none is approved for noncardiac intravenous application in the USA, which has not deterred a relatively large-scale off-label noncardiac use [3]. Similarly, none of the contrast agents are currently approved for use in children, also not in Europe (one single first-generation agent, Levovist (Bayer Schering AG, Germany), was only approved for intraluminal application to detect vesicoureteral reflux (VUR), but has been discontinued by the manufacturer). Especially for children, noninvasive and cost-effective ultrasound technologies offer significant advantages. There is no harmful ionizing radiation and no need for sedation as compared to other imaging modalities such as computed tomography (CT) scan or magnetic resonance imaging (MRI).

The European Federation of Societies for Ultrasound in Medicine and Biology (EFSUMB) has set up an international registry for patients under 18 years of age to accumulate data and prove safety in order to facilitate potential rapid implementation of this exciting technology into clinical pediatric practice (http://www.efsumb.org/education/scientific-corner01.asp).

Adult Applications

In adults, CEUS has been used in clinical practice for more than 25 years with its earliest and most common application in echocardiography. More recently, other intravenous applications have spread. The International Contrast Ultrasound Society (ICUS) was founded in 2008 and adopted the yearly Bubble Conference, which runs already in its 30th year.

S. Scholz (✉)
Division of Pediatric General and Thoracic Surgery, Children's Hospital of Pittsburgh of UPMC, University of Pittsburgh School of Medicine, One Children's Hospital Drive, 4401 Penn Avenue, Pittsburgh, PA 15224, USA
e-mail: stefan.scholz@chp.edu

S. Scholz, M. D. Jarboe (eds.), *Diagnostic and Interventional Ultrasound in Pediatrics and Pediatric Surgery,* DOI 10.1007/978-3-319-21699-7_17

There appears to be great enthusiasm for the potential of this technology in clinical applications utilizing the strengths of ultrasound such as dynamic, real-time imaging, cost-effectiveness, noninvasiveness, and no ionizing radiation. The intravenous microbubble agents are considered safe with no cardio-, hepato-, or nephrotoxic side effects.

Five second-generation microbubble contrast agents are approved for use in adults in various parts of the world. However, intravenous contrast ultrasound agents are only approved for use in echocardiography in the USA (Definity/Luminity, Lantheus Medical Imaging, USA, and Optison, General Electric, USA), but are available for other adult indications in Europe and Canada.

Noncardiac CEUS applications are much more advanced and available in Europe than in the USA, largely due to diverse practice patterns and regulatory aspects. Ultrasound in the USA is done primarily by ultrasound technologists and not by radiologists who receive limited training in this modality. Non-radiographic specialities rarely use ultrasound themselves. Reimbursement for ultrasound is lower than for CT or MRI as is its relative importance under imaging studies.

To facilitate use, EFSUMB recently published international consensus guidelines and recommendations for the clinical practice of CEUS for non-hepatic [4] and hepatic use [5].

Characterizing hepatic lesions is one of the main strengths of CEUS, reliably differentiating hepatocellular carcinoma, liver metastasis, adenoma, hemangioma, and focal nodular hyperplasia. Comparable to CT or MRI, it utilizes the arterial, portal venous and late phases for accurate diagnosis. Radiofrequency ablation or transarterial chemoembolization of liver lesions can be monitored for treatment response, and an accurate volumetric map can depict an adequate perilesion margin after ablation [6].

CEUS can improve imaging quality of post-liver transplant perfusion, especially of the hepatic artery, rendering angiography for detection or thrombosis potentially unnecessary.

In adults, CEUS has been studied for a multitude of clinical problems and applications. Sessa et al. [7] evaluated, retrospectively, 256 consecutive patients with isolated abdominal trauma with conventional focused assessment with sonography in trauma (FAST), CEUS, and CT scan. CT was used as the gold standard and identified 28 liver, 35 spleen, and 21 kidney lesions. Ultrasound alone showed a sensitivity of only 59 %, which could be improved to 96 % with CEUS. As a limitation of the technique, ultrasound contrast agents are not exerted in the urine and therefore cannot detect damage to the urinary excretory system.

Similar to the liver, CEUS is being used to characterize splenic and renal lesions as well as infarcts [4]. Cerebral and cervical vessels can be evaluated for sub-occlusive stenosis missed by Duplex ultrasound. VUR, cholangiography, as well as fistulograms can be performed utilizing contrast agents intraluminally. Endoscopic retrograde cholangiogram under contrast ultrasonography has been reported [8].

Parenchymal perfusion and enhancement dynamics measured by CEUS can be utilized to differentiate between benign and malignant tumors. Initial experiences indicate that CEUS performs as well as blue dye or radioisotope methods performs when used during sentinel node biopsy for breast cancer [9].

Dynamic CEUS enables quantitative assessment of tissue perfusion over time, which means changes in vascularization can be detected already after 1 or 2 weeks of treatment. One of the most promising clinical utilities of CEUS is the prediction of tumor response to chemotherapy within a very short time, shorter than using response evaluation criteria for solid tumors. Other clinical applications where dynamic transit time measurements can add valuable clinical information include quantifying hepatic transit time, evaluation of diabetic kidneys, transplant grafts, or in Crohn's disease. Fröhlich et al. [2] provide a recent literature review over practical applications and clinical use.

EFSUMB has listed emerging and potential applications including interventional diagnosis or guidance, characterization of thyroid nodules, drug and gene delivery, and CEUS-induced thrombolysis [10].

With the accumulation of more data, areas of applications, and design of prospective trials, CEUS has positioned itself to be one of the preferred diagnostic imaging modalities of the future in many clinical settings.

Pediatric Applications

Application of noncardiac intravenous CEUS in children lags significantly behind its use in adults. This may appear surprising since ultrasound technology seemingly offers the most advantages for children. Radiation exposure is a recognized problem in children with an increased additional lifetime risk of malignancy possibly as high as 2.5 in 1000 after a single CT examination [11, 12]. MRI is the imaging modality of choice in neuroimaging but may struggle to be diagnostic in the child's abdomen. It may require anesthesia in younger children and its contrast agent, gadolinium, may lead to nephrogenic systemic fibrosis. CT works best with a layer of fat surrounding abdominal organs, which children may lack. Ultrasound examination thrives on the absence of fat and offers zero radiation exposure. It succeeds as a child-friendly nonintimidating imaging technique, which may also be more cost-effective [13].

To improve the quality of pediatric imaging, often performed in adult centers unfamiliar with the optimal image modality as well as machine settings for children, the Society of Pediatric Radiology (SPR) has created the Alliance for Radiation Safety in Pediatric Imaging. The Image Gently Campaign (http://www.imagegently.org) was created to educate professionals about safe settings for pediatric imaging as well as preferred imaging alternatives such as ultrasound.

Noncardiac CEUS may offer even more diagnostic advantages for children. However, there is no widespread use in pediatric imaging today. Ultrasound contrast agents are not approved for use under 18 years of age in any part of the world and require off-label use, similar to many routine medications used clinically in pediatric patients every day. Many drugs used in children and infants will never achieve Food and Drug Administration (FDA) approval for its current indications. A supporting robust body of medical evidence makes its use possible, even in a litigious medical environment.

Phase three trials with ultrasound contrast agents in children are not economically feasible for pharmaceutical companies. The only historically approved first-generation contrast agent, Levovist (Bayer Schering AG, Germany), which was only approved in Europe for intraluminal application to detect VUR, has been discontinued by the manufacturer. In Europe, SonoVue (Bracco SpA, Milan, Italy) remains the only approved intravenous ultrasound contrast agent for use only in adults.

Most common adult applications, such as detection of liver masses, are rare in children making it difficult to gain experience. The rarity of such a diagnosis and the need for a definite diagnosis routinely trigger a CT scan or MRI, which cannot be replaced by CEUS leaving it looking for its role in the diagnostic algorithm [1]. Despite widespread use in Europe, even pediatric centers, many of which may have replaced voiding cystureterography with contrast-enhanced voiding urosonography (ceVUS) , have often not implemented intravenous CEUS in their routine clinical practice.

EFSUMB recognizes that CEUS for pediatric applications is of critical importance to benefit children. Pediatric practitioners have called for cooperation to achieve adequate patient numbers or multicenter studies to gain approval [1, 13]. To accumulate patient safety data, EFSUMB has set up a registry for pediatric patients (http://www.efsumb.org/education/scientific-corner01.asp).

In a mildly desperate fashion, letters to the editor are calling to also allow pediatric patients to benefit from recent achievements of medicine, based on the "primum non nocere" principle [13, 14]. EFSUMB acknowledges that CEUS is a good example, where strict regulations potentially inhibit the use of a beneficial, safe, and simple technique [4]. Implementing CEUS in pediatric patients poses a real challenge [15].

The SPR has established a Contrast-Enhanced Ultrasound Task Force to promote CEUS, encourage scientific research, coordinate multicenter trials, and to explore ways to develop CEUS as a useful, practical imaging tool (http://www.pedrad.org/Specialties/USContrastEnhanced.aspx#23821750-welcome-). Interested partners have been identified in the pediatric oncology community. Possible multicenter studies could focus on posttreatment follow-up of solid abdominal tumors, evaluation of femoral head perfusion after hip reduction, or posttransplant evaluation of graft perfusion [1].

Several recent publications review intravenous CEUS studies involving pediatric patients, most often with off-label use of SonoVue [15–17].

Safety of Off-Label Use of Intravenous Ultrasound Contrast Agents in Children

In adults, large studies have confirmed a favorable safety profile for SonoVue (Bracco, Milan, Italy) in comparison to CT or MRI agents [18].

The SPR and the ICUS have reviewed the safety of noncardiac CEUS in children [19]. All published studies including 110 patients do not report serious adverse side effects. A European survey of 948 children found only six minor events in five children [20]. For intravesicular use, 15 studies including 2951 children and a European survey of 4131 children reported no adverse events attributed to the contrast agent [20, 21]. The authors conclude that ultrasound contrast agents have an extremely favorable safety profile in children, with no serious and few adverse events overall reported in the literature.

Piskunowicz et al. [22] recently reviewed the safety of an intravenous second-generation ultrasound contrast agent (SonoVue) in children in a single oncology center. SonoVue contains sulfur hexafluoride gas (SF_6) surrounded by a stabilizing thin and flexible shell of phospholipids. With its mean diameter of 2.4 µm, the microbubbles pass through lung capillaries. The lack of reference doses for children has created the need to establish a custom dosing regimen using the principle of minimum effective dose of contrast for the examined body region, similar to the as low as reasonably achievable (ALARA) principle for ionizing radiation. Typical volumes of contrast agent based on patient's age range from 0.1 to 1.8 mL. In a total of 161 patients, the authors did experience one serious anaphylactic reaction, the only reported pediatric case to date. In their review of the limited literature available (five studies), they feel that the lack of uniform monitoring guidelines and standardized regimen does not allow reliable conclusions about the relative risk.

Voiding Urosonography

The American Academy of Pediatrics recommends that renal and bladder ultrasound be used as the primary imaging modality to determine anatomic abnormalities and renal scarring. Due to its risk with radiation exposure, voiding cystourethrography (VCUG) and direct radionuclide cystography (DRNC) are only recommended if abnormalities are detected (Fig. 17.1).

Since the late 1990s, ceVUS has gained widespread acceptance to diagnose VUR in Europe.

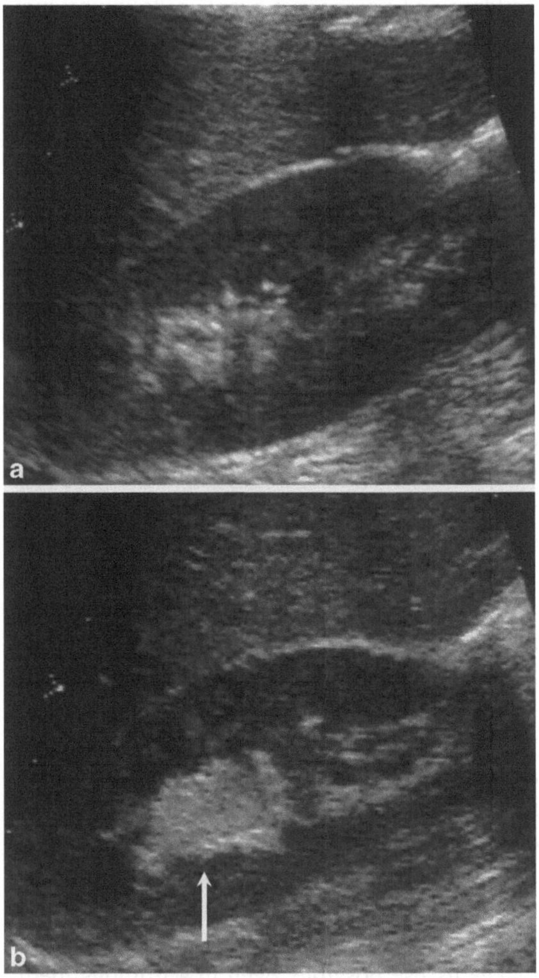

Fig. 17.1 Contrast-enhanced voiding urosonography (ceVUS): Pre- (**a**) and post-intravesical (**b**) administration of ultrasound contrast agent. A duplex kidney on the right with reflux of the ultrasound contrast agent into the upper moiety *(arrow)*. (Courtesy of Kassa Darge, MD, PhD, CHOP, Philadelphia, USA)

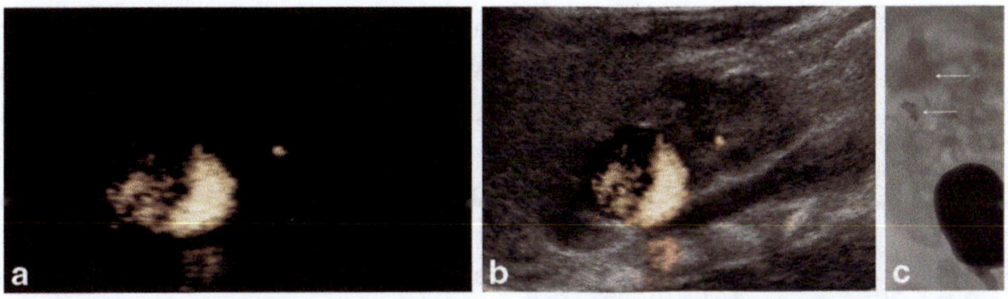

Fig. 17.2 Contrast-enhanced voiding urosonography (ceVUS; **a** and **b**): Images of the right duplex kidney after intravesical administration of ultrasound contrast agent. The scan is a dedicated contrast-specific modality showing a duplex kidney on the right with reflux in both, the upper and lower moieties. For comparison, the voiding cystourethrography (VCUG; **c**) also demonstrates reflux in both moieties in the same patient. (Courtesy of Kassa Darge, MD, PhD, CHOP, Philadelphia, USA)

Using intravesically administered microbubbles, ceVUS can also monitor the filling and voiding functions without harmful radiation. VUR and even infrarenal reflux can be clearly visualized (Figs. 17.2a–c, 17.3). Several recent papers show that transperineal ultrasound during voiding allows for reliable assessment of urethral pathology, indicating that this early restriction for ceVUS has been overcome [23].

The most recent meta-analysis of all the comparative studies of ceVUS with VCUG and DRNC in children included more than 2300 children with more than 4600 pelvi-ureteric units. Using VCUG as the reference method, ceVUS had a sensitivity of 90 % and a specificity of 92 %.

High correlation of reflux grading between the two methods was noticed. Severe and higher-grade VUR is more commonly detected on ceVUS as compared to VCUG [1].

The combination of contrast-enhanced urethrosonography with ceVUS has enabled exquisite depiction of urethral pathologies, including posterior urethral valves [24]. The visualization of intrarenal reflux is easier with ceVUS [15, 25–27].

Promoted by the Uroradiology Task Force of the European Society of Paediatric Radiology (http://www.espr.org/taskforce/uroradiology/), VCUG and DRNC are increasingly being replaced with ceVUS in European pediatric radiology centers.

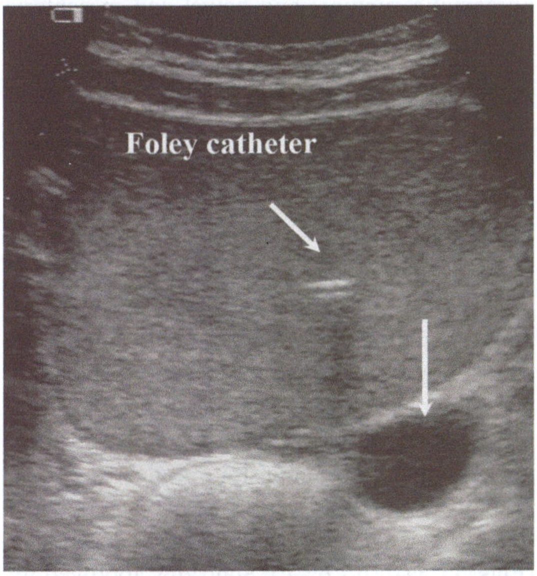

Fig. 17.3 Contrast-enhanced voiding urosonography (ceVUS): the bladder is filled with echogenic ultrasound contrast agent. The left terminal ureter is dilated *(arrow)*. However, there is no reflux of microbubbles into the left ureter. (Courtesy of Kassa Darge, MD, PhD, CHOP, Philadelphia, USA)

Abdominal Trauma

Abdominal ultrasound is commonly used to evaluate blunt abdominal trauma. However, the technique is unreliable for the detection of parenchymal lesions, and intravenous contrast CT imaging remains the mainstay for evaluating serious blunt abdominal trauma in hemodynamically stable patients. Three case reports with four patients are available where pancreatic, hepatic, and splenic injuries were missed on ultrasound alone. In all cases, CEUS correctly identified the organ laceration (Fig. 17.4a, b) [28–30]. Valentino et al. [31]

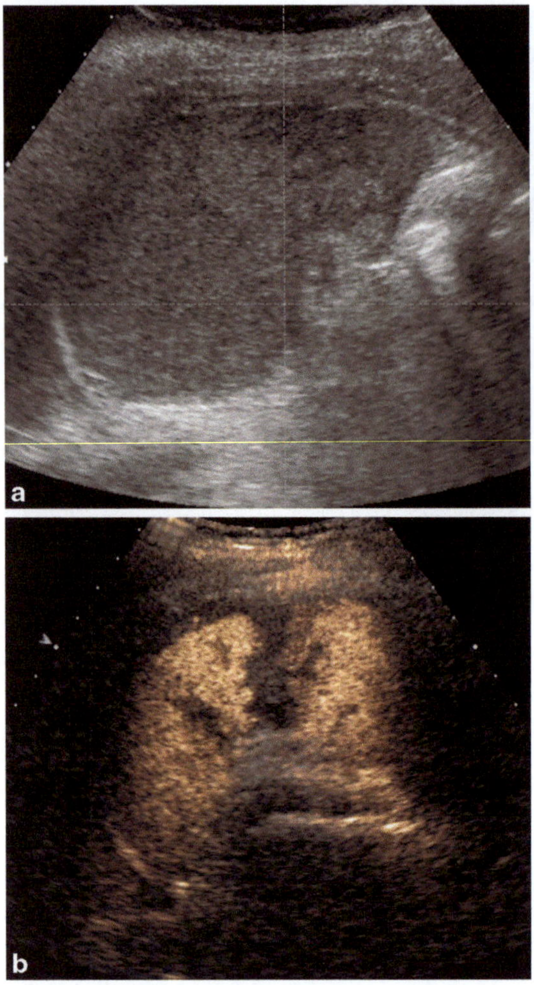

Fig. 17.4 **a** and **b** Contrast-enhanced ultrasound for blunt abdominal trauma. The spleen pre- and post-intravenous ultrasound contrast administration. On the gray scale image, it is difficult to appreciate any laceration of the spleen. However, with intravenous contrast using contrast-specific ultrasound modality, the splenic laceration is clearly depicted. (Courtesy of Kassa Darge, MD, PhD, CHOP, Philadelphia, USA)

reviewed their experience with CEUS for solid organ injuries in 12 children with seven splenic, four liver, one right adrenal gland, and one pancreatic injury as well as 15 children with negative abdominal CT scans. CEUS detected 13 of the 14 lesions with an overall sensitivity and specificity of 92.2 and 93.8 %, respectively (100 % positive and negative predictive values), but missed the right adrenal contusion. In comparison, regular abdominal ultrasound posted a sensitivity and specificity of 57.1 and 68.4 %, respectively. With its improved accuracy, the authors consider CEUS a useful alternative to contrast CT scan for stable abdominal trauma, thus potentially eliminating exposure to radiation.

Menichini et al. [32] retrospectively looked at 73 stable children with abdominal trauma. CT identified 67 lesions to the liver, spleen, and kidneys. CEUS sensitivity, specificity, and accuracy were each 100 %, in difference to ultrasound (38.8, 100, and 44 %, respectively). CEUS identified parenchymal active bleeding in eight cases and partial devascularization in one case. With contrast CT scan, eight additional patients with active parenchymal hemorrhage, two with vascular bleeding, and two with urinoma were identified. The authors conclude that CEUS is almost as sensitive as contrast CT scan to pick up solid organ lesions, but CT scan remains more sensitive and accurate identifying prognostic indicators such as active bleeding and urinoma.

CEUS is considered only part of the trauma algorithm in low-energy trauma in hemodynamically stable patients. Drawbacks include operator competence and reduced panoramic view. Diaphragmatic ruptures and bowel and mesenteric injuries may be missed. CEUS may be valuable for follow-up of solid organ injuries managed nonoperatively, especially in children and pregnant women [33, 34].

Liver Imaging

CEUS offers several advantages over other imaging modalities in evaluation of focal liver lesions. It provides real-time dynamic imaging, permitting visualization of enhancement during the very early or late phases of contrast enhancement. CEUS can demonstrate a clear and consistent washout phase useful to characterize malignant lesions and differentiate benign nodules (Figs. 17.5a–c, 17.6a–c). SonoVue, approved for liver scans in adults in numerous countries (not USA), can be used in patients with renal impairment considered not appropriate candidates for CT or MRI [15].

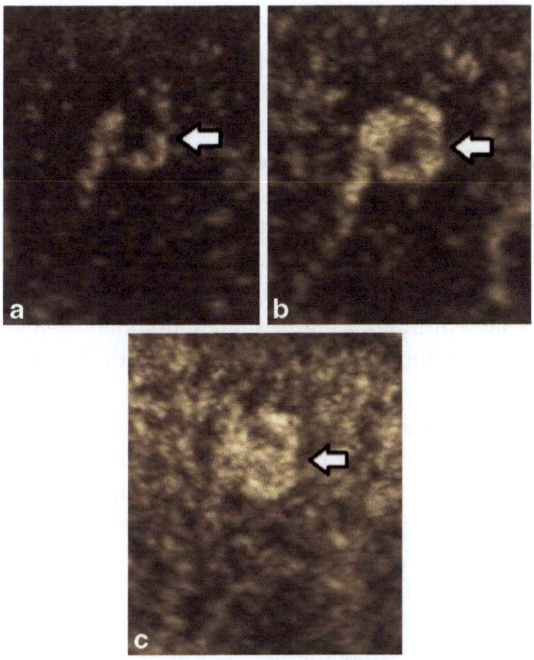

Fig. 17.5 A young man with a hepatic hemangioma. Three sequential CEUS images of the same liver mass *(arrows)*. **a** Early peripheral nodular enhancement. **b** Progressive centripetal contrast enhancement. **c** Near-complete enhancement of the hemangioma. (From [6], with permission from Elsevier, license number 3636550696548)

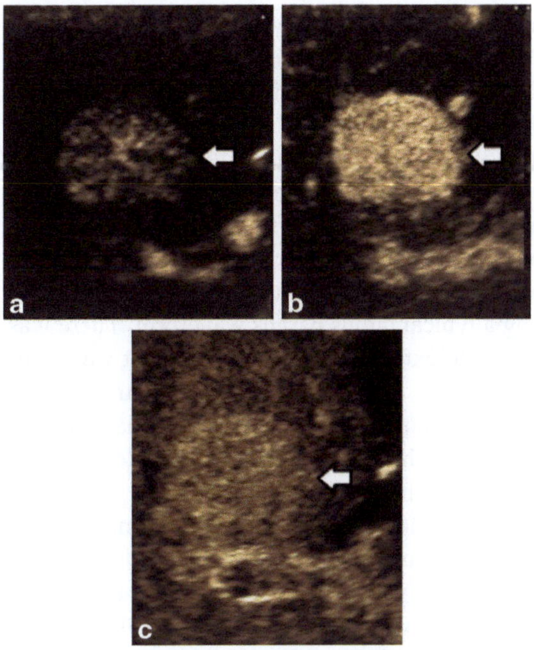

Fig. 17.6 A young woman with focal nodular hyperplasia (FNH). Three sequential CEUS images of the same liver lesion *(arrows)*. **a** Early hypervascular enhancement within the central scar. **b** Progressive centrifugal direction of contrast enhancement. **c** Sustained mild enhancement on the portal venous phase. (From [6], with permission from Elsevier, license number 3636550696548)

There are abundant well-designed studies in the adult literature available, but reports in children remain scarce. There are two single case reports in teenagers where CEUS aided in the diagnosis of rare liver tumors, a primary gastrointestinal stromal tumor of the liver and a fibrolamellar hepatocellular carcinoma [35, 36].

Working at a pediatric liver center, Jacob et al. [37] reviewed 44 children referred for CEUS assessment of a gray scale sonographic indeterminate focal liver lesion over a 5-year period. CEUS examination was compared to consensus interpretation of other imaging and histology. In 29 of 34 cases (85.3 %), reference imaging agreed to CEUS. In the five discordant cases, reference imaging showed no abnormality (four fatty changes and one regenerative nodule on CEUS). In ten cases, no other imaging was performed and histology (seven cases) or follow-up sonography (three cases) confirmed the diagnosis. In one case, all imaging methods were consistent with a malignant lesion, but histology showed a benign hepatocellular adenoma. The specificity of CEUS was 98 % and the negative predictive value 100 %. The authors conclude that CEUS compares favorably with CT scan or MRI to differentiate indeterminate gray scale sonographic liver lesions in children. CEUS could become an important diagnostic tool to reliably characterize focal liver tumors and to avoid radiation, at least in higher-volume pediatric liver centers such as the Pediatric Liver Unit at King's College Hospital, London, UK.

Bonini et al. [38] reviewed 44 liver transplants performed in 40 patients over a 1-year period. In 30 patients, clinical or sonographic signs were suggestive of possible vascular or biliary complications. In all these patients, a second duplex ultrasound with intravenous contrast (SonoVue) was performed. A total of 14 vascular complications were confirmed with CT, angiography, or percutaneous transhepatic cholangiography. CEUS correctly identified four of five cases of hepatic artery thrombosis and all cases of thrombosis involving the portal vein (six) and the hepatic veins (three). It failed to identify one case of hepatic artery thrombosis characterized by collateral circulation arising from the phrenic artery and the single case of hepatic artery stenosis, which was more evident on color Doppler showing a typical tardus parvus waveform. There was also one extensive splenic infarct that was visualized only after infusion of the contrast agent. While biliary leaks were better visualized, the contrast enhancement did not provide any particular diagnostic advantage.

The authors conclude that CEUS improves diagnostic confidence and may reduce the need for more invasive imaging studies in the postoperative follow-up of pediatric liver transplant recipients. CEUS allows accurate assessment of graft vascularization with clear distinction between normally vascularized and hypoperfused areas of the parenchyma and improved visualization of peri-graft collections/leaks as well as bile duct dilatation secondary to anastomotic stenosis.

Other Applications

Other reports about CEUS use in children are rare. Several case reports have been published describing the utility of CEUS to follow up ovarian torsion [39], characterize solid pseudopapillary tumors of the pancreas [40], and diagnose internal iliac vein thrombosis [41] as well as intracardiac masses [42]. Riccabona et al. [43] report on preoperative applications of CEUS for kidney transplants.

Pediatric CEUS may be useful to evaluate femoral head perfusion, arthritis assessment, testicular/ovarian torsion, pyelonephritis, and inflammatory bowel disease [44]. CEUS offers promising applications in pediatric oncology. McCarville et al. [45] from St. Jude Children's Research Hospital in Memphis/TN reported their initial experience in 13 children with CEUS for evaluation of malignant pediatric abdominal and pelvic solid tumors. Post-contrast ultrasound inter-reviewer agreement improved slightly for detection of tumor margins, local tumor invasion, and associated adenopathy.

Two abstracts presented at the Euroson 2013 meeting reported on the initial experience of other centers with CEUS for solid abdominal tumors. Batko et al. [46] presented their experience with 15 children and noted that CEUS examination may be useful for initial diagnosis as well as treatment monitoring of solid abdominal tumors to allow for reduction of imaging with ionizing radiation.

Franke et al. [47] reported their experience with CEUS in six patients with hepatoblastoma and seven with neuroblastoma. Indications in hepatoblastoma patients were initial diagnosis of focal liver lesions, differentiation of uni- or multilocular lesions, evaluation before liver transplantation, and detection of recurrence of the hepatoblastoma in the liver graft. CEUS was also performed in patients with neuroblastomas to evaluate liver or kidney infiltration before and after chemotherapy. The technique was of great benefit for the further management of two unstable, ventilated newborns: one with diffuse stage 4S neuroblastoma not visible on CT scan and a second newborn with rapidly growing hepatoblastoma showing as an initially small and inconclusive lesion on MRI.

Summary

Dynamic CEUS is a promising new technique, which offers cost-effective real-time imaging without ionizing radiation or the need for sedation. Aside from its routine use for echocardiography, CEUS is widely established in adults for differentiation of focal liver lesions and monitoring of tumor response to chemotherapy through parenchymal perfusion and enhancement dynamics. Despite their favorable safety profile, no ultrasound contrast agent has been approved for use in children. In Europe, many pediatric centers have implemented ceVUS as their routine study for evaluation of VUR. Despite promising initial results, other applications such as characterization of focal liver lesions, solid organ injuries in abdominal trauma, and abdominal or pelvic solid tumors have been limited to few pediatric centers. Pediatric experts and societies are calling for collaboration and accumulation of safety data in central registries as well as multicenter studies to minimize the delay of introduction of this promising technique into routine clinical practice.

References

1. Darge K. Contrast-enhanced US (CEUS) in children: ready for prime time in the United States. Pediatr Radiol. 2011;41:1486–8.
2. Fröhlich E, Muller R, Cui XW, Schreiber-Dietrich D, Dietrich DF. Dynamic contrast-enhanced ultrasound for quantification of tissue perfusion. J Ultrasound Med. 2015;34:179–96.
3. Barr RG. Off-label use of ultrasound contrast agents for abdominal imaging in the United States. J Ultrasound Med. 2013;32:7–12.
4. Piscaglia F, Nolsøe C, Dietrich CF, Cosgrove DO, Gilja OH, Bachmann Nielsen M, et al. The EFSUMB guidelines and recommendations on the clinical practice of contrast enhanced ultrasound (CEUS): update 2011 on non-hepatic applications. Ultraschall Med. 2012;33:33–59.
5. Claudon M, Dietrich CF, Choi CI, Cosgrove DO, Kudo M, Nolsøe CP, et al. guidelines and good clinical practice recommendations for contrast enhanced ultrasound (CEUS) in the liver - update 2012. Ultraschall Med. 2013;34:11–29.
6. Malhi H, Grant EG, Duddalwar V. Contrast-enhanced ultrasound of the liver and kidney. Radiol Clin N Am. 2014;52:1177–90.
7. Sessa B, Trinci M, Ianniello S, Menichini G, Galluzzo M, Miele V. Blunt abdominal trauma: role of contrast-enhanced ultrasound (CEUS) in the detection and staging of abdominal traumatic lesions compared to US and CE-MDCT. Radiol Med. 2015;120:180–9.
8. Zuber-Jerger I, Endlicher E, Schölmerich J, Klebl F. Endoscopic retrograde cholangiography with contrast ultrasonography. Endoscopy. 2008;40:E202.
9. Sever AR, Mills P, Jones SE, Cox K, Weeks J, Fish D, Jones PA. Preoperative sentinel node identification with ultrasound using microbubbles in patients with breast cancer. AJR Am J Roentgenol. 2011 Feb;196:251–6.
10. Dietrich CF, Bui XW, Barreiros AP, Hocke M, Ignee A. EFSUMB Guidelines 2011: comment on emergent indications and visions. Ultraschall in Med. 2012;33:S39–47.
11. Brenner D, Elliston C, Hall E, Berdon W. Estimated risks of radiation-induced fatal cancer from pediatric CT. AJR Am J Roentgenol. 2001;176:289–96.
12. Pearce MS, Salotti JA, Little MP, McHugh K, Lee C, Kim KP, et al. Radiation exposure from CT scans in childhood and subsequent risk of leukaemia and brain tumours: a retrospective cohort study. Lancet. 2012;380:499–505.
13. Sellars ME, Deganello A, Sidhu PS. Paediatric contrast-enhanced ultrasound (CEUS): a technique that requires co-operation for rapid implementation into clinical practice. Ultraschall Med. 2014;35:203–6.
14. Piskunowicz M, Kosiak W, Irga N. Primum non nocere? Why can't we use second generation ultrasound contrast agents for the examination of children? Ultraschall Med 2011;32:83–6.(Letter to the editor)
15. Schreiber-Dietrich DG, Cui XW, Piscaglia F, Gilja OH, Dietrich CF. Contrast enhanced ultrasound in pediatric patients: a real challenge. Z Gastroenterol. 2014;52:1178–84.
16. McCarville MB. Contrast-enhanced sonography in pediatrics. Pediatr Radiol. 2011;41:S238–42.
17. Piskunowicz M, Kosiak W, Batko T. Intravenous application of second-generation ultrasound contrast agents in children: a review of the literature. Ultraschall Med. 2012;33:135–40.
18. Piscaglia F, Bolondi L. The safety of SonoVue in abdominal applications: retrospective analysis of 23188 investigations. Ultrasound Med Biol. 2006;32:1369–75.
19. Darge K, Papadopoulou F, Nyoulia A, et al. Safety of contrast-enhanced ultrasound in children for non-cardiac applications: a review by the Society For Pediatric Radiology (SPR) and the International Contrast Ultrasound Society (ICUS). Pediatr Radiol. 2013;43:1063–73.
20. Riccabona M. Application of second-generation ultrasound contrast agent in infants and children—a European questionnaire-based survey. Pediatr Radiol. 2012;42:1471–80.
21. Papadopoulou F, Ntoulia A, Siomou E, Darge K. Contrast-enhanced voiding urosonography with intravesical administration of a second-generation ultrasound contrast agent for diagnosis of vesicoureteral reflux: prospective evaluation of contrast safety in 1010 children. Pediatr Radiol. 2014;44:719–28.
22. Piskunowicz M, Kosiak W, Batko T, Piankoski A, Poczynska K, Adamkeiwicz-Drozynska E. Safety of intravenous s application of second-generation ultrasound contrast agent in children: prospective analysis. Ultrasound Med. 2015;41:1095–9.
23. Riccabona M, Vivier PH, Ntoulia A, Darge K, Avni F, Papadopoulou F, et al. ESPR uroradiology task force imaging recommendations in paediatric uroradiology, part VII: standardised terminology, impact of existing recommendations, and update on contrast-enhanced ultrasound of the paediatric urogenital tract. Pediatr Radiol. 2014;44:1478–84.
24. Duran C, Valera A, Alguersuari A, Ballesteros E, Riera L, Martin C, et al. Voiding urosonography: the study of the urethra is no longer a limitation of the technique. Pediatr Radiol. 2009;39:124–31.

25. Darge K. Voiding urosonography with ultrasound contrast agents for the diagnosis of vesicoureteric reflux in children. I. Procedure. Pediatr Radiol. 2008;38:40–53.
26. Darge K. Voiding urosonography with US contrast agents for the diagnosis of vesicoureteric re-flux in children. II. Comparison with radiological examinations. Pediatr Radiol. 2008;38:54–63.
27. Darge K. Voiding urosonography with US contrast agent for the diagnosis of vesicoureteric reflux in children: an update. Pediatr Radiol. 2010;40:956–62.
28. Oldenburg A, Hohmann J, Skrok J, Albrecht T. Imaging of paediatric splenic injury with contrast-enhanced ultrasonography. Pediatric Radiol. 2004;34:351–4.
29. Valentino M, Galloni SS, Rimondi MR, Gentili A, Lima M, Barozzi L. Contrast-enhanced ultrasound in non-operative management of pancreatic injury in childhood. Pediatric Radiol. 2006;36:558–60.
30. Thorelius L. Emergency real-time contrast-enhanced ultrasonography for detection of solid organ injuries. Eur Radiol. 2007;17:F107–11.
31. Valentino M, Serra C, Pavlica P, Labate AM, Lima M, Baroncini S, Barozzi L. Blunt abdominal trauma: diagnostic performance of contrast-enhanced US in children - initial experience. Radiology. 2008;246:903–9.
32. Menichini G, Sessa B, Trinci M, Galluzzo M, Miele V. Accuracy of contrast-enhanced ultrasound (CEUS) in the identification and characterization of traumatic solid organ lesions in children: a retrospective comparison with baseline US and CE-MDCT. Radiol Med 2015;31:Epub ahead of print.
33. Pinto F, Miele V, Scaglione M, Pinto A. The use of contrast-enhanced ultrasound in blunt abdominal trauma: advantages and limitations. Acta Radiol. 2014;55:776–84.
34. Miele V, Di Giampietro I, Ianniello S, Pinto F, Trinci M. Diagnostic imaging in pediatric polytrauma management. Radiol Med. 2015;120:33–49.
35. Mandry D, Bressenot A, Galloy MA, Chastagner P, Branchereau S, Claudon M. Contrast-enhanced ultrasound in fibro-lamellar hepatocellular carcinoma: a case report. Ultraschall Med. 2007;28:547–52.
36. Luo XL, Liu D, Yang JJ, Zheng MW, Zhang J, Zhou XD. Primary gastrointestinal stromal tumor of the liver: a case report. World J Gastroenterol. 2009;15:3704–7.
37. Jacob J, Deganello A, Sellars ME, Hadzic N, Sidhu PS. Contrast enhanced ultrasound (CEUS) characterization of grey-scale sonographic indeterminate focal liver lesions in pediatric practice. Ultraschall Med. 2013;34:529–40.
38. Bonini G, Pezzotta G, Morzenti C, Agazzi R, Nani R. Contrast-enhanced ultrasound with SonoVue in the evaluation of postoperative complications in pediatric liver transplant recipients. J Ultrasound. 2007;10:99–106.
39. Svensson JF, Larsson A, Uusijärvi J, von Sivers K, Kaiser S. Oophoropexy, hyperbaric oxygen therapy, and contrast-enhanced ultrasound after asynchronous bilateral ovarian torsion. J Pediatr Surg. 2008;43:1380–4.
40. D'Onofrio M, Malagò R, Vecchiato F, Zamboni G, Testoni M, Falconi M, Capelli P, Mucelli RP. Contrast-enhanced ultrasonography of small solid pseudopapillary tumors of the pancreas: enhancement pattern and pathologic correlation of 2 cases. J Ultrasound Med. 2005;24:849–54.
41. de Perrot T, Righini M, Bounameaux H, Poletti PA. Contrast-enhanced sonographic diagnosis of unsuspected internal iliac vein thrombosis. J Clin Ultrasound. 2011;39:553–5.
42. Groth KA, Høyer S, Klaaborg KE, Kim WY, Andersen NH. Get closer to the diagnosis in a flash. Circ Cardiovasc Imaging. 2012;5:280–2.
43. Riccabona M, Avni FE, Damasio MB, Ording-Müller LS, Blickman JG, Darge K, et al. ESPR Uroradiology Task Force and ESUR Paediatric Working Group—Imaging recommendations in paediatric uroradiology, Part V: childhood cystic kidney disease, childhood renal transplantation and contrast-enhanced ultrasonography in children. Pediatr Radiol. 2012;42:1275–83.
44. Chiorean L, Schreiber-Dietrich D, Braden B, Cui XW, Buchhorn R, Chang JM, Dietrich CF. Ultrasonographic imaging of inflammatory bowel disease in pediatric patients. World J Gastroenterol. 2015;21:5231–41.
45. McCarville MB, Kaste SC, Hoffer FA, Khan RB, Walton RC, Alpert BS, et al. Contrast-enhanced sonography of malignant pediatric abdominal and pelvic solid tumors: preliminary safety and feasibility data. Pediatr Radiol. 2012;42:824–33.
46. Batko T, Kosiak W, Piskunowicz M, Polczynska M, Piankowski A. Contrast-enhanced US in assessment of solid tumors vasculature in children - one center experience. Ultraschall Med. 2013;34:S31–2.
47. Franke D, Grigull L. Intravenous contrast-enhanced ultrasound (CEUS) in children with hepatoblastoma and neuroblastoma. Eur J Ultrasound. 2013;34:501.

Part II
Interventional Ultrasound

Ultrasound-Guided Vascular Access

18

Farokh R. Demehri and Marcus D. Jarboe

Introduction

Vascular access remains a cornerstone of pediatric surgical care. Central venous access procedures are among the most common operations performed by pediatric surgeons, and additional vascular access procedures in the perioperative and intensive care settings make up a significant portion of the pediatric surgeon's practice. These procedures include central venous, peripheral venous, and peripheral arterial access, with tunneled and non-tunneled variations depending on the indication.

In this chapter, we cover the technique of ultrasound (US)-guided vascular access. The central message we hope to convey is that safe and reliable US-guided vascular access is not magic. It is a technique guided by the core principles outlined here. With practice and patience, it is within the realm of technical mastery by any pediatric surgeon.

Historically, the use of anatomic landmarks has been a highly successful approach to vascular access, and this remains an essential surgical skill. However, the introduction of US guidance in the 1980s and the subsequent refinement of this technique have increased the safety of vascular access procedures and have thus become the standard of care for central venous access [1]. The *Guidance on the Use of Ultrasound Locating Devices for Placing Central Venous Catheters* from the National Institute of Clinical Excellence, which is endorsed by the American College of Surgeons Committee on Perioperative Care, supports the use of US guidance as the preferred method for insertion of central venous catheters in adults and children [2]. US guidance has been shown to decrease the risk of failed vascular access attempts for the internal jugular (IJ) vein and femoral vein, with decreased complications such as arterial puncture or hematoma with IJ and subclavian venous access. While these recommendations are based largely on adult literature, recent studies suggest similar outcomes in pediatric patients [3–5], with lower rates of IJ vein cannulation failures among infants and children. The benefits of US guidance can be readily extended to peripheral vascular access procedures in children as well [6, 7].

In our experience, US guidance is associated with a decreased risk of injury such as arterial cannulation and pneumothorax. In addition, it allows a higher likelihood of successful vascular cannulation given the ability to directly visualize anatomic landmarks. It also allows detection of abnormalities such as clot or vascular anomalies and gives the surgeon the ability to maneuver around these obstacles in a safe and deliberate

M. D. Jarboe (✉)
Division of Pediatric Surgery, C.S. Mott Children's Hospital, University of Michigan, 1540 E. Hospital Drive, SPC 4211, Ann Arbor, MI 48109-4211, USA
e-mail: marjarbo@med.umich.edu

F. R. Demehri
University of Michigan, 1500 E. Medical Center Drive, Ann Arbor, MI 48109, USA
e-mail: fdemehri@med.umich.edu

S. Scholz, M. D. Jarboe (eds.), *Diagnostic and Interventional Ultrasound in Pediatrics and Pediatric Surgery,* DOI 10.1007/978-3-319-21699-7_18

manner. Finally, with experience, the use of US guidance significantly decreases the time required to obtain vascular access, especially in patients with difficult anatomy. For example, a child under anesthesia may undergo several failed attempts at peripheral venous cannulation before surgical prepping. By applying the principles of US guidance outlined here, the surgeon may rapidly obtain peripheral access, preventing unnecessary "blind" sticks and reducing anesthetic induction time for the patient. This is particularly important for children, where the most significant risk factor for a complication during central venous catheterization is the number of attempts made [8, 9]. For these reasons, our preference is to use US guidance for all central venous access procedures as well as any difficult peripheral venous or arterial access procedures.

This chapter is organized by general principles of US-guided vascular access—equipment, anatomy, setup, technique, and special considerations. We focus on the technique for US-guided initial vascular access—that is, the successful placement of an intravascular guidewire. The subsequent procedure of placing an indwelling catheter via Seldinger technique is no different than non-US-guided procedures and is therefore not covered in depth. Rather than repeating step-by-step instructions for each of the myriad vascular access procedures that may be approached using US guidance, we cover the fundamental techniques of each general vascular approach. This is intended to give the reader a versatile set of skills that may be adapted to each unique vascular access scenario.

Equipment

Pediatric US-guided vascular access requires the following instrumentation:

Ultrasound Machine The surgeon should become familiar with the available portable US machine. Vascular access indications require a linear array high-frequency transducer (7.5–20 MHz). This provides appropriate tissue penetration depth allowing good visualization of vascular structures as well as surrounding anatomic landmarks. A low-frequency transducer (4–5 MHz) provides insufficient image quality at the shallow depths where vessels are usually accessed. The depth provided by a low-frequency probe is not typically required except perhaps in femoral access in the older patient who is morbidly obese. The linear high-frequency probe has a flat, straight head, which facilitates visualization and orientation of the access needle. As larger probes can be difficult to work with, especially for small patients like neonates, we prefer small footprint or "hockey stick" probes.

It is important to ensure correct left/right orientation before beginning the procedure. If the linear probe has a "hockey stick" shape, it will be necessary to keep the handle of the transducer opposite from where the access needle will be inserted. If this is uncomfortable in a given patient setup, using the "invert" or "L&R" toggle button may help by allowing the user to hold the transducer in a comfortable position.

As delineated in other sections of this book, it is important to make appropriate adjustments to obtain high image quality before beginning attempts at vascular access. Settings such as depth, gain, focus, and presets should be optimized. Familiarity with color and Doppler modes can be useful as well.

While not always necessary, color and Doppler modes are sometimes helpful in distinguishing arterial from venous structures or distinguishing cystic from vascular structures. While becoming familiar with US-guided techniques, Doppler imaging can be generously used to verify structures in cases where compression technique cannot distinguish artery from vein. The Doppler mode enables characterization of the flow waveforms of arterial versus venous structures. In vessels that are difficult to visualize, the color mode can highlight areas of flow that reveal the location of the vessel of interest. However, if the vessel is too small, the Doppler or color mode may fail to detect flow, in which case anatomic landmarks are more useful for identification (e.g., the radial artery in a 500-g neonate). If there is a suspected vascular injury or occlusion, continuous Doppler mode may help characterize abnormalities in flow dynamics and quantify the degree of obstruction. In general, after identifying the relevant anatomy, we recommend returning to B-mode when beginning the vascular access procedure, as this usually provides the clearest picture of the needle being inserted.

Fluoroscopy All central venous lines placed in the operating room should be performed on a radiolucent table with fluoroscopy. This will ensure appropriate catheter tip location at the end of the case. Alternatively, practitioners familiar with cardiac US may use this technique to determine the exact location of the catheter tip in a similar fashion as guiding optimal placement of the veno-venous extracorporeal membrane oxygenation (ECMO) catheters in the right atrium or the inferior vena cava (IVC).

Access For most pediatric vascular access indications, a 21- or 22-gauge (g) micropuncture needle is sufficient. Needles smaller than 22 gauge may bend on insertion, may not permit passage of a wire, or might not be visualized well by US. On the other hand, larger bore needles are usually not worth the risk of greater injury if the target is missed. 21- and 22-gauge needles accept a 0.018-in. coaxial wire. We typically use a Cope nitinol mandril 0.018-in. wire guide (Cook Medical, Bloomington, IN). This wire has a stiff shaft which provides a backbone for easy dilator, sheath, or catheter placement while its straight, flexible tip decreases the risk of vascular injury or spasm.

On insertion of this or any other guidewire, it is critical to avoid "pushing through" an obstruction. If at any point the wire does not advance, it should be carefully withdrawn. If the wire does not withdraw easily, the needle should be removed along with the wire. Pulling a stuck guidewire through a needle risks shearing off the tip of the guidewire, which may then embolize.

In general, J- or C-wires should be avoided in pediatric cases. Commonly used for adult central venous access, the preformed curvature in the tips of these wires are meant to form a blunt end after insertion and can be used to guide the wire toward the right atrium from the IJ vein. In the smaller vessels of pediatric patients, however, the radius of the curvature of these tips may exceed the diameter of the vessel. On initial insertion, as the tip of the wire assumes its curve, it very often causes ejection of the needle and wire from the vessel.

Catheters After establishing vascular access with a guidewire, a modified Seldinger technique may be used to directly place the intravascular catheter in the case of peripheral vessels. For central venous catheters, 3–4 dilators (3-French (Fr) dilator inside a 4-Fr dilator which are usually included in the micropuncture kit) can be used to exchange the 0.018-in. guidewire for a more robust 0.035-in. wire. This can be performed in a single maneuver by fitting the 3-Fr dilator within the 4-Fr dilator and placing these together over the 0.018-in. wire. The 3-Fr portion can then be withdrawn along with the guidewire, leaving the 4-Fr dilator in place, which will allow passage of the 0.035-in. wire. This can then be used to allow insertion of additional dilators as indicated for larger catheter insertion. For tunneled central venous catheters, a peel-away sheath is required, which is usually included in the tunneled catheter kit. In general, it is prudent to have a wide range of catheter sizes available.

For peripheral IVs or gaining access on smaller vessels, an angiocath can be helpful. In most cases, a 22-gauge angiocath is ideal, providing a small diameter but accommodating a 0.018-in. diameter wire. It also provides good length if starting a IV in the basilic or brachial vein so that a significant amount of catheter can be left within the vessel to prevent dislodgment during positioning and use. For radial arterial lines on premature neonates, a 24-gauge angiocath can be used. Depending on the taper at the end, it may accommodate a 0.018-in. wire or just a 0.010-in. wire. Angiocaths are readily available and work well for gaining access. The only caveat to be aware of is that walking the angiocath up the lumen of the vessel, as described later in the chapter, is very important. The metal part of the needle will often pierce the vessel giving a flash of blood, but the plastic part of the catheter will drag the vessel wall for some distance (almost

1 cm) before entering the vein itself. Therefore, it is important in this situation to make sure to continue to walk the catheter up the vessel well past the moment when a flash is seen.

Setup

Positioning The patient should be positioned between the surgeon and the US machine. We recommend positioning the patient such that the transducer can be controlled with the dominant hand and the needle with the nondominant hand. This preference is intended to reduce unintentional drift of the transducer during needle insertion as the surgeon focuses on the needle. However, this is not a hard-and-fast rule, and as experience increases, the surgeon will become equally facile with either hand holding the transducer. The supine position is used for most vascular access procedures, with extension of extremities as needed to expose the area of interest. For IJ access, a shoulder roll should be placed, and the head should be turned opposite the side of access. This opens the neck up to allow for more space to work. Trendelenburg positioning is often used to distend the neck vessels and decrease the risk of air embolism, although with US guidance the size of the vessel is rarely a problem. For femoral vein catheterization, the leg should be abducted and externally rotated. For peripheral access, tourniquet use is generally not necessary, although with vessels less than 1 mm in diameter, it can prove helpful. While it may increase the size of a venous target, a tourniquet may also reduce the ability of the vein to be compressed and cause vascular misidentification as both arteries and veins become noncompressible. If one is used, vascular identification should be performed prior to tourniquet application.

Sterile Preparation Standard sterile technique should be used, including chlorhexidine skin preparation, sterile fenestrated drapes, and sterile gown, gloves, mask, and eye protection. If fluoroscopy is being used, appropriate radioprotection should be worn. A sterile US probe cover is required, with nonsterile US gel applied directly to the transducer surface, and a generous amount of sterile US gel placed on the patient. It is well worth the time to ensure no air bubbles are trapped between the transducer and the probe cover prior to applying the rubber band as any residual air will cause shadowing, greatly diminishing image quality.

Anatomy

Before the procedure, a thorough review of the child's history should be performed to evaluate whether prior indwelling vascular catheters have been placed. If the patient has had prior central lines, it may be prudent to perform a bedside vascular US to rule out preexisting thrombosis or stenosis of possible target vessels. For patients with extensive vascular abnormalities, a preoperative magnetic resonance venogram may help identify reasonable targets.

After patient preparation, a thorough anatomic assessment should be performed using US prior to attempting cannulation. This will allow localization of the target vessel, assessment of appropriateness for cannulation, and identification of other structures that may be at risk of injury such as overlying vessels or nerves. This should be performed primarily with the transducer in the transverse orientation such that vessels are viewed in cross section.

Begin by localizing the target vessel and adjusting the US settings to achieve optimal visualization. The gain and depth should be adjusted to bring the target approximately two thirds of the distance down the US screen. The target vessel should be evaluated along its entire length, specifically assessing for thrombosis or stenosis. A vein that appears larger than usual may indicate a down-stream stenosis. For example, a commonly encountered scenario among patients with prior lines is the patent IJ vein with an occlusion at its junction with the subclavian vein.

A key step is differentiating venous from arterial structures. This can be accomplished by compressing or pressing down on the vessels with the transducer. Veins should compress before arteries, while arteries will visibly pulse under compression pressure between systolic and diastolic pressures. Doppler is a useful adjunct that can help characterize the flow waveform. These rules should hold true for all vascular sites but may be unreliable in settings of venous thrombosis, hypovolemia/hypotension, tourniquet use, or structural cardiovascular abnormality such as left-to-right shunt.

Key anatomic considerations for selected vascular sites are shown in Figs. 18.1, 18.2, 18.3, 18.4, 18.5, and 18.6.

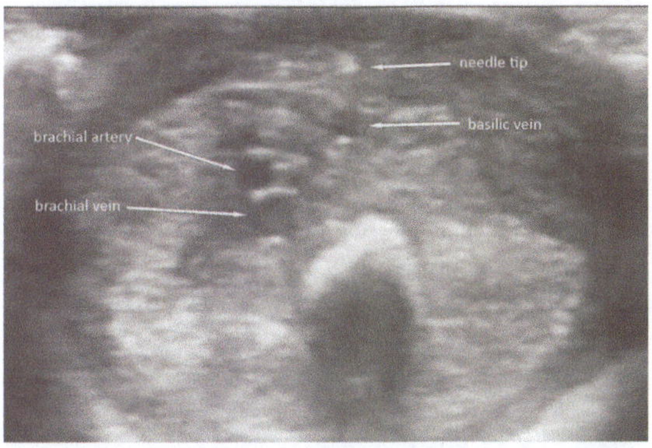

Fig. 18.1 Neonatal peripherally inserted central catheter *(PICC)* access. A common target for placement of a PICC is the *basilic vein.* While an easier target to hit, the cephalic vein is sometimes not ideal for PICC placement as it makes an acute turn as it empties into the subclavian vein, which often makes it difficult to pass the catheter. The *basilic vein,* however, empties directly into the axillary vein without kinking. The *brachial vein* is located more deeply, and it is anatomically just next to the *brachial artery,* making it a more challenging target. Using the transverse transducer orientation, the *needle tip* is visualized in the soft tissue of the upper extremity in a 485-g neonate before it is advanced under direct visualization into the *basilic vein*

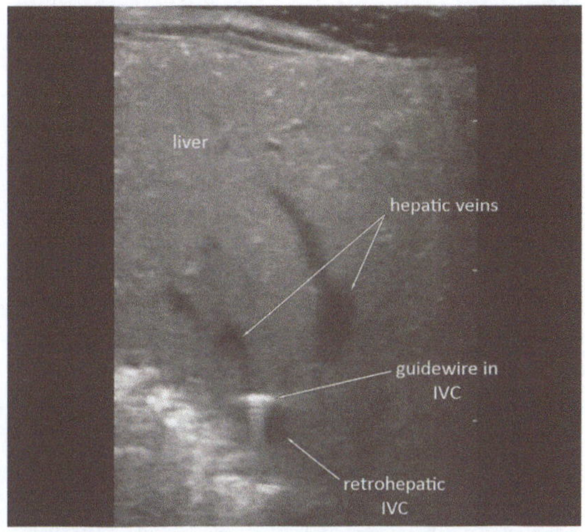

Fig. 18.2 Wire in retrohepatic inferior vena cava *(IVC).* The *guidewire* is seen in the retrohepatic *IVC* after femoral vein cannulation

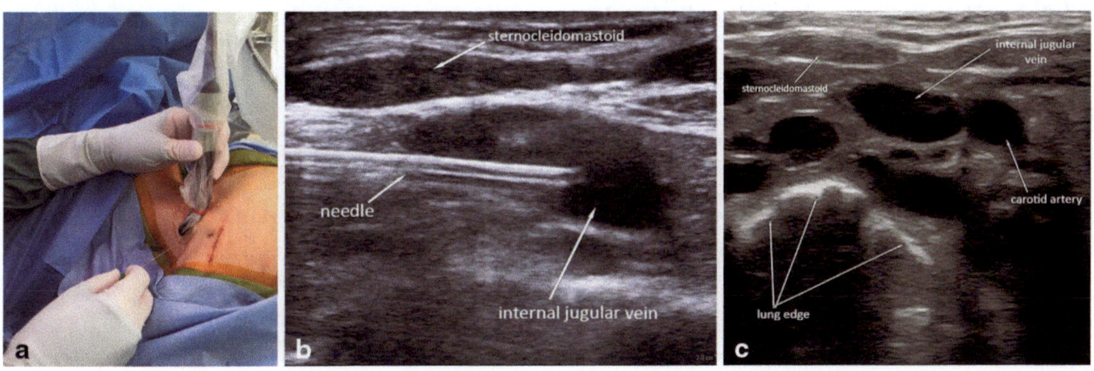

Fig. 18.3 In-line transducer orientation. **a** Using the in-line orientation for internal jugular *(IJ)* vein access, the needle is inserted along the length of the probe, beginning from the end opposite the handle (for a hockey stick probe). **b** This allows excellent longitudinal visualization of the entire length of the *needle,* which is inserted lateral to the *sternocleidomastoid (SCM)* and guided into the IJ vein. **c** The IJ vein is usually anterolateral to the *carotid artery.* The SCM is visible superficially and laterally. The bright outline of the lung is visible deep to the vessels, with loss of signal beyond this in the air-filled lung

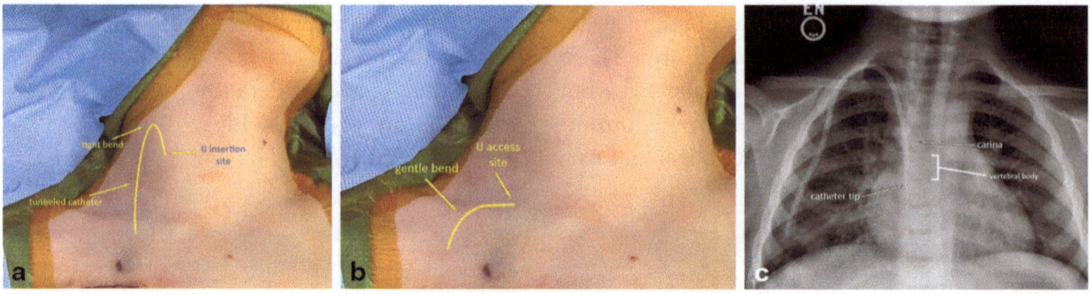

Fig. 18.4 Tunneled internal jugular *(IJ)* catheter placement. **a** The standard ultrasound *(US)*-guided IJ approach uses a transverse US probe orientation and a cranio-caudal needle insertion angle. This produces a high *IJ insertion site* and a tight, 180 ° bend of the *tunneled catheter* high in the neck. **b** The lateral approach uses an in-line US probe orientation low in the neck, just above the clavicle. This allows a low *IJ access site* and a gentle, 90° bend of the tunneled catheter. **c** A post-procedure chest X-ray shows a gradual curve of the tunneled catheter just above the clavicle, without kinking. The *tip of the catheter* rests approximately 1.7 *vertebral bodies* below the *carina,* corresponding to the cavo-atrial junction

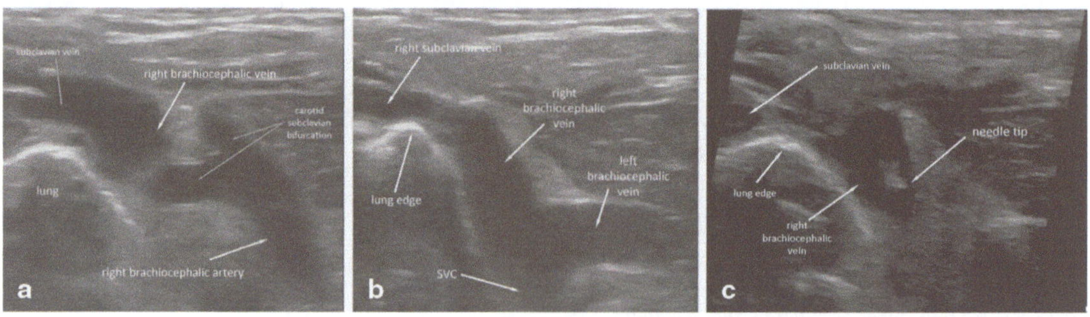

Fig. 18.5 Brachiocephalic access. **a** The ultrasound *(US)* probe is placed low above the clavicle and directed caudally to visualize the *right brachiocephalic vein* and *artery.* Medially, the *bifurcation* of the brachiocephalic artery into the carotid and subclavian arteries is clearly visualized. The subclavian–IJ venous junction is seen laterally, just above the apical *lung.* **b** With a slight adjustment in transducer position, the junction of the *right* and *left brachiocephalic veins* can be visualized, as well as the beginning of the superior vena cava *(SVC).* **c** The *needle* is directed under US guidance directly into the right *brachiocephalic vein*

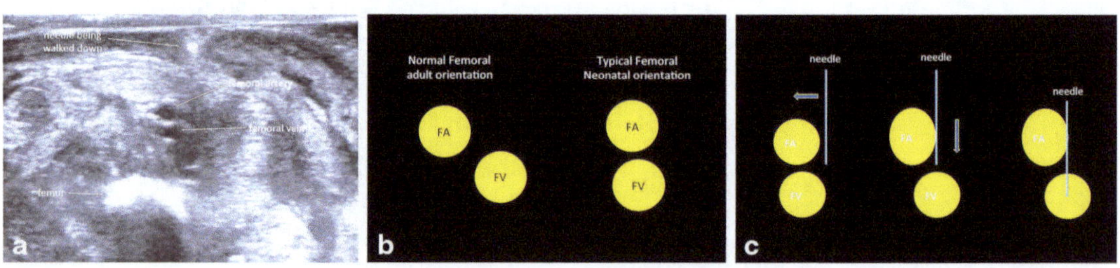

Fig. 18.6 Femoral access. **a** The *femoral vein (FV)* of a neonate commonly lies directly deep to the *femoral artery (FA)*, which can obstruct needle access. **b** This is in contrast to adults and older children, who typically have the classic anatomic relationship of the *FV* lying medially to the *FA*. **c** Under US guidance, the *needle* can be placed just medial to the *FA* and moved laterally to push the artery aside, allowing *FV* cannulation

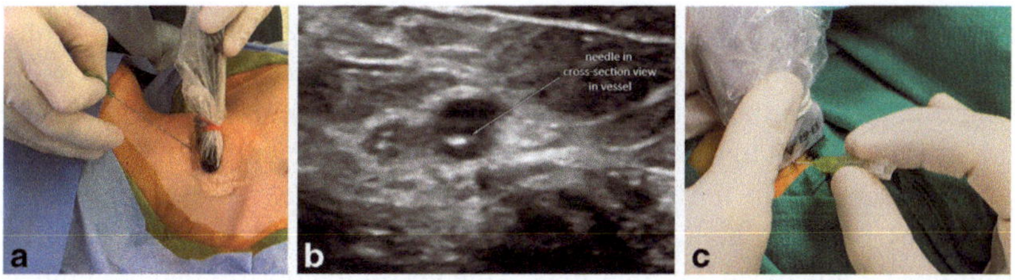

Fig. 18.7 Transverse transducer orientation. **a** Using the transverse orientation for internal jugular *(IJ)* access, the probe is placed perpendicular to the underlying vessel, and the needle is placed under the middle of the probe. **b** The *needle* is seen in cross section in the vessel when the transverse orientation is used. **c** Using the transverse orientation for peripheral access, the needle is oriented at a 45° angle to the skin with the transducer held so that the needle is positioned at the middle of the transducer

Technique

Transducer Orientation: A "Third-Dimension" Problem A linear US probe displays a planar image that includes depth along the vertical axis and the linear orientation of the probe along the horizontal axis. At any given time, the probe is only able to display a "slice" of a target vessel and the needle—either in cross section or longitudinally. Therefore, the *x*–*y* plane of the two-dimensional screen is excellent, but the *z*-axis (in and out of the screen) requires moving the transducer and manually processing the image information in the operator's/surgeon's mind. This training takes effort and time in order to be comfortable and effective at it. Given that limitation, the two US transducer orientations relative to the needle are *transverse* and *in-line.* By becoming versatile in changing the transducer orientation and location, one can accurately map out the course of a target vessel and accurately visualize the needle during the entire course of cannulation. This provides the fundamental safety benefit of US-guided vascular access—at no point during the procedure is the tip of the needle not visualized.

Transverse Orientation (Peripheral Access, Femoral Access, Arterial Access) The *transverse* orientation is classically used most frequently. The transducer head is oriented perpendicular to the needle axis, creating a cross-sectional image of the vessel and needle (Fig. 18.7a, b). This creates a clear picture of the relationship of the vessel to other structures. During needle insertion, it provides excellent left-to-right spatial resolution, though it is difficult to establish the location of the needle tip. In general, if the target vessel is very small, the *transverse* orientation provides the best approach and, in general, is most useful for vascular access in all scenarios except supraclavicular central venous access.

When using the *transverse* orientation during needle insertion, extra care must be taken to ensure proper localization of the needle tip. To safely gain intravascular access using the *transverse* US orientation, the needle is placed at an approximately 45 ° angle perpendicular to the transducer at the midway point (Fig. 18.7c). The needle is then advanced through the skin, and as it is advanced through the subcutaneous tissues, the US probe is used to "walk" down the needle to find the tip at regular intervals. The goal is to be able to identify the exact location of the needle tip, which in cross section can only be identified by moving the transducer down the needle until it disappears. Then, while keeping the needle still, the transducer is moved back until the tip reappears, confirming its location. The transducer is then moved slightly past the tip, and the needle is advanced into the field of view while keeping the transducer stationary. The needle is thus advanced slowly, regularly verifying the tip location, until the tip is watched as it enters the target vessel. Figure 18.1 shows the needle tip in soft tissue in the upper extremity of a 485-g neonate as the needle is being walked down to the target vessel.

On needle insertion into the target vessel, one may encounter significant "tenting" of the vessel if it is a vein, especially in the setting of low venous pressure. It is important to note the shape and location of the venous wall through which the needle is being inserted. If it invaginates significantly during needle advancement, one may not actually be intraluminal although the needle position appears this way. In this case, a short but aggressive push of the needle to "pop" through the venous wall can be helpful. If the needle is inadvertently advanced completely through the vessel, then the needle can be carefully withdrawn until the tip returns to the vessel lumen. Alternatively, instead of the aggressive push, the needle can simply be walked further up the lumen of the vessel for a centimeter or so and the same "pop" will occur as the needle tip becomes intraluminal. This is described below.

During vessel access with US guidance, it is preferable to avoid placing a syringe on the needle. The syringe adds weight and decreases fine touch and manipulation. Furthermore, in a small vessel, aspiration collapses the vessel around the tip, causes spasm, and will not result in blood return even when in the lumen of the vessel. In addition, the needle can be very easily dislodged from the lumen of a very small vessel when removing the syringe from the needle. Lastly, whether the needle is in the lumen or not is almost always visible via the US, making confirmation with aspiration unnecessary.

After the needle tip has been successfully maneuvered into the vessel lumen, it is important to advance it further until it is well clear of the site of vessel entry. We usually advance the needle under US guidance until it is 1–2 cm into the vessel before advancing the guidewire (Fig. 18.7b). The reason for this lies with the fact that vessels in the pediatric population, especially newborns, have a tendency to spasm. This is not limited to arteries but also occurs in veins. If the vein is entered with the needle but the needle is left at the puncture site, the vein will tend to spasm at the site of the venipuncture and not allow passage of the wire. This advancement of the needle also ensures intraluminal position and reduces the risk of inadvertent needle ejection with premature guidewire advancement. This strategy has been shown to decrease the risk of extravasation injury for peripheral venous access [10]. Once the needle is sufficiently advanced, the guidewire is placed into the vessel under US visualization. After the guidewire is inserted, move the probe up the vessel to confirm that the guidewire is within the vessel lumen. Sequential catheterization or guidewire exchange can then be performed as needed. Figure 18.2 shows the guidewire in the retrohepatic IVC after femoral vein cannulation.

In-line Orientation (Internal Jugular Access) The *in-line* transducer orientation (Fig. 18.3a) is ideal for IJ central venous access. The transducer is placed parallel to needle axis, allowing visualization of the entire length of the needle during insertion. The needle can be placed *in-line* with the transducer and slowly advanced directly under the transducer into the skin. The full length of the needle can then be visualized in the subcutaneous tissues, with excellent appreciation of the depth of the needle tip relative to surrounding structures (Fig. 18.3b). The primary benefit of this orientation is the ability to visualize the full needle length and confidently locate the needle tip depth as it relates to major structures in the vicinity such as the lung and the carotid artery (Fig. 18.3c). In general, if vessel spasm is not a concern because of the large size of the vessel and the vessel can be approached from the side, the *in-line* orientation is best.

Position and alignment are very important in using the *in-line* technique. If it is a hockey stick transducer, the needle should be inserted at the end opposite the probe handle (but with that said, comfort and maneuverability are the most important considerations). The needle is then advanced into the subcutaneous tissues directly underneath and aligned with the transducer, which should allow visualization of the entire needle as it is further advanced (Fig. 18.3b). Under direct visualization, the needle tip is then advanced into the underlying target vessel. Applying the principles outlined above to avoid vessel wall invagination, the needle is advanced well into the vessel lumen prior to guidewire placement.

When using the *in-line* orientation during needle insertion, it is imperative to see the full length of the needle itself, rather than just the movement of tissue in response to the needle. This latter phenomenon may assist in locating the needle, but relying on it alone is imprecise and will lead to misplacement of the needle tip. Maintaining view of the needle requires patience but will ensure accurate placement. If it is difficult to locate the needle, keep the needle and transducer steady and look down at both. Ensure the transducer is directly over and in-line with the path of the needle. Once they are lined up, make small corrections with the transducer until the full needle comes into view.

Special Considerations

Tunneled Catheter Placement Tunneled IJ venous catheter placement is the most common pediatric vascular access procedure we perform in the operating room. This procedure involves creating a subcutaneous tunnel from the point of venous access, coursing laterally over the clavicle, and then inferiorly to the chest wall to either an external catheter hub or a subcutaneous port. The course of the tunneled catheter is critical as an acute bend may cause the catheter to kink and occlude. In addition, a tunnel that rises high in the neck may cause the catheter to pull back significantly during head turning, leading to malposition of the catheter tip. The lateral approach keeps the catheter at the base of the neck and provides a gentle curve in the tunneled catheter (Fig. 18.4a, b, c). As the course of the tunneled catheter may vary significantly depending on the point and angle of initial vascular access, it is important to plan accordingly when performing the initial US-guided needle insertion. We have adopted a lateral approach to the tunneled IJ access, as shown in Figs. 18.3 and 18.4.

In this approach, the hockey stick linear transducer is placed low, directly above the clavicle (Fig. 18.3a). The handle of the transducer is held medially, exposing the lateral end of the transducer for needle alignment, parallel to the clavicle. The IJ vein is seen via US, with the carotid artery lying medially. The needle is inserted *in-line,* beginning just lateral to the sternocleidomastoid (SCM) while being careful not to injure the nearby external jugular vein. The needle is advanced medially, below the SCM, directly into the IJ vein, while maintaining *in-line* full needle visualization throughout (Fig. 18.3b).

Once the needle is in the vein, the guidewire is placed. The wire will go through the needle and tangentially hit the far wall of the IJ and direct itself down into the superior vena cava (SVC). On occasion, the IJ is accessed at a precisely perpendicular orientation, and the wire either does not pass or goes cephalad into the cranial portion of the IJ. If this occurs, first check with US that the needle is still in the IJ, and if it is, tilt the needle to guide the tip down toward the brachiocephalic and SVC. The wire will then easily pass in the appropriate direction.

After guidewire placement, the subcutaneous tunnel is made from the chest wall incision to the neck incision. In planning this tunnel, it is important to avoid any acute turns or extensive subcutaneous courses high in the neck. Using a low, lateral initial access site allows the creation of a gradual curve over the clavicle when creating the tunnel (Fig. 18.4).

Before feeding the catheter through the sheath, it is necessary to cut the catheter to the appropriate length to ensure proper tip location at the cavo-atrial junction. This can be performed by first tunneling the catheter to the vascular access site on the skin, then draping the catheter on the patient's chest in line with the wire that is sitting in the SVC using fluoroscopy. Fluoroscopy can be used to mark the location of the cavo-atrial junction on the catheter, at which point it can be cut. A useful anatomic landmark for estimating the depth of the cavo-atrial junction is approximately 1.5–2.0 vertebral bodies below the carina as seen on an anteroposterior X-ray or fluoroscopy (Fig. 18.4c).

Brachiocephalic Venous Access One of the advantages of using US guidance is the ability to visualize thrombus or stenosis and change plans accordingly. This is a common encounter in patients with a history of prior central venous catheters. For example, if a proximally occluded IJ vein is encountered, the contralateral side may have a more favorable anatomy. Occasionally, a patient will present for a tunneled catheter with bilaterally unfavorable IJ veins due to multiple prior catheters. In this case, direct brachiocephalic catheterization can be safely performed under US guidance. This is best performed only after gaining comfort with the lateral US-guided IJ approach, as it requires excellent needle control and patience.

To perform direct brachiocephalic venous access, the linear transducer is placed in the same position as for IJ access—directly above the clavicle—but with a more inferior angle, pointing toward the mediastinum. The confluence of the subclavian and IJ veins can be seen, with the brachiocephalic vein running next to the apical lung (Fig. 18.5b). Care should be taken at this point to ensure proper identification of the anatomy and differentiate the brachiocephalic vein from the artery (Fig. 18.5a). The needle can then be inserted in a lateral-to-medial direction using an *in-line* transducer orientation just as in the IJ access. This is critical to prevent inadvertent arterial puncture or pneumothorax. With continuous full needle visualization, the brachiocephalic vein can be safely cannulated by turning the needle caudally toward the heart while changing the transducer angle to follow the tip of the needle (Fig. 18.5c). A considerable amount of patience is needed for this maneuver to be safe. This is not an entry-level procedure given a small error or lack of visualization/identification can lead to catastrophic outcomes.

Femoral Venous Access The femoral vein is often accessed in acute resuscitation scenarios, for ECMO cannula placement or in patients with limited upper central venous access. Although not supported by as robust of a body of literature as IJ access, evidence does favor use of US guidance for femoral access as well [11]. With US experience, the initial success rate of femoral venous cannulation can be improved, especially for neonates and other difficult access scenarios.

The femoral vein can be approached with either a *transverse* or an *in-line* transducer orientation. In most cases, we use a *transverse* approach as this provides good visualization of both the artery and vein in one plane and is better suited for small babies. In neonates, it is important to thoroughly characterize the femoral vascular anatomy before beginning needle access as the orientation of the femoral vessels is notably different than that of adults. Specifically, the neonatal femoral artery is often directly anterior to the femoral vein (Fig. 18.6a, b). Using US guidance, the artery can be avoided by carefully placing the needle just medially alongside the artery. Then, with a lateral movement of the needle, the artery can be pushed out of the way, exposing the anterior surface of the vein for the needle tip (Fig. 18.6c).

Neonatal Vascular Access Achieving adequate vascular access is particularly challenging for neonatal patients. US guidance, however, is especially useful in these patients as palpable landmarks can be difficult to appreciate and vascular targets are often a millimeter or less in diameter. Even with B-mode US examination, vessels can be difficult to distinguish given their small size and toggling to color or Doppler mode can reveal the location of a diminutive artery or vein. With practice, US guidance can be used to successfully access peripheral vessels even in the smallest patients (Fig. 18.1).

In addition to having smaller vascular targets, neonates are prone to significant vasospasm. This can create the scenario where intravascular needle placement is successful but guidewire placement fails due to spasm and occlusion of the vessel just beyond the needle tip. By advancing the needle far into the vessel after cannulation, the needle tip can reach an intravascular location far from the injured cannulation site, which is most prone to spasm. The guidewire can then be advanced freely into this less traumatized area.

Peripheral Vascular Access US-guided peripheral vascular catheterization is becoming increasingly popular, especially in children with difficult access [10, 12]. A similar technique should be used for either peripheral arterial (i.e., radial artery) or peripheral venous access. In these cases, a *transverse* transducer orientation is usu-

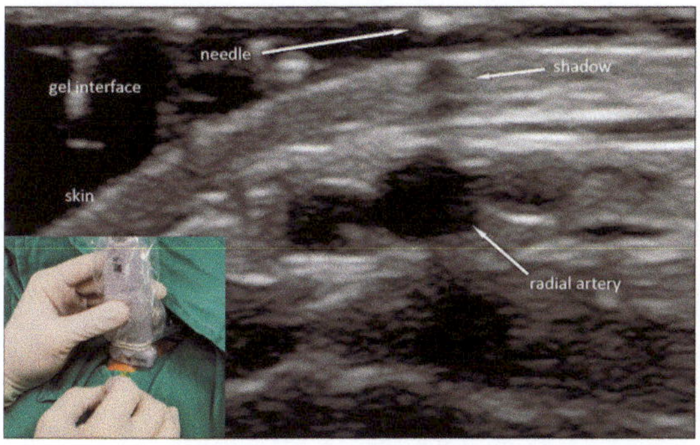

Fig. 18.8 Peripheral access: Using a transverse orientation, the *needle* can be placed flat against the *skin* directly under the probe to create a *shadow,* which can help align the *needle* over the target peripheral vessel

ally most effective as it allows precise left-to-right alignment of the needle tip with the vessel. A useful technique is applying a general amount of gel between the transducer and the skin and placing the needle directly underneath the transducer flat against the skin. This creates a shadow under the needle that can be used to align the needle directly above the vessel (Fig. 18.8). Once the left-to-right location of the vessel is marked in this manner, the needle can be angled down and inserted superficially into the subcutaneous tissues. At this point, the needle can be "walked" down to the vessel as described previously in the chapter. It is important to ensure that the needle insertion entry angle is approximately 45° as a more acute angle may lead to a kink in the catheter and difficulty visualizing the needle tip. An angle less than 45° may increase the distance to reach the lumen of the vessel and therefore leave a short length of catheter inside the vein. This frequently results in catheter dislodgment and infiltration if the catheter is not exchanged to a longer one. Employing this technique, it is possible to achieve successful peripheral vascular access even in extremely small patients (Fig. 18.1).

Summary

While vascular access procedures have long played an important role in pediatric surgical care, the use of US guidance has become the standard of care by improving the safety and success rate with the diverse array of access procedures. Keys to success include practicing with both the *transverse* and *in-line* orientations of the high-frequency linear transducer probe, a thorough anatomic survey prior to attempting cannulation, anticipating vasospasm, and full needle visualization throughout the procedure. In the case of tunneled catheter placement, the use of US guidance allows the surgeon to create a consistent, gradual subcutaneous course for the catheter via a lateral approach. In summary, for standard access procedures, US guidance provides an increased level of safety, and for difficult scenarios, US guidance allows for success where traditional methods are unreliable. With practice and patience, the use of US guidance can become a useful tool for any pediatric surgeon.

References

1. O'Grady NP, Alexander M, Burns LA, Dellinger EP, Garland J, Heard SO, et al. Guidelines for the prevention of intravascular catheter-related infections. Am J Infect Control. 2011;39(4 Suppl 1):S1–S34.
2. (NICE). NIfCE. Guidance on the Use of Ultrasound Locating Devices for Placing Central Venous Catheters. NICE [Internet]. 2002; Technology appraisal guidance no. 49.
3. Bruzoni M, Slater BJ, Wall J, St Peter SD, Dutta S. A prospective randomized trial of ultrasound- vs landmark-guided central venous access in the pediatric population. J Am Coll Surg. 2013;216(5):939–43. Epub 2013/03/13.
4. Hind D, Calvert N, McWilliams R, Davidson A, Paisley S, Beverley C, et al. Ultrasonic locating devices for central venous cannulation: meta-analysis. BMJ. 2003;327(7411):361. Epub 2003/08/16.
5. Sigaut S, Skhiri A, Stany I, Golmar J, Nivoche Y, Constant I, et al. Ultrasound guided internal jugular vein access in children and infant: a meta-analysis of published studies. Paediatr Anaesth. 2009;19(12):1199–206.
6. Ishii S, Shime N, Shibasaki M, Sawa T. Ultrasound-guided radial artery catheterization in infants and small children. Pediatr Crit Care Med. 2013;14(5):471–3.
7. Tang L, Wang F, Li Y, Zhao L, Xi H, Guo Z, et al. Ultrasound guidance for radial artery catheterization: an updated meta-analysis of randomized controlled trials. PloS ONE. 2014;9(11):e111527.
8. Karapinar B, Cura A. Complications of central venous catheterization in critically ill children. Pediatr Int. 2007;49(5):593–9.

9. Johnson EM, Saltzman DA, Suh G, Dahms RA, Leonard AS. Complications and risks of central venous catheter placement in children. Surgery. 1998;124(5):911–6.
10. Costantino TG, Parikh AK, Satz WA, Fojtik JP. Ultrasonography-guided peripheral intravenous access versus traditional approaches in patients with difficult intravenous access. Ann Emerg Med. 2005;46(5):456–61.
11. Brass P, Hellmich M, Kolodziej L, Schick G, Smith AF. Ultrasound guidance versus anatomical landmarks for subclavian or femoral vein catheterization. Cochrane Database Syst Rev. 2015;1:CD011447.
12. Dargin JM, Rebholz CM, Lowenstein RA, Mitchell PM, Feldman JA. Ultrasonography-guided peripheral intravenous catheter survival in ED patients with difficult access. Am J Emerg Med. 2010;28(1):1–7.

Core Biopsy of Masses and Solid Organs

19

Kushal Parikh, Joseph J. Gemmete and Ranjith Vellody

Introduction

Portability, accessibility, lack of radiation, relatively low cost, and real-time imaging, makes ultrasound an ideal modality for mass or solid organ biopsies. Ultrasound-guided biopsy in adults is a well-established technique and there are well-established guidelines that outline the indications, contraindications, pre- and post-biopsy care, etc. [1, 2]. In pediatric patients, however, such guidelines are scant and not widely accepted. Historically, there has also been significant variance in the patient care and referral patterns among referring pediatricians [3]. In this chapter, the existing literature on ultrasound-guided biopsy of masses and solid organs in pediatric patients is reviewed, which can serve as a guide for an interventionalist practice. Biopsies of the thyroid lesions are discussed in a separate chapter.

R. Vellody (✉)
Department of Radiology, Childrens National Medical Center, 111 Michigan Ave NW, Washington, DC 20010, USA
e-mail: Rvellody@childrensnational.org

K. Parikh · J. J. Gemmete
Department of Radiology, University of Michigan, 1500 E. Medical Center Drive Room UH B1-0502, Ann Arbor, MI 48109, USA
e-mail: pkushal@med.umich.edu

J. J. Gemmete
e-mail: gemmete@med.umich.edu

Pre-procedural Workup

Professional societies have created basic practice parameters for image-guided percutaneous needle biopsies as well as for periprocedural hematologic management that the practitioner should be familiar with [4, 5]. Paramount among these parameters is that the interventionalist should confirm that the indication for the biopsy is appropriate. Suitable indications include confirming the nature of a lesion, staging a patient with a known malignancy, guiding future treatments, obtaining microbiologic analysis, or determining the nature and extent of parenchymal disease. Common absolute contraindications include severe uncorrectable coagulopathy, poor sonographic visualization of the lesion and lack of a safe pathway to the lesion. Poor cardiopulmonary reserve, hemodynamic instability, or the lack of cooperation from the patients or the caretakers are relative contraindications and may be able to overcome by the type of anesthesia administered. There may be additional contraindications unique to each patient and thus concerted decision-making with the referring physicians is a must. A pre-procedural review of the imaging and consultation with a pediatric radiologist are essential for determining whether the lesion is accessible by ultrasound. Often, a mass initially found on CT or MRI is amenable to ultrasound-guided biopsy and a pre-procedural ultrasound examination may also be helpful for confirmation (Fig. 19.1).

Prior to the procedure, a discussion with the pathologist may be needed to determine the

S. Scholz, M. D. Jarboe (eds.), *Diagnostic and Interventional Ultrasound in Pediatrics and Pediatric Surgery,* DOI 10.1007/978-3-319-21699-7_19

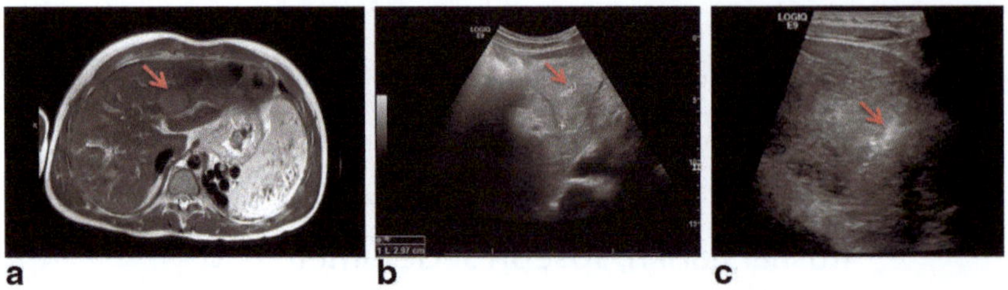

Fig. 19.1 MR-US correlation of a solid, indeterminate hepatic mass. **a** Demonstrates a T2-hyperintense mass *(arrow)* in the *left* lobe of the liver. Ultrasound examination of the same area demonstrates an approximately 3 cm echogenic lesion *(arrow)* as seen in (**b**). Given the adequate visualization and lack of intervening large vasculature (Doppler image not provided), this mass was successfully biopsied percutaneously using an 18G needle *(arrow)*

appropriate biopsy type and specimen handling. The specimen can be obtained either by fine needle aspiration (FNA) or core needle biopsy. Traditionally, core needle biopsies (as well as surgical biopsies) have been preferred over FNA due to the perceived limitation of the FNA in obtaining adequate sample sizes. This limitation may delay care in cases of suspected small blue round cell tumors such as neuroblastoma, Wilms' tumor, hepatoblastoma, or Ewing's sarcoma since the small sample sizes preclude the use of histopathological studies [6]. However, some have argued that even in these cases, FNA can be useful as it can either "rule in" or "rule out" round-cell diagnostic categories [7]. If the decision is made to perform an FNA, presence of an on-site pathologist should be requested to ensure adequate cellularity of the sample. Specimen handling techniques such as formalin fixation, paraffin block, or sterile saline media should also be discussed.

Informed consent should be obtained in all cases from the legal guardian. The consent should at least explain the indications, alternative options, expected risks and benefits, possibility of a non-diagnostic sample, and the post-procedural care [8, 9]. There may be additional factors to consider depending on the individual case. As with most adult interventional procedures, pediatric patients require some level of anesthesia ranging from sedation to general endotracheal anesthesia [10]. While a trained anesthesiologist provides general anesthesia, any privileged provider may administer sedation. The institution and local trends usually determine the type of anesthesia given and who provides it. In the hands of a capable provider, sedation-related complications remain exceeding low [11]. A preoperative consultation with anesthesia can alleviate some of the parents' and patient's anxiety and improve patient satisfaction [12, 13].

Indications

Solid Masses

The majority of solid mass and tumor biopsies in children not associated with the liver or kidney are related to abnormal lymph nodes or suspected hematologic and musculoskeletal tumors. Historically, open surgical biopsy has been the primary way of obtaining biopsies in children in order to obtain larger samples. Minimally invasive surgical approaches have also been tried [14–16]. However, many laparoscopic cases have to be converted to "open" due to poor visibility or bleeding. Similar concerns may also hinder a percutaneous approach; but in most cases, the benefits of the percutaneous approach outweigh the hypothetical risks. Research on ultrasound-guided biopsies of solid pediatric masses so far is relatively scant [17–22], but promising.

Liver Abnormalities

Common indications for liver biopsy include cholestasis, hepatomegaly, liver mass, suspected infection, portal hypertension, or biomarker abnormalities [23–25]. In patients with liver transplantation, additional indications may include suspected graft dysfunction, staging and grading of graft dysfunction, or suspected recurrent malignant disease. Options for obtaining liver specimens include the percutaneous approach with or without image guidance, transjugular approach, and surgery. Samples obtained from the percutaneous approach are usually adequate for making the diagnosis. Core needle biopsies are almost always preferred over the FNA.

As in adults, severe coagulopathy is an absolute contraindication to obtaining a liver biopsy. Other liver-specific contraindications include extrahepatic biliary obstruction or cholangitis [25]. Extremely small sizes of premature children and Morbid obesity are also considered relative contraindications for some, although in our experience, they are not usually an issue when using an ultrasound-guided percutaneous approach. Some practitioners may also consider ascites as a contraindication due to the increased risk of peritonitis and bleeding be further subdivided. However, a paracentesis can be performed prior to performing the biopsy. In these cases, the liver should be scanned again after the paracentesis to confirm a safe window. Alternatively, referral to an interventional radiologist for a transjugular biopsy may be used in cases of refractory ascites. The transjugular route may also be used in cases where there is uncorrectable coagulopathy or if indirect portal manometry measurments are required.

Renal Abnormalities

Some of the common indications for renal biopsy in native kidneys include nephrotic syndrome, hematuria, proteinuria, or renal failure [26–29]. Graft dysfunction-related indications may also be present in patients with renal transplant. It is important to note that many believe that percutaneous biopsy in renal masses, especially in suspected Wilms' tumor, is contraindicated due to potential tumor spread [30]. Recent research, however, remains controversial on this topic.

Percutaneous renal biopsies are likely not as common as liver biopsies in most practices; however, they still remain one of the more relevant procedures for a pediatric interventionalist. Similar to liver biopsies, options for obtaining renal specimens include the percutaneous approach, transjugular approach, and surgery [29]. The transjugular approach is far less common, however, and is reserved for the patients with contraindications to the percutaneous approach (i.e., coagulopathy).

Instruments and Techniques

In the procedure suite, the patient should be placed in the positioning that will allow for the best access to the location of interest. For liver biopsies, the patient's should be supine and the right arm may need to be abducted. For renal biopsies, the patient may be placed in a prone, lateral or lateral oblique position. Subsequently, the area of interest should be rescanned to confirm the continued presence of the suspected abnormality and presence of a safe biopsy window. Infrequently, such as in the cases of reactive lymph nodes, the previously seen abnormality may no longer be present. Additionally, small, tortuous adjacent vasculature may have been missed on other imaging modalities. Doppler interrogation can help detect these vasculature. This pre-procedural scan can also be used to measure the distance from the skin surface to the lesion.

It is also important to predetermine the needle type and size before the procedure. For FNA, smaller needles, 21 gauge or less, are commonly utilized. For core biopsies, the main types of needles are cutting needles and suction needles. Cutting needles can be further subdivided into spring loaded and non-spring loaded varieties. Suction needles include Menghini, Jamshidi or Klatsin needles [25, 31, 32]. Cutting needles are generally preferred over the suction needles due to decreased fragmentation of the tissue, supposed bigger specimen size, and increased diagnostic yield. Tru-Cut is the most commonly used non-spring loaded cutting needle. Some operators prefer the spring-loaded type of cutting needles, which may be further subdivided into controlled-fire or noncontrolled fire. Spring-loaded cutting needles essentially automate the cutting movement once triggered. If you choose to use the spring-loaded cutting needles , it is also important to understand the "throw length." This is a measurement of how much the needle will be advanced from the device once it is triggered. As such, if the abnormality is sized only 1 cm, a needle with a 2 cm throw may not be optimal. Similarly, if there is vasculature abutting the lesion at its posterior acoustic wall, a longer throw may lead to unnecessary complications. The controlled-fire variety allows the practitioner to control the length of the throw.

The proceduralist should also understand the difference between coaxial and noncoaxial methods [33]. The coaxial method employs a larger needle (introducer needle) that creates a tract to the lesion and has another needle that passes through it to obtain the actual specimen while the outer larger needle remains in place (Fig. 19.2). The advantages include creation of only a single skin puncture wound and a single trans-capsular puncture in the case of an organ biopsy. Introducer needles also allow for multiple samples at different angles from the single insertion site. Hemostatic agents can also be delivered to the lesion or the capsule of the organ through the introducer needle. The major disadvantages are that the puncture wound is larger than the size of the core specimen and a needle remains within the patient for nearly the entire procedure. As such, patient cooperation or immobilization is essential. Noncoaxial systems, on the other hand, create smaller puncture wounds and remain within the patient a shorter period of time. However, multiple punctures may be needed to obtain sufficient samples. Since pediatric biopsies require multiple samples (upwards of 10–15 samples per lesion in some cases), coaxial systems are preferred.

For superficial lesions, scanning should be attempted with high-frequency linear transducers (5–15 MHz). Higher frequency waves are easily attenuated and produce a degraded image of the deeper lesions. Conversely, the image quality of the superficial lesions is much better. For deeper lesions, lower frequency curved transducers (2.5–5 MHz) should be used. Additionally, color Doppler examination may be useful for real-time evaluation of any nearby vasculature (Fig. 19.3). After the confirmation of the lesion and administration of the pre-determined sedation, the region of interest should be cleaned and draped in a sterile fashion. The ultrasound transducer should be covered with gel and a sterile cover. Additional gel should be used on the top of the cover. The region of interest should be rescanned under sterile conditions. At this point, if available and desired, an in-plane needle guide can be used to confirm the path and alignment of the needle. These needle guides are biopsy needle brackets that can be snapped onto the transducer and show the expected path of the needle. However, it should be noted that guides restrict freedoms of motion of the needle and may not always be useful, particularly if the operator is already experienced with percutaneous ultrasound-guided biopsies. Once confirmed, the skin should be infiltrated with local anesthetic.

In the case of non-coaxial systems , the needle is advanced to the lesion under ultrasound guidance, making sure to leave room for the throw of the needle. For coaxial core needle devices, the

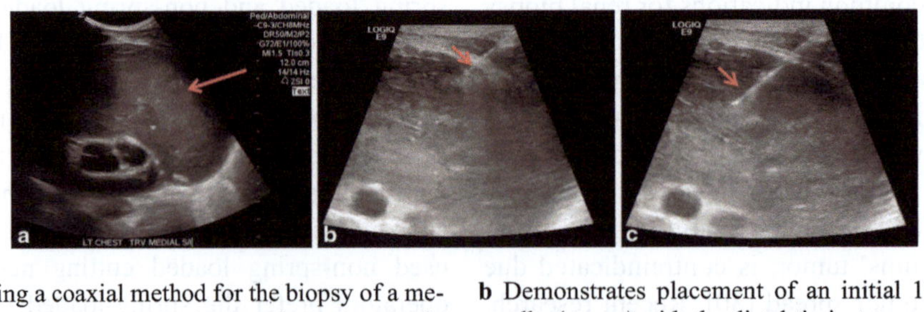

Fig. 19.2 Using a coaxial method for the biopsy of a mediastinal mass. **a** Demonstrates a large, echogenic mass in the anterosuperior mediastinum *(arrow)*. Given the location of the lesion adjacent to vascular organs and need for multiple samples, the coaxial system was preferred. **b** Demonstrates placement of an initial 17G introducer needle *(arrow)* with the distal tip just traversing the outer margin of the lesion. **c** An 18G biopsy needle *(arrow)* is seen traversing the lesion further obtaining a sample

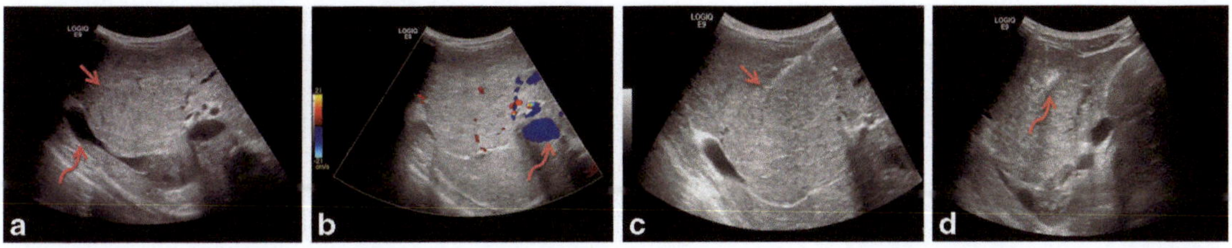

Fig. 19.3 Assessing vascularity using a pre-biopsy scan. **a** Demonstrates an isoechoic hepatic lesion *(straight arrow)* with mass effect on the adjacent inferior vena cava *(curved arrow)*. **b** Demonstrates color Doppler examination of the same mass demonstrating an additional large vessel medially *(curved arrow)*. Given these adjacent vessels, the coaxial biopsy system, an 18G needle with a 17G introducer *(arrow)*, was placed more superficially as seen in **c**. The post-biopsy image in **d** demonstrates the gelfoam *(curved arrow)* that was placed to reduce the risk of bleeding

introducer needle is parked proximal to or just at the periphery of the lesion thus allowing the biopsy needle throw to traverse the lesion. Once the needle or the device is positioned, samples can be taken with or without breath-hold depending on the location of the lesion, level of sedation, and patient cooperation. After each sample acquisition, an image demonstrating the tip of the needle should be taken for documentation. The samples should be placed in the appropriate transport media (formalin, paraffin block, or sterile saline) before obtaining the next sample. Up to 10–15 core samples may be required in certain cases.

When enough samples are obtained, the biopsy needle is removed. For the biopsies involving vascular organs or masses with a coaxial system, some prefer to embolize the tract to reduce the risk of post-procedural bleeding. As the introducer needle is removed, one may inject collagen slurry or gelfoam. Gelfoam may be administered as a pledget directly with a syringe or as a slurry after it has been cut into small (less than 1–2 mm) cubes and mixed with saline through a 3-way stopcock. Under ultrasound, these appear more heterogeneous and echogenic compared to the surrounding parenchyma, especially when there has been a small amount of bleeding (Fig. 19.4).

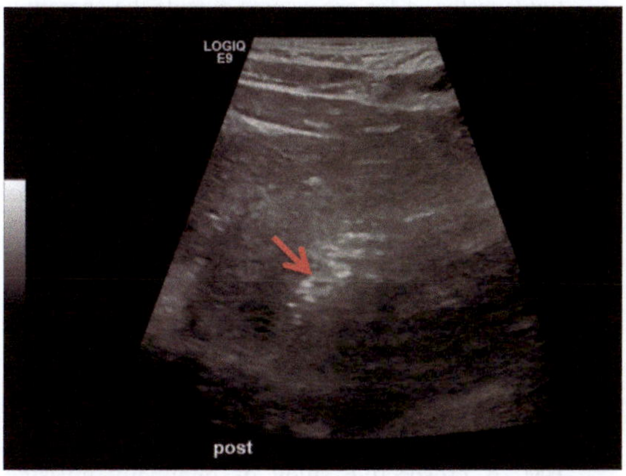

Fig. 19.4 After the biopsy of the lesion seen in Fig. 19.4, the tract was embolized using gelfoam *(arrow)*, which appears echogenic on the ultrasound images

Post-procedural Care and Complications

Following the biopsy, the patient should be transferred to a post-procedural holding area for several hours of observation prior to discharge or transfer back to the floor. A complete blood count (CBC) draw is recommended at 4–6 h post-procedure to document any change in hematocrit. Post-procedural bedside ultrasound examination can also be obtained to evaluate for any complications including hematoma formation.

Complications following percutaneous biopsies remain low. Biopsy-site related bleeding remains one of the most common complications [17–25, 27–29]. In at least one study, increased risk of bleeding post-liver biopsy was associated with younger age and lower weight [34]. Other complications may include pain at the site, hemothorax, pneumothorax, hemoperitoneum (Fig. 19.5), cholangitis, or sedation-related complications. There have been scattered case reports of arterivenous fistula formation, bile

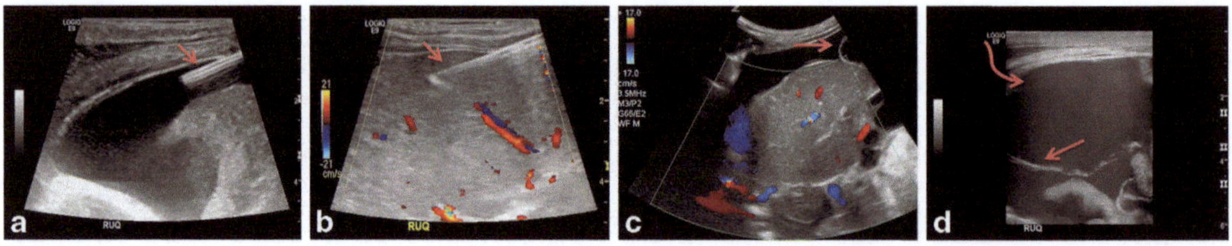

Fig. 19.5 Paracentesis and random liver biopsy in a patient resulting in hemorrhagic ascites. **a** Shows placement of an 18G drainage catheter with subsequent random liver biopsy with a coaxial biopsy system consisting of an 18G biopsy needle through a 17G introducer *(arrow)* in (**b**). Follow-up ultrasound 2 days later, **c** Showed recurrence of ascites with septations *(arrow)*. An ultrasound obtained the day after (3 days post-procedure), **d** Demonstrated large amount of fluid *(curved arrow)* throughout the abdomen with septations *(straight arrow)* and increased echogenicity. The repeat paracentesis yielded dark bloody fluid compatible with old hemorrhage

leak, or deaths following liver biopsies [24]. Arteriovenous fistula formation may occur following renal biopsies as well [28]. In such cases, possible embolization should be considered. Patient death or needle tract seeding remains exceedingly rare.

Summary

Percutaneous ultrasound-guided biopsy of solid organs and masses in children is a safe and efficient procedure that has a very high diagnostic yield. It is important to better understand the role and technique of the percutaneous approach as it becomes more widely used, possibly replacing the surgical approach in many cases.

References

1. Rockey DC, Caldwell SH, Goodman ZD, Nelson RC, Smith AD. American association for the study of liver diseases. Liver biopsy. Hepatology. 2009;49(3):1017–44.
2. Grant A, Neuberger J. Guidelines on the use of liver biopsy in clinical practice. British Society of Gastroenterology. Gut. 1999;45(Suppl 4):IV1–11.
3. Banerjee S, Bishop.W, Valim C, Mahoney LB, Lightdale JR. Percutaneous liver biopsy practice patterns among pediatric gastroenterologists in North America. J Pediatr Gastroenterol Nutr. 2007;45(1):84–9.
4. ACR Interventional Radiology Practice Parameters. ACR-SIR-SPR practice parameter for the performance of image-guided percutaneous needle biopsy (PNB). www.acr.org (2015). Accessed 7 Feb 2015.
5. Patel IJ, Davidson JC, Nikolic B, et al. Consensus guidelines for periprocedural management of coagulation status and hemostasis risk in percutaneous image-guided interventions. J Vasc Interv Radiol. 2012;23(6):727–36.
6. Layfield LJ, Glasgow B, Ostrzwga N, et al. Fine-needle aspiration cytology and the diagnosis of neoplasms in the pediatric age group. Diagn Cytopathol. 1991;7(5):451–61.
7. Howell LP. Changing role of fine-needle aspiration in the evaluation of pediatric masses. Diagn Cytopathol. 2001;24(1):65–70.
8. American College of Surgeons. Informed Consent. www.facs.org/education/patient-education/patient-resources/informed-consent (2015). Accessed 8 Feb 2015.
9. ACR Interventional Radiology Practice Parameters. ACR-SIR Practice Parameter on informed consent for image-guided procedures. www.acr.org (2015). Accessed 8 Feb 2015.
10. Mason KP. Pediatric procedures in interventional radiology. Intl Anesthesiol Clin. 2009;47(3):35–43.
11. Cravero JP, Blike GT, Beach M, et al. Incidence and nature of adverse events during pediatric sedation/anesthesia for procedures outside the operating room: report from the pediatric sedation research consortium. Pediatrics. 2006;118(3):1087–96.
12. Zuwala R, Barber KR. Reducing anxiety in parents before and during pediatric anesthesia induction. AANA J. 2001;69(1):21–5.
13. McEwen A, Moorthy C, Quantock C, et al. The effect of videotaped preoperative information on parental anxiety during anesthesia induction for elective pediatric procedures. Paediatr Anesth. 2007;17(6):534–9.
14. Malkan AD, Loh AH, Sandoval JA. Minimally invasive surgery in the management of abdominal tumors in children. J Pediatr Surg. 2014;49(7):1171–6.
15. Warmann S, Fuchs J, Jesch NK, Schrappe M, Ure BM. A prospective study of minimally invasive techniques in pediatric surgical oncology: preliminary report. Med Pediatr Oncol. 2003;40(3):155–7.

16. Waldhausen JH, Tapper D, Sawin RS. Minimally invasive surgery and clinical decision-making for pediatric malignancy. Surg Endosc. 2000;14(3):250–3.
17. Hassan SF, Mathur S, Magliaro TJ, et al. Needle core vs open biopsy for diagnosis of intermediate- and high-risk neuroblastoma in children. J Pediatr Surg. 2012;47(6):1261–6.
18. Shin HJ, Amaral JG, Armstrong D, Chait PG, et al. Image-guided percutaneous biopsy of musculoskeletal lesions in children. Pediatr Radiol. 2007;37(4):362–9.
19. Sebire NJ, Roebuck DJ. Pathological diagnosis of paediatric tumours from image-guided needle core biopsies: a systemic review. Pediatr Radiol. 2006;36(5):426–31.
20. Sköldenberg EG, Jakobson AA, Elvin A, et al. Diagnosing childhood tumors: a review of 147 cutting needle biopsies in 110 children. J Pediatr Surg. 2002;37(1):50–6.
21. Willman JH, White K, Coffin CM. Pediatric core needle biopsy: strengths and limitations in evaluation of masses. Pediatr Dev Pathol. 2001;4(1):46–52.
22. Garrett KM, Fuller CE, Santana VM, et al. Percutaneous biopsy of pediatric solid tumors. Cancer. 2005;104(3):644–52.
23. Ovchinsky N, Moreira RK, Lefkowitch JH, et al. Liver biopsy in modern clinical practice: a pediatric point-of-view. Adv Anat Pathol. 2012;19(4):250–62.
24. Dezőfi A, Baumann U, Dhawan A, Durmaz O, et al. Liver biopsy in children: position paper of the ESPGHAN hepatology committee. J Pediatr Gastroenterol Nutr. 2014; Epub ahead of print.
25. Dezőfi A, Knrisely AS. Liver biopsy in children 2014; who, whom, what, when, where, why? Clin Res Hepatol Gastroenterol. 2014;38(4):395–8.
26. Bakr A, Eid R, Sarhan A, et al. Fifteen years of kidey biopsies in children: a single center in Egypt. Saudi J Kidney Dis Transpl. 2014;25(6):1321–7.
27. Feneberg R, Schaefer F, Zieger B, et al. Percutaneous renal biopsy in children: a 27-year experience. Nephron. 1998;79(4):438–46.
28. Franke M, Kramarczyk A, Taylan C, et al. Ultrasound-guided percutaneous renal biopsy in 295 children and adolescents: role of ultrasound and analysis of complications. PLoS ONE. 2014;9(12):e114737 eCollection.
29. Brachemi S, Bollée G. Renal biopsy practice: what is the gold standard? World J Nephrol. 2014;3(4):287–94.
30. Zoeller G, Pekrun A, Lakomek M, et al. Wilms' tumor: the problem of diagnostic accuracy in children undergoing preoperative chemotherapy without histological tumor verification. J Urol. 1994;151(1):169–71.
31. Colombo M, Del Ninno E, de Franchis R, et al. Ultrasound-assisted percutaneous liver biopsy: superiority of the Tru-Cut over the menghini needle for diagnosis of cirrhosis. Gastroenterology. 1988;95(2):487–9.
32. Goldner F. Comparison of the Menghini, Klatskin and Tru-Cut needles in diagnosing cirrhosis. J Clin Gastroenterol. 1979;1(3):229–31.
33. Hatfield MK, Beres RA, Sane SS, et al. Percutaneous imaging-guided solid organ core needle biopsy: coaxial versus noncoaxial method. AJR Am J Roentgenol. 2008;190(2):413–7.
34. Short SS, Papillon S, Hunter CJ, et al. Percutaneous liver biopsy: pathologic diagnosis and complications in children. J Pediatr Gastroenterol Nutr. 2013;57(5):644–8.

Fine Needle Aspiration (FNA) of the Thyroid Gland

20

Ranjith Vellody

Introduction

Thyroid cancer is the most common endocrine malignancy in children [1] and is increasing in both incidence and prevalence. Risk factors for thyroid cancer in children are radiation exposure (such as prior therapy for lymphoma), female gender, and family history [2]. Children have the same types of thyroid cancer as seen in adults (papillary, follicular, medullary, anaplastic); however, children often present with more advanced disease [2]. Data have shown that thyroid nodules in children are more likely to be malignant than adults. In spite of this, children have a better prognosis. Factors which worsen the prognosis include male sex, nonsurgical treatment, non-papillary type cancer, and patients with distant metastases [3].

Guidelines from Society of Radiologists in Ultrasound (SRU) and the American Association of Clinical Endocrinologists do not specifically mention the management of thyroid nodules in children [4, 5]. However, the revised 2009 guidelines from the American Thyroid Association do suggest that the management of pediatric thyroid nodules should be the same as adults [3].

The original version of this chapter was revised.
An erratum to this chapter can be found at
DOI 10.1007/978-3-319-21699-7_25

R. Vellody (✉)
Department of Radiology, University of Michigan,
1500 E. Medical Center Drive, Room UH B1-0502,
Ann Arbor, MI 48109, USA
e-mail: ranjithv@med.umich.edu

A detailed clinical history and physical examination are performed with an emphasis on detecting signs and symptoms of thyroid disease. Laboratory values including a serum TSH are then drawn. If TSH levels are normal or high, a diagnostic ultrasound may be performed. Several ultrasound characteristics of the thyroid gland are important to evaluate. These include whether the disease process is diffuse versus focal, the number and size of the lesions present, and whether lesions are solid, cystic, or mixed (Fig. 20.1 and 20.2). In addition, the presence of calcifications, colloid, associated vascularity, and levels of pathologically enlarged lymph nodes should be documented. Typically, descriptors in the thyroid ultrasound report suggesting that a process may not be benign include the presence of macrocalcifications or microcalcifications, absence of a halo, increased vascularity, solid composition, and irregular margins (Figs. 20.3, 20.4 and 20.5).

Based on the SRU consensus statement, fine needle aspiration (FNA) is suggested for a thyroid nodule of 1.0 cm or larger if microcalfcifications are present, 1.5 cm or larger if the nodule is solid with coarse calcifications, 2 cm with mixed solid and cystic components, or nodules that have substantial growth over an interval period [6]. As reflected in the SRU guidelines, ultrasound characteristics are more important than size when determining whether a nodule should be sampled.

The cytopathology result of the FNA determines whether observation, repeat FNA, or surgery should be performed. With respect to the cytopathology result, the Bethesda Classification System for Reporting Thyroid Cytopathology

S. Scholz, M. D. Jarboe (eds.), *Diagnostic and Interventional Ultrasound in Pediatrics and Pediatric Surgery,* DOI 10.1007/978-3-319-21699-7_20

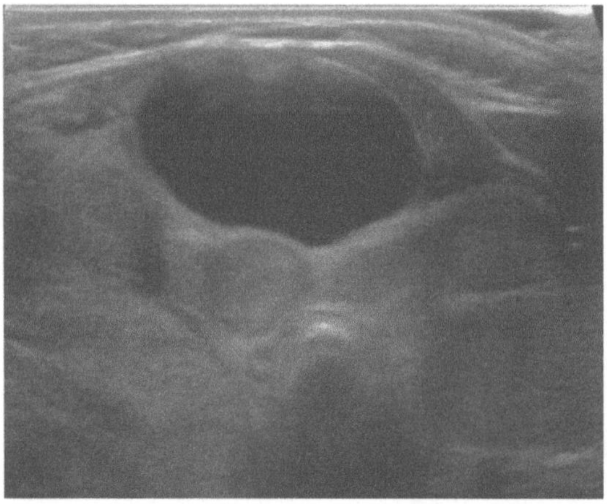

Fig. 20.1 Transverse ultrasound image of the right lobe demonstrates a thin-walled anechoic structure with posterior acoustic enhancement in the thyroid gland. This is a simple benign cyst

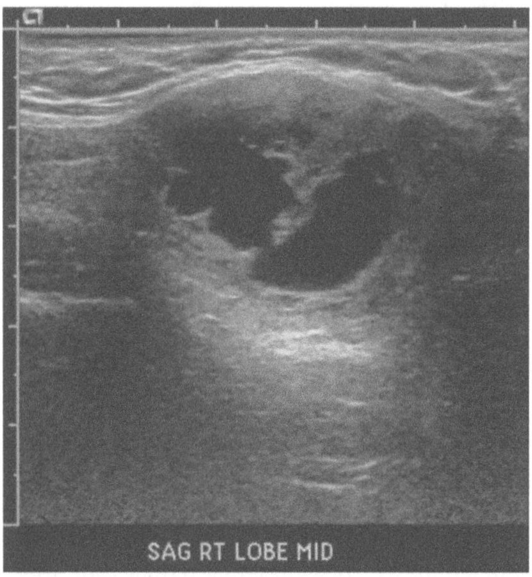

Fig. 20.2 Transverse ultrasound image of the right lobe of the thyroid demonstrating a mixed solid and cystic nodule. Targeted FNA of the solid portion of the lesion revealed papillary thyroid carcinoma

allows for standardization which in turn dictates management [7]. Every FNA report groups the cytopathology into six distinct categories. Each category has an associated risk for malignancy and a recommended management scheme (Table 20.1).

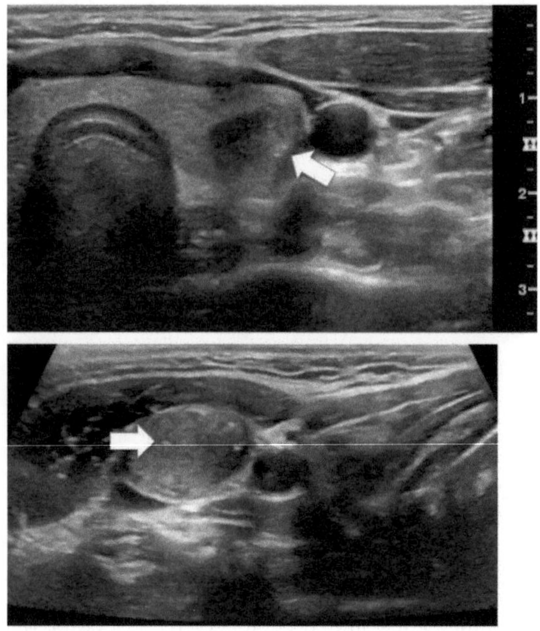

Fig. 20.3 **a** Transverse thyroid ultrasound image reveals microcalcifications *(arrow)* within a solid nodule in the left lobe of the thyroid. Fine needle aspiration of the lesion was significant for papillary thyroid carcinoma. **b** Transverse image of lymph node in the right neck adjacent to the carotid artery in the same patient. Note the similar sonographic appearance to the primary thyroid lesion *(arrow)*

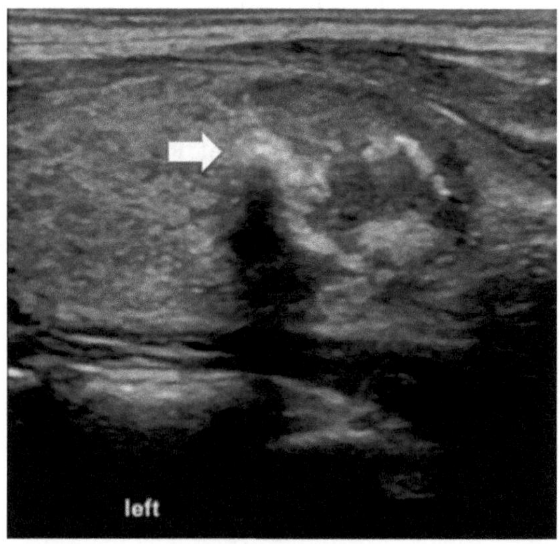

Fig. 20.4 Coarse calcifications within a thyroid nodule. Note the posterior shadowing from the calcifications *(arrow)*. FNA revealed papillary cancer

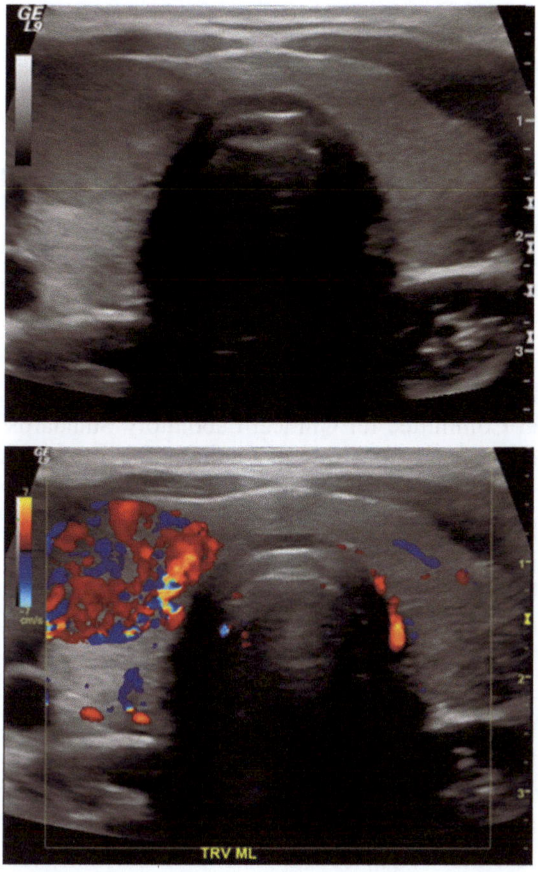

Fig. 20.5 **a** Transverse ultrasound images of the thyroid in a 10-year-old female. A dominant nodule path proven to be papillary thyroid carcinoma is noted within the right lobe of the thyroid. **b** *Color Doppler* demonstrates hypervascularity of the lesion

FNA in children presents a unique challenge as opposed to adults. While most adults can lie still for an FNA, children may require local anesthesia, intravenous conscious sedation, or even general anesthesia. Anesthesia does carry inherent risks and every case should undergo an appropriate risk/benefit analysis. However, it is best to err on the side of increased patient comfort and hence decreased patient motion as adjacent structures can be inadvertently damaged even with a small-gauge needle.

Some practitioners perform FNA of thyroid without ultrasound. Although ultrasound guidance may add slightly to the cost and length of the procedure, it is felt to provide more accurate diagnostic information. This is particularly true when nodules cannot be palpated, when there is some alteration in anatomy, and when a specific thyroid nodule needs to be sampled in the setting of multiple nodules. Additionally, ultrasound allows for targeting of the solid components of a lesion that has mixed solid and cystic characteristics and allows for the visualization of larger vasculature that should be avoided.

Pre-procedural Management

The most important aspect of pre-procedural management is confirming that there is a documented indication for the biopsy. All prior imaging studies should be reviewed. Most practitioners agree that anticoagulants, including antiplatelet agents, should be held for 4–7 days prior to the FNA procedure. In some instances, antiplatelet agents may be difficult to hold. Thyroid lesions can still be safely biopsied in this clinical setting as long as the procedure is meticulously performed. Informed consent with documentation of the risks of the procedure should be obtained from the patient or legal guardian. It is also prudent to discuss each case individually with the

Table 20.1 The Bethesda classification system for thyroid malignancy

Classification	Risk of malignancy (%)	Management
Nondiagnostic	1–4	Repeat FNA
Benign	<5	Follow up ultrasound in 6–18 months
Follicular lesion of uncertain significance	5–15	Follow up ultrasound +/− repeat FNA in 3–6 months
Follicular neoplasm, Hürthle cell neoplasm	20–30	Surgical lobectomy
Suspicious for papillary thyroid cancer	60–75	Thyroid lobectomy/total thyroidectomy
Papillary thyroid cancer	98	Total thyroidectomy

FNA Fine needle aspiration

anesthesia provider to determine whether local anesthetic alone, intravenous sedation, or general endotracheal anesthesia will be required. If the institution has the capability, having an on-site cytopathologist during the procedure can eliminate unnecessary needle passes through the thyroid lesion and limit the amount of nondiagnostic biopsies.

Technique

Once the child is in the procedure room, patient verification is performed. A preliminary thyroid ultrasound should be performed at this time to document the continued presence of the lesion that is to be biopsied. The patient should then be anesthetized according to the previously determined plan. The patient is positioned with their neck in extension, usually with a rolled towel or small pillow underneath the shoulder blades [8].

With a high frequency probe (7.5–15 MHz), the nodule of interest is identified and an overview of the surrounding anatomy is obtained [4]. Using color Doppler, large surrounding vascular structures are noted. An appropriate path for the biopsy needle is determined to avoid vascular structures and traverse as little as normal tissue as possible. The neck is prepped and draped in standard sterile fashion. At this point, the ultrasound probe should be covered with a sterile probe cover containing ultrasound gel.

Although many ultrasound-guided procedures require the use of ultrasound gel on the outside of the probe cover in order to maximize image quality, gel can get stuck in the needle bore and can interfere with the cytology assessment by causing precipitation on Wright staining [9]. For this reason and because the thyroid is a superficial structure, FNA can be performed in an alternative manner using only an antiseptic solution such as betadine to achieve adequate skin contact with the ultrasound probe. It should be noted that ultrasound gel can still be used as long as the operator is aware of the potential downsides.

Because the thyroid gland is highly vascular, a small gauge needle is recommended for aspiration. There are different recommendations for the gauge of a needle ranging between 22 and 27 gauge [4, 9, 10, 12]. Any needle gauge less than 27 is too small, given that the diameter of the follicular cell nucleus is in the 200 μm range and the inside diameter of a 25- and 27-gauge needle is between 191 and 241 μm [9]. Furthermore, core biopsies of the thyroid gland are not part of routine practice and are rarely performed due to the potential increased risk of bleeding complications.

While operators at many institutions use local anesthesia, it is not recommended by the National Committee for Clinical Laboratory Standards because it can cause more pain than the FNA itself. Moreover, it can obscure cellular detail on pathology and anatomic detail during instillation [11]. However, local anesthesia does offer the benefit of pain relief during and after the procedure, allowing for a better patient experience. Typically, this is done using a 25-gauge needle and should be used in the subcutaneous fat, not the reticular dermis, to infiltrate dermal nerves [9]. The amount of anesthetic that can be administered varies depending upon the type of medication used, whether it is mixed with epinephrine, and the weight of the patient. Additionally, an anesthetic cream such as EMLA cream, a spray formulation or ice can be used as an anesthetic. The former has a vasoconstrictor effect and leads to less hemodilution of the aspirate [9, 12].

Under ultrasound guidance, utilizing the free hand technique or an ultrasound guide, the needle is slowly advanced toward the superficial margin of the nodule. Several forward and back oscillations are made with the needle through the lesion (Fig. 20.6). This motion allows for more material to enter the bore of the needle and become trapped for extraction. The intralesional dwell time during this portion of the procedure should be 2–5 s. Suction can be applied to the needle with a syringe during the aspiration but is not necessary as there is already native suction provided by the existing surface tension in the nodule [13, 14]. The literature suggests that suction is more convenient, however, it is not does not provide a better diagnostic yield when compared to using no suction [13, 14].

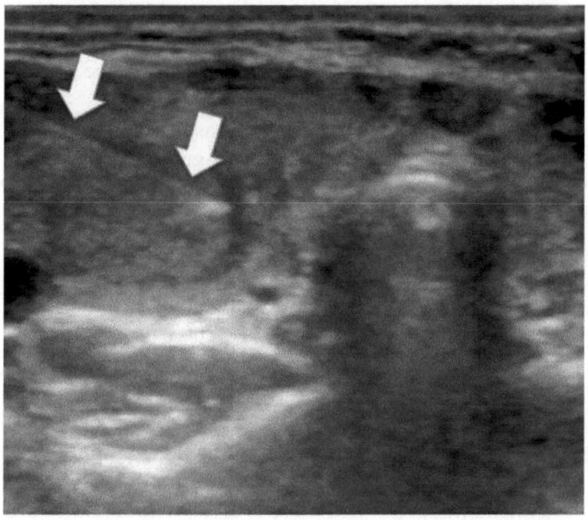

Fig. 20.6 Intraprocedural transverse ultrasound image of a thyroid fine needle aspiration. Note the echogenic 25-gauge needle *(arrow)* within a dominant right thyroid nodule

Some operators feel more needle passes through the lesion can increase the diagnostic yield. However, there is some literature to suggest that more than ten needle passes during sampling can increase the risk of hematoma formation [10]. If blood is identified within the needle during sampling the operator should not be alarmed, since this only means that the lower-viscosity blood has preferentially entered the needle over the higher-viscosity material. Blood identified within the needle can be due to excessive suction or a long dwell time of the needle within the lesion [9, 11].

The nodule of interest is sampled and the needle is given to the cytopathologist for analysis. Typically, three to five passes are performed at the beginning of the procedure and given to the cytopathologist at one time, since preparation of the material for viewing under the microscope can take a few minutes. If no cytopathologist is present, the needle can be placed bevel down and the aspirate smeared onto a slide and submitted to cytopathology [11]. When preparing your own slides, using a one step method is preferable by using one slide to hold the sample and the second to spread it. It can be difficult to know when enough material is present for diagnosis when an on-site cytopathologist is not present.

A thorough ultrasound of the neck is performed after the procedure to look for a hematoma [10]. An ice pack or acetaminophen is the preferred method of analgesia post procedure. Discharge instructions should include notifying the clinician for any signs of neck swelling, shortness of breath, redness, or discharge from the FNA site [10].

Post-procedural Complications

Complications that can be seen after a thyroid FNA include pain, bruising, and hematoma around the FNA site. Rarely, an infection may be encountered. Allergic reactions to local anesthetics are rare and the main treatment is antihistamines. The recurrent laryngeal nerve is within the region of the thyroid, therefore puncture is possible, however this is extremely rare [11, 15]. Large blood vessel transgression can occur with the needle, but with good ultrasound imaging and color Doppler this is also extremely rare. Another rare complication is tumor seeding which has been noted in 12 cases [16]. Tumor seeding may be prevented by limiting the number of needle passes, making sure the needle does not transgress deep to the lesion and using smaller needles for the FNA.

The main cause of inadequate samples is other substances such as ultrasound gel or blood predominating the sample. This can be minimized by limiting the use of ultrasound gel or suction and having on-site cytopathologist to review the sample. Other causes include performing a biopsy on a predominantly cystic or excessively vascular nodule. Although studies evaluating the efficacy of FNA of the thyroid in children are not well established, many centers find that diagnostic samples can be obtained in over 90 % of patients. Some authors have concluded that the efficacy is less for nodules less than 5 mm [17].

Summary

FNA of suspicious thyroid nodules in children is an important part in the medical evaluation of these patients. As research continues to evolve, it is important for clinicians to know what constitutes best practice with respect to technique. Doing so will allow for maximum yield, less discomfort to the patient, and less inconvenience to the patient's family.

References

1. Hogan A. The incidence of pediatric thyroid cancer is increasing and is higher in girls than in boys and may have an adverse outcome. Clin Thyroidol. 2009;21(10):10–2.
2. Önder A. Approach to thyroid nodules in children and adolescents. Turk J Pediatr. 2014;56:219–25.
3. Cooper D, et al. Revised American thyroid association management guidelines for patients with thyroid nodules and differentiated thyroid cancer. Thyroid. 2009;19(11):1167–214.
4. Kim M, et al. US-guided fine-needle aspiration of thyroid nodules: indications, techniques, results. Radiographics. 2008;28(7):1869–86.
5. Frates M. Management of thyroid nodules detected at US society of radiologists in ultrasound consensus conference statement. Ultrasound Q. 2006;22(4):231–40.
6. Frates M. Management of thyroid nodules detected at us: society of radiologists in ultrasound consensus conference statement. Radiology. 2005;237(3):794–800.
7. Cibas E, Ali S The bethesda system for reporting thyroid cytopathology. Thyroid. 2009;19:1159–1165.
8. Dhurandhar N, et al. Fine needle aspiration biopsy (FNAB) techniques; approved guideline-second edition. Clinical and Laboratory Standards Institute. 2003;23(27):3.
9. Pitman M, et al. Techniques for thyroid FNA: A synopsis of the national cancer institute thyroid fine-needle aspiration state of the science conference. Diagn Cytopathol. 2008;36(6):407–24.
10. Dogra V, Saad W. Fine-needle aspiration biopsy of thyroid nodules. In: Ultrasound-guided procedures. 2nd ed. New York: Thieme; 2010. pp. 67–72.
11. NCCLS. Fine Needle Aspiration Biopsy (FNAB) Techniques; Approved Guideline-Second Edition. NCCLS document GP20-A2 [ISBN 1-56238-509-7]. NCCLS, 940 West Valley Road, Suite 1400, Wayne, Pennsylvania 19087-1898 USA, 2003.
12. Oertel Y. Fine-needle aspiration of the thyroid: technique and terminology. Endocrinol Metab Clin North Am. 2007;36:737–51.
13. Pothier D, Narula A. (2006). Should we apply suction during fine needle cytology of thyroid lesions? A systematic review and meta-analysis. Ann R Coll Surg Engl. 88(7):643–45.
14. Maurya AK, Mehta A, Mani NS, Nijhawan VS, Batra R. Comparison of aspiration vs non-aspiration techniques in fine-needle cytology of thyroid lesions. J Cytol/Indian Acad Cytol. 2010;27(2):51–4. doi:10.4103/0970-9371.70737.
15. Tomoda C, Takamura Y, Ito Y, Miya A, Miyauchi A. Transient vocal cord paralysis after fine-needle aspiration biopsy of thyroid tumor. Thyroid. 2006;16(7):697–9.
16. Polyzos S, et al. A systematic review of cases reporting needle tract seeding following thyroid fine needle biopsy. World J Surg. 2010;34:844–51.
17. Kim D, et al. Ultrasound-guided fine-needle aspiration biopsy of thyroid nodules: comparison in efficacy according to nodule size. Thyroid. 2009;19(1):27–31.

21 Diagnostic and Therapeutic Drainage

Samir K. Gadepalli

Introduction

There are many different types of collections of fluid (e.g., those in a cavity, those after surgery, those that are congenital); the approach to diagnosis or therapy may be different based on the type and location. Being able to categorize fluid collections by type and location in the body is the first step. These fluid collections can occur at any part of the body and knowing your anatomy is a key way to avoid any complications.

The next step is preparation which leads to a series of questions: Do I have all the equipment, does this need to be sterile, does the primary team managing the patient want the fluid sent for special things including cultures, is this a recurrence, do we need to perform a sclerosis, is this in conjunction with a biopsy, is ultrasound the correct image guidance modality for this instance. Knowing the history and doing a thorough physical checkup is still important prior to picking up the ultrasound. A patient with allergies, having severe anxiety to the procedure, or just after a meal, could seriously hinder the ability to perform an ultrasound. As interventional ultrasound is an adjunct to clinical care—the provider caring for the patient and the person performing the ultrasound-guided procedure may be different—leading to a fragmentation in care that could lead to communication issues.

Finally, technical considerations, such as having more than one ultrasound probe, are essential. The diagnostic and therapeutic probes used for ultrasound do not have to be the same. For example, identifying the collection may be better with a curved probe, but following the needle into the cavity may be better with a linear probe. Furthermore, having a range of drainage catheters, guidewires, and dilators is crucial to the success of a drainage procedure. Moreover, the path to the collection does not have to be directly percutaneous and may need to traverse an organ. For example, accessing the gallbladder through the liver parenchyma or a pelvic collection through a transrectal approach often is superior to other options. Finally, having the ability to inject the collection with contrast and monitoring this using fluoroscopy should not be underestimated.

In this chapter, we focus on general principles as briefly outlined above, then focus on a transrectal approach to drainage, after which we discuss special circumstances where there is literature to support a specific strategy. For example with ascites, make sure to have albumin available or know if the patient has significant liver disease; or with a pleural effusion, use of tissue plasminogen activator (TPA) to prevent a recurrence versus needing to send samples to rule out malignancy.

S. K. Gadepalli (✉)
Division of Pediatric Surgery, Department of Surgery, C.S. Mott Children's Hospital, 1540 East Hospital Drive, SPC 4211, Ann Arbor, MI 48108, USA
e-mail: samirg@med.umich.edu

S. Scholz, M. D. Jarboe (eds.), *Diagnostic and Interventional Ultrasound in Pediatrics and Pediatric Surgery,* DOI 10.1007/978-3-319-21699-7_21

General Principles

Fluid collections can be differentiated into various types based on history and anatomic location. Categorizing them based on history and location helps with management by using a diagnostic or therapeutic algorithm. The following is an example of various ways a collection can be categorized:

1. Collections in general: unknown, malignant, infectious, lymphatic
2. Abscesses: postoperative, chest, mediastinal, abdominal, pelvic
3. Gastrointestinal (GI): pancreatic, splenic, foregut/duplication, chronic cholecystitis, hydatid cyst
4. Urologic: hydronephrosis, suprapubic catheter placement

Prior to drainage of a collection, the indications must be reviewed, coagulopathy must be excluded or treated, and the appropriate imaging modality must be chosen [1]. The diagnostic approach to fluid collections starts with a good history and location of the lesion. If the patient has a history of malignancy or risk factors that increase the risk for a malignancy, the identification of a collection, such as a pleural effusion, can be a marker of the malignancy. Furthermore, qualities of a collection, such as the percentage of solid material, can differentiate a cystic collection. Knowing the likelihood of a malignancy is important in the approach to drainage of a collection as the tract used to sample the fluid can be a potential pathway for the spread of the disease.

Similarly, the sampling of the collection can be diagnostic, therapeutic, or both. Therefore, having a general framework to approach the fluid is useful to prevent additional procedures or anesthetics. As there is always a risk in the aspiration of a collection, combining procedures into one setting can mitigate further risks. For example, injection of a sclerosant into the cavity during drainage of a lymphatic collection prevents recurrence of the collection and, concomitantly, an additional procedure.

Drainage of a fluid collection should only be performed when there is [2]: a suspicion of infection, a need for fluid characterization, or symptoms that warrant drainage. "The basic indication for needle aspiration is to confirm the radiological diagnosis of an abscess because the radiological signs may not distinguish amongst various types of fluid collection including abscess, hematoma, urinoma, biloma, lymphocele, seroma, and loculated ascites. The main indications for catheter drainage include treatment or palliation of sepsis associated with an infected fluid collection, and alleviation of the symptoms that may be caused by fluid collections by virtue of their size, like pancreatic pseudocele or lymphocele" [1]. Figure 21.1 demonstrates needle entry into a fluid collection of unknown etiology for diagnostic purposes.

Informed consent following a thorough discussion with the patient is mandatory for any invasive procedure. Rarely are the procedures emergent and the expectations of the patients and primary-care providers need to be assessed prior to performing the procedure. Identification of the indications, approach to drainage, choosing the appropriate imaging modality, specific diagnostic tests on the drainage, and therapeutic options should all be discussed at this time.

In diagnostic or therapeutic drainage, the steps are fairly simple though difficult to execute without sufficient practice. The collection is identified using an ultrasound probe (as mentioned earlier, the probe used to initially find the collection and that used for targeting drainage may be different). Using ultrasound guidance, the collec-

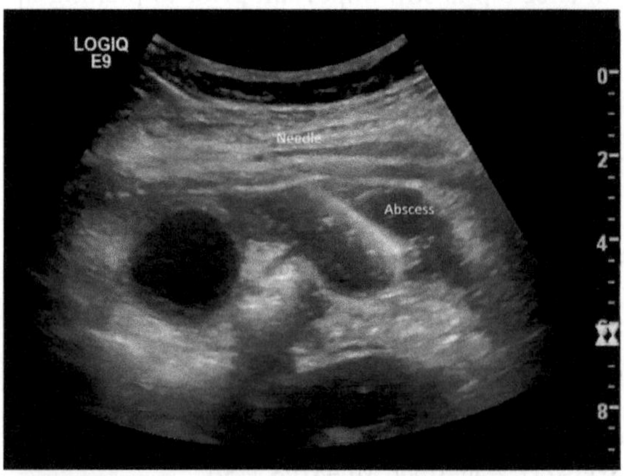

Fig. 21.1 Figure represents needle entry into a collection of unknown etiology using a curved probe for guidance

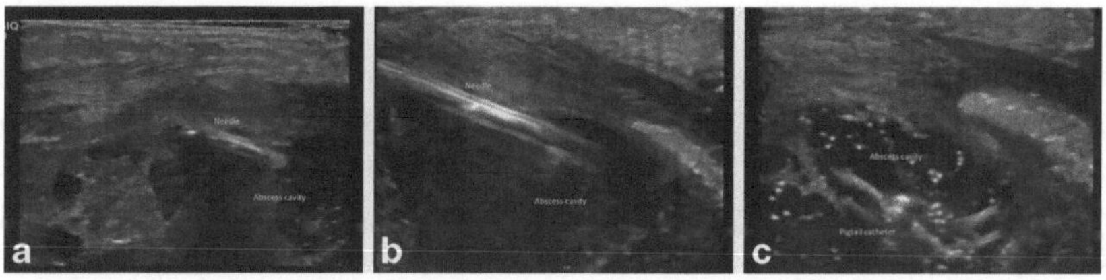

Fig. 21.2 **a** Figure represents needle entry into a loculated abscess cavity with multiple septations. **b** Figure represents needle connecting multiple loculated collections by breaking up the septations under visualization. **c** Figure represents abscess cavity being drained by the pigtail catheter that is now in place. The abscess is irrigated with saline and collapsed down at the end of the procedure

tion is approached using an 18- or 22-gauge entry needle based on the depth and size of the fluid. Advancing the needle in line with the ultrasound transducer provides excellent visualization of the entire needle and the target collection simultaneously. This improves safety and maneuverability in advancing the needle. If purulent fluid is aspirated, it is sent for culture; of note, immunocompromised patients may have bacteria or fungal collections without evidence of an immune response. Keep in mind that a Gram stain may fail to grow any organisms if the patient has already received antimicrobial therapy. Furthermore, use of a needle without the syringe attached can be a useful technique to facilitate guiding the needle into the cavity without the added weight of the syringe. The syringe can be attached once entry into the cavity can be confirmed by imaging. Based on the thickness of the fluid, the needle may need to be "upsized" prior to drainage of the contents.

To "upsize" the needle, a guidewire can be inserted with serial dilation over the guidewire using a Seldinger technique. A 0.010- or 0.018-in. wire can be placed through the 22-gauge needle whereas a 0.035 guidewire can be inserted through an 18-gauge entry needle. When using larger dilators, we routinely exchange a thinner guidewire to a larger diameter and stiffer wire to provide a stiff backbone for the dilator to travel over preventing dislodgment and errant passage of the dilator. Furthermore, the needle and guidewire exchange is easier to accomplish with the cavity filled with fluid as there is more resistance on the wall to prevent dislodgement as well as prevent inadvertent entry through the opposite wall. If the fluid within a cavity has already been evacuated for diagnosis, irrigation with saline can be used to refill the area and help with the needle and guidewire exchange. Once a drainage cathether has been inserted into the cavity, we routinely use ultrasound to confirm adequate drainage of the cavity and assess for additional located collections that were not initially noted or were inadequately drained. Although, the largest possible drainage catheter is generally used, there is no difference in recurrence, drainage time, and complications [3]. Figure 21.2 demonstrates evacuation of a loculated abscess by breaking up septations using the needle and placement of a pigtail for irrigation and drainage.

The management of a drain when placed should be standard for each institution. Drains can be placed to bulb or gravity drainage based on the expected quality and quantity of output. They should be ideally flushed with saline daily and removed in about 1–3 days when the output is less than 10 ml/day or 5 ml/day in infants [2]. While a drain is in place, antibiotics should be considered if there is a risk of translocation based on host factors, if there is adjacent foreign material such as an implant, or if the output is presumptively infectious.

Ultrasound has become the imaging modality of choice for many interventions with the advent of high-resolution, wide-angle probes. Ultrasound also offers the unique advantages of portability, immediate availability, and flexibility, owing in part to the wide range of transducers now available. Ultrasound probes have been specifically designed to guide the biopsy of small lesions, allow precise control of biopsy instruments, and provide direct, real-time visualization of successful target lesion biopsies. Moreover, ultrasound avoids ionizing radiation—an important concern especially when imaging the organs of the pelvis, namely the gonads [4].

Transrectal Drainage

A transrectal approach can be used for drainage of an abscess or fluid collection in the pelvis. As the bowel can obscure the collection and prevent a transabdominal approach to the collection, a transrectal access can be more direct. Also, this approach may be less painful than transgluteal as it does not traverse any muscles. A transgluteal approach requires the catheter to be placed close to the sacrum/coccyx to avoid injury to the sciatic nerve and gluteal vessels; this approach can cause pelvic and leg pain if it passes through the piriformis muscle or near the sacral plexus [4]. Securing the catheter using the transrectal approach may be more difficult though, therefore, a pigtail is recommended. Figure 21.3 demonstrates the use of real-time ultrasound to access a pelvic abscess using the transrectal approach.

One study recommends having all patients who are having transrectal or transvaginal drainage of an abscess be started on antibiotics at least 2 h in advance to achieve adequate systemic levels [5]. A bowel preparation is considered unnecessary for transrectal drainage; however a gentle enema—if not contraindicated—using saline or Fleet's may help clear out remnant stool, making the procedure easier and cleaner to perform.

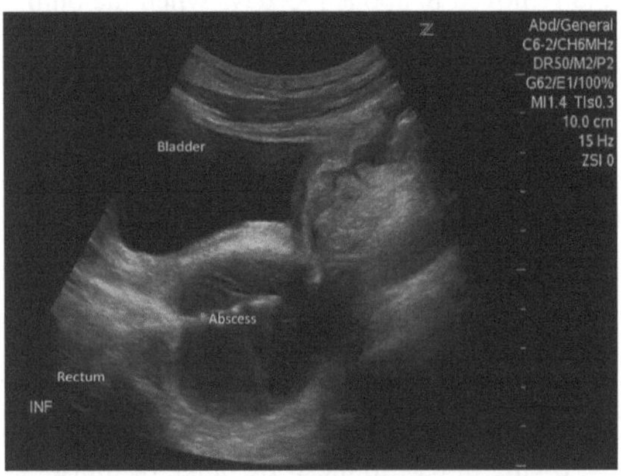

Fig. 21.3 Figure represents needle entry into a pelvic abscess using a transrectal approach. The needle enters the cavity under direct visualization. The probe (curved) was placed in a longitudinal orientation on the abdominal wall visualizing the bladder and rectum while accessing the abscess cavity

For teenagers, a transrectal probe with guide can be used since their anal sphincter complex can accommodate the probe without damage. However, in both older and younger children, a curved transducer in a sagittal orientation placed just above the pubic bone can provide excellent transabdominal guidance for transrectal abscess drainage. In this method the bladder acts as an acoustic window so that catheterizing the bladder to fill with saline augments visualization [5]. Leaving a pigtail catheter in the abscess is preferred to solely draining an abscess when transrectal approach is used. Furthermore, daily irrigation should be performed approximately every 8 h with 5–10 mL of sterile saline to flush both the abscess cavity and the associated tubing [4].

Transrectal techniques are also used in assessment of male infertility, hemospermia, and azospermia. Seminal vesicle, ejaculatory duct, and midline cysts can be aspirated under transrectal ultrasound guidance and analyzed for semen and sperm motility. Aspiration of ejaculatory duct cysts may improve obstructive azospermia and improve paternity rates [4].

Furthermore, the transrectal technique is a safe, adequate, and effective treatment for prostate abscess [6].

The rest of the chapter focuses on diagnostic and therapeutic approaches that should be considered for various anatomic locations.

Head and Neck

Drainage of a fluid collection in the head and neck region can be required for an infection with subsequent abscess formation, hemorrhage into an existing cyst, or a postoperative complication [7]. As the oral cavity is closely intertwined with head and neck anatomy, several sources of bacterial translocation can occur. As these anaerobic organisms spread, they can lead to a retropharyngeal abscess or those that track anteriorly into the mediastinum. Early drainage can identify these organisms and allow for aggressive treatment, preventing later complications [8].

Peritonsillar cellulitis and abscess can present similarly with edema, trismus, and erythema [9]. Usage of ultrasound improves the diagnostic accuracy and ability to drain the collection. As the carotid artery can be near the posterior extent of the abscess, an ultrasound can be used to guide the needle while limiting the potential injury to adjacent structures. In one study, ultrasound was used to diagnose and drain the collection in the emergency room, facilitating an earlier discharge home without complications [10].

Cysts in the head and neck region can be fairly common, arising from the thyroid origin as a thyroglossal duct cyst—a dermoid cyst confined to the superficial tissues or laterally as branchial cleft cysts. These cysts ultimately may require surgical excision; however, infection or hemorrhage can occur at initial presentation or postoperatively requiring ultrasound-guided drainage for management. The most important concepts to consider in the head and neck region include: (1) the use of anatomic landmarks and identification of important vascular and air-filled structures that course over a small area and (2) weighing the risks of drainage for diagnostic purposes versus an earlier more aggressive surgical approach for therapy. Alternatively, use of sclerotherapy after drainage of cysts in the thyroid, parathyroid, and salivary glands has been shown to be successful to prevent recurrence [11]. Figure 21.4 demonstrates entry into a thyroid cyst for diagnostic sampling.

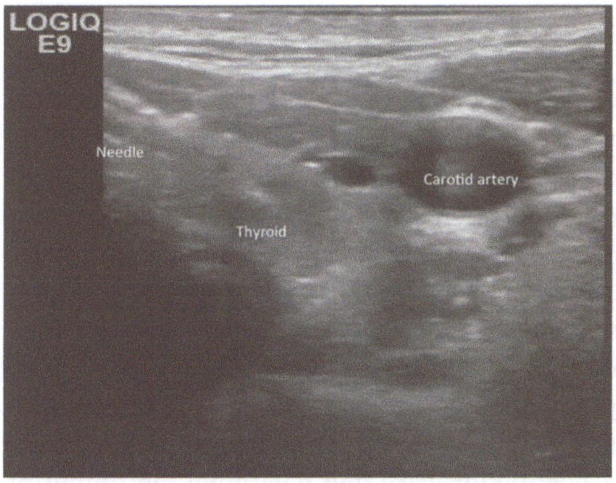

Fig. 21.4 Figure represents needle entry into a cyst in the thyroid. Note the adjacent vascular structures and how well they can be visualized and avoided using ultrasound

Chest

Pleural effusions or fluid collections in the chest can occur for a variety of reasons—infectious, malignant, lymphatic, or idiopathic. Classically, drainage of the fluid has been used for diagnosis—classifying effusions as transudative versus exudative. The Light criteria can be used to define the type of effusion [12]: pH <7.2, lactate dehydrogenase >1000 U, glucose <40 mg/dL, or $<25\,\%$ blood glucose, Gram stain, or culture positive and with loculations or septations proven with imaging indicating an exudative or complex collection. In future studies, an exudative effusion was most definitively confirmed with a low pH [13–15]. Figure 21.5 demonstrates the use of ultrasound to drain a pleural fluid collection.

Parapneumonic effusions occur during or after a bout of bacterial pneumonia, with translocation of the bacteria into the pleural space from the interstitial. The fluid starts as clear with some mild particulate matter, thickening over time, until it

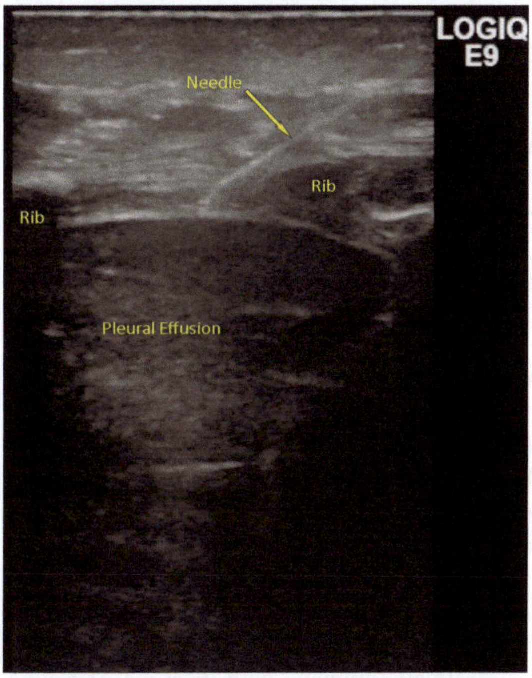

Fig. 21.5 Figure represents needle entry into the pleural cavity using a linear probe. Note the image quality below each rib causing a shadow to appear. The needle usually "disappears" in this shadow and reappears on the other side. The lung is collapsed and therefore seen better than usual when fully filled with air

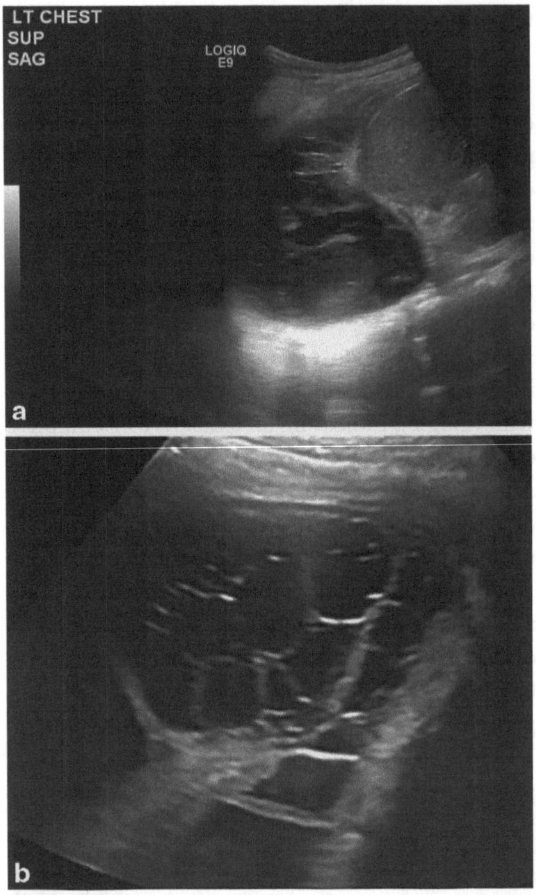

Fig. 21.6 **a** and **b** The pictures show possible sonographic findings in the setting of an advanced parapneumonic pleural effusion or empyema. Treatment options include ultrasound-guided placement of pigtail chest tube with TPA(tissue plasminogen activator) applications or VATS (video-assisted thoracoscopic surgery) with decortication

reaches a fibrotic nature, compromising the lung volume by trapping the lung in various areas (Fig. 21.6a and b). Drainage of the fluid alone has been used for treatment, but has a high recurrence rate. Surgical approaches with or without using minimally invasive techniques have been advocated to decorticate the fibrotic bands and release trapped lung; however, this carries morbidity of the surgery and an increase in cost. Alternatively, drainage with insertion of a lytic agent has been proposed to decrease the recurrence rate without the morbidity or cost associated with surgery [16]. Placement of the drainage catheter can be performed using an ultrasound to target the area of fluid more precisely.

On patients on a ventilator, drainage of simple or complex pleural effusions in mechanically ventilated patients appears to improve oxygenation and is safe [17]. A pleural effusion was detected in critically ill patients in 60 % of patients in one intensive care unit (ICU) with over 40 % present on admission [18]. These effusions can be the result of heart failure, atelectasis, malignancy, pneumonia, hypoalbuminemia, and even positive-pressure ventilation [18, 19]. In any patient where drainage of an effusion is considered, there is a risk of an iatrogenic pneumothorax with intervention. Therefore, the use of an ultrasound should be considered mandatory for the drainage of pleural effusions in this population of patients that has minimal reserve at baseline.

Malignant pleural effusions affect more than 175,000 people each year in the USA, with lung cancer contributing to 30 % of the cases [20]. Thoracentesis or drainage of the pleural fluid can be used for diagnostic and therapeutic purposes when a malignant effusion is suspected. Unfortunately, nearly a third of these procedures may be associated with a complication when performed without an ultrasound, with a third of these complications being a pneumothorax [21]. In contrast, an ultrasound-guided thoracentesis, especially when performed by an experienced operator, can have a less than 3 % rate of any of the following complications: pain, pneumothorax, bleeding or hematoma, shortness of breath, or re-expansion pulmonary edema [22].

Accumulation of fluid in the pericardial sac can cause cardiac compression and tamponade from elevated pressure. Classically, Beck's triad of low blood pressure, distended neck veins (jugular venous distension), and muffled heart sounds represents cardiac tamponade. In reality however, the right ventricle and atrium have thinner walls and decreased pressures, therefore they collapse first and findings of low systemic blood pressure or cardiac output can be a late presentation. Furthermore, the rate and volume of fluid accumulation vary and determine the timing of hemodynamic compromise.

Ultrasound can be used to diagnose and drain a pericardial effusion in a timely manner with decreased risk. The following is an approach to diagnosis of tamponade adapted from Chandraratna et al. [23]: (1) Rarely is isolated right atrial collapse seen without right ventricular diastolic collapse (RVDC), (2) RVDC, best observed in the most compressible part—the right ventricle outflow tract—is a sensitive sign of cardiac tamponade because the right ventricular (RV) pressure is lowest in early diastole, (3) RVDC, occurs initially in early diastole and in more advanced tamponade, is seen throughout diastole, and (4) A dilated non-pulsatile inferior vena cava, nonspecific for tamponade, indicates marked elevation of right atrial (RA) pressure.

To drain the fluid, a subxiphoid or apical approach can be used. For the subxiphoid approach, the ultrasound probe is placed at the cardiac apex to obtain an apical four-chamber view; while for the apical approach, the transducer is placed at the left sternal border for monitoring. For a subxiphoid approach, a long needle is inserted under the xiphoid process and directed toward the left shoulder at a 15–30° angle to the skin between the xiphoid and left costal margin [23]. For the apical approach, an 18-gauge needle with a syringe, under constant negative pressure and attached to a 3-way stopcock, is passed through the rib space until fluid is aspirated [23]. Complications for either include "arrhythmias, coronary or left internal mammary artery puncture, hemothorax, pneumothorax, and hepatic injury" [23].

Ultrasound-guided interventions in the chest are limited by the bony ribs, spine and sternum exteriorly and the air-filled trachea, esophagus, and lungs interiorly but adequate windows can be gotten with sufficient practice and the use of acoustic windows from the neck, through the liver, or into the mediastinum and pleura between the ribs. These can be used to guide diagnostic and therapeutic procedures in the setting of bedside procedures or those requiring real-time visualization. In many instances, cross-sectional imaging may provide adequate diagnostic detail, curtailing the need for ultrasound and these should be considered based on the patient and procedure risk profiles.

Abdomen and Pelvis

Abdominal and pelvic abscesses may occur from solid organs such as spleen, kidney, or pancreas, or an enteric source such as those from post-surgery, appendicitis, diverticulitis, or Crohn's disease[24]. Percutaneous drainage could potentially eliminate the need for surgical drainage altogether–whether the abscess is simple or complex and multiloculated. Approach to drainage can be through the abdominal wall, transgastric, transrectal, transvaginal, transperineal, or transgluteal [24]. Occasionally, a catheter cannot be placed and only a drainage with sampling of the fluid is performed, especially if the abscess is not large or loculated [25].

In children, the most common cause of abdominal abscess is appendicitis [2]. Other common etiologies for intra-abdominal collections in children include "cerebrospinal fluid pseudocysts, post-traumatic collections, pancreatic fluid collections, acalculous cholecystitis, and abscesses due to Crohn's disease or necrotizing enterocolitis" [2]. Furthermore, in children, the use of ultrasound is ubiquitous due to the increased radiation risk with computed tomography (CT) scans and the difficulty with prolonged sedation required for magnetic resonance imaging (MRI) for diagnosis and therapy of an abdominal source. Therefore, the algorithm for children with a fluid collection in the abdomen includes the early use of ultrasound-guided drainage for diagnosis or for therapy.

An enteric source of an abscess in the abdomen can be addressed via percutaneous intervention guided by ultrasound as a temporizing measure [1] addressing the acute bacterial infection; however, the underlying source must eventually be addressed as a general principle. For example, a perforated appendicitis, diverticulitis, or an ileopsoas abscess secondary to Crohn's can be addressed with drainage of the abscess but eventually may require an appendectomy, colon resection, or ileocolic excision, respectively. Postoperative abscess secondary to an enteric source is another common indication for percutaneous drainage. Depending on the location, however, a CT-guided approach may be needed or preferred [26].

Occasionally, a patient presents with idiopathic ascites and part of the workup involves drainage of the fluid for diagnosis or for therapy. It is important to communicate extensively with the primary team to identify the specific indications, risks of bleeding secondary to liver disease, portal hypertension and venous congestion, and next steps with worsening patient status. When a large volume is identified on ultrasound, the drainage should be done in steps with protein-rich replacement to prevent severe hypotension. Patient access for transfusion and fluid resuscitation should be identified prior to starting a paracentesis. Finally, drainage of the ascites might occasionally identify chylous output (potentially indicating a malignancy from lymphatic congestion, an underlying lymphatic abnormality, or an undiagnosed malrotated state of the bowel requiring emergent operative detorsion).

An enteric source must be quickly identified and addressed for most abdominal and pelvic collections. Occasionally, an abdominal or pelvic collection can be secondary to a solid organ such as liver, pancreas, spleen, ovary, or kidney.

A liver abscess can be single or multiple, occurring more commonly in the right lobe or bilaterally, respectively. Various diseases that may lead to pyogenic liver abscesses include prior abdominal surgery, trauma, neoplastic disease, biliary tract disease, or bacteremia in immune-compromised patients [1]. A single abscess can be drained using ultrasound guidance but multiple usually require CT guidance with several catheters inserted. Furthermore, it is imperative that pyogenic abscesses are differentiated from amebic as these are treated with antimicrobials. Other conditions such as tumors, secondary abscesses, and hydatic cysts may present similarly and need to be differentiated as the management options differ drastically.

Pancreatic pseudocysts can develop 1–4 weeks from a bout of pancreatitis. These collections of fluid can be sterile or infected. Immature collections are usually observed unless an infection is suspected on imaging and a sample needs to be obtained. These cysts, once mature, are usually treated surgically or endoscopically, although a percutaneous approach can be used when patient condition prohibits a more definitive intervention. An ultrasound-guided intervention is rarely done due to the location of these cysts and bowel gas obscuring an adequate window for drainage.

Splenic cysts can be congenital, posttraumatic, or idiopathic. Rarely, these cysts can be complex and represent an abscess, presenting with a classic triad of left upper quadrant pain, fever, and leukocytosis [1]. Percutaneous drainage can be used for diagnosis and therapy of the cyst, with surgical excision used for recurrence. Multilocular abscesses and rupture with bleeding are considered relative contraindications with medical therapy reserved for fungal abscess [1].

Ultrasound is the workhorse and preferred imaging modality for the female pelvis: widely available, noninvasive, cheap, does not use ionizing radiations, and is able to provide definitive diagnostic information in heterogeneous clinical situations [27]. An abdominal approach is usually used initially to study the female anatomy; however, a transvaginal approach can be used to provide additional details and for therapeutic interventions. A filled bladder can act as an acoustic window augmenting the transabdominal view but can impede a transvaginal approach due to pressure anteriorly.

Simple cysts are the most common asymptomatic pelvic mass in a female patient. These can be observed and followed using ultrasound with larger lesions (greater than 5–6 cm) having a higher risk of being malignant [27] or requiring intervention to prevent torsion [28]. Hemorrhagic and ruptured cysts can be managed similarly with observation. Any cyst with solid components should have a workup for malignancy—ascites alone is not an accurate predictor of malignancy. Mature cystic teratomas are the most common ovarian tumors in children and adolescents and represent half of all tumors [28]; whereas in adults, epithelial tumors represent 70 % of all ovarian malignancies [27].

Pelvic inflammatory disease is a common cause of acute pelvic pain. A transvaginal approach can be used to diagnose and drain a tubo-ovarian abscess. Sampling of fluid to target antimicrobial therapy can also be a useful adjunct. Furthermore, use of ultrasound can be helpful to

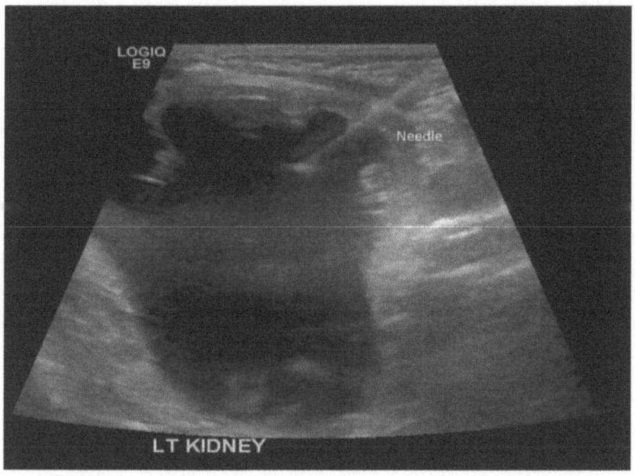

Fig. 21.7 Figure represents needle entry into an enlarged collecting system in the left kidney. Following entry into the collecting system, the needle is replaced by a guidewire, dilator, and drain to evacuate the congenital hydronephrosis

exclude alternate pathology causing pelvic pain such as ectopic pregnancy, appendicitis, or endometriosis.

In the setting of percutaneous nephrostomy, ultrasound is valuable for accessing the renal pelvis for interventional procedures and for drainage. Indications include "urinary diversion for urinary tract obstruction, nephrolithiasis, urinary tract infections, urinary fistulas, providing access for subsequent ureteral interventions, such as stent placement, nephroscopy, and ureteroscopy" [29]. These procedures can be performed on native and transplanted kidneys. The most important contraindication is severe coagulopathy. Figure 21.7 demonstrates drainage of a congenital hydronephrosis using ultrasound guidance.

The most common indication is for urinary obstruction from congenital anomalies, from urinary calculi or from a malignancy. Hydronephrosis can also form without an obstruction, such as in pregnancy, over hydration, and diabetes insipidus [29]. Important pre-procedure concepts to consider include abnormal orientation or location of the kidney, presence of a duplicated collecting system, cysts, diverticula and tumors that increase the complexity and difficulty of a procedure, need for lithotripsy prior to or in conjunction with the procedure, and residual contrast that may obscure or eliminate the need for retrograde injection [29].

Infection can occur in the setting of urinary reflux, an obstruction from calculi, or susceptible transplanted kidneys. A renal abscess can rupture externally, presenting as a perinephric abscess, or it can rupture into the collecting system or vascular structures [1]. Percutaneous drainage of a renal or perinephric abscess may be enough, although additional drainage of the collecting system may be necessary if the abscess is associated with urinary obstruction.

Ultrasound can also be used for placement of suprapubic catheters for urinary retention after urethral trauma and in patients needing long-term catheterization for bladder dysfunction in neurological conditions, for example, multiple sclerosis, spinal cord injury [30]. Using an ultrasound, the bladder can be accessed and serially dilated to allow placement of a Foley or alternate catheter. The catheter can be secured to the skin and left in place for a prolonged time period. Once a tract has formed, routine removal and catheterization can be accomplished.

Soft Tissue and Extremities

Similar to head and neck, the soft tissue of the trunk and extremities may exhibit an indication of ultrasound-guided drainage for diagnosis and therapy of an infection, hemorrhage, or a postoperative complication. Use of ultrasound for percutaneous aspiration of breast abscess can be simple, performed as an outpatient, with a low recurrence rate, and improved cosmetic outcomes [31]. Other cysts, abscesses, and superficial collections can similarly be drained percutaneously with ultrasound, limiting morbidity and cosmetic disfigurement.

In extremities, joint aspiration can be augmented with the use of ultrasound with improved diagnostic and therapeutic capability. Systematically screening for soft-tissue infections, including abscesses and bursal fluid collections, before joint aspiration is imperative. Ultrasound use prior to aspiration can lessen the risk of delayed or missed diagnoses and can decrease the risk of joint aspiration by preventing seeding of superficial infection into a sterile joint [32]. Finally,

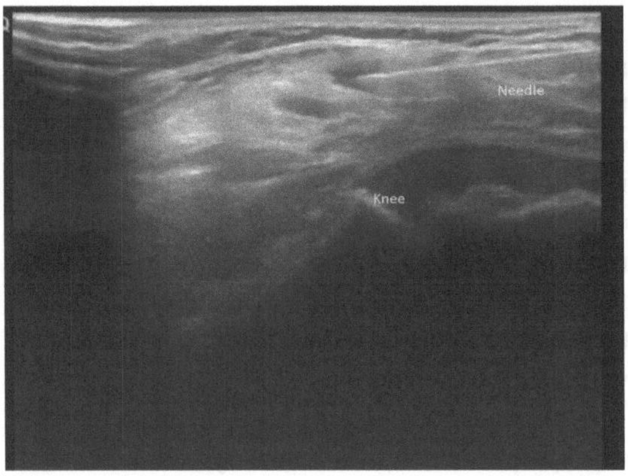

Fig. 21.8 Figure represents needle entry into a cyst anterior to the knee. Similarly, joint effusions can also be drained using ultrasound guidance to minimize complications

using ultrasound guidance to access the fluid collection can prevent injury to normal or aberrant neurovascular structures. Figure 21.8 demonstrates drainage of a cyst on the anterior knee.

Summary

Diagnostic and therapeutic drainage of fluid collections throughout the body using ultrasound guidance should be standard of care. The availability, flexibility, and real-time guidance provided by ultrasound can decrease complications, improve cosmesis, and increase the success of a procedure. Clarifying the indications and understanding the anatomic landmines are essential in completing the procedure with minimal complication. Technical skills are simple in concept but complex in practice and require meticulous care and dedicated training. Finally, thorough preparation including equipment readiness, understanding the disease process and patient's history, and communication with primary care providers will provide ultimate satisfaction with this approach.

References

1. Men S, Akhan O, Köroğlu M. Percutaneous drainage of abdominal abcess. Eur J Radiol. 2002;43:204–18.
2. Hogan MJ, Hoffer FA. Biopsy and drainage techniques in children. Tech Vasc Interv Radiol. 2010;13:206–13.
3. Röthlin MA, Schöb O, Klotz H, Candinas D, Largiadèr F. Percutaneous drainage of abdominal abscesses: are large-bore catheters necessary? Eur J Surg Acta Chir. 1998;164:419–24.
4. Ganguli S, Brennan D. Transanorectal interventions. Semin Ultrasound CT MR. 2008;29:483–91.
5. Sudakoff GS, Lundeen SJ, Otterson MF. Transrectal and transvaginal sonographic intervention of infected pelvic fluid collections: a complete approach. Ultrasound Q. 2005;21:175–85.
6. Arrabal-Polo MA, Jimenez-Pacheco A, Arrabal-Martin M. Percutaneous drainage of prostatic abscess: case report and literature review. Urol Int. 2012;88:118–20.
7. Smith RB. Ultrasound-guided procedures for the office. Otolaryngol Clin North Am. 2010;43:1241–54.
8. Chang K-P, Chen Y-L, Hao S-P, Chen S-M. Ultrasound-guided closed drainage for abscesses of the head and neck. Otolaryngol Head Neck Surg. 2005;132:119–24.
9. Ramirez-Schrempp D, Dorfman DH, Baker WE, Liteplo AS. Ultrasound soft-tissue applications in the pediatric emergency department: to drain or not to drain? Pediatr Emerg Care. 2009;25:44–8.
10. Lyon M, Blaivas M. Intraoral ultrasound in the diagnosis and treatment of suspected peritonsillar abscess in the emergency department. Acad Emerg Med. 2005;12:85–8.
11. Lohela P. Ultrasound-guided drainages and sclerotherapy. Eur Radiol. 2002;12:288–95.
12. Light RW. Parapneumonic effusions and empyema. Clin Chest Med. 1985;6:55–62.
13. Padman R, King KA, Iqbal S, Wolfson PJ. Parapneumonic effusion and empyema in children: retrospective review of the duPont experience. Clin Pediatr (Phila). 2007;46:518–22.
14. Picard E, et al. Predictive factors of morbidity in childhood parapneumonic effusion-associated pneumonia: a retrospective study. Pediatr Infect Dis J. 2010;29:840–3.
15. Wong KS, Lin TY, Huang YC, Chang LY, Lai SH. Scoring system for empyema thoracis and help in management. Indian J Pediatr. 2005;72:1025–8.
16. St Peter SD, et al. Thoracoscopic decortication vs tube thoracostomy with fibrinolysis for empyema in children: a prospective, randomized trial. J Pediatr Surg. 2009;44:106–111; discussion 111.
17. Goligher EC, et al. Utility and safety of draining pleural effusions in mechanically ventilated patients: a systematic review and meta-analysis. Crit Care Lond Engl. 2011;15:R46.
18. Mattison LE, Coppage L, Alderman DF, Herlong JO, Sahn SA. Pleural effusions in the medical ICU: prevalence, causes, and clinical implications. Chest. 1997;111:1018–23.
19. Soni N, Williams P. Positive pressure ventilation: what is the real cost? Br J Anaesth. 2008;101:446–57.

20. Bennett R, Maskell N. Management of malignant pleural effusions. Curr Opin Pulm Med. 2005;11:296–300.
21. Kastelik JA. Management of malignant pleural effusion. Lung. 2013;191:165–75.
22. Jones PW, et al. Ultrasound-guided thoracentesis: is it a safer method? Chest. 2003;123:418–23.
23. Chandraratna PA, Mohar DS, Sidarous PF. Role of echocardiography in the treatment of cardiac tamponade. Echocardiography. 2014;31:899–910.
24. Fulcher AS, Turner MA. Percutaneous drainage of enteric-related abscesses. Gastroenterologist. 1996;4:276–85.
25. Lorentzen T, Nolsøe C, Skjoldbye B. Ultrasound-guided drainage of deep pelvic abscesses: experience with 33 cases. Ultrasound Med Biol. 2011;37:723–8.
26. Gazelle GS, Mueller PR. Abdominal abscess. Imaging and intervention. Radiol Clin North Am. 1994;32:913–32.
27. Derchi LE, Serafini G, Gandolfo N, Gandolfo NG, Martinoli C. Ultrasound in gynecology. Eur Radiol. 2001;11:2137–55.
28. Hayes-Jordan A. Surgical management of the incidentally identified ovarian mass. Semin Pediatr Surg. 2005;14:106–10.
29. Saad WEA, Moorthy M, Ginat D. Percutaneous nephrostomy: native and transplanted kidneys. Tech Vasc Interv Radiol. 2009;12:172–92.
30. Jacob P, Rai BP, Todd AW. Suprapubic catheter insertion using an ultrasound-guided technique and literature review. BJU Int. 2012;110:779–84.
31. Karstrup S, et al. Acute puerperal breast abscesses: US-guided drainage. Radiology. 1993;188:807–9.
32. Hadduck TA, et al. Value of ultrasound before joint aspiration. AJR Am J Roentgenol. 2013;201:W453–9.

Sclerotherapy of Vascular Malformations

22

Joseph J. Gemmete and Ranjith Vellody

Introduction

In 1982, John Mulliken and Julie Glowacki proposed a classification of vascular anomalies based on the clinical behavior, histology, and histochemistry [1]. The International Society for the Study of Vascular Anomalies (ISSVA) accepted this classification in 1992 [2–4]. The classification divides vascular anomalies into two groups: tumors (e.g., hemangiomas), in which the etiology is one of endothelial cell proliferation, and vascular malformations, in which the developmental error has resulted in abnormally formed vascular channels. The tumor group will not be discussed in this chapter. Vascular malformations can be further subdivided into lesions consisting of arterial, capillary, lymphatic, venous, and fistulous networks. Furthermore, they can be further subdivided functionally based on the flow characteristics, i.e., high-flow versus low-flow lesions [5]. In this chapter, we discuss the clinical features, natural history and epidemiology, and diagnostic imaging features of vascular malformations. We then concentrate on the percutaneous/endovascular treatment for each of the vascular malformations briefly describing additional treatment options. Finally, we discuss the clinical outcomes of the main forms of treatment.

Venous Malformations

Clinical Features

Venous malformations (VMs) can occur anywhere in the body, but are most frequently located in the head and neck. They can be solitary, small, well circumscribed, large, superficial, or infiltrative involving multiple tissue planes. The lesion is nonpulsatile, may have a light blue to deep purple color, and can be associated with telangiectasias, varicosities, or ecchymosis. The mass may increase in size in a dependent position, with a tourniquet, or during a Valsalva maneuver. Superficial lesions are soft and compressible and can usually be emptied of blood. Patients usually present with pain associated with compression on the surrounding nerves or thrombosis of a portion of the mass. An elevated D-dimer has been determined to be highly specific for a VM and can help to distinguish VMs form lymphatic malformations (LMs) and slow-flow Klippel–Trenaunay (KT) syndrome from high flow Parks Weber syndrome [6].

VMs are usually isolated findings; however, they may be associated with the following syndromes (Table 22.1):

J. J. Gemmete (✉) · R. Vellody
Department of Radiology, University of Michigan, 1500 E. Medical Center Drive, Room UH B1D 328, Ann Arbor, MI 48109, USA
e-mail: gemmete@med.umich.edu

R. Vellody
e-mail: ranjithv@med.umich.edu

S. Scholz, M. D. Jarboe (eds.), *Diagnostic and Interventional Ultrasound in Pediatrics and Pediatric Surgery,* DOI 10.1007/978-3-319-21699-7_22

Table 22.1 Syndromes associated with vascular anomalies

Syndromes	Vascular malformations			
	Venous	Capillary	Lymphatic	Arterial or arteriovenous
PHACES				
LUMBAR				•
Kasabach–Merritt			•	
Maffucci	•		•	
Klippel–Trenaunay	•	•	•	•
Gorham–Stout	•	•	•	
Proteus	•	•	•	
Parkers Weber	•	•		•
Sturge–Weber	•	•		
CM-AVM	•			•
Familial cerebral VM	•			
Familial cutaneomucosal VM	•			
Blue rubber bleb nevus	•			
Bockenheimer	•			
Cobb		•		•
Osler–Weber–Rendu		•		•
Beckwith–Wiedemann		•		
Louis–Barr		•		
Down			•	
Turner			•	
Wyburn–Mason				•
Dandy–Walker				
Von Hippel–Lindau				

This table is intended to generalize common associations. For example, there are at least six case reports of AVM in PHACES syndrome, but the association is uncommon, and thus is not included in the table. Syndromes with multiple malformations subtypes (e.g., Proteus) often involved mixed-type malformations

CM capillary malformation, *AVM* arteriovenous malformation, *VM* venous malformation

Klippel–Trenaunay (KT) syndrome
Blue rubber bleb nevus (BRBN) syndrome
Mucocutaneous familial VMs
Glomuvenous malformation
Maffacci's syndrome
Proteus syndrome
Bannayan–Riley–Ruvalcaba syndrome
CLOVES/S syndrome

Natural History/Epidemiology

VMs are present at birth. They are clinically not always apparent and tend to grow in proportion to the growth of the child. The growth is most pronounced during puberty and pregnancy. These are congenital lesions that affect boys and girls of equal frequency with a reported incidence of 1–2 per 100,000 births and a prevalence of 1% [7].

Most VMs (95%) are sporadic, but can be seen in a number of heritable conditions. The molecular basis for sporadic is yet to be discovered, however there are familial cases where the genetic defect has been localized on a specific chromosome. In 1994–1995, two families were identified to have autosomal dominant inherited cutaneous and mucosal VMs. Genetic analysis mapped a locus for both of these families to the chromosome 9p21 [8, 9]. These families shared a mutation resulting in an arginine to tryptophan substitution R849W in the gene that encodes the kinase domain of the endothelial cell receptor Tie2 [10]. In 1999, four more families with autosomal dominant inherited VMs were identified [11]. Only one of those families shared the same mutation as the previous two reports. The second family had a novel hyperphosphorylating Y897S mutation in the *TIE2* gene. The other families showed no evidence of linkage to 9p21, which suggests genetic heterogeneity. Multifocal VMs are most commonly seen in the familial forms of VM, including the following: Blue rubber bleb nevus (BRBN) syndrome, Mucocutaneous familial VMs, Glomovenous malformation, and Maffucci's syndrome [12].

Diagnostic Imaging

Ultrasound: On gray-scale imaging, VMs usually are hypoechoic to anechoic with the shape of tubular structures [13]. Some lesions can have a heterogeneous echotexture if phleboliths or different forms of thrombus are present within the lesion. Doppler ultrasound is usually a monophasic low-velocity waveform. Sometimes flow can only be seen with compression and release of the lesion [14].

Computed tomography: On non-contrast CT, VMs are usually hypoattentuating, however, they can be heterogeneous depending on the amount of fatty tissue within the lesion. Phleboliths or dystrophic calcifications can be seen within the lesion. After the administration of contrast, the lesion usually enhances at the periphery and then fills in centrally on the delay images [14]. CT is excellent at looking for boney involvement from the lesion. MRI is better at characterizing the lesions relationship to the surrounding soft tissue structures.

MRI: VMs appear usually as hypointense to isointense on T1-weighted imaging. They can however have areas of bright signal on T1-weighted images if the lesion has fat, subacute blood products, or certain types of calcifications contained within the lesion [15]. On T2-weighted images, VMs have high signal intensity. Gradient echo sequence usually shows areas of low signal corresponding to calcification, hemosiderin, or thrombus. The best sequence to determine the fully extent of the lesion and its relationship to surrounding soft tissue structures is the T2-weighted sequence [16]. On T1-weighted post contrast imaging, the lesions usually demonstrates early peripheral enhancement that later fills in centrally on delayed imaging [17].

Diagnostic venography: Contrast venography is helpful in the anatomical characterization of a VM. It is performed to determine the fully extent of the malformation and its draining veins. It is also helpful in confirming patency of the deep venous system in the extremity. Venography is also performed to determine the volume of contrast needed to fill the malformation before empties into normal draining veins.

Based on the pattern of venous drainage Dubois and Puig divided VMs into four types [18–20]. This drainage pattern is a reflection of the response to the treatment and rates of complications. Types I and II respond best to sclerotherapy with a better control rate and a lesser number of sessions to achieve control. Types III and IV have a higher rate of complications [20].

Type I :isolated malformation without disconcernible venous drainage
Type II :lesion draining into normal veins
Type III :lesion draining into dysplastic veins
Type IV :lesion consists primary of venous ectasia

Treatment

VMs can be treated percutaneously by injecting a sclerosing agent. The most commonly described sclerosing agents (Table 22.2) included: alcohol, sodium tetradecol, ethibloc, polidocanol, and bleomycin [19, 21–24]. The procedure is performed under general anesthesia, since injection of the sclerosing agent can be extremely painful. A foley catheter is placed in the bladder to monitor urine output and color, since some patients

Table 22.2 Common sclerosing agents

Alcohol
Sodium tetradecol
Bleomycin
Doxycycline
Alcoholic solution of zein (Ethibloc)
Polidocanol
OK-432 (Picibanil)

may develop a hemoglobinuria. This is most likely to happen in younger patients and in patients with large lesions. In addition, if an extremity is being treated, we start an IV distal to the lesion to infusion saline and heparin overnight to flush out the sclerosing agent and prevent acute deep venous thrombosis [12]. Sclerotherapy is performed by cannulating the lesion percutaneously under ultrasound or fluoroscopy. Contrast material is injected to define the extent of the lesion, determine the flow rate within the lesion and the communication with normal veins, the presence of a possible arterial component, and to give an estimate of the volume of sclerosing agent needed to fill the lesion. If a large draining vein is visualized, these can be treated with embolization utilizing coils, liquid embolic agents, or with temporary balloon occlusion to increase the contact time of the sclerosing agent with the VM and to prevent egress of the agent into the systemic circulation [12]. This may also be performed with a tourniquet, blood pressure cuff, or manual compression. The VM is accessed with ultrasound guidance and the sclerosant is then injected under fluoroscopic guidance to decrease the risk of extravasation, overfilling of the lesion, and limit undesired egress of the sclerosing agent into the normal deep veins (Fig. 22.1). Overfilling of the lesion may also be prevented by the two-needle access technique, which allows

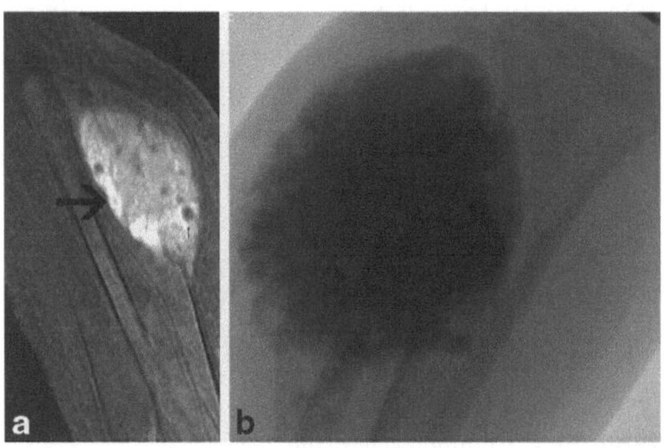

Fig. 22.1 A 4-year-old boy who complains of pain and swelling within his left calf from a venous malformation. **a** Coronal post contrast fat saturation T1-weighted MRI image shows an enhancing mass within the left calf *(black arrow)* with a few scattered areas of round low signal within it *(small black arrow)*, consistent with pheboliths. **b** Frontal spot fluoroscopic image shows the venous malformation filled with alcohol mixed with contrast

decompression of the lesion through the second needle access. Cone beam CT can be performed to evaluate the anatomical distribution of the administered sclerosant and compare the distribution to the preprocedure imaging [25]. After the needles are removed, a 20–30 mmHg compression stocking is placed over the area of concern so that the veins do not refill with blood. This allows maximum contact of the damage circumference endothelium of the vein walls, promoting fibrosis and scarring. The procedure is then repeated at 8–10 weeks intervals, until there is no recanalization, swelling, or pain from the lesion. Diffuse VMs are much more difficult to treat. The area of maximum symptomatology is usually targeted, since these lesions cannot be completely obliterated.

After sclerotherapy, the lesion should feel firm to palpation. Swelling is generally maximum 24 h after the procedure. We recommend placing a custom fitted class II compression garment over the lesion as soon as possible. If the lesion involves the airway, the patient may need to be kept intubated overnight in the ICU. The patient is given IV steroids in the hospital and then sent home on a tapered dose pack. The affected area is kept elevated above the heart with ice packs applied to minimize swelling. Patients receive IV fluids twice the maintenance dose before, during, and after the sclerotherapy for 24 h. Urine output is closely monitored for hemoglobinuria. Appropriate IV and oral analgesics and anti-inflammatory agents are prescribed in the hospital and post discharge for 7 days afterwards.

Patients with extensive limb lesions should be instructed from childhood in the proper use of compression garments. Compression helps to decrease the discomfort associated with the lesion, protects the overlying skin, limits swelling, and improves localized intravascular coagulation.

In patients with extensive VMs in whom a low fibrinogen is present, the use of low molecular weight heparin is recommended for 2 weeks pretreatment and possible cryoprecipitate transfusion if still low on the day of the procedure. This therapy will reduce the consumptive coagulopathy of the extensive VM and potentially lower the recanalization rate [12].

Sclerosant Drugs

Absolute ethanol (95–98 %) is probably the most common agent used for sclerotherapy. It is the most effective sclerosant agent available, however it is also the most toxic [12]. Ethanol works by causing instant precipitation of endothelial cell proteins and rapid thrombosis (Fig. 22.2). It may also cause transmural vessel necrosis resulting in diffusion into the surrounding tissues. Serious side effects from ethanol injection include: massive swelling, tissue necrosis, hypoglycemia, peripheral nerve injury, CNS depression, hemolysis, pulmonary vasospasm, cardiac arrhythmias, and electromechanical disassociation [26–33]. Given the serious side effects, patients must be closely monitored during ethanol procedures. Some practitioners even suggest monitoring of pulmonary artery pressure during and for a short while after the procedure. Ethanol blood levels correlate directly with the amount of ethanol injected [34]. Mason et al. demonstrated that a level of >1 ml/kg may put patients at increased risk of respiratory depression, cardiac arrhythmias, seizures and rhabdomyolysis [35]. A total dose of 1 ml/kg (or 60 ml) per session should never be exceeded. In pediatric patients, a maximum dose of 0.5 mg/kg per single session is recommended. Ethanol can be injected in an undiluted form, which we feel is dangerous since the agent cannot be identified under fluoroscopy. We usually dilute alcohol with water-soluble

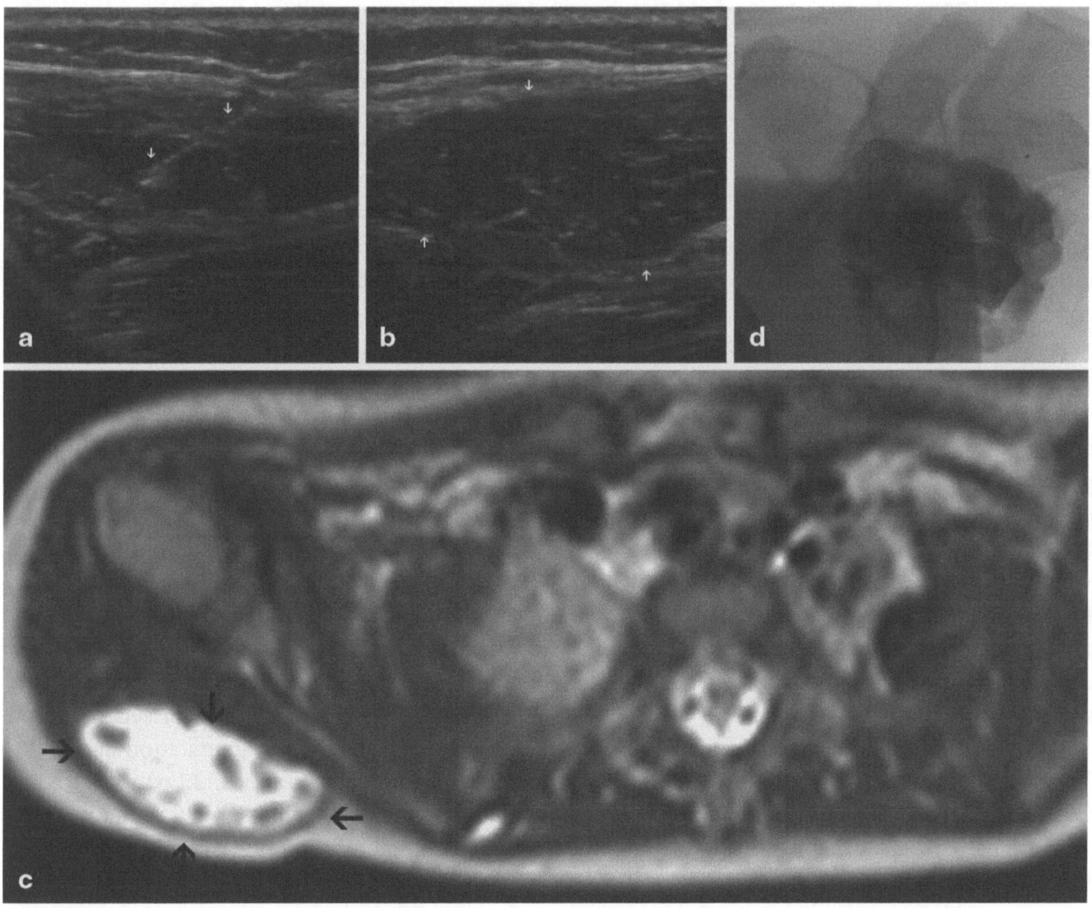

Fig. 22.2 A 3-year-old girl who complains of pain and swelling along with a bluish discoloration within the posterior right shoulder. **a** Gray-scale ultrasound image obtained with a liner 10 MHz transducer of the posterior right shoulder demonstrates a hypoechoic mass just below the cutaneous soft tissue *(white arrows)*. **b** Ultrasound image shows an angiocatheter entering the mass *(white arrows)*. **c** Axial T2-weight MRI image of the shoulder demonstrates a high-signal intensity mass with a few areas of low signal within it involving the soft tissue of the posterior right shoulder *(black arrow)*. **d** Spot fluoroscopic image shows the venous malformation filled with alcohol mixed with contrast

liquid or oily contrast medium during injection. Alcohol should not be mixed with Visipaque since this will cause precipitation of the contrast medium. In a series of 60 patients with VM involving the head and neck treated with ethanol, Su et al. reported a 68 % complete response (>90 % volume reduction), 25 % marked response (>50 % volume reduction), and a 7 % moderate response (<50 % volume decrease) with a 10 % complication rate [36]. In a series of 158 patients with VM, 16 % of patients had a good response defined by a clinical examination and a ≥30 % decrease in the size of MRI, unfortunately 27 % of these patients experienced a complication [37]. In another series of 87 patients with craniofacial VMs treated with ethanol sclerotherapy, 32 % had an excellent response (>75 % volume reduction), 52 % a good response (>25 % volume reduction), and a 16 % a poor response (25 % volume decrease) with a 5 % complication rate [38].

Detergents

Detergents used for sclerotherapy of VM include sodium tetradecyl sulfate (STS), polidocanol, sodium morrhuate, and ethanolamine [39–43]. STS is approved in the USA for the treatment of varicose veins [44]. Polidocanol has an FDA approval for sclerosis of spider and reticular veins [45]. Similar to ethanol, all of the drugs damage the endothelial cells, resulting in thrombosis and fibrosis. Detergents may be mixed with water soluble or oily contrast medium prior to injection. These agents are thought to have a low rate of complications when compared to ethanol, but a greater tendency towards recanalization. Reported complications include cardiovascular collapse, skin pigmentation, skin necrosis, anaphylaxis, and hemoglobinuria [46]. Foaming the sclerosant by mixing the drug with air has also become popular [42, 47]. The theory is that the foam probably results in better contact between the drug and vein wall along with prolonged displacement of the blood with the lesion. Air can be made easily by mixing 10 cc of sclerosant with 3 cc of Ethiodol and 5–10 cc of air through a three-way stopcock. Patient receiving large volumes of detergent sclerosants may need aggressive hydration and alkalization of the urine to treat hemoglobinuria [39]. In prospective randomized controlled trial comparing foamed versus liquid polidocanol or ethanolamine in 89 patients with VMs, 90 % of patients had partial or complete response in the foamed group versus 63 % in the liquid group ($p=0.002$) [48]. In another series of 50 patients with VMs treated with polidocanol foam resulted in complete resolution in 38 % of patients, size reduction of ≥50 % in 30 % of patients, and a size reduction of 0–50 % in 26 % of patients, and no change in 8 % of the patients [49]. Reported complications were noted in 8 % of the patients. Furthermore, in a series involving 26 patients with VM using ethanolamine oleate showed 49 % excellent, 39 % good, 12 % fair, and 0 % poor results based on the clinical examination [50].

Bleomycin

Bleomycin is an antibiotic and antitumor agent originally derived from *Streptomyces verticillus* in 1966, which causes an inflammatory response in endothelial cells [21]. Bleomycin can be mixed with water-soluble liquid or oily contrast medium. There is some concern with the use of this agent due to the association with pulmonary fibrosis in the setting of chemotherapy. The threshold dose for pulmonary fibrosis and interstitial fibrosis is 450 units, whereas doses for sclerotherapy are typically 0.5–1 units/kg for pediatric patients and 1–15 units in adults [21]. Reported complications include skin ulceration, skin pigmentation, laryngeal edema, flu-like symptoms, cellulitis, nausea and vomiting, and focal alopecia [21, 51]. In a series of 31 patients with VM treated with percutaneous injection of bleomycin resulted in 0 % complete resolution, 34 % marked (≥50 %) decrease in size, 31 % minimal (≤50 %) decrease in size, 34 % stable size, and 0 % increase in size on post procedure MRI [51]. Complications were seen in 12.5 % of patients comprised predominantly of transient skin pigmentation and cellulitis. Muir in another series of 32 patients treated with percutaneous bleomycin sclerotherapy showed complete resolution of the lesion in 32 % of patients and significant improvement in 52 % of patient by clinical examination [21].

Liquid Embolic Agents

N-butyl-2-cyanoacrylate (n-BCA) has a limited role in the treatment of vascular malformations because of its high cost, limited reabsorption, and formation of a hard mass after injection that may last for many months. Burrows et al. suggest this form of treatment for preoperative embolization prior to surgical resection [12]. This is most common in the treatment of intra-articular VMs where injection of a sclerosing agent could cause possible damage to the articular cartilage. This form of treatment has also been described for an orbital VM [52]. Ethylene vinyl alcohol copolymer (Onyx), a newer liquid polymer may also be useful for preoperative embolization of VMs prior to resection.

Other Forms of Treatment

Endovascular diode laser therapy has been reported in a small series of VMs with a good response rate at 14-month follow-up [53]. In patients with Klippel–Trenaunay syndrome, endovenous laser ablation of the marginal vein may be a useful alternative therapy. Percutaneous, interstitial (nonendovascular) laser photocoagulation of VM using the diode or Nd:YAG lasers via a fiber optic delivery system has also been reported with reasonable success [54–58]. Because of the controlled delivery of energy, and with external cooling, this modality may be of use in extensive superficial cutaneous/subcutaneous lesions or isolated anatomic locations such as the digit or tongue where sclerosis or embolization may carry a higher risk of surrounding tissue necrosis.

Surgical resection of VM is indicated only when complete resection without a resulting functional or anatomical deficit is possible. Surgery plays a limited role in the management of extremity lesion, but if performed localized coagulopathy must be controlled before surgery [19, 59, 60]. Surgery may also help in avoiding joint distention from repeat hemarthrosis, if joint involvement with the VM of the synovium is present.

Lymphatic Malformation

Clinical Features

LMs are present at birth and are composed of abnormal dilated lakes of lymphatic tissue that result from a defective embryological development of the primordial lymphatic channels. LMs can be classified radiographically as macrocystic (cysts ≥2 cm), microcystic (cysts <2 cm), or mixed, which has important implications for treatment. Macrocystic lesions are most commonly located in the neck, axilla, and chest wall and when large may interfere with the birth process. Microcystic lesions usually present as diffuse soft tissue thickening, often associated with vesicles of the skin and mucosa with an overlying capillary malformation (CM). The lesions grow in proportion to the patient. They may undergo periodic swelling often associated with signs of inflammation, which may be spontaneous or related to a regional infection. Acute swelling of the lesion may also be related to hemorrhage or lymphatic obstruction. Symptoms due to LMs are typically related to the localized mass effect on adjacent structures. On physical examination, LMs are mobile and have a boggy or cystic consistency. The lesions cannot be decompressed and do not distend with the Valsalva maneuver like VMs. The presence of lymphatic endothelium can be confirmed by staining with D2-40 antibody [61].

Infection is usually common in suprahyoid LMs with mucosal involvement. Patient with airway involvement can present with stridor and sleep apnea. In one series, tracheostomy placement occurred in 5 % of patients with airway compromise at birth. Orbit LM can present with pain, swelling, proptosis, blepharoptosis, and emblyopia. An underlying cerebral developmental anomaly is seen in 45 % of patients with orbital involvement.

Natural History/Epidemiology

LMs are present at birth. Developmental defects during embryonic lymphangiogenesis result in LMs [7, 62]. They tend to grow in proportion to the growth of the child. The growth is most pronounced during puberty and pregnancy. The incidence is reported at between 0.02 and 0.05 %, and represents approximately 3 of 100,000 hospital admissions [63, 64]. Greater than 50 % of LMs are identified at birth, with 80–90 % usually identified by 2 years of age [65]. Approximately 75 % of the lesions occur in the head and neck region [64]. Spontaneous regress is rare and has been report in <4 % of the cases [63, 66]. Multiple genes have been described in the process of lymph angiogenesis including: VEGFR3, VEGFC, Ang2, Lyve1, Nrp2, podoplanin [7]. No evidence exists for a heritable LM. Cervical LM do occur in association with Klippel–Trenaunay, Turner, and Noonan syndromes, as well as Trisomy 13 and 18 [67].

Diagnostic Imaging

Ultrasound: Macrocystic lesions appear on gray-scale imaging as multiple anechoic or hypoechoic, cystic spaces with internal septations and debri. Microcystic lesions appear as an ill-defined hyperechoic mass on gray-scale imaging [68].

CT: LMs appear as fluid filled low attenuation lesions, with occasion fluid/fluid levels that represent hemorrhage into the cystic structure. Peripheral enhancement of the walls may occur, however there is no central filling of the lesion on delayed images like a VM [69]. The internal septations are commonly not seen.

MRI: Macrocystic LMs appear as fluid-filled lesions with a single locule or multiple loculations, displaying high signal on T2-weighted imaging and low signal on T1-weighted images [70]. Occasionally, a fluid/fluid level can be seen in the setting of internal hemorrhage. Post-gadolinium T1-weighted images show minimal or absent septal enhancement. Microcystic lesions demonstrate intermediate signal intensity on T1 and T2-spin echo sequences [18].

Treatment

Multiple sclerosing agents have been used effectively for the treatment of LMs, including absolute alcohol, STS, doxycycline, ethibloc, OK-432, and bleomycin [71–76].

The technique for sclerotherapy of LMs consists of cannulation of each cyst with a standard angiocatheter under ultrasound guidance (Fig. 22.3). Fluid is aspirated as much as possible from the cyst. Contrast is injected under fluoroscopic guidance to identify the size of the lesion. The sclerosing agent is mixed with a contrast medium and the cyst is injected under fluoroscopic guidance. Smaller macrocystic lesions can be treated with aspiration and sclerotherapy without catheter drainage [76]. For large lesions, a pigtail catheter may be placed into the cysts and the lesion drained and injected over several days. Microcystic lesions are a challenge to treat and generally require multiple injections. Treatment is continued until imaging identifies no treatable cysts or the patient is satisfied with the clinical outcome.

Doxycycline

Doxycycline is generally instilled into the cyst as a solution of 10 mg/ml. The dose of doxycycline can range from 150 to 1000 mg depending on the size of the lesion. In neonates, the maximum recommended dose at one time is 150 mg, because higher doses may cause hemolytic anemia, hypoglycemia, and metabolic acidosis [77]. Blood glucose is monitored 2 h post procedure in neonates. If the patient develops hypoglycemia, IV dextrose can be administered. A few small series have described a 93–100 % complete radiographic response for the treatment of macrocystic LMs [73, 78]. Lower response rates are noted for microcystic LMs.

Detergents

There is a limited literature on the used of detergents as sclerosant agents for LMs. One study described the use of 98 % ethanol and 3 % STS with a 100 % complete radiographic response rate [73]. A second series described the use of foamed STS for the treatment of 6 intraorbital LMs with a reduction in lesion size in all patients [79].

OK-432 (Picibanil)

OK-432 (Picibanil) is a lyophilized mixture of group A *Streptococcus pyogenes*, initially developed as an immunotherapeutic agent in the treatment of gastric and lung carcinoma with its first use as a sclerosant in the treatment of a LM described in a case report in 1987 [80]. Ok-432 is not approved in the USA. Direct injection of the solution into a LM has been shown to increase intralesional cytokine levels, namely tumor necrosis factor, interleukin 6 (Il-6), IL-8, interferon alpha, and vascular endothelial growth factor in patients with a response to treatment with Ok-432 [81, 82]. A review of the literature by Poldervaart

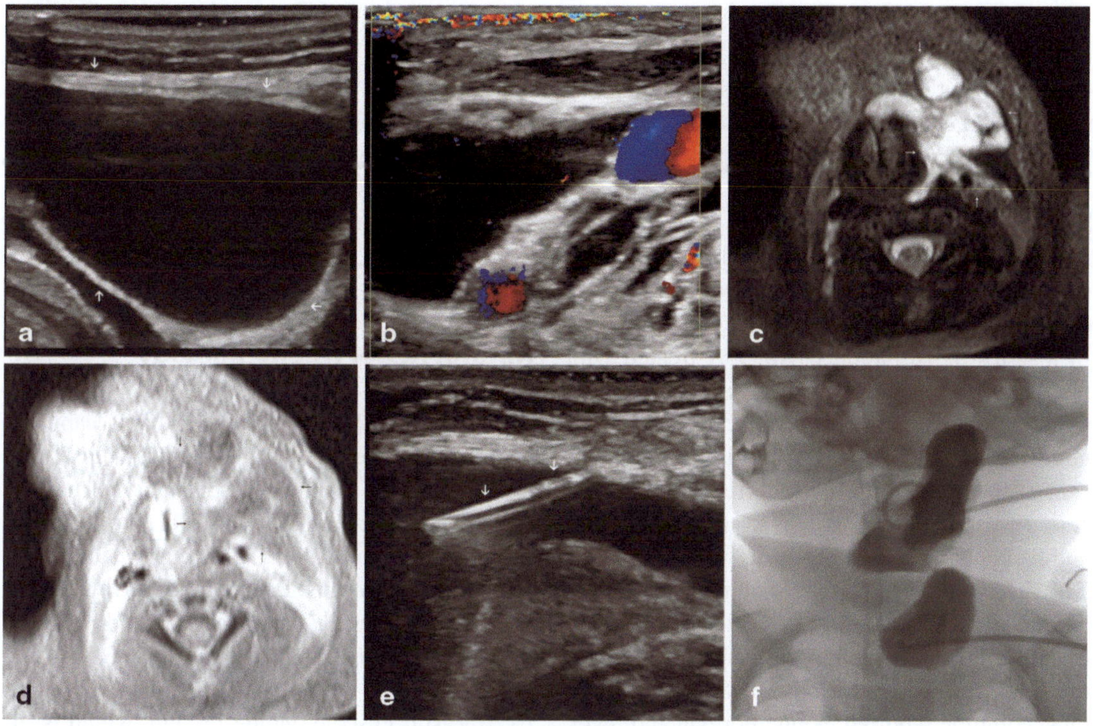

Fig. 22.3 A 3-month-old boy who presents with pain and swelling within his left neck. **a** Gray-scale ultrasound image shows large cyst within the soft tissues of the left neck consistent with a macrocystic lymphatic malformation *(white arrow)*. **b** Color Flow Doppler ultrasound image of the large cyst within the soft tissues of the left neck demonstrates no vascular flow within the lesion. **c** Axial fat saturation T2-weighted MRI image of the neck, demonstrates an infiltrative area of an abnormal high signal within the soft tissues of the left neck *(white arrows)*. **d** Corresponding axial fat saturation post contrast T1-weighted images shows that these areas have a peripheral rim of enhancement with a central area of low signal, consistent with a macrocystic lymphatic malformation *(black arrows)*. **e** Gray-scale ultrasound image shows an angiocatheter entering the cyst *(white arrows)*. **f** Spot fluoroscopic image shows two pigtail catheters in the cysts with contrast mixed with doxycycline

et al. showed an 88 % excellent response rate for macrocystic lesions [83]. Microcystic lesions demonstrated an excellent response rates in 27 %, good in 33 %, and poor in 40 % of cases [83]. Adverse side effects were mild and consisted on fever, lethargy, and local inflammation. A phase II trial was conducted in the USA on 182 patients with LMs. In this trial, 94 % of the patient with macrocystic disease had a response to treatment, 63 % of the patients with mixed macrocystic/microcystic disease had a response to treatment, and 0 % of the patients with microcystic disease responded to treatment [66]. In two other series, complete response rates of 76 % and 83.5 % were noted [82, 84].

Alcohol Solution of Zein

Alcoholic solution of zein (Ethibloc; Ethicon, Norderstedt, Germany) is a biodegradable thrombogenic solution consisting of a combination of zein (corn protein), sodium diaatrizoate, and oleum in ethanol. It has been used in Canada and Europe, but is currently not approved in the USA. Dubois et al. reported >95 % volumetric regression by CT in 64 % of lesions and>50 % in the remainder of both macrocystic and microcystic lesions [75]. Reported complications in this series included a minor local inflammatory reaction and an initial increase in size of the lesion in all patients. In another study of 65 patients with LMs treated with Ethibloc equal to 10 % of the lesion volume, 49% achieved excellent results, 355 satisfactory results, and 16% had poor results [85]. Complications included a localized inflammatory reaction and self-limiting external leakage of the Ethiobloc at a mean of 2 months post-therapy.

Bleomycin

Bleomycin is also used for sclerotherapy of LMS. The previous discussion related to the use of bleomycin for VMs also hold true for LMs. In a series of 70 patients with LM treated with intralesional injection of bleomycin, 47% of the patients achieve excellent results, 36% achieved good results, and 17% poor results. Seven percent of the group suffered recurrence [86]. Mild side effects consisted of fever, pain, swelling, and leukopenia. In another series of 200 patients with LM treated with intralesional injection of bleomycin-A5, 87% of the patients demonstrated complete lesion resolution with a recurrence rate of 13% [87]. Complications were mild with the most common reported being anorexia and fever.

Laser Therapy

Laser therapy is generally reserved for lesion with superficial cutaneous/mucosal vesicles. Microcystic lesions of the oral cavity and tongue have also been treated with the carbon dioxide laser and the Nd-YAG with success [54, 88].

Radiofrequency Ablation

Grimmer et al. in a series of 11 patients reported a response rate of 62% with radiofrequency ablation in patients with microcystic lesions of the lips, tongue, buccal mucosa, and floor of the mouth [89].

Surgery

Surgery is usually performed after an attempt at sclerotherapy. Depending on the location of the lesion, removal can be disfiguring with a high incidence of recurrence.

Capillary Malformations (CMs)

Clinical Presentation

CM is present at birth and grows commensurately with the child. CMs may be single or multiple, involve only the dermis, are well demarcated, and appear pink in infancy and may become dark purple with age [90]. Symptoms related to sporadic CM are primarily cosmetic although they can develop severe bleeding following minor trauma [44]. CMs can associated with overgrowth of the affected limb or face with certain syndromes [91].

Natural History/Epidemiology

CM, also termed as port-wine stain, capillary hemangioma, nevus flammeus, angel's kiss, and stork's bite, are common vascular malformations with an incidence of 0.3% [44, 90]. CM is usually sporadic, but families with a dominant inheritance pattern with incomplete penetrance have been reported. CM-arteriovenous malformation (AVM) syndrome has been link to chromosome 5q14-21, with a defect in the RASA1 gene, that encodes a p120 RasGTPase-activating protein, which is involved in cell adhesion and angiogenesis [92, 93]. The majority of CMs in the head and neck occur in the V1 and V2 distribution of the trigeminal nerve. Approximately 8% of the CMs are associated with Sturge–Weber syndrome and unilateral glaucoma [94]. CMs are also associated with Klippel–Trenaunay, Parkes Weber, macrocephaly CM, and CM-AVM syndromes [7].

Diagnostic Imaging

There is a little role for imaging except to exclude more serious disorders associated with CMs such as in Sturge–Weber syndrome. Ultrasound you may see areas of hyperechogenicity on gray scale with minimal flow on Doppler imaging. Given the superficial location of these lesions, a high-frequency ultrasound probe (> 10 MHz) is necessary to fully characterize the lesion. CT imaging findings are usually minimal even with extensive disease. On MRI, the skin may appear thickened with abnormal signal in the superficial soft tissue. The lesion may enhance after intravenous contrast administration. The value of CT and MRI in diagnosing CM is in ruling out more serious syndromes.

Treatment

Photocoagulation with pulsed dye laser (PDL) has been shown to be effective in improving the appearance of CMs [95–97]. Controversy, however, does exist whether PDL provides long-term benefit [96, 97].

There is no indication for embolization of these lesions, except in the reconstruction of a hyperemic facial skeleton. Preoperative particulate embolization of the lesion may decrease blood loss during surgical reconstruction.

Arterial Venous Malformations (AVMs)

Clinical Presentation

An AVM consists of an abnormal nidus of vascular channels with feeding arteries and draining veins with no normal intervening capillary network. Except for rare high-flow lesions, which may present with cardiac overload in neonates and infants, a majority of the AVMs are asymptomatic in the first two decades of life. On physical examination, an AVM may show local erythema and hyperthermia with prominent pulsations, a palpable thrill, and an audible bruit. Growth of these lesions is often precipitated by hormonal factors (puberty, pregnancy, and hormone therapy), trauma, infection, or iatrogenic causes (surgery, embolization). If venous hypertension develops, this may result in tissue ischemia leading to pain and skin ulceration, often associated with bleeding. In 1990, the Schobinger clinical staging system documenting the natural history of AVMs was introduced at the International Workshop for the Study of Vascular Anomalies in Amsterdam [98].

Natural History/Epidemiology

AVMs can be detected at birth in 40% of the cases and most commonly occur in the pelvis or extremities [7]. Rapid growth is not the characteristic of the lesions natural history. AVMs are usually sporadic with no genetic predisposition. There is a relationship between CMs and high-flow lesions like arterial venous fistulas and AVMs, and Parkes Weber syndrome associated with RASA-1 mutations [92].

There are also numerous reports in the literature of phosphatase and tension homologue (PTEN) mutations associated with cerebral and peripheral AVMs. PTEN is a tumor suppressive gene located on chromosome 10q. Mutations of this gene are associated with various syndromes including Bannayan–Riley–Ruvalcaba syndrome and Cowden syndrome [99–101]. Screening of patients with this mutation is recommended.

Mutations in endoglin and activin receptor-like kinase 1 (ALK1) are associated with hereditary hemorrhagic telangiectasia (HHT). AVMs in HHT can be seen in the brain, liver, lung, and gastrointestinal tract [102].

Diagnostic Imaging

AVMs are high-flow lesions without a normal capillary bed between the arteries and veins. These features contribute to their imaging characteristics.

Ultrasound: Gray–scale ultrasound shows a poorly defined heterogeneous structure. Fat is often seen around the AVM. Doppler ultrasound shows a network of multiple arteries with increased diastolic flow and arterialized draining veins with a biphasic waveform [68].

CT: AVMs appear as multiple enlarged enhancing feeding arteries filling a cluster of grapes like structures (i.e., the nidus) with enlarged surrounding draining veins. CT may show hypertrophy of the adjacent bone. It is important in delineating skeletal involvement of the axial skeleton, mandible, maxilla, skull base, and orbits.

MRI: MRI is the imaging modality of choice to image an AVM, given its excellent soft tissue resolution and ability to characterize the flow characteristics and hemodynamics. T2-weighted spin echo sequence shows multiple flow voids from the enlarged feeding arteries, the AVM nidus, and the draining outflow veins. In contrast enhanced gradient-echo images, the corresponding flow voids show enhancement [68].

4D-TRAKS can give an idea of the flow characteristics and hemodynamics of the lesion [103].

Angiography: Angiography is only necessary when intervention is considered or MRI/MRA examination is equivocal. The classic angiographic appearance of an AVM is that of multiple enlarged feeding arteries rapidly shunting into a nidus and then into dilated draining veins. Direct arteriovenous fistulous components and intralesional aneurysms may be identified.

Treatment

Treatment of AVMs is difficult. Endovascular embolization is often the first treatment option with or without surgical resection. The main goal of any form of treatment is to eradicate the nidus. From an endovascular approach, this can be performed from a transarterial approach, a direct percutaneous puncture of the nidus, or a retrograde transvenous approach.

Flow reduction techniques can be used to increase the concentration of the embolic agent within the AVM nidus. This can be performed using balloon catheters to temporary occlude the arterial inflow or venous outflow. If the lesion involves an extremity, a tourniquet or pneumatic cuff can be placed upstream or downstream from the lesion. In addition, coils or liquid adhesive agents may be placed in the draining vein to assist in flow reduction.

Cho et al. proposed an angiographic classification of AVMs based on the nidal morphology with implications for therapeutic approach and outcomes [104].

- Type I —arteriovenous fistulae
- Type II —arteriolovenous fistulae
- Type IIIa —arteriolovenulous fistulae with nondilated fistula
- Type IIIb —arteriolovenulous fistulae with dilated fistula

Eradication of the nidus is necessary for the proper treatment of an AVM (Fig. 22.4). This requires placement of a permanent agent within the nidus. Surgical ligation or occlusion of the feeding artery with coils should not be performed, since the lesion will develop collateral arterial feeders that will make the treatment of the lesion more difficult. The authors also feel that polyvinyl alcohol (PVA) particles have a very limited role in the embolization of an AVM, because of their non-permanent nature.

Alcohol

Alcohol is an agent most often used for the embolization of peripheral AVMs, given that it is permanent and probably the most effective. The maximum recommended volume is 1.0 ml/kg, however, Mason et al. in his report suggested that the dose should be reduced to 0.5 ml/kg, given the increased serum alcohol levels and potential negative side effects [35]. Success rates of up to 68 % have been published with multiple treatment sessions and complications noted in 52 % of the patients [105]. Response rates of up to 82 % have been reported with extremity bone AVMs [106]. Cho et al. in a series of 66 AVMs found alcohol

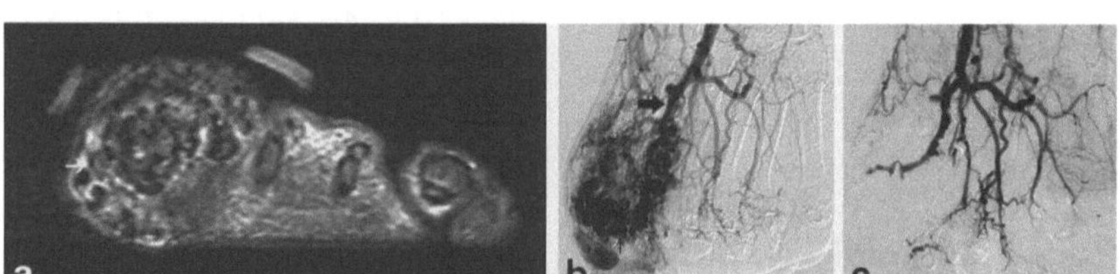

Fig. 22.4 A 55-year-old female with a thrill and a non-healing ulcer involving her first toe. **a** Axial fat saturation T2-weighted MRI image shows multiple flow voids within the soft tissues of the first toe *(white arrow)*. **b** Frontal dorsal pedal arteriogram shows a high-flow lesion with an abnormal tangle of vessels *(medium size black arrow)* within the soft tissues of the first toe, consistent with an AVM. The arterial supply is of multiple hypertrophied vessels *(large black arrow)* of the dorsal pedal artery with the main venous outflow through a hypertrophied vein along the medial foot *(small black arrow)*. **c** Frontal dorsal pedal arteriogram after the injection of alcohol into the AVM shows no arterial filling of the AVM

to be most effective for type II (100 %), and more effective for type IIIb (83 %) than for type IIIa, or mixed types (<or=50 %) [104]. Despite the use of the transarterial approach, direct puncture and transvenous approaches were more relevant for treating type II AVMs. Only the transarterial approach was used for treating type IIIa; both direct puncture and transarterial approaches were used for treating the other types. In a retrospective review of absolute alcohol use in soft tissue AVMs in a series of 32 patients (142 total sessions), Shin et al. concluded that dose limitations of <0.5–1 mg/kg and a maximum dose per injection of 10 ml does not cause an overall increase in pulmonary artery pressures [105]. The most common complications reported with alcohol include the skin and peripheral nerve injury. Less common complications include cardiopulmonary collapse, end organ damage, and renal failure [104–107].

N-butyl-2-cyanoacrylate (n-BCA)

n-BCA belongs to a group of cyanoacrylates or adhesive glues. Since n-BCA is a clear substance, it is mixed with ethiodol and tantalum to provide radiopacity during fluoroscopic injection. The amount of ethiodol mixed with the glue controls the rate of polymerization. When the glue is exposed to the anions in blood, it polymerizes and forms a cast, which is adherent to the vessel wall. To prevent polymerization within the catheter D5W is infused prior to the injection. Once the glue refluxes retrograde around the tip of the microcatheter, it is removed to prevent gluing of the catheter within the vessel. The glue causes an acute fibrotic inflammatory reaction that progress over several weeks as a foreign body giant cell granulomatous reaction. There are limited reports in the literature describing its use in peripheral AVMs. A majority of its use has been reported in the embolization of cerebral AVMs [108]. Complications of its use include pulmonary embolism, catheter retention, formation of a glue mass that can be a source of infection, tissue erosion, or muscle dysfunction [107, 109, 110].

Ethylene Vinyl Alcohol (Onyx)

Ethylene vinyl alcohol copolymer (Onyx) is a nonadhesive liquid embolic agent. It is dissolved in dimethyl sulfoxide (DMS0). Tantalum powder is added to the mixture for fluoroscopic visualization. The risk of catheter retention is less than with n-BCA, given the nonadhesive properties of the mixture. A plug is initially formed around the tip of the microcatheter acting as a backstop to allow the mixture to be pushed into the AVM. The concentration of Onyx chosen is based on the rapidity of the flow within the tumor vasculature. Embolization is continued until the desired degree of tumor penetrance or the maximal degree of Onyx reflux along the microcatheter is reached. Suction is then applied, followed by the withdrawal of the microcatheter. Embolization of other feeding pedicles then proceeds in a similar manner. A majority of its use has been reported in the embolization of cerebral AVMs. There are a few small case series on its use in peripheral AVMs [111]. The published literature reports rates for cerebral AVM lesion up to 24 %, average lesion volume reduction of 70 % with 3.8 % morbidity, and 2.5 % mortality [112, 113]. Complications of its use include pulmonary embolism, catheter retention, and nerve injury.

Gamma Knife

Stereotactic radiosurgery with a cobalt x-ray source (Gamma knife) may be successful in obliterating intracranial AVM in up to 80 % of the cases, with greater success in lesions under 4 cm [114–116]. However, there is a lack of certainty of obliteration with this method.

Surgery

Surgery alone is not generally effective for the treatment of AVM, with significant risk of recurrence. When surgery is indicated, embolization of the lesion and/or feeding vessels 48–72 h prior to resection may be helpful to reduce intraoperative blood loss.

Summary

Vascular malformations are congenital lesions secondary to errors in the development of arteries, capillaries, veins, or lymphatics. The majority of these lesions are sporadic, however, a certain percentage can present with a syndrome which the treating physician should be aware of. These lesions are best treated from a multidisciplinary team comprising pediatricians, plastic surgeons, dermatologists, radiologists, otolaryngologists, and oral maxillary facial surgeons. Minimal invasive percutaneous therapies play a vital role in the treatment of vascular malformations, as a sole therapy of choice, or as an adjunct to surgery. Currently, a wide variety of embolic agents are utilized as seen in this chapter in the treatment of vascular malformations, however to date there are no published, randomized, control trials comparing the efficacy of the different agents. Further, animal and clinical studies are needed to help optimize the treatment for each type of vascular malformation.

References

1. Mulliken JB, Glowacki J. Classification of pediatric vascular lesions. Plast Reconstr Surg. 1982;70(1):120–1.
2. Legiehn GM, Heran MK. Venous malformations: classification, development, diagnosis, and interventional radiologic management. Radiol Clin N Am. 2008;46(3):545–97, vi.
3. Tucci FM, De Vincentiis GC, Sitzia E, Giuzio L, Trozzi M, Bottero S. Head and neck vascular anomalies in children. Int J Pediatr Otorhinolaryngol. 2009;73 Suppl 1:S71–6.
4. Burrows PE, Mulliken JB, Fellows KE, Strand RD. Childhood hemangiomas and vascular malformations: angiographic differentiation. AJR Am J Roentgenol. 1983;141(3):483–8.
5. Mulliken JB, Glowacki J. Hemangiomas and vascular malformations in infants and children: a classification based on endothelial characteristics. Plast Reconstr Surg. 1982;69(3):412–22.
6. Dompmartin A, Ballieux F, Thibon P, Lequerrec A, Hermans C, Clapuyt P, et al. Elevated D-dimer level in the differential diagnosis of venous malformations. Arch Dermatol. 2009;145(11):1239–44.
7. Brouillard P, Vikkula M. Genetic causes of vascular malformations. Hum Mol Genet. 2007;16 Spec No. 2:R140–9.
8. Boon LM, Mulliken JB, Vikkula M, Watkins H, Seidman J, Olsen BR, et al. Assignment of a locus for dominantly inherited venous malformations to chromosome 9p. Hum Mol Genet. 1994;3(9): 1583–7.
9. Gallione CJ, Pasyk KA, Boon LM, Lennon F, Johnson DW, Helmbold EA, et al. A gene for familial venous malformations maps to chromosome 9p in a second large kindred. J Med Genet. 1995;32(3): 197–9.
10. Vikkula M, Boon LM, Carraway KL 3rd, Calvert JT, Diamonti AJ, Goumnerov B, et al. Vascular dysmorphogenesis caused by an activating mutation in the receptor tyrosine kinase TIE2. Cell. 1996;87(7):1181–90.
11. Calvert JT, Riney TJ, Kontos CD, Cha EH, Prieto VG, Shea CR, et al. Allelic and locus heterogeneity in inherited venous malformations. Hum Mol Genet. 1999;8(7):1279–89.
12. Burrows PE, Mason KP. Percutaneous treatment of low flow vascular malformations. J Vasc Interv Radiol. 2004;15(5):431–45.
13. Trop I, Dubois J, Guibaud L, Grignon A, Patriquin H, McCuaig C, et al. Soft-tissue venous malformations in pediatric and young adult patients: diagnosis with Doppler US. Radiology. 1999;212(3):841–5.
14. Dubois J, Soulez G, Oliva VL, Berthiaume MJ, Lapierre C, Therasse E. Soft-tissue venous malformations in adult patients: imaging and therapeutic issues. Radiographics. 2001;21(6):1519–31.
15. Moukaddam H, Pollak J, Haims AH. MRI characteristics and classification of peripheral vascular malformations and tumors. Skeletal Radiol. 2009;38(6):535–47.
16. Fayad LM, Hazirolan T, Carrino JA, Bluemke DA, Mitchell S. Venous malformations: MR imaging features that predict skin burns after percutaneous alcohol embolization procedures. Skeletal Radiol. 2008;37(10):895–901.
17. van Rijswijk CS, van der Linden E, van der Woude HJ, van Baalen JM, Bloem JL. Value of dynamic contrast-enhanced MR imaging in diagnosing and classifying peripheral vascular malformations. AJR Am J Roentgenol. 2002;178(5):1181–7.
18. Puig S, Casati B, Staudenherz A, Paya K. Vascular low-flow malformations in children: current concepts for classification, diagnosis and therapy. Eur J Radiol. 2005;53(1):35–45.
19. Dubois JM, Sebag GH, De Prost Y, Teillac D, Chretien B, Brunelle FO. Soft-tissue venous malformations in children: percutaneous sclerotherapy with Ethibloc. Radiology. 1991;180(1):195–8.
20. Puig S, Aref H, Chigot V, Bonin B, Brunelle F. Classification of venous malformations in children and implications for sclerotherapy. Pediatr Radiol. 2003;33(2):99–103.
21. Muir T, Kirsten M, Fourie P, Dippenaar N, Ionescu GO. Intralesional bleomycin injection (IBI) treatment for haemangiomas and congenital vascular malformations. Pediatr Surg Int. 2004;19(12): 766–73.
22. Lee BB. New approaches to the treatment of congenital vascular malformations (CVMs)–a single centre experience. Eur J Vasc Endovasc Surg. 2005;30(2):184–97.
23. O'Donovan JC, Donaldson JS, Morello FP, Pensler JM, Vogelzang RL, Bauer B. Symptomatic hemangiomas and venous malformations in infants, children, and young adults: treatment with percutaneous injection of sodium tetradecyl sulfate. AJR Am J Roentgenol. 1997;169(3):723–9.

24. Chen Y, Li Y, Zhu Q, Zeng Q, Zhao J, He X, et al. Fluoroscopic intralesional injection with pingyangmycin lipiodol emulsion for the treatment of orbital venous malformations. AJR Am J Roentgenol. 2008;190(4):966–71.
25. Wallace MJ, Kuo MD, Glaiberman C, Binkert CA, Orth RC, Soulez G. Three-dimensional C-arm cone-beam CT: applications in the interventional suite. J Vasc Interv Radiol. 2008;19(6):799–813.
26. Berenguer B, Burrows PE, Zurakowski D, Mulliken JB. Sclerotherapy of craniofacial venous malformations: complications and results. Plast Reconstr Surg. 1999;104(1):1–11; discussion 2–5.
27. Lee BB, Do YS, Byun HS, Choo IW, Kim DI, Huh SH. Advanced management of venous malformation with ethanol sclerotherapy: mid-term results. J Vasc Surg. 2003;37(3):533–8.
28. Mason KP, Neufeld EJ, Karian VE, Zurakowski D, Koka BV, Burrows PE. Coagulation abnormalities in pediatric and adult patients after sclerotherapy or embolization of vascular anomalies. AJR Am J Roentgenol. 2001;177(6):1359–63.
29. Wong GA, Armstrong DC, Robertson JM. Cardiovascular collapse during ethanol sclerotherapy in a pediatric patient. Paediatr Anaesth. 2006;16(3):343–6.
30. Donnelly LF, Bisset GS 3rd, Adams DM. Marked acute tissue swelling following percutaneous sclerosis of low-flow vascular malformations: a predictor of both prolonged recovery and therapeutic effect. Pediatr Radiol. 2000;30(6):415–9.
31. Anadon MJ, Almendral J, Gonzalez P, Zaballos M, Delcan JL, De Guevara JL. Alcohol concentration determines the type of atrial arrhythmia induced in a porcine model of acute alcoholic intoxication. Pacing and clinical electrophysiology. PACE. 1996;19(11 Pt 2):1962–7.
32. Chi LM, Wu WG. Mechanism of hemolysis of red blood cell mediated by ethanol. Biochim Biophys Acta. 1991;1062(1):46–50.
33. Behnia R. Systemic effects of absolute alcohol embolization in a patient with a congenital arteriovenous malformation of the lower extremity. Anesth Analg. 1995;80(2):415–7.
34. Hammer FD, Boon LM, Mathurin P, Vanwijck RR. Ethanol sclerotherapy of venous malformations: evaluation of systemic ethanol contamination. J Vasc Interv Radiol. 2001;12(5):595–600.
35. Mason KP, Michna E, Zurakowski D, Koka BV, Burrows PE. Serum ethanol levels in children and adults after ethanol embolization or sclerotherapy for vascular anomalies. Radiology. 2000;217(1):127–32.
36. Su L, Fan X, Zheng L, Zheng J. Absolute ethanol sclerotherapy for venous malformations in the face and neck. J Oral Maxillofacial Surg Off J Am Assoc Oral Maxillofacial Surg. 2010;68(7):1622–7.
37. Yun WS, Kim YW, Lee KB, Kim DI, Park KB, Kim KH, et al. Predictors of response to percutaneous ethanol sclerotherapy (PES) in patients with venous malformations: analysis of patient self-assessment and imaging. J Vasc Surg. 2009;50(3):581–9, 9 e1.
38. Lee IH, Kim KH, Jeon P, Byun HS, Kim HJ, Kim ST, et al. Ethanol sclerotherapy for the management of craniofacial venous malformations: the interim results. Korean J Radiol. 2009;10(3):269–76.
39. de Lorimier AA. Sclerotherapy for venous malformations. Journal of pediatric surgery. 1995;30(2):188–93; discussion 94.
40. Gelbert F, Enjolras O, Deffrenne D, Aymard A, Mounayer C, Merland JJ. Percutaneous sclerotherapy for venous malformation of the lips: a retrospective study of 23 patients. Neuroradiology. 2000;42(9):692–6.
41. Siniluoto TM, Svendsen PA, Wikholm GM, Fogdestam I, Edstrom S. Percutaneous sclerotherapy of venous malformations of the head and neck using sodium tetradecyl sulphate (sotradecol). Scand J Plast Reconstr Surg Hand Surg. 1997;31(2):145–50.
42. Cabrera J, Cabrera J Jr, Garcia-Olmedo MA. Sclerosants in microfoam. A new approach in angiology. Int Angiol. 2001;20(4):322–9.
43. Yamaki T, Nozaki M, Fujiwara O, Yoshida E. Duplex-guided foam sclerotherapy for the treatment of the symptomatic venous malformations of the face. Dermatol Surg Off Publ Am SocDermatol Surg [et al]. 2002;28(7):619–22.
44. Choi DJ, Alomari AI, Chaudry G, Orbach DB. Neurointerventional management of low-flow vascular malformations of the head and neck. Neuroimaging Clin N Am. 2009;19(2):199–218.
45. Hussar DA, Stevenson T. New drugs: Denosumab, dienogest/estradiol valerate, and polidocanol. J Am Pharm Assoc (Wash DC). 2010;50(5):658–62.
46. Marrocco-Trischitta MM, Guerrini P, Abeni D, Stillo F. Reversible cardiac arrest after polidocanol sclerotherapy of peripheral venous malformation. Dermatol Surg Off Publ Am SocDermatol Surg [et al]. 2002;28(2):153–5.
47. Tessari L, Cavezzi A, Frullini A. Preliminary experience with a new sclerosing foam in the treatment of varicose veins. Dermatol Surg Off Publ Am SocDermatol Surg [et al]. 2001;27(1):58–60.
48. Yamaki T, Nozaki M, Sakurai H, Takeuchi M, Soejima K, Kono T. Prospective randomized efficacy of ultrasound-guided foam sclerotherapy compared with ultrasound-guided liquid sclerotherapy in the treatment of symptomatic venous malformations. J Vasc Surg. 2008;47(3):578–84.
49. Cabrera J, Cabrera J Jr, Garcia-Olmedo MA, Redondo P. Treatment of venous malformations with sclerosant in microfoam form. Arch Dermatol. 2003;139(11):1409–16.
50. Kaji N, Kurita M, Ozaki M, Takushima A, Harii K, Narushima M, et al. Experience of sclerotherapy and embolosclerotherapy using ethanolamine oleate for vascular malformations of the head and neck. Scand J Plast Reconstr Surg Hand Surg. 2009;43(3):126–36.
51. Spence J, Krings T, terBrugge KG, da Costa LB, Agid R. Percutaneous sclerotherapy for facial venous malformations: subjective clinical and objective MR imaging follow-up results. AJNR Am J Neuroradiol. 2010;31(5):955–60.
52. Lacey B, Rootman J, Marotta TR. Distensible venous malformations of the orbit: clinical and hemo-

dynamic features and a new technique of management. Ophthalmology. 1999;106(6):1197–209.
53. Sidhu MK, Perkins JA, Shaw DW, Bittles MA, Andrews RT. Ultrasound-guided endovenous diode laser in the treatment of congenital venous malformations: preliminary experience. J Vasc Interv Radiol. 2005;16(6):879–84.
54. Werner JA, Lippert BM, Gottschlich S, Folz BJ, Fleiner B, Hoeft S, et al. Ultrasound-guided interstitial Nd: YAG laser treatment of voluminous hemangiomas and vascular malformations in 92 patients. Laryngoscope. 1998;108(4 Pt 1):463–70.
55. Chang CJ, Fisher DM, Chen YR. Intralesional photocoagulation of vascular anomalies of the tongue. Br J Plast Surg. 1999;52(3):178–81.
56. Vesnaver A, Dovsak DA. Treatment of vascular lesions in the head and neck using Nd:YAG laser. J Craniomaxillofac Surg. 2006;34(1):17–24.
57. Scherer K, Waner M. Nd:YAG lasers (1,064 nm) in the treatment of venous malformations of the face and neck: challenges and benefits. Lasers Med Sci. 2007;22(2):119–26.
58. Sarig O, Kimel S, Orenstein A. Laser treatment of venous malformations. Ann Plast Surg. 2006;57(1):20–4.
59. Enjolras O, Mulliken JB. The current management of vascular birthmarks. Pediatr Dermatol. 1993;10(4):311–3.
60. Burrows PE, Fellows KE. Techniques for management of pediatric vascular anomalies. In: Current techniques in interventional radiology. Philadelphia: McGraw-Hill Professional; 1995. pp. 11–7.
61. Al-Adnani M, Williams S, Rampling D, Ashworth M, Malone M, Sebire NJ. Histopathological reporting of paediatric cutaneous vascular anomalies in relation to proposed multidisciplinary classification system. J Clin Pathol. 2006;59(12):1278–82.
62. North PE, Waner M, Buckmiller L, James CA, Mihm MC Jr. Vascular tumors of infancy and childhood: beyond capillary hemangioma. Cardiovasc Pathol. 2006;15(6):303–17.
63. Smith RJ. Lymphatic malformations. Lymphat Res Biol. 2004;2(1):25–31.
64. Perkins JA, Manning SC, Tempero RM, Cunningham MJ, Edmonds JL Jr, Hoffer FA, et al. Lymphatic malformations: review of current treatment. Otolaryngol Head Neck Surg Off J Am Acad Otolaryngol Head Neck Surg. 2010;142(6):795–803, e1.
65. de Serres LM, Sie KC, Richardson MA. Lymphatic malformations of the head and neck. A proposal for staging. Arch Otolaryngol Head Neck Surg. 1995;121(5):577–82.
66. Smith MC, Zimmerman MB, Burke DK, Bauman NM, Sato Y, Smith RJ. Efficacy and safety of OK-432 immunotherapy of lymphatic malformations. Laryngoscope. 2009;119(1):107–15.
67. Abernethy LJ. Classification and imaging of vascular malformations in children. Eur Radiol. 2003;13(11):2483–97.
68. Dubois J, Alison M. Vascular anomalies: what a radiologist needs to know. Pediatr Radiol. 2010;40(6):895–905.
69. Dubois J, Garel L. Imaging and therapeutic approach of hemangiomas and vascular malformations in the pediatric age group. Pediatr Radiol. 1999;29(12):879–93.
70. Burrows PE, Laor T, Paltiel H, Robertson RL. Diagnostic imaging in the evaluation of vascular birthmarks. Dermatol Clin. 1998;16(3):455–88.
71. Mathur NN, Rana I, Bothra R, Dhawan R, Kathuria G, Pradhan T. Bleomycin sclerotherapy in congenital lymphatic and vascular malformations of head and neck. Int J Pediatr Otorhinolaryngol. 2005;69(1):75–80.
72. Shiels WE 2nd, Kenney BD, Caniano DA, Besner GE. Definitive percutaneous treatment of lymphatic malformations of the trunk and extremities. J Pediatr Surg. 2008;43(1):136–9, discussion 40.
73. Shiels WE 2nd, Kang DR, Murakami JW, Hogan MJ, Wiet GJ. Percutaneous treatment of lymphatic malformations. Otolaryngol Head Neck Surg Off J Am Acad Otolaryngol Head Neck Surg. 2009;141(2):219–24.
74. Okazaki T, Iwatani S, Yanai T, Kobayashi H, Kato Y, Marusasa T, et al. Treatment of lymphangioma in children: our experience of 128 cases. J Pediatr Surg. 2007;42(2):386–9.
75. Dubois J, Garel L, Abela A, Laberge L, Yazbeck S. Lymphangiomas in children: percutaneous sclerotherapy with an alcoholic solution of zein. Radiology. 1997;204(3):651–4.
76. Alomari AI, Karian VE, Lord DJ, Padua HM, Burrows PE. Percutaneous sclerotherapy for lymphatic malformations: a retrospective analysis of patient-evaluated improvement. J Vasc Interv Radiol. 2006;17(10):1639–48.
77. Cahill AM, Nijs EL. Pediatric vascular malformations: pathophysiology, diagnosis, and the role of interventional radiology. Cardiovasc Intervent Radiol. 2011;34(4):691–704.
78. Nehra D, Jacobson L, Barnes P, Mallory B, Albanese CT, Sylvester KG. Doxycycline sclerotherapy as primary treatment of head and neck lymphatic malformations in children. J Pediatr Surg. 2008;43(3):451–60.
79. Svendsen PA, Wikholm G, Rodriguez M, Enoksson P, Frisen L, Stromland K, et al. Direct puncture and sclerotherapy with sotradecol ((r)). Orbital lymphatic malformations. Interv Neuroradiol J Perith Neuroradiol Surg Proced Relat Neurosci. 2001;7(3):193–9.
80. Ogita S, Tsuto T, Tokiwa K, Takahashi T. Intracystic injection of OK-432: a new sclerosing therapy for cystic hygroma in children. Br J Surg. 1987;74(8):690–1.
81. Ogita S, Tsuto T, Nakamura K, Deguchi E, Tokiwa K, Iwai N. OK-432 therapy for lymphangioma in children: why and how does it work? J Pediatr Surg. 1996;31(4):477–80.

82. Ohta N, Fukase S, Watanabe T, Ito T, Aoyagi M. Effects and mechanism of OK-432 therapy in various neck cystic lesions. Acta Otolaryngol. 2010;130(11):1287–92.
83. Poldervaart MT, Breugem CC, Speleman L, Pasmans S. Treatment of lymphatic malformations with OK-432 (Picibanil): review of the literature. J Craniofac Surg. 2009;20(4):1159–62.
84. Yoo JC, Ahn Y, Lim YS, Hah JH, Kwon TK, Sung MW, et al. OK-432 sclerotherapy in head and neck lymphangiomas: long-term follow-up result. Otolaryngol Head Neck Surg Off J Am Acad Otolaryngol Head Neck Surg. 2009;140(1):120–3.
85. Emran MA, Dubois J, Laberge L, Al-Jazaeri A, Butter A, Yazbeck S. Alcoholic solution of zein (Ethibloc) sclerotherapy for treatment of lymphangiomas in children. J Pediatr Surg. 2006;41(5):975–9.
86. Niramis R, Watanatittan S, Rattanasuwan T. Treatment of cystic hygroma by intralesional bleomycin injection: experience in 70 patients. Eur J Pediatr Surg Off J Austrian Assoc Pediatr Surg [et al]= Z Kinderchir. 2010;20(3):178–82.
87. Zhong PQ, Zhi FX, Li R, Xue JL, Shu GY. Long-term results of intratumorous bleomycin-A5 injection for head and neck lymphangioma. Oral Surg Oral Med Oral Pathol Oral Radiol Endod. 1998;86(2):139–44.
88. Wiegand S, Eivazi B, Zimmermann AP, Neff A, Barth PJ, Sesterhenn AM, et al. Microcystic lymphatic malformations of the tongue: diagnosis, classification, and treatment. Arch Otolaryngol Head Neck Surg. 2009;135(10):976–83.
89. Grimmer JF, Mulliken JB, Burrows PE, Rahbar R. Radiofrequency ablation of microcystic lymphatic malformation in the oral cavity. Arch Otolaryngol Head Neck Surg. 2006;132(11):1251–6.
90. Elluru RG, Azizkhan RG. Cervicofacial vascular anomalies. II. Vascular malformations. Semin Pediatr Surg. 2006;15(2):133–9.
91. Geronemus RG, Ashinoff R. The medical necessity of evaluation and treatment of port-wine stains. J Dermatol Surg Oncol. 1991;17(1):76–9.
92. Eerola I, Boon LM, Mulliken JB, Burrows PE, Dompmartin A, Watanabe S, et al. Capillary malformation-arteriovenous malformation, a new clinical and genetic disorder caused by RASA1 mutations. Am J Hum Genet. 2003;73(6):1240–9.
93. Frech M, John J, Pizon V, Chardin P, Tavitian A, Clark R, et al. Inhibition of GTPase activating protein stimulation of Ras-p21 GTPase by the Krev-1 gene product. Science. 1990;249(4965):169–71.
94. Tallman B, Tan OT, Morelli JG, Piepenbrink J, Stafford TJ, Trainor S, et al. Location of port-wine stains and the likelihood of ophthalmic and/or central nervous system complications. Pediatrics. 1991;87(3):323–7.
95. Geronemus RG, Quintana AT, Lou WW, Kauvar AN. High-fluence modified pulsed dye laser photocoagulation with dynamic cooling of port-wine stains in infancy. Arch Dermatol. 2000;136(7): 942–3.
96. van der Horst CM, Koster PH, de Borgie CA, Bossuyt PM, van Gemert MJ. Effect of the timing of treatment of port-wine stains with the flash-lamp-pumped pulsed-dye laser. N Engl J Med. 1998;338(15):1028–33.
97. Cordoro KM, Speetzen LS, Koerper MA, Frieden IJ. Physiologic changes in vascular birthmarks during early infancy: Mechanisms and clinical implications. J Am Acad Dermatol. 2009;60(4):669–75.
98. Enjolras O, Mulliken JB. Vascular tumors and vascular malformations (new issues). Adv Dermatol. 1997;13:375–423.
99. Srinivasa RN, Burrows PE. Dural arteriovenous malformation in a child with Bannayan-Riley-Ruvalcaba Syndrome. AJNR Am J Neuroradiol. 2006;27(9):1927–9.
100. Naidich JJ, Rofsky NM, Rosen R, Karp N. Arteriovenous malformation in a patient with Bannayan–Zonana syndrome. Clin Imaging. 2001;25(2):130–2.
101. Tan WH, Baris HN, Burrows PE, Robson CD, Alomari AI, Mulliken JB, et al. The spectrum of vascular anomalies in patients with PTEN mutations: implications for diagnosis and management. J Med Genet. 2007;44(9):594–602.
102. Seki T, Yun J, Oh SP. Arterial endothelium-specific activin receptor-like kinase 1 expression suggests its role in arterialization and vascular remodeling. Circ Res. 2003;93(7):682–9.
103. Taschner CA, Gieseke J, Thuc V L, Rachdi H, Reyns N, Gauvrit JY, et al. Intracranial arteriovenous malformation: time-resolved contrast-enhanced MR angiography with combination of parallel imaging, keyhole acquisition, and k-space sampling techniques at 1.5 T. Radiology. 2008;246(3):871–9.
104. Cho SK, Do YS, Shin SW, Kim DI, Kim YW, Park KB, et al. Arteriovenous malformations of the body and extremities: analysis of therapeutic outcomes and approaches according to a modified angiographic classification. J Endovasc Ther. 2006;13(4):527–38.
105. Shin BS, Do YS, Lee BB, Kim DI, Chung IS, Cho HS, et al. Multistage ethanol sclerotherapy of soft-tissue arteriovenous malformations: effect on pulmonary arterial pressure. Radiology. 2005;235(3):1072–7.
106. Do YS, Park KB, Park HS, Cho SK, Shin SW, Moon JW, et al. Extremity arteriovenous malformations involving the bone: therapeutic outcomes of ethanol embolotherapy. J Vasc Interv Radiol. 2010;21(6):807–16.
107. Yakes WF, Rossi P, Odink H. How I do it. Arteriovenous malformation management. Cardiovasc Intervent Radiol. 1996;19(2):65–71.
108. N-butyl cyanoacrylate embolization of cerebral arteriovenous malformations: results of a prospective, randomized, multi-center trial. AJNR Am J Neuroradiol. 2002;23(5):748–55.

109. Pollak JS, White RI Jr. The use of cyanoacrylate adhesives in peripheral embolization. J Vasc Interv Radiol. 2001;12(8):907–13.
110. De Luca D, Piastra M, Pietrini D, Rollo M, Conti G. "Glue lung": pulmonary micro-embolism caused by the glue used during interventional radiology. Arch Dis Child. 2008;93(3):263.
111. Arat A, Cil BE, Vargel I, Turkbey B, Canyigit M, Peynircioglu B, et al. Embolization of high-flow craniofacial vascular malformations with onyx. AJNR Am J Neuroradiol. 2007;28(7):1409–14.
112. Panagiotopoulos V, Gizewski E, Asgari S, Regel J, Forsting M, Wanke I. Embolization of intracranial arteriovenous malformations with ethylene-vinyl alcohol copolymer (Onyx). AJNR Am J Neuroradiol. 2009;30(1):99–106.
113. Loh Y, Duckwiler GR. A prospective, multicenter, randomized trial of the Onyx liquid embolic system and N-butyl cyanoacrylate embolization of cerebral arteriovenous malformations. Clinical article. J Neurosurg. 2010;113(4):733–41.
114. Pollock BE, Flickinger JC, Lunsford LD, Maitz A, Kondziolka D. Factors associated with successful arteriovenous malformation radiosurgery. Neurosurgery. 1998;42(6):1239–44, discussion 44–7.
115. Pollock BE, Gorman DA, Coffey RJ. Patient outcomes after arteriovenous malformation radiosurgical management: results based on a 5- to 14-year follow-up study. Neurosurgery. 2003;52(6):1291–6, discussion 6–7.
116. Friedman WA. Radiosurgery versus surgery for arteriovenous malformations: the case for radiosurgery. Clin Neurosurg. 1999;45:18–20.

Regional Blocks for Postoperative Pain Control

23

Mihaela Visoiu

Introduction

Pediatric regional anesthesia is challenging but is effective and becoming more widely used. Central neuroaxial block (CNB) techniques are commonly used for pediatric pain relief after a wide variety of surgical procedures. They produce excellent analgesia and the complications rate is low, but the risk of some serious complications such as paraplegia are more prevalent than is often realized [1–5]. Recently, there is a trend towards an increased use of peripheral nerve blocks (PNBs). They produce effective pain relief and have a low risk of morbidity [1, 6–11]. However, PNBs as a sole agent for pediatric anesthesia are still underutilized.

Trunk blocks such as paravertebral (PVB), transversus abdominis plane (TAP), rectus sheath (RS), and ilioinguinal/iliohypogastric IIG/IIH are becoming a very popular means to provide analgesia for thoracic and abdominal procedures. In neonates, infants, and small children these PNBs are very challenging secondary to anatomy that is miniscule and difficult to manipulate. The introduction of ultrasound guidance improves accuracy, efficacy, and safety of these PNBs and also decreases the amount of local anesthetic injected [12, 13]. The ability to visualize pleura, bone structures, relevant musculature, and fascial layers with ultrasound offers many advantages over the subjective conventional "pops" technique upon the penetration into fascial compartment.

M. Visoiu (✉)
Department of Anesthesiology, Children's Hospital of Pittsburgh of University of Pittsburgh Medical Center, Children's Hospital Drive, 4401 Penn Avenue, Pittsburgh, PA 15224, USA
e-mail: visoium@upmc.edu

Equipment Overview

Ultrasound equipment with high frequency (15/13–6 Hz), linear probe or a hockey stick, small print, and minimal penetrance probes are ideal for PNBs in this age group. A larger probe of lower frequency, linear or curved, may be more desirable for children with increased weight and deep structures. Given the diminutive structures of pediatric patients and the close proximity of many vital structures, an in-plane ultrasound technique where the advancing needle is continuously visualized is recommended. Resistance to skin and fascia in face of these small distances should to be carefully considered to avoid peritoneal or visceral puncture. As an attempt to reduce puncture size, pain, or bruising a small echogenic needle (e.g., 24 G, 40 mm or less) is recommended for neonates, small infants, and children (weight 20–30 kg). A sharp enough needle to pierce fascial planes is recommended for TAP, RS, and IIG/IIH blocks. A blunt Tuohy tip needle is recommended for PVB blocks.

There are many considerations when performing PNBs in the pediatric population. First, the placement of all types of regional anesthetic

S. Scholz, M. D. Jarboe (eds.), *Diagnostic and Interventional Ultrasound in Pediatrics and Pediatric Surgery,* DOI 10.1007/978-3-319-21699-7_23

techniques under deep sedation or general anesthesia is considered the standard of care in the pediatric population [14]. The second consideration is the local anesthetic. Options are ropivacaine up to the maximum allowed dose of 3 mg/kg or bupivacaine and levo-bupivacaine up to the maximum dose of 2–2.5 mg/kg. Concentrations of 0.5−0.2% for ropivacaine, 0.25% for bupivacaine, and 0.25% levobupivacaine are recommended based on the patient's age, weight, surgical procedure, and desired duration of analgesia. For bilateral blocks, the volume should be divided between the two blocks and more diluted local anesthetic such as 0.1% ropivacaine should be used for neonates and very small children. The dose should be reduced in neonates and infants younger than 6 months or if local anesthetic was previously administered. Single injection nerve blocks have a limited duration and the patients can benefit from the infusion of local anesthetic via catheters. The use of peripheral nerve block catheters is becoming more prevalent in the inpatient and outpatient settings [7, 8, 15–17].

In summary, an experienced pediatric regional anesthetist can safely perform pediatric regional anesthesia in appropriately selected patients and PNBs should be used instead of CNBs as often as possible. This chapter will review a variety of single injection trunk blocks that can be performed with ultrasound guidance for postoperative pain control.

PVB Nerve Blocks

Introduction The PVB blocks consist of anesthetizing the spinal nerve after they exit from the spinal foramen in transit to becoming the intercostal and subsequently the thoracoabdominal nerves. PVBs are ideal blocks for surgeries of the thorax and abdomen and offer an alternative to epidural blocks in pediatric patients [9, 18]. PVBs may be classified as cervical, thoracic, or lumbar.

Anatomy The PVB space is wedge shaped and bounded by the anterior surface of the transverse process (TP) and intercostal membrane (posterior), parietal pleura (anterior), posterolateral aspect of the vertebral body, intervertebral disc, and the lateral aspect of the spinal canal (medial). It contains the spinal nerves, dorsal ramus, intercostal vessels, rami communicants, and the sympathetic chain. The PVB space communicates medially with the epidural space and can communicate with the contralateral PVB space through the prevertebral or epidural space.

Indication Thoracic procedures: thoracotomy, video assisted thoracoscopy, pleurodesis, Nuss procedure, rib resection and fracture, breast surgery; Abdominal procedures: bowel resection, cholecystectomy, appendectomy, nephrectomy, ventral and inguinal hernia repair, orchidopexy; Other: iliac crest bone graft.

Ultrasound Technique In-plane.

Ultrasound Probe High-frequency linear probe (15/13−6 MHz), 5 cm footprint. A small footprint (2.5 cm) is recommended for patients less than 20–30 kg. A 3.8 cm curved probe, 5−10 MHz is recommended for morbidly obese patients.

Patient Position Sitting, if the blocks are done under sedation. If the blocks are done under general anesthesia, lateral with the operative/block side up for single block, and either full prone or "sloppy lateral" (initially positioned lateral and shoulders rotated forward forming an approximate 45° angle with the bed to allow access to both sides of the back) (Fig. 23.1).

Step-by-Step Technique

The appropriate thoracic level is identified using landmarks and marked. The ultrasound probe is placed in a transverse orientation over the midline of the back at the designated dermatomal level and the spinous process identified by the characteristic hyperechoic inverted V shape with an acoustic shadow beneath. The probe is moved lateral and rotated to a slightly oblique orientation (lateral probe edge slightly caudal) until the

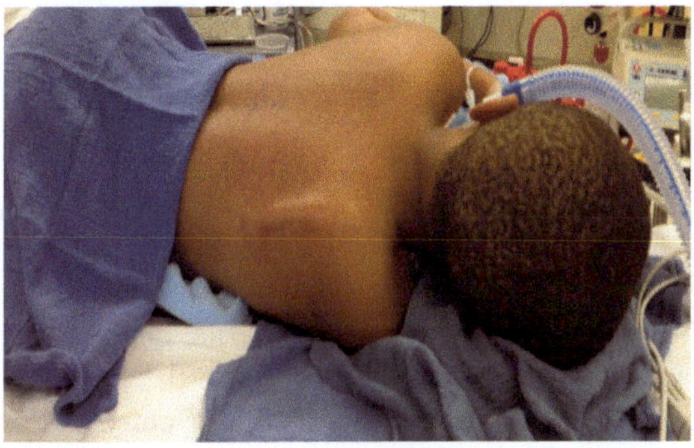

Fig. 23.1 "Sloppy lateral" position for insertion of bilateral paravertebral nerve block catheters

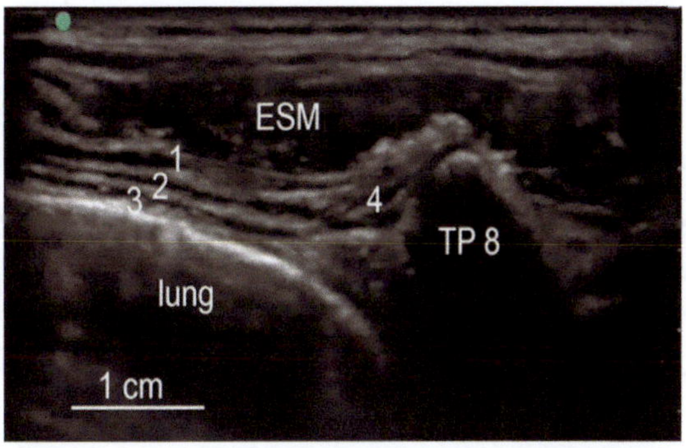

Fig. 23.3 Ultrasound anatomy of paravertebral nerve block: *1* external intercostal muscle; *2* internal intercostal muscle; *3* innermost intercostal muscle; *4* internal intercostal membrane *(IICM)*. *ESM* erector spinae muscle, *TP8* 8th transverse process

tip of the TP is seen in the same view as the parietal pleura (Fig. 23.2). The internal intercostal membrane (IICM), the membranous extension of the internal intercostals muscle, is identified as a hyperechoic structure connecting the edge of the internal intercostal muscles to the lower edge of the TP (Fig. 23.3).

An echogenic needle is introduced, bevel up and in-plane, at the lateral edge of the probe and advanced from lateral to medial until the needle tip is through the IICM in the space between the parietal pleura and the acoustic shadow of the overlying TP (Fig. 23.4). Correct position within the PVB space is confirmed by real-time ultrasound visualization of anterior displacement of the pleura with an injection of a few milliliter of saline solution (Fig. 23.5). Once the paravertebral space is identified, and after a negative aspiration for blood and CSF, local anesthetic is injected.

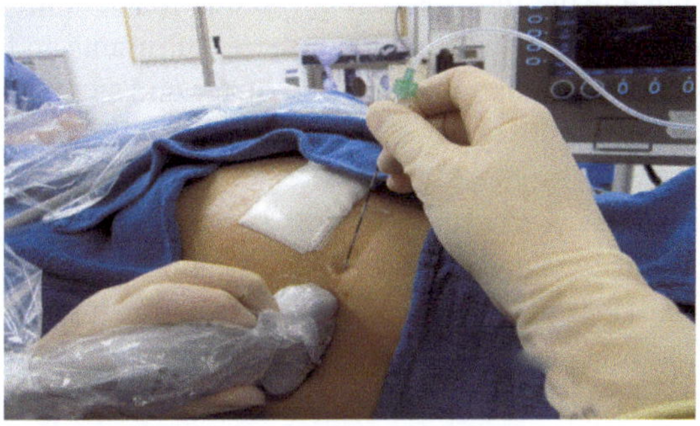

Fig. 23.4 Lateral to medial needle orientation for paravertebral block

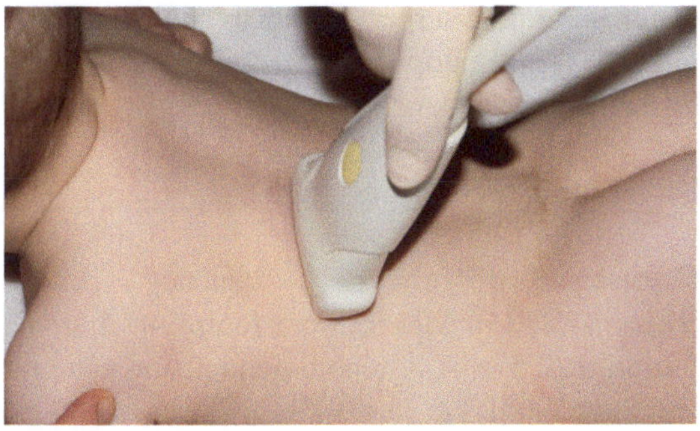

Fig. 23.2 Lateral and slightly oblique orientation of probe for paravertebral blocks

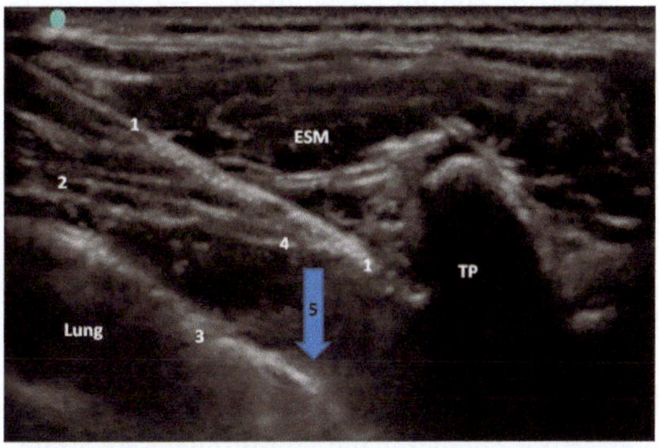

Fig. 23.5 Needle position in paravertebral space: *1* Tuohy needle; *2* intercostal muscles; *3* parietal pleura; *4* internal intercostal membrane; *5* downward displacement of parietal pleura. *TP* transverse process, *ESM* erector spinae muscle

Medication A maximum of 0.5 ml/kg of local anesthetic for a unilateral thoracic block can be injected. A single injection of 0.5 ml/kg in children may be expected to cover at least four dermatomal segments [19]. A single injection of 0.2–0.3 ml at T12 level can be enough to cover T10-L1 segments [20].

Complications Pneumothorax, pleural puncture, vascular puncture, tenderness at injection site, unilateral or bilateral Horner syndrome, hypotension, and spinal anesthesia.

Scientific Literature in Children

Boretsky et al. found that a lateral in-plane technique is the most reliable technique for continuous needle visualization in a series of infants and children as young as 6 months of age and as small as 6 kg [7].

Important Points If the rib is seen, the probe is slid cephalad a few millimeter until the pleura and TP are visualized with no overshadowing rib. The superior costotransverse ligament should not be visible on the ultrasound image, since it spans between the TP and the rib. If the tip of the needle is placed below the IICM (the lateral continuation of the superior costotransverse ligament) and an anterior movement of the pleura is visualized during injection of local anesthetic the block can technically be considered correctly performed.

TAP Blocks

Introduction The TAP blocks are increasingly being used to provide analgesia after pediatric surgeries involving the abdominal wall [21]. TAP blocks reduce opioids consumption, improve pain scores compared with traditional pain strategies, and are alternatives to neuroaxial analgesia [22].These blocks require injection of local anesthetic between the internal oblique and transversus abdominis muscles. Evidence suggests that midaxillary and subcostal injections result in a predominantly anterior spread of local anesthetic and the sensory blockade produced is relatively patchy [23]. Therefore, TAP blocks should be performed as posterior as possible [24].

Anatomy The innervation of the abdominal wall is from the anterior divisions of the T6-L1. The nerves run between the internal oblique and transversus abdominis muscle into the transversus abdominis plane. The points of entry of the anterior branches into the TAP and the distance that these nerves travel in this plane are variable [23]. The nerves have a perforator branch that innervates the anterolateral portion of the abdominal wall. A posterior injection may block T6-L1 nerves in close proximity to one another before they bifurcate. This is clinically significant because the blocks should be performed as posterior as possible to include these nerves, improve the spread of local anesthetic, cover several dermatomes, and improve the block success.

Indication Using the classic midaxillary procedure, these blocks work well for procedures below the T10 dermatome (urology and gynecologic procedures, varicocelectomy, hydrocelectomy, ureteral reimplantation). Lateral, posterior, or quadratus lumborum TAP block techniques are recommended for surgeries at the T10 dermatome (colectomy, colostomy, ileostomy creation and take down, inguinal hernia repair, laparoscopic procedures such as appendectomy). More studies should be done to assess whether these blocks can cover as high as the T8 dermatome. Alternative techniques are recommended for upper abdominal surgeries such as cholecystectomies, Nissen fundoplications, and G tube placements (subcostal TAP).

Ultrasound Techniques In-plane.

Ultrasound Probe High-frequency linear probes (15/13–6 MHz), 5 cm footprint. A small footprint (2.5 cm) is recommended for patients less than 20–30 kg.

Patient Position Supine.

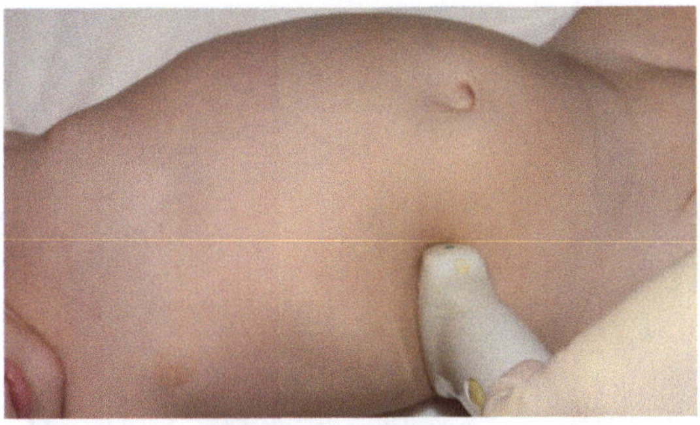

Fig. 23.6 Ultrasound probe position for transversus abdominis plane block

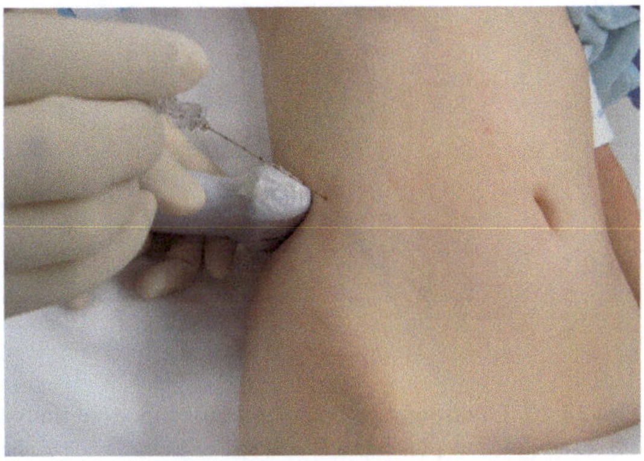

Fig. 23.8 Medial to lateral needle orientation for transverses abdominis and quadratus lumborum plane blocks

Step-by-Step Technique

Place the probe in a transverse plane with the medial end of probe over the umbilicus and obtain an image of the rectus abdominis muscle. Slide the probe laterally across the abdominal wall with the goal to have the probe in the anterior axillary line, between the costal margin and iliac crest, until three muscle layers are present (Fig. 23.6). The most superficial one is the external oblique followed by the internal oblique and the transversus abdominis muscle. Continue to move the probe laterally until the transversus abdominis muscle terminates on the screen (Fig. 23.7). The site of injection is between the internal oblique and transversus abdominis muscles, close to the termination of transversus abdominis muscle. The needle is advanced from anterior to posterior direction through adipose tissue, external, and internal oblique muscles (Fig. 23.8). Correct needle position within the TAP is confirmed by real-time ultrasound visualization of saline hydrodissecting the plane between the two muscle layers (Fig. 23.9). Once proper needle location is confirmed local anesthetic is injected.

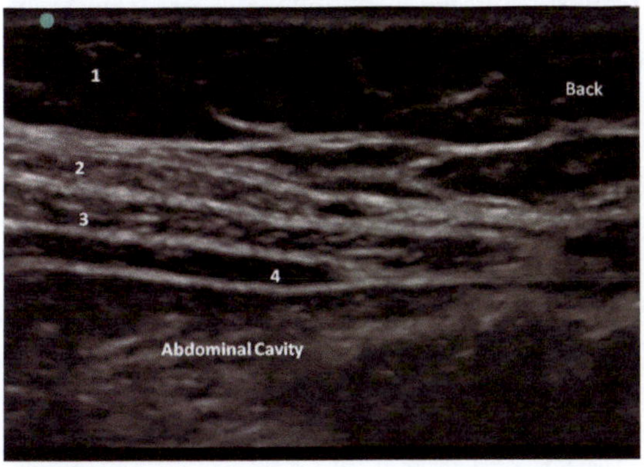

Fig. 23.7 Ultrasound anatomy of transversus abdominis plane block: *1* adipose tissue; *2* external oblique muscle; *3* internal oblique muscle; *4* transversus abdominis muscle

Alternate Techniques

To obtain analgesia above the umbilicus, a subcostal TAP block is necessary. The probe should be placed parallel to the costal margin and

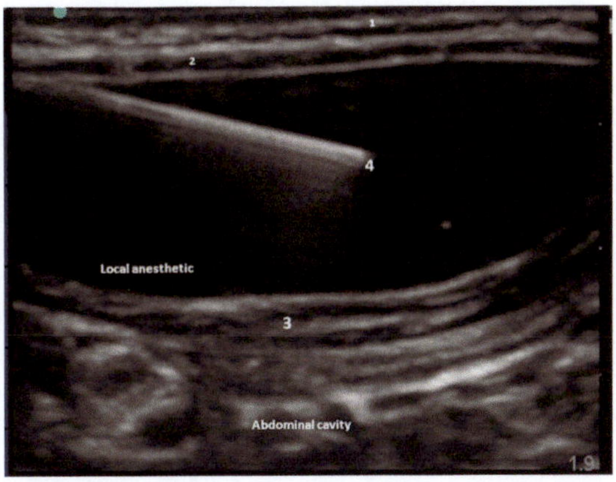

Fig. 23.9 Local anesthetic hydrodissecting transversus abdominis plane in a neonate: *1* external oblique muscle; *2* internal oblique muscle; *3* transversus abdominis muscle; *4* needle

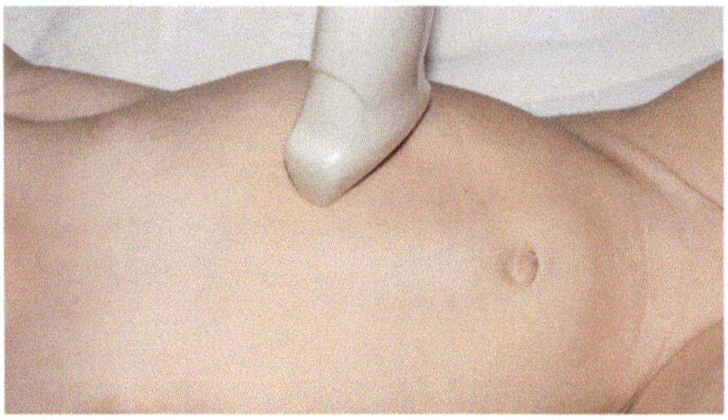

Fig. 23.10 Ultrasound probe position for subcostal transversus abdominis plane block

move medially just inferior to the costal margin (Fig. 23.10). Transversus abdominis muscle can be seen extending behind the rectus abdominis muscle (Fig. 23.11). The needle should be inserted in a medial to lateral direction beneath the costal margin (Fig. 23.12) and the medication should be seen hydrodissecting the plane above the transversus abdominis muscle.

In order to reach as many dermatomes as possible, a quadratus lumborum block can be performed. A lateral position with the operative side up (Fig. 23.13) or "sloppy lateral" (positioned supine with the body rotated towards the opposite side to have access to the patient's back at the block site) (Fig. 23.1). The probe should be placed between the costal margin and iliac crest and moved as posterior as possible until quadratus lumborum muscle is identified (Fig. 23.14).

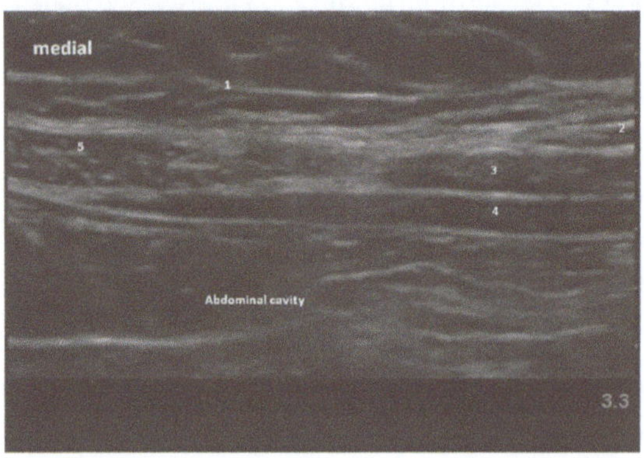

Fig. 23.11 Ultrasound anatomy of subcostal transversus abdominis plane blocks: *1* adipose tissue; *2* external oblique muscle; *3* internal oblique muscle; *4* transversus abdominis muscle; *5* rectus muscle

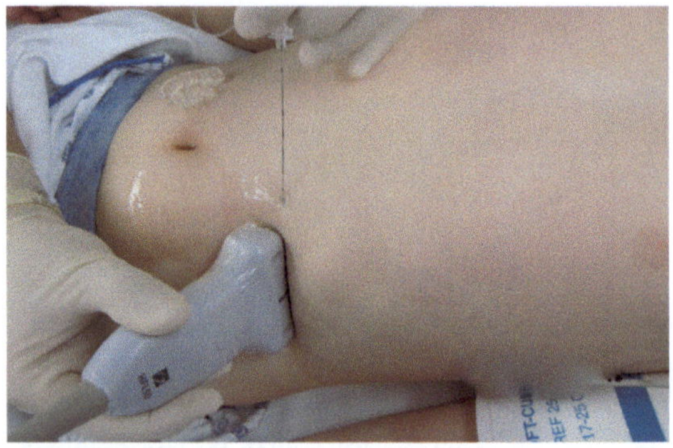

Fig. 23.12 Medial to lateral needle orientation for subcostal transversus abdominis plane block

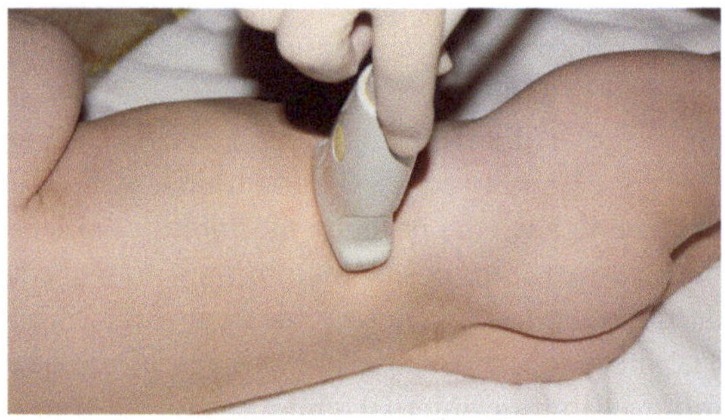

Fig. 23.13 Patient position for posterior and quadratus lumborum transversus abdominis plane block

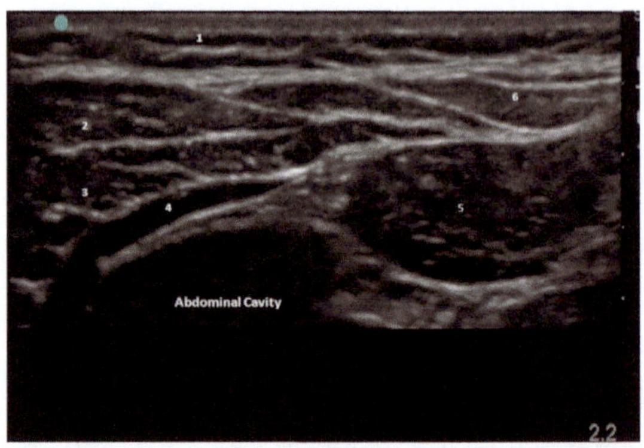

Fig. 23.14 Ultrasound anatomy of quadratus lumborum block: *1* adipose tissue; *2* external oblique muscle; *3* internal oblique muscle; *4* transversus abdominis muscle; *5* quadratus lumborum muscle; *6* latissimus dorsi muscle

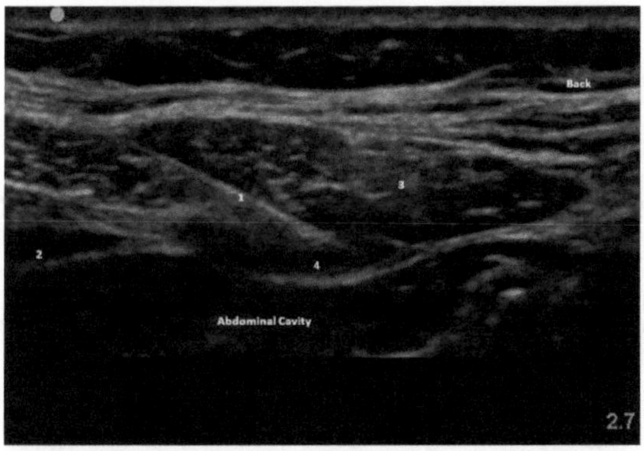

Fig. 23.15 Needle position under the anterior border of quadratus lumborum muscle: *1* needle; *2* transversus abdominis muscle; *3* quadratus lumborum muscle; *4* local anesthetic

The needle is inserted in a medial to lateral direction beneath the anterior border of quadratus lumborum muscle (Fig. 23.15). This block may be very challenging because the muscle is not always easy to identify and is difficult to keep the needle in the correct tissue plane as the body curves laterally.

Medication 0.25 ml/kg of local anesthetic, for a maximum of 0.5 ml/kg/per site can be injected.

Complications Skin bruises, hematoma, intravascular and intraperitoneal injection, perforation of liver, abdominal perforations, femoral block.

Scientific Literature in Children Long et al. showed that overall complications associated with TAP blocks in children are very low (0.3 %) [6].

Important Points TAP blocks do not cover the peritoneal or visceral pain. A posterior ultrasound TAP approach and injection under the anterior border of quadratus lumborum muscle results in a posterior spread of local anesthetic with longer duration of analgesia [25, 26].

RS Nerve Blocks

Introduction The RS blocks are effective for midline abdominal incisions. This procedure aims to block the terminal branches of the 9th, 10th, and 11th intercostal nerves within the posterior RS. The ultrasound use improves successful placement of local anesthesia.

Anatomy The RS is formed by aponeurosis of the transversus abdominis, the external and internal oblique muscles. There is a variation of these layers from the xyphoid to the symphysis pubis. It contains the rectus abdominis muscles that run vertically next to the midline from the lower anterior ribs to the pubis. The RS consists of two compartments: the anterior and posterior RSs. Beneath the posterior RS lie the transversalis fascia, peritoneum, and abdominal content.

Indications Umbilical, epigastric, and ventral hernia repair, ileocecetomy with small midline incisions, pyloromiotomy, laparoscopic and robotic surgeries such as cholecystectomy, appendectomy, nephrectomy, oophorectomy, Nissen procedure, and gastric tube placement to provide analgesia at umbilicus instrument site.

Ultrasound Technique In-plane.

Ultrasound Probe High-frequency linear probe (15/13–6 MHz), small footprint for patients less than 20–30 kg.

Patient Position Supine.

Step-by-Step Technique

The transducer is positioned just lateral to the umbilicus and moved laterally a few centimeters until the lateral border of the rectus muscle is visualized (Fig. 23.16). Moving more laterally, the muscle is seen as a narrow white band of tissue and the transversus abdominis muscle appears. Move the probe back, the optimal site for injection is at the lateral border of the rectus muscle (Fig. 23.17). Deep to the muscle, identify

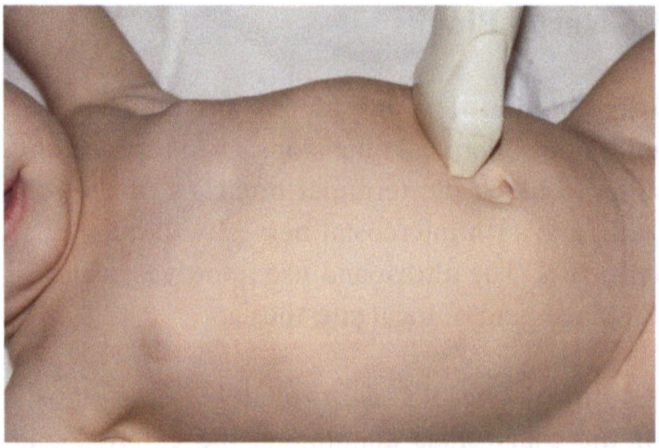

Fig. 23.16 Ultrasound probe position for rectus sheath block

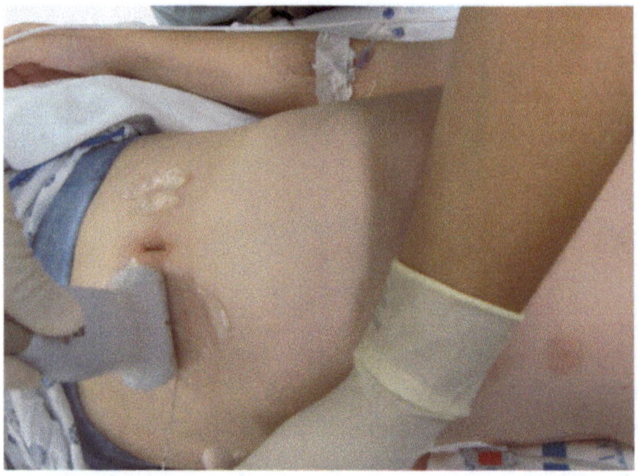

Fig. 23.18 Lateral to medial needle orientation for rectus sheath nerve block

the bright white (hyperechoic) layer of fascia. An echogenic needle is advanced from lateral to medial direction, through the adipose tissue under the muscle (Fig. 23.18). A few milliliters (ml) of saline solution are injected until the spread of medication is visualized in the correct location, deep to the rectus muscle, superficial to the posterior aspect of the RS, hydrodissecting the plane between rectus muscle and posterior aspect of the RS (Fig. 23.19). Be careful not to inject too deep under the deepest hyperechoic line that moves with breathing. The procedure should be repeated on the other side.

Medication 0.1–0.2 ml/kg of 0.2 % or 0.5 %ropivacaine, 0.25 % bupivacaine, or 0.25 % levobupivacaine based on the patient's age, weight, and the surgical procedure, for a maximum of 10 ml/side. Concentration of 0.5 % for ropivacaine is recommended for longer duration of analgesia.

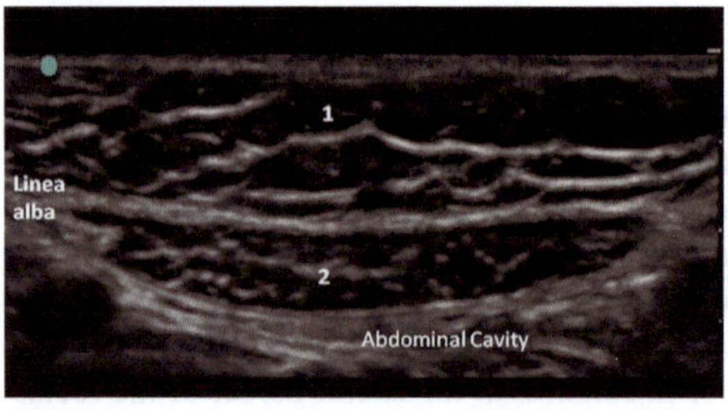

Fig. 23.17 Ultrasound anatomy of rectus sheath block: *1* adipose tissue; *2* rectus muscle

Complications Skin bruises, hematoma, intravascular and intraperitoneal injection, perforation of stomach, colon, puncture of mesenteric vessels, retroperitoneal hematoma.

Scientific Literature in Children Willschke et al. described the considerable advantages of ultrasound over the conventional landmark techniques for RS blocks performed for umbilical hernia repair [27].

Important Points The bilateral single injection RS blocks should not be used for postoperative analgesia for midline abdominal incisions from the xyphoid superiorly to the symphysis pubis inferiorly. If RS blocks are desired, mul-

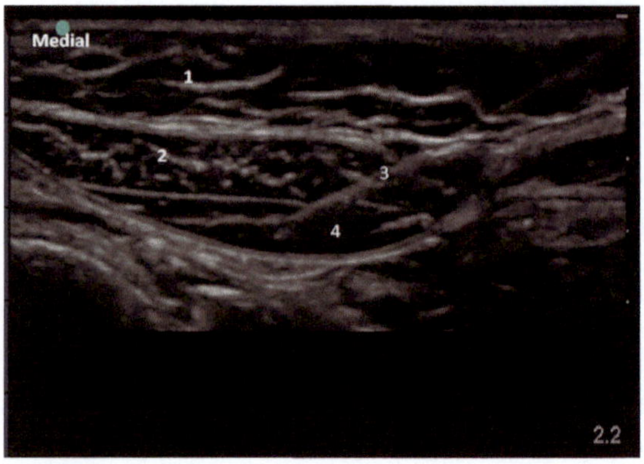

Fig. 23.19 Local anesthetic hydrodissecting posterior rectus sheath: *1* adipose tissue; *2* rectus muscle; *3* needle; *4* local anesthetic

tiple injections should be performed instead, at the same level as the incision, just lateral to the incision. These blocks do not provide anesthesia of peritoneum and viscera. They do not provide analgesia for the lateral abdomen, but can be combined with TAP blocks.

Ilioinguinal/Iliohypogastric Nerve Blocks

Introduction Ilioinguinal/iliohypogastric nerve blocks provide ipsilateral analgesia in the inguinal area. A relatively high failure rate of 10–25 % has been reported with a conventional "pop" technique.

Anatomy Ilioinguinal (L1) and Iliohypogastric (T12-L1) are branches of the lumbar plexus. They exit the neuroaxis between the iliacus and psoas muscle. They pierce the transversus abdominis muscle to run in the TAP plane. The iliohypogastric then pierce the internal oblique muscle and run under the external oblique muscle, superior to the inguinal canal. The ilioinguinal nerve continues in the inguinal canal.

Indication Inguinal hernia repair, orchidopexy, hydrocelectomy, and varicelectomy.

Ultrasound Techniques In-plane.

Ultrasound Probe High-frequency linear probe (15/13–6 MHz), small footprint for patients less than 20–30 kg.

Patient Position Supine.

Step-by-Step Technique:

The probe is placed over the bony prominence of the anterior superior iliac spine (ASIS) and rotated so the one side rests on the ASIS and the other side points at the umbilicus (Fig. 23.20). The bony iliac crest is maintained on the lateral part of the ultrasound image and the probe is moved cranial and caudal until the layers of abdominal wall

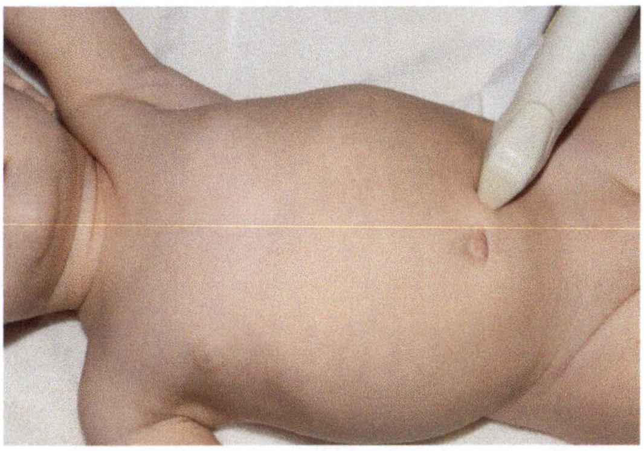

Fig. 23.20 Ultrasound probe position for ilioinguinal/iliohypogastric nerve block

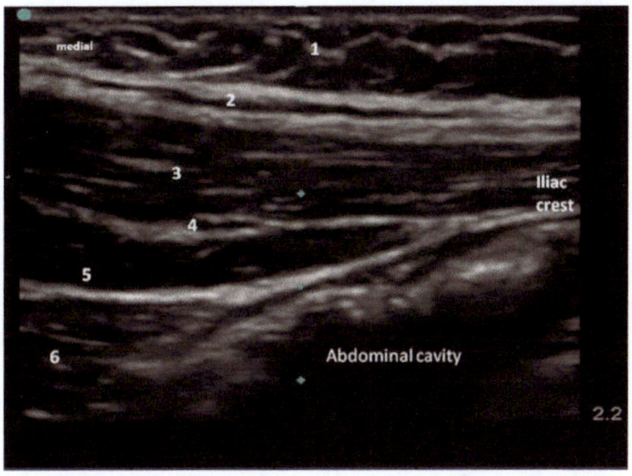

Fig. 23.21 Ultrasound anatomy of ilioinguinal, iliohypogastric nerves: *1* adipose tissue; *2* external oblique muscle; *3* internal oblique muscle; *4* ilioinguinal and Iliohypogastric nerves; *5* transversus abdominis muscle; *6* iliacus muscle

can be identified. The first muscle layer is the external oblique, next lies the internal oblique, and deep is the transversus abdominis. The nerves are located between the internal oblique and the transversus abdominis (Fig. 23.21). They are very closely related to the iliac crest and sometimes appear as a hypoechoic (dark) with bright covering and sometimes as bright (hyperechoic) thickness between the two muscle layers. The needle is advanced from medial to lateral, or from lateral to medial, until it enters the fascial plane between the internal oblique and the transversus abdominis (Fig. 23.22). Inject the medication in this

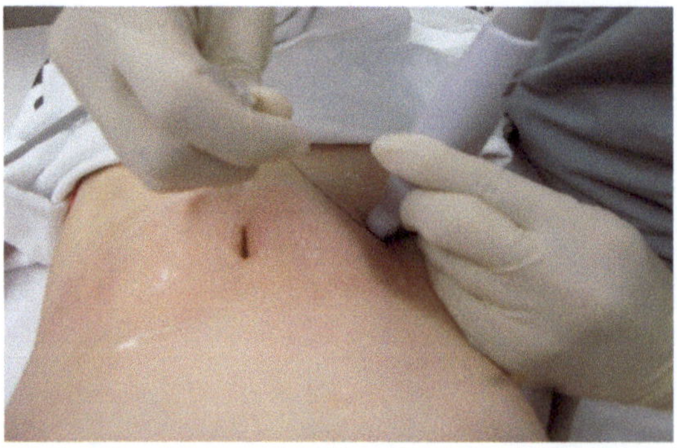

Fig. 23.22 Medial to lateral needle orientation for ilioinguinal/iliohypogastric nerve block

plane. Due to the depth of these nerves, an out-of plane can be utilized. The target structures should be placed in the middle of the ultrasound probe.

Medication 0.1–0.2 ml/kg of 0.2 % or 0.5 % ropivacaine, 0.25 % bupivacaine, or 0.25 % levobupivacaine based on the patient's age, weight, and the surgical procedure.

Complications Visceral perforation, femoral nerve blockade; abdominal wall puncture hematoma, and infections.

Scientific Literature in Children Weintraud et al. showed that accurate placement of local anesthetic around the ilioinguinal/iliohypogastric nerves is seldom possible when landmark-based techniques are used [28].

Important Points There is high inter-individual rate variability in nerve location and the nerves are closer to the ASIS than previously described [29]. Attempt to do these blocks as lateral possible. These blocks do not abolish visceral pain due to traction of spermatic cord.

Summary

Children experience significant postoperative pain and effective analgesia is necessary for optimal recovery. A multimodal approach that includes ultrasound guided PNBs is a better therapeutic regimen by simultaneously improving analgesia and reducing side effects from opioid use.

In addition, PNBs, a form of regional analgesia, improves quality of care, increases satisfaction and saves health care costs. Furthermore, ultrasound technology improves accuracy and efficacy, decreases the amount of local anesthetic, and offers additional safety benefits.

References

1. Polaner DM, Taenzer AH, Walker BJ, Bosenberg A, Krane EJ, Suresh S, Wolf C, Martin LD. Pediatric Regional Anesthesia Network (PRAN): a multi-institutional study of the use and incidence of complications of pediatric regional anesthesia. Anesth Analg. 2012;115(6):1353–64.
2. Meyer MJ, Krane EJ, Goldschneider KR, Klein NJ. Case report: neurological complications associated with epidural analgesia in children: a report of 4 cases of ambiguous etiologies. Anesth Analg. 2012;115(6):1365–70.
3. Allison CE, Aronson DC, Geukers VG, van den Berg R, Schlack WS, Hollmann MW. Paraplegia after thoracotomy under combined general and epidural anesthesia in a child. Paediatr Anaesth. 2008;18(6):539–42.
4. Ecoffey C, Lacroix F, Giaufré E, Orliaguet G, Courréges P, Association des Anesthésistes Réanimateurs Pédiatriques d'Expression Française (ADARPEF). Epidemiology and morbidity of regional anesthesia in children: a follow-up one-year prospective survey of the French-Language Society of Paediatric Anaesthesiologists (ADARPEF). Paediatr Anaesth. 2010;20(12):1061–9.
5. Llewellyn N, Moriarty A. The national pediatric epidural audit. Paediatr Anaesth. 2007;17(6):520–33.
6. Long JB, Birmingham PK, De Oliveira GS Jr, Schaldenbrand KM, Suresh S. Transversus abdominis plane block in children: a multicenter safety analysis of 1994 cases from the PRAN (Pediatric Regional Anesthesia Network) database. Anesth Analg. 2014;119(2):395–9.
7. Boretsky K, Visoiu M, Bigeleisen P. Ultrasound-guided approach to the paravertebral space for catheter insertion in infants and children. Paediatr Anaesth. 2013;23(12):1193–8.
8. Visoiu M, Boretsky KR, Goyal G, Cladis FP, Cassara A. Postoperative analgesia via transversus abdominis plane (TAP) catheter for small weight children-our initial experience. Paediatr Anaesth. 2012;22(3):281–4.
9. Hall Burton DM, Boretsky KR. A comparison of paravertebral nerve block catheters and thoracic epidural catheters for postoperative analgesia following the Nuss procedure for pectus excavatum repair. Paediatr Anaesth. 2014;24:516–20.

10. Taenzer AH, Walker BJ, Bosenberg AT, Martin L, Suresh S, Polaner DM, Wolf C, Krane EJ. Asleep versus awake: does it matter?: Pediatric regional block complications by patient state: a report from the Pediatric Regional Anesthesia Network. Reg Anesth Pain Med. 2014;39(4):279–83.
11. Bhalla T, Sawardekar A, Dewhirst E, Jagannathan N, Tobias JD. Ultrasound-guided trunk and core blocks in infants and children. J Anesth. 2012;27:109–23.
12. Oberndorfer U, Marhofer P, Bosenberg A, Willschke H, Felfernig M, Weintraud M, Kapral S, Kettner SC. Ultrasonographic guidance for sciatic and femoral nerve blocks in children. Br J Anaesth. 2007;98(6):797–801.
13. Barrington MJ, Kluger R. Ultrasound guidance reduces the risk of local anesthetic systemic toxicity following peripheral nerve blockade. Reg Anesth Pain Med. 2013;38(4):289–97.
14. Taenzer A, Walker BJ, Bosenberg AT, Krane EJ, Martin LD, Polaner DM, Wolf C, Suresh S. Interscalene brachial plexus blocks under general anesthesia in children: is this safe practice?: A report from the Pediatric Regional Anesthesia Network (PRAN). Reg Anesth Pain Med. 2014;39(6):502–5.
15. Visoiu M. Outpatient analgesia via paravertebral peripheral nerve block catheter and On-Q pump-a case series. Paediatr Anaesth. 2014;24:875–8.
16. Ganesh A, Rose JB, Wells L, Ganley T, Gurnaney H, Maxwell LG, DiMaggio T, Milovcich K, Scollon M, Feldman JM, Cucchiaro G. Continuous peripheral nerve blockade for inpatient and outpatient postoperative analgesia in children. Anesth Analg. 2007;105(5):1234–42.
17. Gurnaney H, Kraemer FW, Maxwell L, Muhly WT, Schleelein L, Ganesh A. Ambulatory continuous peripheral nerve blocks in children and adolescents: a longitudinal 8-year single center study. Anesth Analg. 2014;118(3):621–7.
18. Qi J, Du B, Gurnaney H, Lu P, Zuo Y. A prospective randomized observer-blinded study to assess postoperative analgesia provided by an ultrasound-guided bilateral thoracic paravertebral block for children undergoing the Nuss procedure. Reg Anesth Pain Med. 2014;39:208–13.
19. Naja ZM, El-Rajab M, Al-Tannir MA, Ziade FM, Tayara K, Younes F, Lonnqvist PA. Thoracic paravertebral block: influence of the number of injections. Reg Anesth Pain Med. 2006;31(3):196–201.
20. Albokrinov AA, Fesenko UA. Spread of dye after single thoracolumbar paravertebral injection in infants. A cadaveric study. Eur J Anaesthesiol. 2014;31(6):305–9.
21. Suresh S, Chan VW. Ultrasound guided transversus abdominis plane block in infants, children and adolescents: a simple procedural guidance for their performance. Paediatr Anaesth. 2009;19(4):296–9.
22. Mai CL, Young MJ, Quraishi SA. Clinical implications of the transversus abdominis plane block in pediatric anesthesia. Paediatr Anaesth. 2012;22(9): 831–40.
23. Abdallah FW, Chan VW, Brull R. Transversus abdominis plane block: a systematic review. Reg Anesth Pain Med. 2012;37(2):193–209.
24. Abdallah FW, Laffey JG, Halpern SH, Brull R. Duration of analgesic effectiveness after the posterior and lateral transversus abdominis plane block techniques for transverse lower abdominal incisions: a meta-analysis. Br J Anaesth. 2013;111(5):721–35.
25. Carney J, Finnerty O, Rauf J, Bergin D, Laffey JG, Mc Donnell JG. Studies on the spread of local anaesthetic solution in transversus abdominis plane blocks. Anaesthesia. 2011;66(11):1023–30.
26. Visoiu M, Yakovleva N. Continuous postoperative analgesia via quadratus lumborum block—an alternative to transversus abdominis plane block. Paediatr Anaesth. 2013;23(10):959–61.
27. Willschke H, Bosenberg A, Marhofer P, Johnston S, Kettner SC, Wanzel O, Kapral S. Ultrasonography-guided rectus sheath block in paediatric anaesthesia—a new approach to an old technique. Br J Anaesth. 2006;97(2):244–9.
28. Weintraud M, Marhofer P, Bosenberg A, Kapral S, Willschke H, Felfernig M, Kettner S. Ilioinguinal/iliohypogastric blocks in children: where do we administer the local anesthetic without direct visualization? Anesth Analg. 2008;106(1):89–93.
29. van Schoor AN, Boon JM, Bosenberg AT, Abrahams PH, Meiring JH. Anatomical considerations of the pediatric ilioinguinal/iliohypogastric nerve block. Paediatr Anaesth. 2005;15(5):371–7.

An Introduction to Intraoperative Ultrasound

24

Marcus M. Malek and Marcus D. Jarboe

Introduction

Surgeons use many tools in the operating room. These surgical tools help with dissection, ligation, exposure, visualization, and other aspects of the operation. Different situations call for different tools for different surgeons. Ultrasound is one such tool that can have countless uses in the operating room. If a surgeon is comfortable using intraoperative ultrasound, it can provide incredibly valuable information that has a significant impact on the operation. In the adult literature, diagnostic laparoscopy with laparoscopic ultrasound has been shown to be valuable in many settings (Figs. 24.1 and 24.2) [1, 2]. For example, intraoperative ultrasound has had a significant effect on the treatment of adult gastric cancer. As many as 40% of patients are upstaged by diagnostic laparoscopy with ultrasound, and about 25% are spared a laparotomy in cases where the disease was previously thought to be resectable [3–6]. There is no limit to the uses of ultrasound

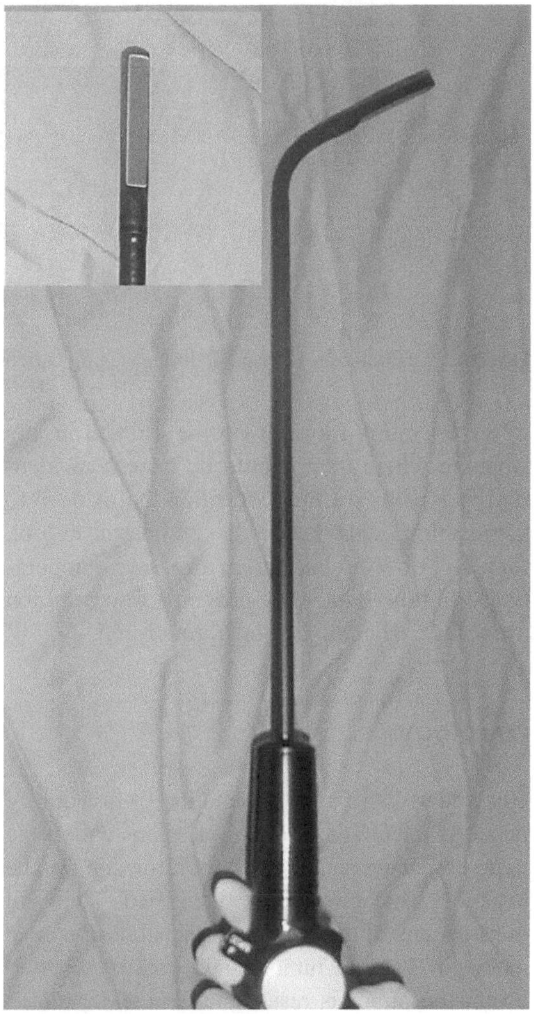

Fig. 24.1 Laparoscopic ultrasound probe. Notice that the angle of the probe can be adjusted to allow for easier positioning during laparoscopy. The ultrasound sensor is highlighted in the *inset* [1]

M. M. Malek (✉)
Department of Surgery, Pediatric Surgery Oncology, Children's Hospital of Pittsburgh of UPMC, University of Pittsburgh School of Medicine, 4401 Penn Ave, Pittsburgh, PA 15237, USA
e-mail: marcus.malek@chp.edu

M. D. Jarboe
Division of Pediatric Surgery, C.S. Mott Children's Hospital, University of Michigan, 1540 E. Hospital Drive., SPC 4211, Ann Arbor, MI 48109-4211, USA

S. Scholz, M. D. Jarboe (eds.), *Diagnostic and Interventional Ultrasound in Pediatrics and Pediatric Surgery,* DOI 10.1007/978-3-319-21699-7_24

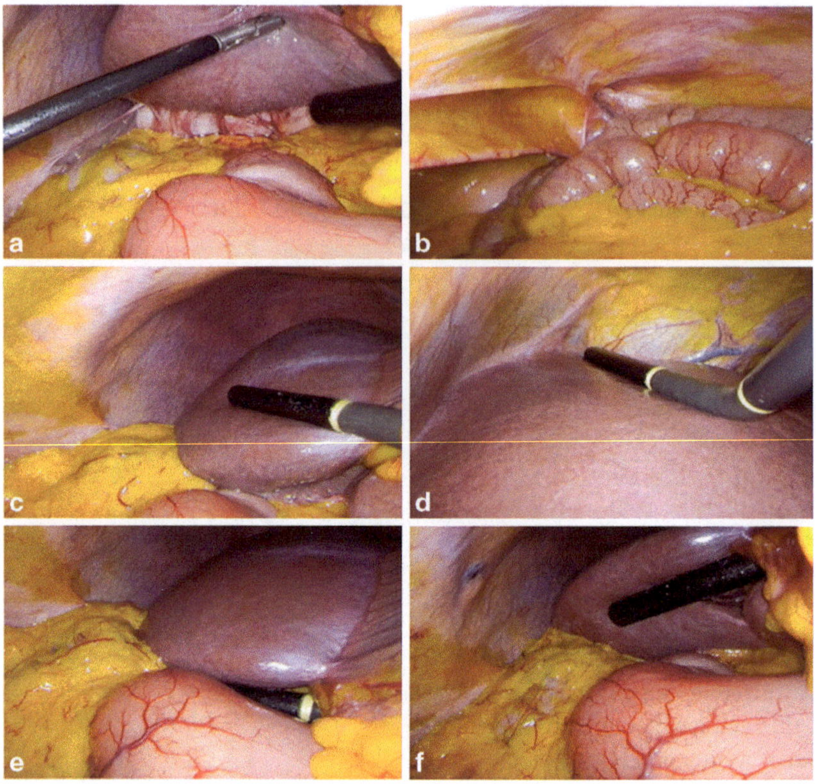

Fig. 24.2 Laparoscopic ultrasound during staging laparoscopy for adult gastric cancer [2]

in the operating room. It can be utilized in any situation where there would be benefit in identifying a lesion or fluid collection that is deep to the visible tissues. It can also be helpful to look for blood flow or clots within a vessel intraoperatively. In this chapter, we present a few common uses of ultrasound in the operating room.

Oncology

Ultrasound can have tremendous utility during pediatric oncological surgery. Lesions within the liver parenchyma and their relationship to the hepatic vasculature can be identified. This will dictate many of the important decisions one must make for hepatic tumors, specifically whether or not the tumor is resectable, and if so, which vessels will need to be taken to get an adequate resection. The pretreatment extent of disease (PRETEXT) is the staging system currently used to guide therapy for hepatoblastoma (Fig. 24.3). Defining the PRETEXT stage is based on knowing the liver sectors which are defined by the portal and hepatic vein branches. The PRETEXT stage also contains modifiers which identify how close the tumor is to the hepatic veins, inferior vena cava (IVC), or portal vein branches [7, 8]. Understanding these relationships is critical to planning your resection. In the operating room, identifying this relationship will define which vessels need to be taken to get an adequate resection. Once you understand which vessels need to be taken for the tumor resection, you will know whether a standard left or right hepatic lobectomy will be sufficient, or if a trisegmentectomy or central hepatectomy are required. It is also important to note that intraoperative ultrasound may provide more up to date information than preoperative imaging. It may also more clearly identify some of the anatomic relationships of the tumor, which may actually lead to performing a differ-

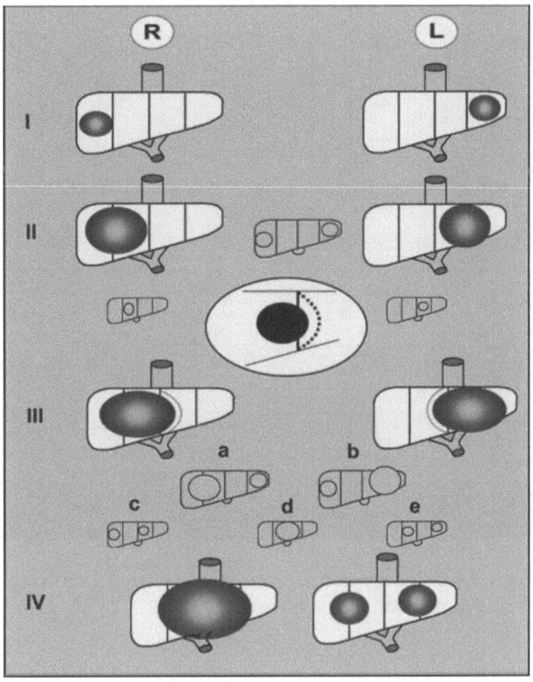

Fig. 24.3 PRETEXT stages. The liver is divided into four sectors defined by the hepatic veins. PRETEXT stage is defined by the number of uninvolved sectors. (1) PRETEXT 1 tumors have three contiguous uninvolved sectors. (2) PRETEXT 2 tumors have two contiguous uninvolved sectors. (3) PRETEXT 3 tumors have one contiguous uninvolved sector. (4) PRETEXT 4 tumors have no uninvolved sectors [7]

ent operation than was planned pre-operatively (Figs. 24.4 and 24.5) [9].

For Wilms' tumor, the role of ultrasound to identify tumor thrombus in the renal vein and IVC has already been well established [10]. Intravascular extension of tumor thrombus occurs in 4–11 % of children with Wilms' tumor [11, 12]. Intraoperative ultrasound can be used to confirm the extent of tumor thrombus in the operating room, or alternatively to confirm the lack of tumor thrombus before ligating and transecting the renal vein. This point is important, because accidental encounter of renal vein tumor thrombus during vessel ligation and transection will upstage the patient to a local stage III tumor, which necessitates flank radiation and the addition of doxorubicin and its inherent risk for cardiac toxicity. Conversely, the presence of intravascular extension does not affect the prognosis if it is successfully resected [13]. Identifying tumor thrombus while ligating the renal vein has been previously reported, and can be avoided with the intraoperative use of ultrasound [14].

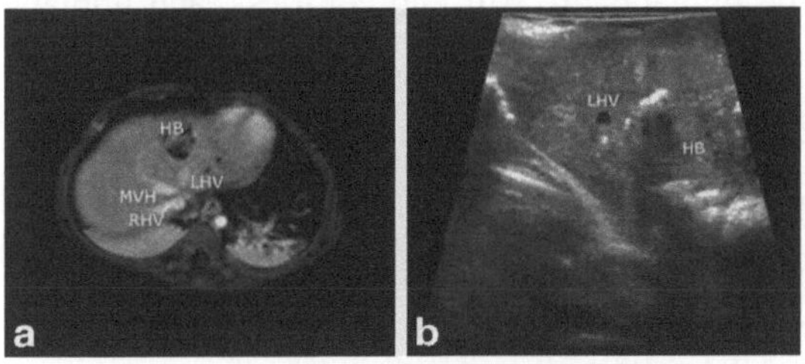

Fig. 24.4 Findings on intraoperative ultrasound. **a** Preoperative MRI showed extension of hepatoblastoma into segment IVa. **b** Intraoperative ultrasound showed tumor extending near but not beyond the left hepatic vein, meaning there was no segment IVa involvement. This allowed an adequate resection with a left lateral segmentectomy as opposed to the original plan for a left hemihepatectomy [9]

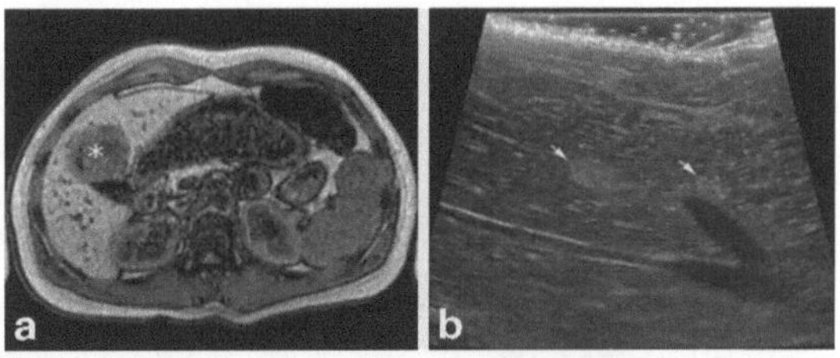

Fig. 24.5 Findings on intraoperative ultrasound. **a** Single adenoma *(asterisk)* identified on preoperative MRI. **b** Intraoperative ultrasound identified multiple additional adenomas *(arrows)*. This patient was diagnosed with diffuse adenomatosis and will require biannual ultrasound surveillance [9]

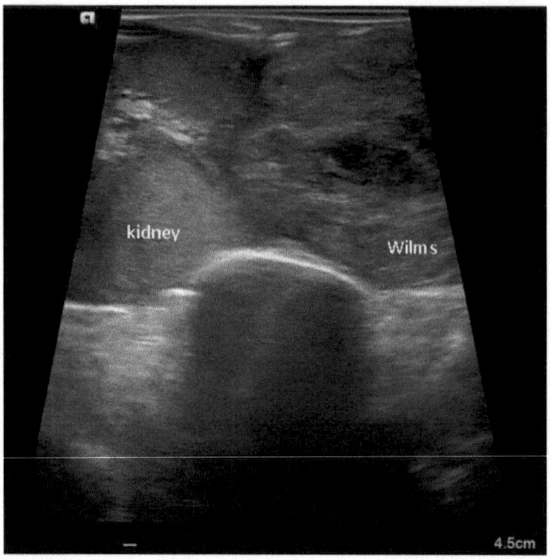

Fig. 24.6 Intraoperative renal ultrasound showing Wilms' tumor for margin planning

In bilateral Wilms, partial nephrectomy is the treatment option [15, 16]. Sparing some of each kidney often allows retention of adequate renal function to avoid dialysis. Obtaining appropriate margins is important and these margins are not always obvious from visual inspection. Intraoperative ultrasound can guide resection margins for the partial nephrectomy and is becoming the standard of care today (Fig. 24.6).

Foreign Body

Fluoroscopy has proven to be an invaluable adjunct in the localization of radiopaque foreign bodies and is utilized extremely often for this purpose. In the case of foreign bodies that cannot be seen on X-ray, surgeons are often forced to rely on palpation to locate the object. The lack of imaging guidance can make these cases extremely challenging and certainly decrease the success rate of foreign body removal. Ultrasound is an excellent tool in this situation, as the foreign body will typically have a different echogenicity than the soft-tissue and will therefore be easily visible on ultrasound (Fig. 24.7a and b). If planning to use ultrasound intraoperatively to locate a foreign body, it is best to have a preoperative ultrasound to confirm that the foreign body can be visualized. Once that is confirmed, the ultrasound will be very valuable in the operating room. Wooden splinters are notoriously difficult to find, and cannot be identified with fluoroscopy. Ultrasound is typically able to identify wooden splinters and has been used to aid in their removal [17–19].

Supprelin implants are subdermal implants utilized for long-term delivery of the gonadotropin-releasing hormone analog histrelin in patients with central precocious puberty. These implants allow hormone delivery without the need for frequent intramuscular injections and are the preferred method for patients and families. The implants need to be removed and replaced at regular intervals. Removal can be challenging as the implants are soft and colorless, and implant

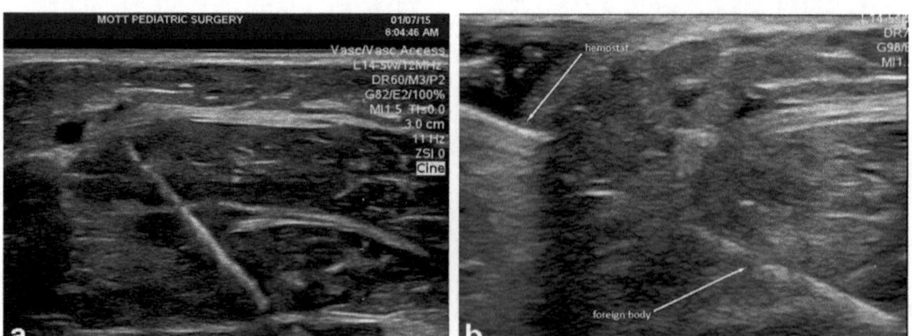

Fig. 24.7 Foreign body in soft tissue. **a** Foreign body seen in intraoperative ultrasound. **b** Ultrasound guidance of instrument (hemostat) to foreign body

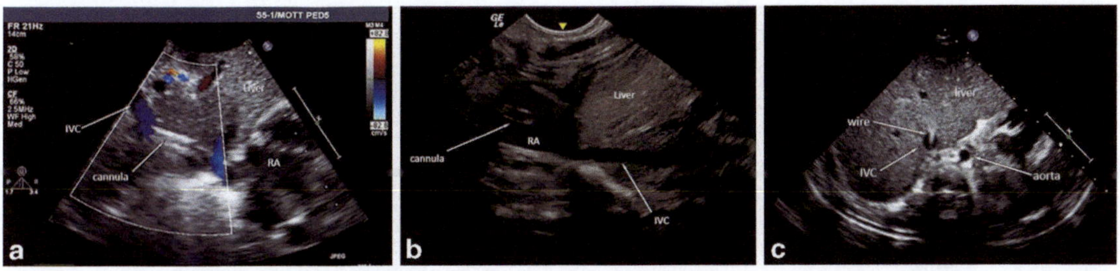

Fig. 24.8 Ultrasound-guided placement of percutaneous ECMO cannulas. **a** Placement of an veno-venous Avalon cannula with tip in the inferior vena cava (*IVC*). The proximal hole is lined up with the tricuspid valve. **b** Placement of a single lumen venous cannula with the tip in the right atrium (*RA*). **c** *Wire* in retrohepatic *IVC*

fracture is not an uncommon event. Ultrasound can be used in this situation to find the fractured implant and assist in its removal [20].

Extracorporeal Membrane Oxygenation (ECMO) Cannula Placement

Percutaneous placement of ECMO cannulas has become more common, in part due to the excellent visualization afforded by echocardiogram. Proper positioning of the cannula is critical to maintain good flows on the ECMO circuit. Cardiac ultrasound is used to identify the position of the cannula and guide its placement. Ultrasound guidance can be used for placement of a single double-lumen cannula for veno-venous ECMO such as the Avalon cannula (Fig. 24.8a) as well as for placement of a single lumen venous cannula that will be used for either veno-venous or arterio-venous ECMO (Fig. 24.8b). These are typically placed in the internal jugular vein. Correct positioning can be a challenge, as the cannulas are large and often will have a hard time traversing through the right atrium and into the IVC, which often reaches the heart at an angle. A guidewire is essential, and can be seen on ultrasound (Fig 24.8c) and confirmed with fluoroscopy. Once the guidewire has passed down the IVC, you can thread the cannula over the wire and watch the tip of the cannula pass down the IVC as well. In the case of the Avalon cannula, it is critical that the catheter is placed in the proper position as the more proximal hole will need to be oriented to face toward the tricuspid valve. Incorrect placement can lead to cardiac perforation. Catheter tip position can be determined with cardiac ultrasound or transabdominal ultrasound.

Vascular Access

Intraoperative ultrasound is invaluable for vascular access. Ultrasound provides consistency and safety in vascular access and allows very good assessment of key anatomy while gaining access (Fig. 24.9). Needle guidance in to vascular structures is discussed extensively in other chapters.

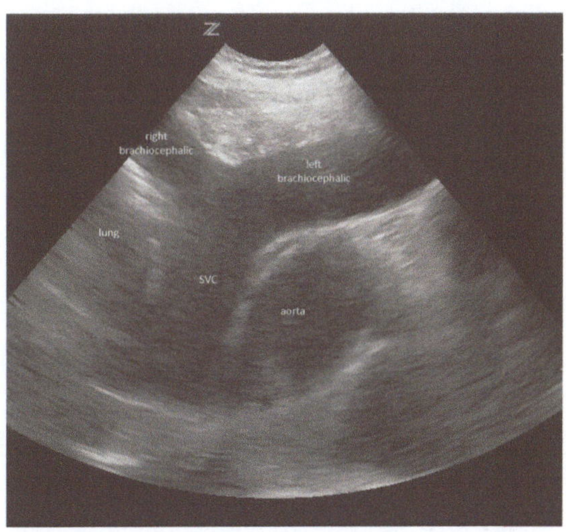

Fig. 24.9 View of great vessels with ultrasound placement just above the clavicles and the probe aimed in the caudal direction

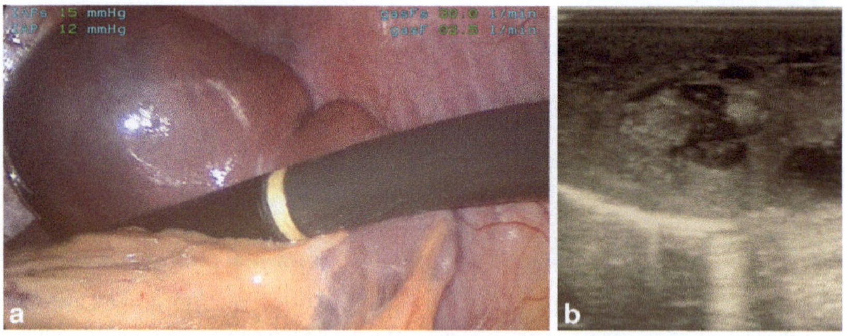

Fig. 24.10 **a** Laparoscopic view of spleen with cyst and ultrasound probe. **b** Ultrasound image very near to the margin of the cyst from laparoscopic probe

Splenic Cysts

Partial splenectomy for cysts can be challenging when attempting to determine the margin for resection. Laparoscopic partial splenectomy is well described and the minimally invasive approach can result in favorable postoperative coarse in comparison to open resection. That challenge only increases in the case of laparoscopic partial splenectomy [21]. Intraoperative ultrasound can provide excellent guidance when determining the resection margin (Fig. 24.10).

Perirectal Fistula and Abscesses

Crohn's disease is a common and challenging disease process seen in the pediatric population. Perirectal Crohn's is especially difficult to treat with the recurrent fistulas and abscesses. Given the inflammatory nature of the disease process, seton drainage of the fistulas and abscesses is often preferred over straight forward incision and drainage. Endorectal ultrasound is a very useful tool in both evaluating the perirectal area for seton placement and abscess drainage [22]. Endosonography can be used to locate fistulas and abscesses in the rectal canal and ultrasound can even be used to guide precise seton placement through fistulas that wax and wane in their patency (Fig. 24.11).

Fetal Interventions

In twin-twin transfusion syndrome (TTTS), fetoscopic laser ablation of communicating vessels is standard therapy [23]. In twins with monochorionic/diamniotic pregnancy, one twin shunts blood to the other through communicating vessels. With a standard posterior placenta this procedure is relatively straightforward and is performed through the mother's anterior abdominal wall with standard ultrasound. With an anterior placenta this maneuver is much more complex. Uterine entry must be posterior enough to avoid the placenta and enable visualization of the communicating vessels on the placenta surface. Several methods are described but using maternal laparoscopy with laparoscopic ultrasound probe enables laparoscopic manipulation of the uterus and also visualization of the fetus while entering with a needle (CO_2 inflation of abdomen precludes useful transabdominal ultrasound) [24]. The needle in the uterus allows wire passage and ultimately trocar placement over the wire (Fig. 24.12).

Summary

Intraoperative ultrasound is a powerful tool that has a wide spectrum of utility. This chapter reviews a few common uses and shows that the ultrasound can be very helpful and has a signifi-

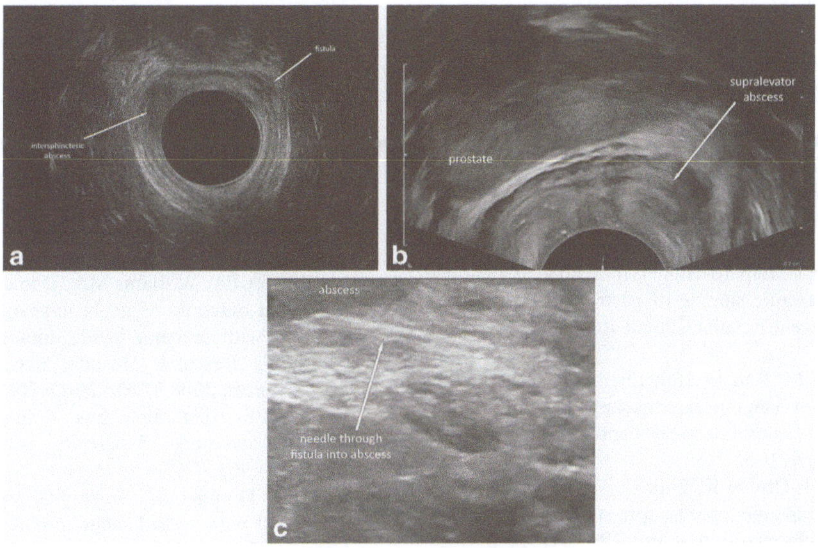

Fig. 24.11 **a** Endorectal ultrasound demonstrating intersphincteric abscess and a fistula. **b** Endorectal ultrasound demonstrating a Crohn's supralevator abscess. **c** Ultrasound-guided needle placement through fistula and abscess

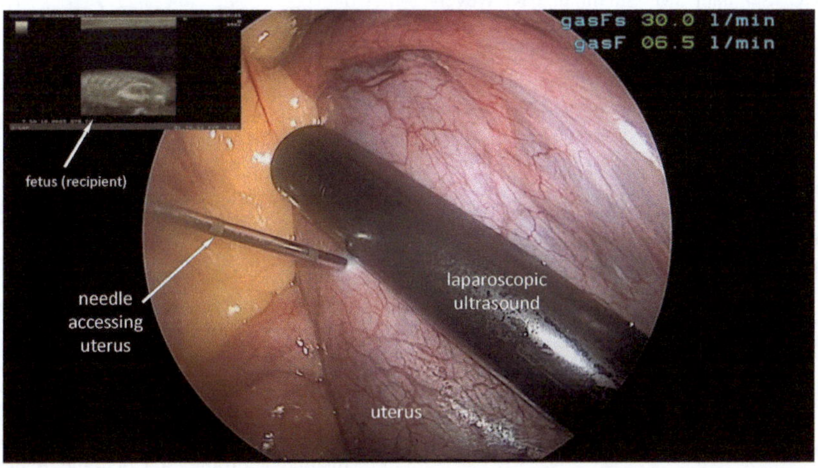

Fig. 24.12 Laparoscopic ultrasound assisted access of the uterus in twin-twin transfusion syndrome laser ablation with anterior placenta

cant impact on an operation. In certain cases, it enables the surgeon to perform an operation in a more effective or efficient manner. In other cases, the ability of ultrasound to clarify anatomy and relationships may change the operative plan in real time. We are likely underutilizing intraoperative ultrasound at this point; its use will surely increase as surgeons become more adept with the technology and identify additional situations in which it can provide valuable information.

References

1. Wadan AA, Eissa M, Senebani JA, Al Saadi A. Laparoscopic ultrasound feasibility and effectiveness. WebmedCentral LAPAROSCOPY 2010;1(10):WMC001025. doi:10.9754/journal.wmc.2010.001025.
2. http://www.datasurg.net/2013/05/04/images-in-operative-ultrasound/10_n2_small/.
3. Rau B, Hünerbein M, Reingruber B, Hohenberger P, Schlag PM. Laparoscopic lymph node assessment in pretherapeutic staging of gastric and esophageal cancer. Recent Results Cancer Res. 1996;142:209–15.
4. Hünerbein M, Rau B, Hohenberger P, Schlag PM. The role of staging laparoscopy for multimodal therapy of gastrointestinal cancer. Surg Endosc. 1998;12(7):921–5.
5. Feussner H, Omote K, Fink U, Walker SJ, Siewert JR. Pretherapeutic laparoscopic staging in advanced gastric carcinoma. Endoscopy. 1999;31(5):342–7.
6. Stein HJ, Kraemer SJ, Feussner H, Fink U, Siewert JR. Clinical value of diagnostic laparoscopy with laparoscopic ultrasound in patients with cancer of the esophagus or cardia. J Gastrointest Surg. 1997;1(2):167–72.
7. Aronson DC, Schnater JM, Staalman CR, Weverling GJ, Plaschkes J, Perilongo G, Brown J, Phillips A, Otte JB, Czauderna P, MacKinlay G, Vos A. Predictive value of the pretreatment extent of disease system in hepatoblastoma: results from the International Society of Pediatric Oncology Liver Tumor Study Group SIOPEL-1 study. J Clin Oncol. 2005;23(6):1245–52.
8. Roebuck DJ, Aronson D, Clapuyt P, Czauderna P, de Ville de Goyet J, Gauthier F, Mackinlay G, Maibach R, McHugh K, Olsen OE, Otte JB, Pariente D, Plaschkes J, Childs M, Perilongo G. International Childrhood Liver Tumor Strategy Group. 2005 PRETEXT: a revised staging system for primary malignant liver tumours of childhood developed by the SIOPEL group. Pediatr Radiol. 2007; 37(2):123–32.
9. Felsted AE, Shi Y, Masand PM, Nuchtern JG, Goss JA, Vasudevan SA. Intraoperative ultrasound for liver tumor resection in children. J Surg Res. 2015. [Epub ahead of print].
10. Ohtsuka Y, Takahashi H, Ohnuma N, Tanabe M, Yoshida H, Iwai J. Detection of tumor thrombus in children using color Doppler ultrasonography. J Pediatr Surg. 1997;32(10):1507–10.
11. Shamberger RC. Renal tumors. In: Carachi R, Grosfeld JL, Azmy AF, editors. The surgery of childhood tumors. Berlin: Springer; 2008. p. 171–99.
12. http://www.cancer.gov/types/kidney/hp/wilms-treatment-pdq#link/_898_toc.
13. Ritchey ML, Kelalis PP, Breslow N, Offord KP, Shochat SJ, D'Angio GJ. Intracaval and atrial involvement with nephroblastoma: Review of National Wilms' Tumor Study-3. J Urol. 1988;140:1113–8.
14. Kanojia RP, Mishra A, Rao KLN. Surgical misadventure of transecting tumor infiltrated infrarenal vena cava in a patient of Wilms tumor. Indian J Cancer. 2010;47(3):349.
15. Davidoff AM, Giel DW, Jones DP, Jenkins JJ, Krasin MJ, Hoffer FA, Williams MA, Dome JS. The feasibility and outcome of nephron-sparing surgery for children with bilateral Wilms tumor. The St Jude Children's Research Hospital experience: 1999–2006. Cancer. 2008;112(9):2060–70.
16. Ehrlich PF. Bilateral Wilms' tumor: the need to improve outcomes. Expert Rev Anticancer Ther. 2009;9(7):963–73.
17. Teng M, Doniger SJ. Subungual wooden splinter visualized with bedside sonography. Pediatr Emerg Care. 2012;28(4):392–4.
18. Graham DD Jr. Ultrasound in the emergency department: detection of wooden foreign bodies in the soft tissues. J Emerg Med. 2002;22(1):75–9.
19. Leung A, Patton A, Navoy J, Cummings RJ. Intraoperative sonography-guided removal of radiolucent foreign bodies. J Pediatr Orthop. 1998;18(2):259–61.
20. Monroe BJ, Fallon SC, Brandt ML. Intraoperative sonographic localization of a fractured Supprelin implant in a pediatric patient: a case report. J Pediatr Endocrinol Metab. 2012;25(1–2):167–9.
21. Keckler SJ, Peter SD, Tsao K, Holcomb GW. Laparoscopic excision of splenic cysts: a comparison to the open approach. Eur J Pediatr Surg. 2010;20(5):287–9.
22. Rosen MJ, Moulton DE, Koyama T, Morgan WM 3rd, Morrow SE, Herline AJ, Muldoon RL, Wise PE, Polk DB, Schwartz DA. Endoscopic ultrasound to guide the combined medical and surgical management of pediatric perianal Crohn's disease. Inflamm Bowel Dis. 2010;16(3):461–8.
23. Roberts D, et al. Interventions for twin-twin transfusion syndrome: a Cochrane review. Ultrasound Obstet Gynecol. 2008;31(6):701–11.
24. Jarboe MD, Berman DR, Wright T, Treadwell MC, Mychaliska GB. Novel application of laparoscopic ultrasound for fetoscopic laser ablation in twin-twin transfusion syndrome with complete anterior placenta. Fetal Diagn Ther (in press).

Erratum to: Fine Needle Aspiration (FNA) of the Thyroid Gland

Ranjith Vellody

Erratum to: S. Scholz, M. D. Jarboe (eds.), *Diagnostic and Interventional Ultrasound in Pediatrics and Pediatric Surgery*, DOI 10.1007/978-3-319-21699-7_20

The Publisher regret that in chapter 20 only one author was listed as chapter and corresponding author i.e. Ranjith Vellody. However, there are additional two co-authors contributed in this chapter. The details of those two authors are as follows:

Matthew Hermann, MD
Department of Radiology
University of Michigan
Ann Arbor, MI, USA

Joseph J. Gemmete
Department of Radiology,
University of Michigan,
Ann Arbor, MI, USA

The correct order of the authors for chapter opening page will be:

Matthew Hermann, Joseph J. Gemmete and Ranjith Vellody

The online version of the original chapter can be found under
http://dx.doi.org/10.1007/978-3-319-21699-7_20

R. Vellody (✉)
Department of Radiology , University of Michigan,
1500 E. Medical Center Drive, Room UH B1-0502,
Ann Arbor , MI 48109 , USA
e-mail : ranjithv@med.umich.edu

S. Scholz, M. D. Jarboe (eds.), *Diagnostic and Interventional Ultrasound in Pediatrics and Pediatric Surgery,* DOI 10.1007/978-3-319-21699-7_25

Index

S. Scholz, M. D. Jarboe (eds.), *Diagnostic and Interventional Ultrasound in Pediatrics and Pediatric Surgery,* DOI 10.1007/978-3-319-21699-7

MIX
Papier aus verantwortungsvollen Quellen
Paper from responsible sources
FSC® C105338

If you have any concerns about our products,
you can contact us on
ProductSafety@springernature.com

In case Publisher is established outside the EU,
the EU authorized representative is:
Springer Nature Customer Service Center GmbH
Europaplatz 3, 69115 Heidelberg, Germany

Printed by Libri Plureos GmbH
in Hamburg, Germany

SpringerBriefs in Economics

For further volumes:
http://www.springer.com/series/8876

Vikram Dayal

The Environment in Economics and Development

Pluralist Extensions of Core Economic Models

Springer

Vikram Dayal
Institute of Economic Growth
Delhi
India

ISSN 2191-5504 ISSN 2191-5512 (electronic)
ISBN 978-81-322-1670-4 ISBN 978-81-322-1671-1 (eBook)
DOI 10.1007/978-81-322-1671-1
Springer New Delhi Heidelberg New York Dordrecht London

Library of Congress Control Number: 2013951506

Printed on acid-free paper

Springer is part of Springer Science+Business Media (www.springer.com)

For Varsha

Preface

This brief is about economic models—theoretical and statistical—that address environmental issues in developing countries. The brief aims to simplify exposition, beginning each of Chaps. 3–7 with a very simple core model of environmental economics, and then discussing extensions to these core models. An intermediate level of mathematics is used only in the last section or an appendix of Chaps. 3–7. Chapter 2 is an exposition of several types of models and frameworks. Chapter 1 provides an introduction and overview around graphs of select world development indicators.

This brief discusses important problems of developing countries that are not stressed as much as they should be in books on environmental economics: traditional pollution; livelihoods and the commons; biological invasions; and complex ecology. The brief looks at old questions from different angles; the overall philosophy is of careful methodological pluralism, advocated by Richard Norgaard. First, I bring in perspectives from institutional economics. Second, I pay careful attention to issues of causality. Third, I emphasize equity as much as efficiency.

The brief aims to cater to those with a curiosity about environment and development economics—students who have not studied economics previously, economists who work in other areas but are interested in environmental issues, and perhaps even environmental economists interested in a different treatment. The treatment here is brief and selective, not detailed or comprehensive.

I am grateful to the Institute of Economic Growth, where I work, and to my colleagues at the Institute who have stimulated my thinking. I am grateful to the South Asian Network for Development and Environmental Economics (SANDEE) for the Partha Dasgupta Fellowship. This fellowship helped me visit the Workshop in Political Theory and Policy Analysis in Bloomington, Indiana, where I reflected on several issues presented in the brief. Professor Kanchan Chopra, who has influenced my thinking and encouraged me over the years, commented on a draft of the brief. At Springer, Ms. Sagarika Ghosh was very supportive.

My family and friends saw me through a difficult time while this was being written. They are too numerous to mention individually, but most immediately

Deepu, Ranu, Ma, and Papa will be happy to see this brief published, for diverse reasons.

This brief is for Varsha, for her health and happiness.

Delhi, 29 July 2013 Vikram Dayal

Contents

Chapter 1
Context and Overview of Environment and Development Economics

Abstract I provide an overview of the brief and discuss pluralism briefly. I explore environmental indicators (using the World Bank's World Development Indicators) with statistical graphs related to Chaps. 3–7 of the brief. I plot time series for certain select countries as well as scatter plots for all countries. For modern pollution I explore the indicator ambient concentration of fine particulate matter and for traditional pollution I explore the indicator access to an improved water source. Both indicators have been improving over the last few decades. The percentage of population that is rural indicates the population in developing countries who tend to depend on rural commons; this has been declining. Countries have attempted to preserve complex ecosystems by setting aside land as protected areas—often with a period of rapid growth in such areas followed by leveling off. Carbon dioxide emissions have followed economic growth closely. Finally, I explore the World Bank's adjusted net national savings estimates, which are intended to be indicators of sustainable development.

Keywords Environment · Development · Pluralism · Environmental indicators

In 1997, Partha Dasgupta and Karl-Goran Maler published a paper that I consider a manifesto for environment and development economics: "The dependence of poor countries on their natural resources ... should be self evident .... Until very recently, environmental resources made but perfunctory appearances in government planning models, and were cheerfully ignored in most of what goes by the name development economics. This was harmful not only for public economics and the economics of development, but also for environmental economics." Since then, Environment and Development Economics has matured and Economics in general has developed in diverse directions—for example, there is more careful attention to causality and institutions.

I believe that we in developing countries should not only take a given theoretical framework (often developed in the developed countries) to data,

V. Dayal, *The Environment in Economics and Development*,
SpringerBriefs in Economics, DOI: 10.1007/978-81-322-1671-1_1, © The Author(s) 2014

but develop theory while doing empirical work, with the context of developing countries influencing the theory.

The environment is often controversial, and there are several discourses with different adherents (Dryzek 2005). Economists also see things differently—Environmental Economists tend to look at environmental issues as market failures which they will address with economic valuation and market signals (Tietenberg and Lewis 2009); Ecological Economists point to the limitations of valuation and the limits to growth (Daly and Farley 2010); and institutionally minded economists stress the legal structure and norms (Vatn 2005). Economists often use models to support their arguments.

1.1 A Pluralist Approach

Here, following Norgaard (1989), I adopt a pluralist approach. According to Norgaard (1989, p. 37), 'all the aspects of complex systems can only be understood through multiple methodologies.' In 1992, forty-four leading economists—including four Nobel Laureates—published an advertisement in the American Economic Review, pleading for pluralism in economics, 'involving critical conversation and tolerant communication between different approaches' (Hodgson et al. 1992, p. xxv).

Rather than discuss the philosophy of pluralism, in this brief I present the core economic models of environment and development and then extend them in diverse directions—including, for example, perspectives from ecology and political science. In a sense, I am adopting the approach of the fox who knows many small things rather than the hedgehog who knows one big thing—Berlin (1953) had argued that famous thinkers such as Aristotle and Plato had adopted the contrasting styles of the fox and the hedgehog. Although I will not be looking at predictions in this brief, Tetlock (2005) empirically established that analysts who were like foxes made more accurate predictions than those who were like hedgehogs. He asked the analysts to respond to statements to measure their cognitive style. One example was: 'Even after I have made up my mind about something, I am always eager to consider a different opinion,' with the fox agreeing and the hedgehog disagreeing.

I begin each of Chaps. 3–7 by discussing a core economic model in a simple way, and then extend the core model in different theoretical and empirical directions. For example, in the chapter on pollution, I start with a simple economic model of externalities. I then (1) suggest that developing countries suffer not just modern but traditional pollution, (2) look at how the effects of pollution on health can be established statistically, and (3) re-interpret a theoretical and empirical model of air pollution. Thus, the chapter on pollution begins with standard neoclassical environmental economics, then moves to issues of causality, and finally suggests that we should consider institutions and identity.

1.2 Statistical Graphs of Key Indicators

To get a sense of the context of developing countries, I will look at statistical graphs of select world development indicators while providing an overview of the chapters in this brief. An indicator suggests rather than finds out something, and a statistical indicator's integrity depends on the quality of the data. It is difficult to assess data quality unless there are alternative estimates. Pandit et al. (2006) did such alternative estimation—they examined deforestation trends in the Indian Himalayas during 1970–2000 using diverse sources of data. They estimated an overall decrease at the rate of $-0.54\ \%$ per year in the total forest area in the Indian Himalayas, in contrast with a rise at the rate of $0.17\ \%$ per year indicated by the Indian Agricultural Statistics dataset.

I view the statistical graphs here as descriptive indicators of the macro context of developing countries. I want to make comparisons across countries of levels and changes, and I point out outlier countries that depart from the average. I am exploring data, not doing a formal 'Environmental Kuznets Curve' analysis.

The literature on the Environmental Kuznets Curve (EKC) is large. In the World Bank's World Development Report of 1992 (p. 11), which made the EKC popular, several curves were plotted based on regressions with data for different countries in a given year. The regressions fitted quadratic curves. The graph for sulphur dioxide concentrations versus per capita income was inverse U-shaped. Environmental economists saw this as a general description of how the environment varied with income, whereas advocates of growth went further, suggesting that growth would help improve the environment. In Chap. 2, we shall see that regressions can be viewed descriptively or causally. According to Stern (2004, p. 1420), 'most of the EKC literature is econometrically weak .... When we do take diagnostic statistics and specification tests into account and use appropriate techniques, we find that the EKC does not exist.'

1.3 Gross Domestic Product per Capita

Economic growth is a key indicator; it shapes issues of environment and development. In 1972, Meadows et al. (2005) in their famous 'Limits to Growth' study drew attention to the dilemma of exponential growth in a finite world. In general, economists were critical of the study. However, several decades later, in 1996, the Nobel Laureate Kenneth Arrow, other economists, and ecologists, accepted that the resource base was finite and stressed that environmental policy should accompany growth. We look at the indicator gross domestic product (GDP) per capita, (in purchasing power parity and constant 2005 international dollars). The time series of the logarithm of GDP per capita for select countries is plotted from 1980 to 2010 in Fig. 1.1. China, India and Indonesia grew fast; Egypt, USA and Brazil grew at lower rates; Russia experienced a fall and then picked up; Kenya and Mexico were flat.

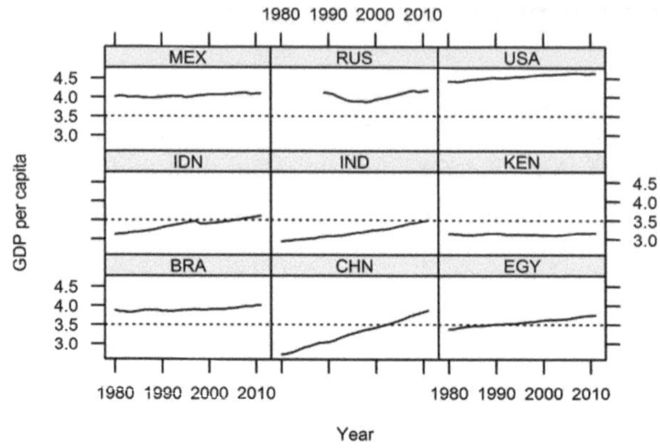

Fig. 1.1 Time series of logarithm of GDP (gross domestic product) per capita (Purchasing Power Parity, constant 2005 international $) from 1980 to 2010. China, India and Indonesia grew fast. Egypt, USA and Brazil grew at lower rates. Russia experienced a fall and then picked up. Kenya and Mexico were flat. *Source* World Development Indicators, World Bank (2012)

The distribution of GDP per capita across countries in 2010 is graphed with the aid of a boxplot (Fig. 1.2). The lower quartile was about 2,300, median was about 7,400, and the upper quartile was about 17,200. The distribution was positively skewed. The boxplot of change in GDP per capita across countries between 1980

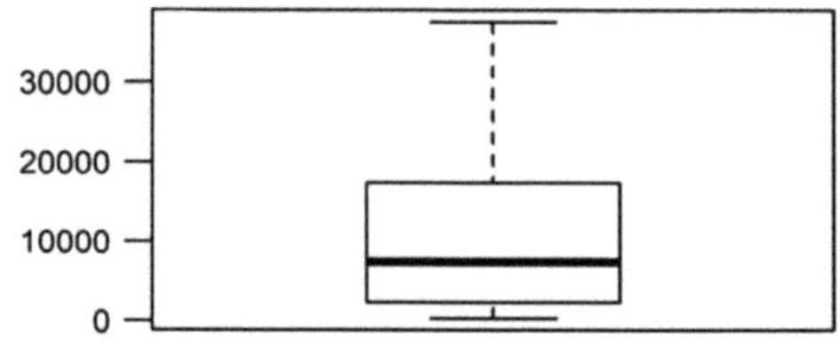

Fig. 1.2 Boxplot of GDP per capita for all countries (for which data were reported in the World Development Indicators) in PPP (constant 2005 international $) in 2010. The lower quartile was about 2,300, median was about 7,400, and the upper quartile was about 17,200. The distribution was positively skewed. *Source* World Development Indicators, World Bank (2012)

and 2010 is shown in Fig. 1.3. The lower quartile was about 400, the median was about 2,500, and the upper quartile was about 7,900. The distribution was positively skewed (Fig. 1.3).

1.4 Traditional and Modern Pollution

Pollution—one of the key topics in environmental economics—is thought to be correlated with urbanization and industrialization. PM10 (fine particulate matter) in micrograms per cubic meter of air is an indicator of air pollution. Time series of

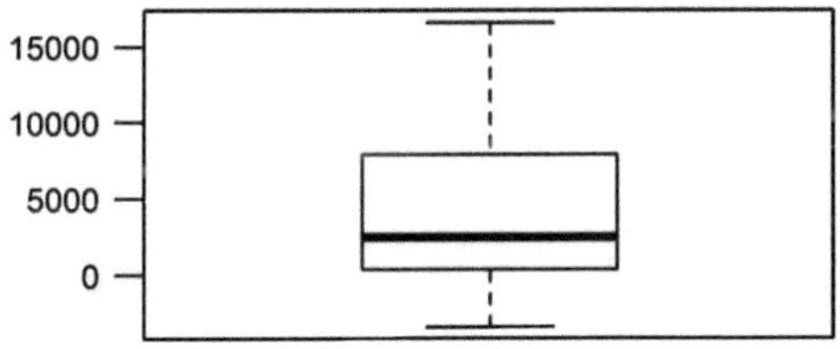

Fig. 1.3 Boxplot of change in GDP per capita across countries between 1980 and 2010, in PPP (constant 2005 international $). The lower quartile was about 400, the median was about 2500, and the upper quartile was about 7,900. The distribution was positively skewed. *Source* World Development Indicators, World Bank (2012)

PM10 concentration for a few select countries are plotted for the years 1990 to 2009 in Fig. 1.4. PM10 fell for all countries and most rapidly for Egypt. Yet, levels of air pollution continue to be high in several cities in developing countries—Egypt, China, Indonesia and India were above or close to the 50 mark in 2009. Figure 1.5 shows the scatter plot of PM10 versus logarithm of per capita GDP in 2009. The line is almost flat and the variation in PM10 appears to go down with income (Fig. 1.5). Uruguay (URY), Sudan (SDN) and Bangladesh (BGD) had very high levels of PM10; Saudi Arabia (SAU) and Kuwait (KWT) had high levels even though their per capita GDP levels were high. The boxplot shows that the lower quartile of PM10 in 2009 was 18, the median was about 30 and the upper quartile was 50. The distribution was highly positively skewed. Figure 1.6 shows the scatter plot for the change in PM10 for countries between 1990 and 2009 versus the change in logarithm of per capita GDP in the same period. The line is flat, correlation is low. The lower quartile of change in PM10 was −52, the median was −27, and the upper quartile was −15. SDN (Sudan), GEO (Georgia) and ARE

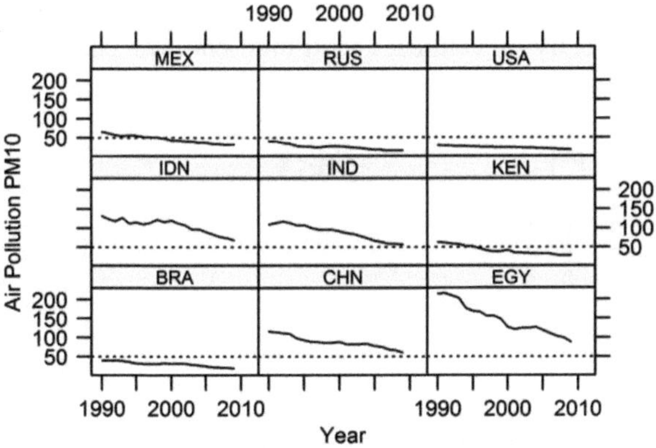

Fig. 1.4 Time series of PM10 (fine particulate matter), in micrograms per cubic meter of air, for the years 1990–2009. PM10 fell for all countries and most rapidly in Egypt. Egypt, China, Indonesia and India were above or close to the 50 mark in 2009. *Source* World Development Indicators, World Bank (2012)

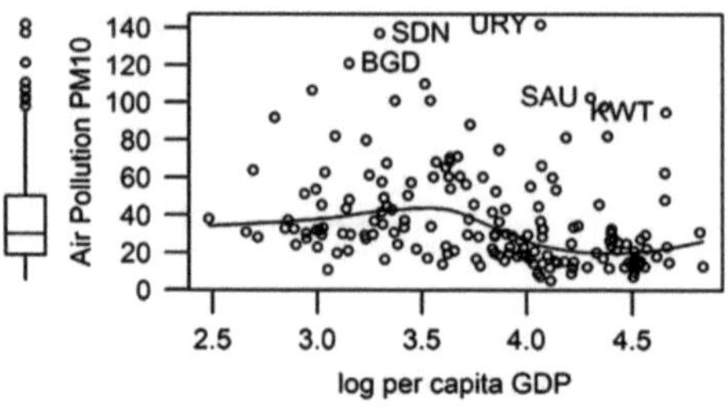

Fig. 1.5 Scatter plot of PM10 versus the logarithm of per capita GDP in 2009. The *line* is almost flat and the variation in PM10 appears to go down with income. Uruguay (URY), Sudan (SDN) and Bangladesh (BGD) had very high levels; Saudi Arabia (SAU) and Kuwait (KWT) had high levels even though their per capita GDP levels were high. The boxplot (on the *left* of the scatter plot) shows that the lower quartile of PM10 in 2009 was 18, the median was about 30 and the upper quartile was 50. The distribution was highly positively skewed. *Source* World Development Indicators, World Bank (2012)

(United Arab Emirates) saw large falls in PM10. The distribution was highly negatively skewed.

Developing countries experience not only modern pollution but also traditional pollution. An indicator of improvement in traditional pollution is percentage of population with access to improved water source. Time series for the years 1990–2010 are plotted in Fig. 1.7. Kenya, Indonesia, India, and China start low and increase rapidly. Mexico, Russia and Brazil start high and continue up.

Improved water source is correlated with the logarithm of per capita GDP (Fig. 1.8); the variation in its distribution between countries also goes down with income (Fig. 1.8). Comoros (COM) had a high percentage of reported improved water source relative to per capita GDP in contrast to Ethiopia (ETH), Angola (AGO) and Papua New Guinea (PNG). The boxplot indicates that the median in 2010 was high but the distribution was negatively skewed (Fig. 1.8). In Fig. 1.9, if one disregards the outlying countries with high and low changes in logarithm of

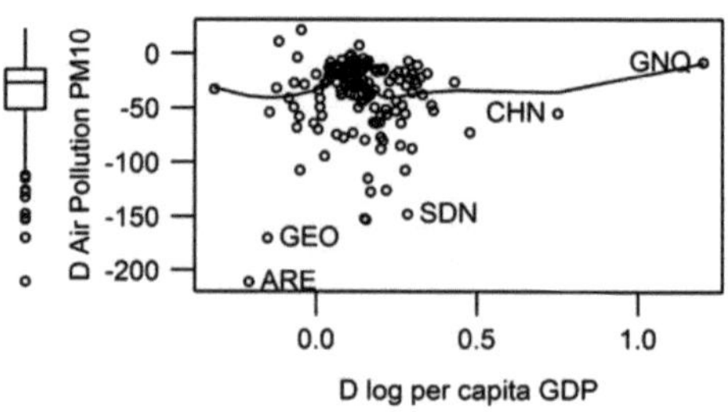

Fig. 1.6 Scatter plot for the change (D) in PM10 for countries between 1990 and 2009 versus the change in logarithm of GDP per capita in the same period. The *line* is flat, correlation is low. In the boxplot to the *left* of the scatter plot, the lower quartile of change in PM10 was −52, the median was −27, and the upper quartile was −15. Sudan (SDN), Georgia (GEO) and United Arab Emirates (ARE) saw large falls in PM10. The distribution was highly negatively skewed. *Source* World Development Indicators, World Bank (2012)

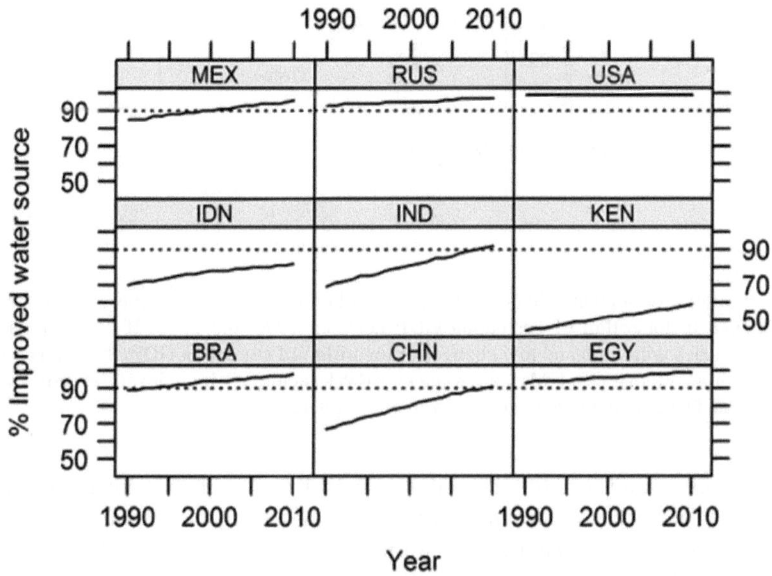

Fig. 1.7 Time series for the years 1990–2010 of percentage of population with access to improved water source. Kenya, Indonesia, India, and China start low and increase rapidly. Mexico, Russia and Brazil start high and continue up. *Source* World Development Indicators, World Bank (2012)

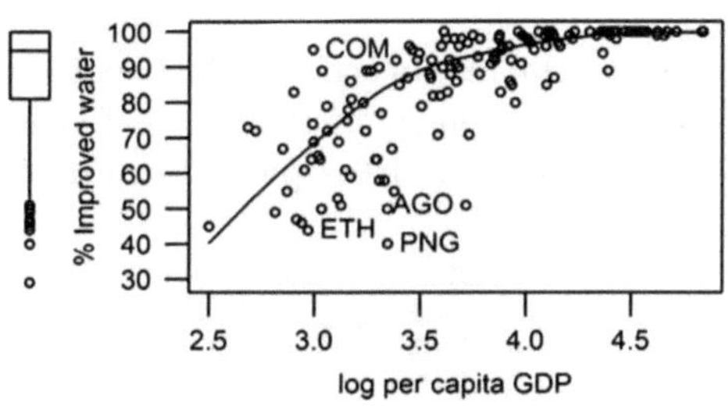

Fig. 1.8 Scatter plot of percentage of population with access to improved water source versus logarithm per capita GDP in 2010. The upward slope tapers off as countries reach 100 %. Improved water source is correlated with logarithm of per capita GDP. Comoros (COM) had a high percentage of reported improved water source relative to per capita GDP in contrast to Ethiopia (ETH), Angola (AGO) and Papua New Guinea (PNG). The boxplot indicates that the median in 2010 was high but the distribution was negatively skewed. *Source* World Development Indicators, World Bank (2012)

per capita GDP, the line is flat, with low correlation between change in improved water source and change in logarithm of per capita GDP. Vietnam (VNM) and Malawi (MWI) achieved high levels of improvement (Fig. 1.9).

We have seen that countries have found ways of reducing particulate matter concentration and poor countries are overcoming traditional pollution. Economists use the core economic model to persuade us to look at the issue of pollution in

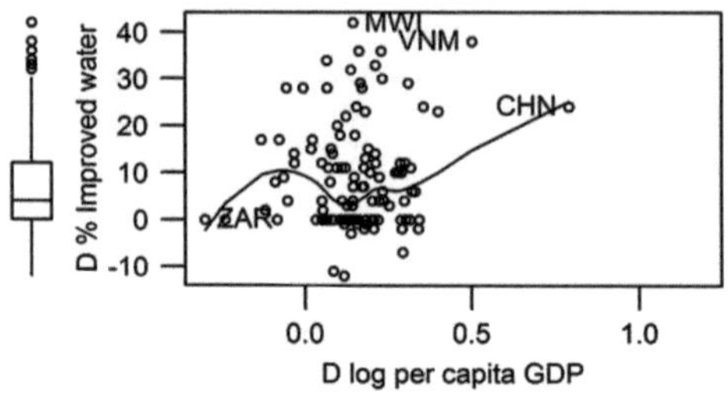

Fig. 1.9 Scatter plot of change in percentage of population with access to improved water source versus change in logarithm of per capita GDP between 1990 and 2010. If one disregards the outlying countries with high and low changes in logarithm of per capita GDP, the *line* is flat, with low correlation. Vietnam (VNM) and Malawi (MWI) achieved high levels of improvement. *Source* World Development Indicators, World Bank (2012)

terms of its costs and benefits. How do we establish the causal effects of pollution on health? When we use economic models to value air pollution in rural areas in developing countries, what role do norms—who does which tasks in a household—play in the analysis? We look at the issues of traditional and modern pollution in Chap. 3.

1.5 Commons and Livelihoods

In several countries in the world, half or more of the population lives in rural areas (Figs. 1.10, 1.11, 1.12) depending on commons such as forests. The time series for % Rural Population from 1962 to 2010 is plotted in Fig. 1.10. After 1980, the

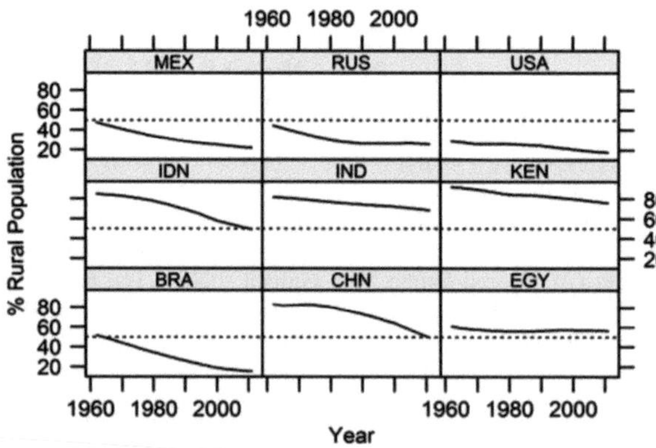

Fig. 1.10 Time series for % Rural population from 1962 to 2010. After 1980, the decline in China's rural population accelerated. Indonesia also saw a large fall in its rural population over this period. Brazil, Mexico and Russia, already below the 50 % reference line in 1960 saw rapid declines. Kenya and India saw moderate declines, while the curve for Egypt was flat. *Source* World Development Indicators, World Bank (2012)

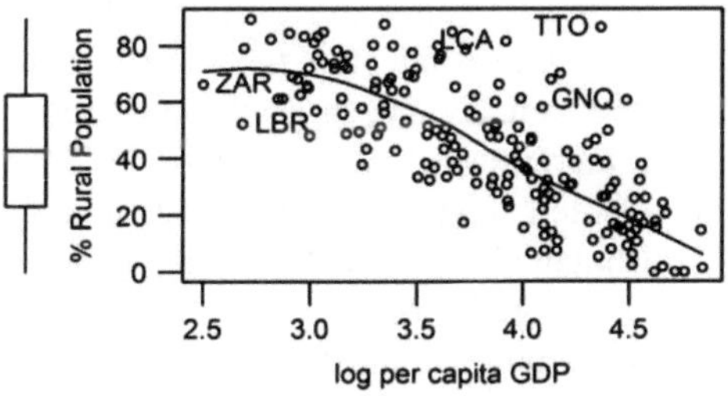

Fig. 1.11 Scatter plot of % Rural Population versus logarithm of per capita GDP in 2010. There is a clear negative correlation between % Rural population and logarithm of per capita GDP. In several countries in the world half or more of the population still lives in rural areas. Trinidad and Tobago (TTO) had a surprisingly high % Rural population; Equatorial Guinea (GNQ) had a high level. *Source* World Development Indicators, World Bank (2012)

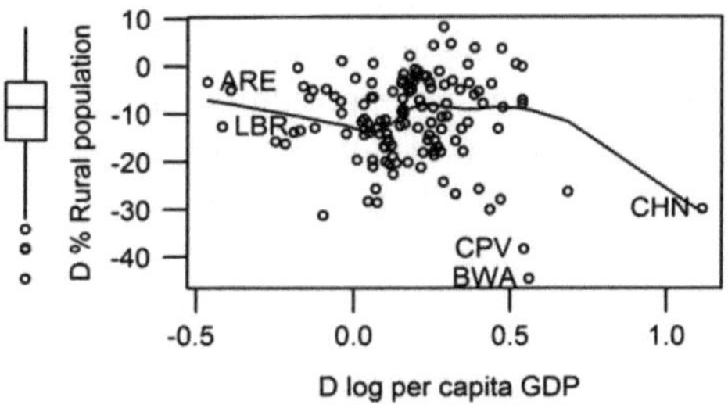

Fig. 1.12 Scatter plot of change in % Rural Population versus change in logarithm of per capita GDP from 1980 to 2010. Most countries experienced a fall in % Rural population, but there is no correlation between change in % Rural population and change in logarithm of per capita GDP if we ignore China. Cape Verde (CPV) and Botswana (BWA) saw huge falls. *Source* World Development Indicators, World Bank (2012)

decline in China's rural population accelerated. Indonesia also saw a large fall in its rural population over this period. Brazil, Mexico and Russia, already below the 50 % reference line in 1960, saw rapid declines. Kenya and India saw moderate declines, while the curve for Egypt was flat. There is a clear negative correlation between % Rural population and logarithm of per capita GDP. In several countries in the world half or more of the population still lives in rural areas. Trinidad and Tobago (TTO) had a surprisingly high % Rural population; Equatorial Guinea (GNQ) had a high level (Fig. 1.11). Most countries experienced a fall in % Rural population, but there is no correlation between change in % Rural population and change in logarithm of per capita GDP if we ignore China; Cape Verde (CPV) and Botswana (BWA) saw huge falls (Fig. 1.12).

Rural households in developing countries are very different from their urban counterparts in both developing and developed countries—in their dependence on local commons, in the organization of their households, in their production and consumption activities, in their vulnerability to traditional pollution, and in the institutions that underpin their daily lives.

Surprisingly there is not much change in forest area. However, the composition of forests may have changed over time. For the indicator forest area (% of land area) for most countries the trend is flat, at a level that reflects geography. India and China show modest increases, Brazil and Indonesia decreases (Fig. 1.13). There is no correlation between % land area under forest and the logarithm of per capita GDP (Fig. 1.14). Bhutan (BTN) and Vietnam (VNM) show large increases in % land area under forest (Fig. 1.15).

Forests are one kind of commons, and forest area is a somewhat coarse indicator—it does not inform us about access, for instance. The Environmentalism of the Poor arose from struggles to keep the commons intact (Guha 2005). A scholarly tradition central to environment and development economics also arose from studies of the commons. Instead of a remorseless tragedy of the commons we now have detailed studies of the management of the commons. How do we establish the causal effect of state or village management on forest cover? When we study the dependence on the commons by rural households, we can use microeconomic models to guide the empirical analysis—when a villager covers a certain distance on foot she incurs an opportunity cost. But is the microeconomic model leaving out the co-evolution of norms and local ecology? We examine the issue of the commons and livelihoods in Chap. 4.

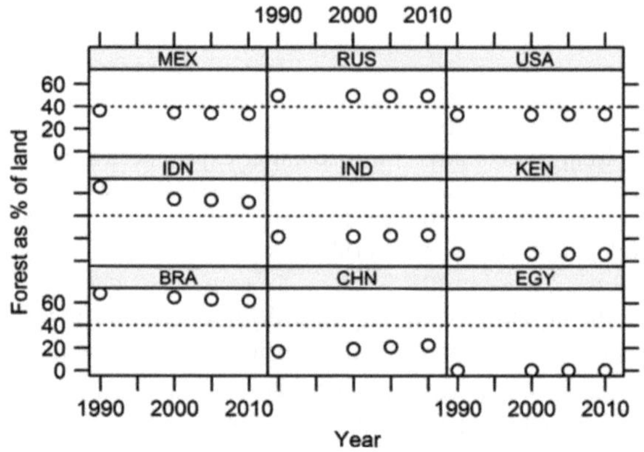

Fig. 1.13 Forest area (% of land area) for select countries from 1990 to 2010. For most countries the trend is flat, at a level that reflects geography. India and China shows modest increases, Brazil and Indonesia decreases. *Source* World Development Indicators, World Bank (2012)

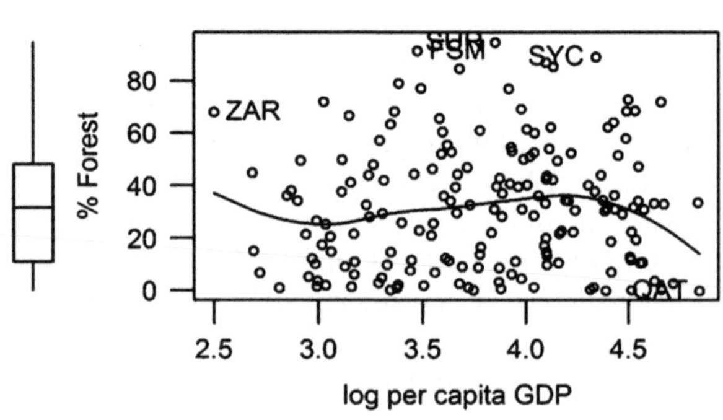

Fig. 1.14 Scatter plot of % Forest Area versus logarithm of per capita GDP in 2010. There is no correlation between % forest area and logarithm of per capita GDP. *Source* World Development Indicators, World Bank (2012)

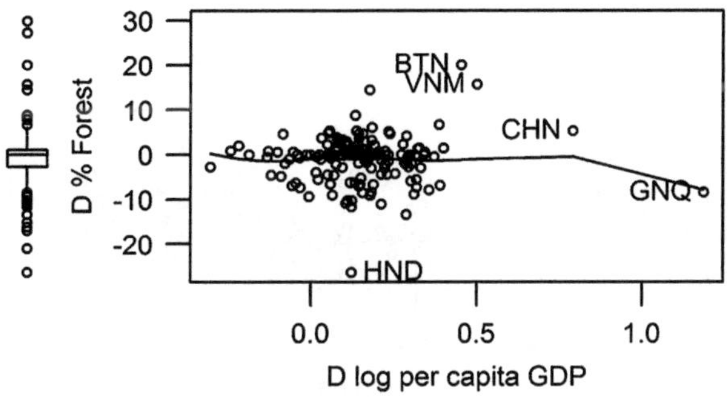

Fig. 1.15 Scatter plot of change in % Forest area versus change in logarithm of per capita GDP between 1990 and 2010. Again no correlation. Bhutan (BTN) and Vietnam (VNM) show large increases in % forest. The median level of change is zero; there are several countries with large positive and negative changes. *Source* World Development Indicators, World Bank (2012)

1.6 Complex Ecology

Ecology is complex. In an attempt to keep ecosystems intact different countries have designated protected areas (PAs) (Figs. 1.16, 1.17, 1.18). In developing countries the interaction of ecology and the livelihoods of rural people who live next to these protected areas is complex. We look at the issue of complex ecology in Chap. 5.

In Fig. 1.16, time series for terrestrial protected areas as percentage of total land area are graphed. Mexico, Russia, Indonesia, Brazil and Egypt saw substantial increases in areas demarcated as PAs (Fig. 1.16). There is no correlation between % area under protected areas and the logarithm of per capita GDP (Fig. 1.17). Venezuela (Ven) and Brunei Darussalam (BRN) have large areas as PAs (Fig. 1.17). Most countries had little or no change in PAs (Fig. 1.18).

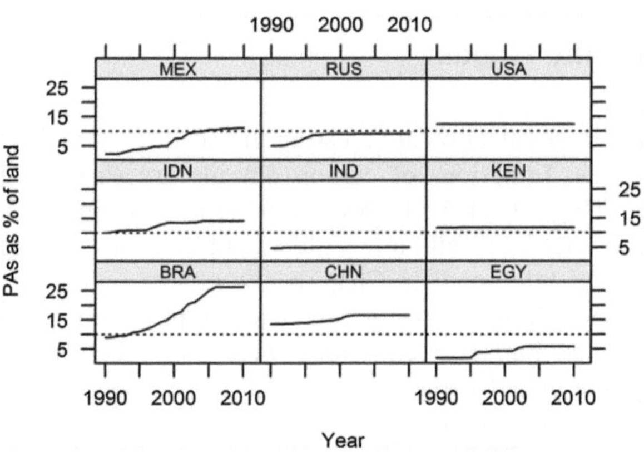

Fig. 1.16 Terrestrial protected areas as % of total land area for select countries from 1990 to 2010. Mexico, Russia, Indonesia, Brazil and Egypt saw substantial increases in areas demarcated as PAs. *Source* World Development Indicators, World Bank (2012)

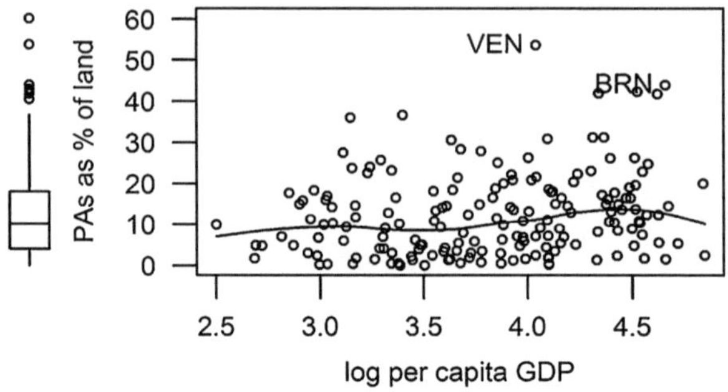

Fig. 1.17 Scatter plot of PAs as % of land area versus logarithm of per capita GDP in 2010. There is no correlation. VEN (Venezuela) and BRN (Brunei Darussalam) have large areas as PAs. Although the median % PA area is modest, the distribution is positively skewed, with a few countries having % PA area at a third or more of land area. *Source* World Development Indicators, World Bank (2012)

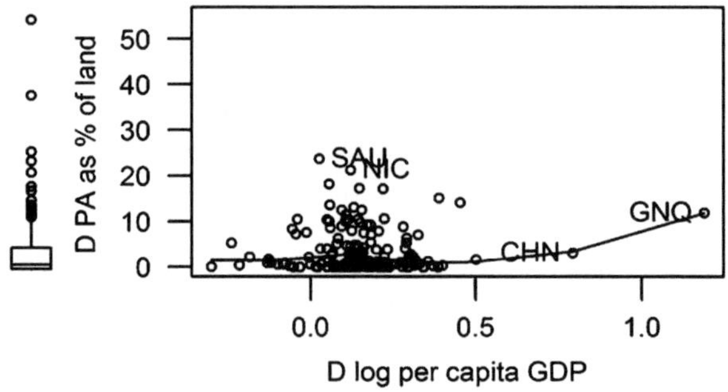

Fig. 1.18 Scatter plot of change in PAs as % of land area versus change in logarithm of per capita GDP from 1990 to 2010. No correlation. Most countries made little or no change in their land area designated as PAs. *Source* World Development Indicators, World Bank (2012)

1.7 Global Public Goods

Globalization and modernization are creating the need for global action to provide global public goods. Emissions of carbon dioxide are strongly correlated with economic growth (Figs. 1.20, 1.21). Merchandise trade (Figs. 1.22, 1.23, 1.24) is associated with another less well known global public good—biological invasions. We address global public goods in Chap. 6.

Mexico, Indonesia, India, Brazil, China, and Egypt saw large increases in CO_2 emissions per capita, but their emissions were still much lower than the US emissions per capita in 2010 (Fig. 1.19). Of all the environmental indicators discussed in this chapter, CO_2 emissions per capita is the most highly correlated with logarithm of per capita GDP (Fig. 1.20). Even the change in logarithm of CO_2 emissions per capita is correlated with the change in logarithm of per capita GDP (Fig. 1.21).

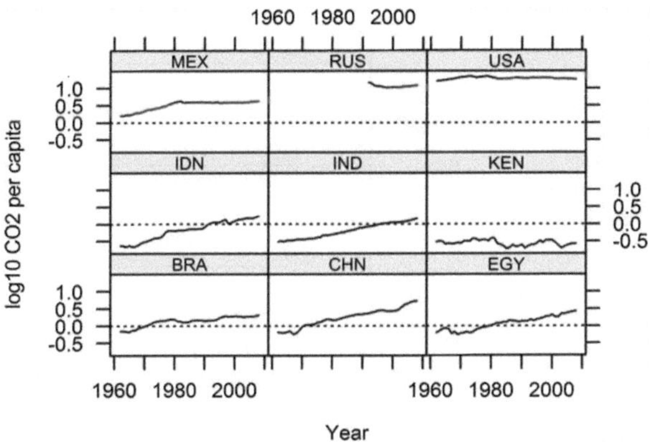

Fig. 1.19 Logarithm of CO_2 emissions per capita (metric tonnes per capita) for select countries from 1962 to 2008. Mexico, Indonesia, India, Brazil, China, and Egypt saw large increases in CO_2 emissions per capita, but their emissions were still much lower than US emissions per capita in 2010. *Source* World Development Indicators, World Bank (2012)

Fig. 1.20 Scatter plot of logarithm of CO_2 emissions per capita versus logarithm of per capita GDP in 2008—we see a high correlation. *Source* World Development Indicators, World Bank (2012)

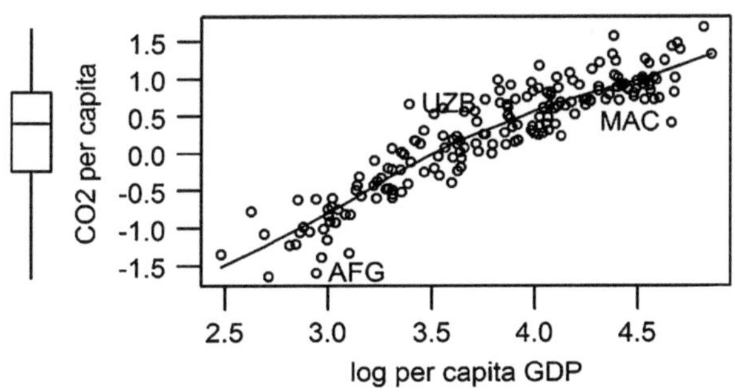

Fig. 1.21 Scatter plot of the change in logarithm of CO_2 emissions per capita versus the change in logarithm of CO_2 per capita from 1962 to 2008. *Source* World Development Indicators, World Bank (2012)

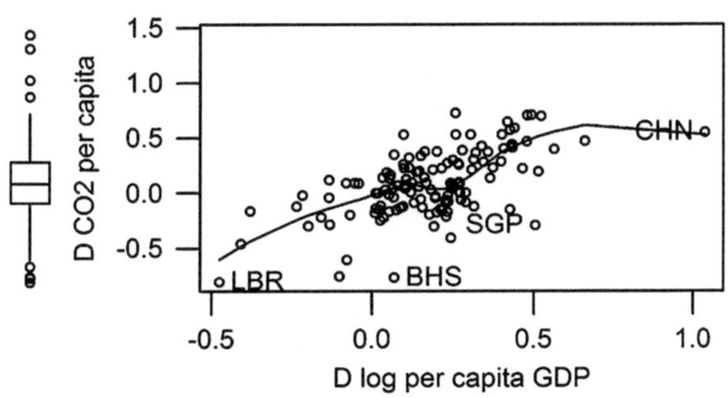

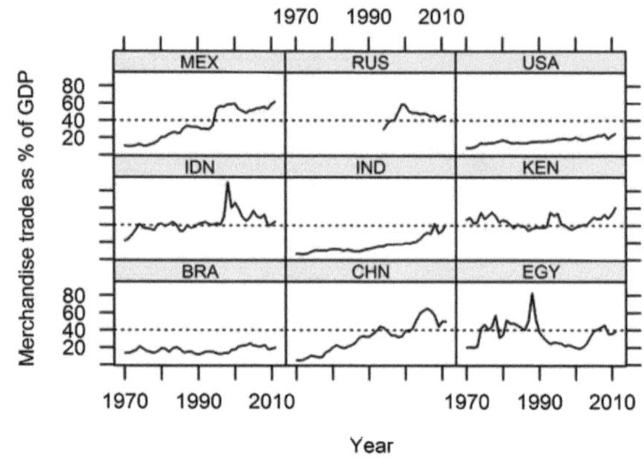

Fig. 1.22 Merchandise trade (% of GDP) from 1970 to 2010. Mexico, China and India saw sustained increases; Russia, Indonesia, Egypt, Kenya saw fluctuations. *Source* World Development Indicators, World Bank (2012)

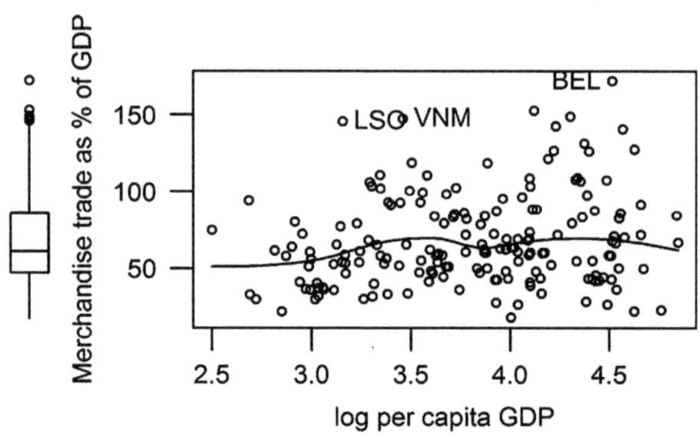

Fig. 1.23 Scatter plot of merchandise trade as % of GDP and logarithm of per capita GDP in 2010—no correlation. *Source* World Development Indicators, World Bank (2012)

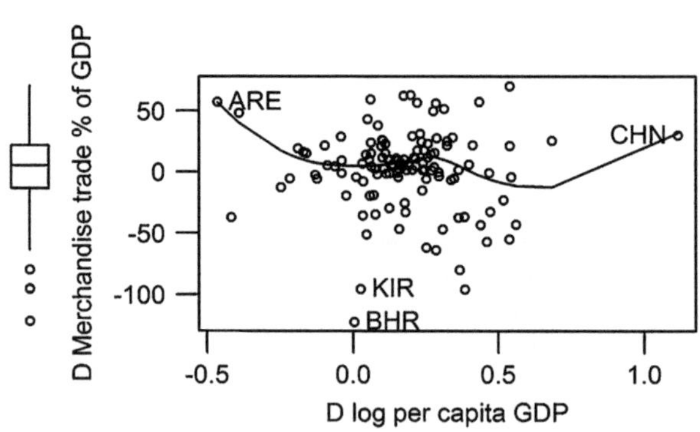

Fig. 1.24 Scatter plot of change in merchandise trade as % of GDP versus change in logarithm of per capita GDP from 1970 to 2010—no correlation. Almost no change in merchandise trade as % of GDP for most countries from 1970 to 2010. *Source* World Development Indicators, World Bank (2012)

Climate change is an environmental issue that has been studied by a large number of economists. A starting point for analyzing climate change is a game theoretic model of public goods. A key issue in climate change and in resource economics in general is the choice of the discount rate, where economists enjoy something like a monopoly of expertise, but disagree among themselves. In developing countries, climate change links up with issues of livelihoods.

Mexico, China and India saw sustained increases in merchandise trade as a % of GDP; Russia, Indonesia, Egypt, Kenya saw fluctuations (Fig. 1.22). Merchandise trade was not correlated with income in 2010 (Fig. 1.23). There was almost no change in merchandise trade as % of GDP for most countries from 1970 to 2010 (Fig. 1.24).

1.8 Sustainable Development

In addressing the issue of sustainable development, economists have focused on correcting the major target of economic policy—gross domestic product. One attempt by the World Bank to correct for environmental depreciation—adjusted net national savings—is notable because it is now computed on an annual basis for most countries (Figs. 1.25, 1.26, 1.27).

China's adjusted net national savings rate rose to almost amazing levels—its large investment in physical capital was much larger than the estimated dissavings due to resource depletion and environmental damages; Russia and India too saw increases; Egypt and the US saw a fall (Fig. 1.25). There is no correlation between adjusted net national savings and the logarithm of per capita GDP. Worryingly several countries have zero or negative levels of adjusted savings (Fig. 1.26). The change in adjusted net savings was adverse for several countries (Fig. 1.27).

Is evaluation for sustainable development not only an issue of the correct application of the right techniques and models, but also about deliberative democracy? Does talk of democracy make some of us feel good, whereas in reality

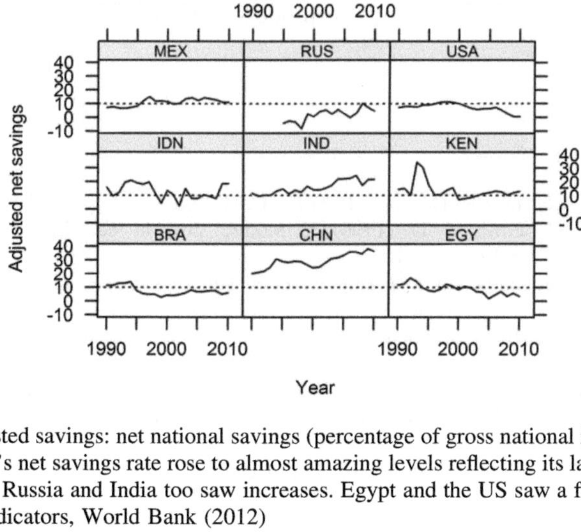

Fig. 1.25 Adjusted savings: net national savings (percentage of gross national income) for select countries. China's net savings rate rose to almost amazing levels reflecting its large investment in physical capital. Russia and India too saw increases. Egypt and the US saw a fall. *Source* World Development Indicators, World Bank (2012)

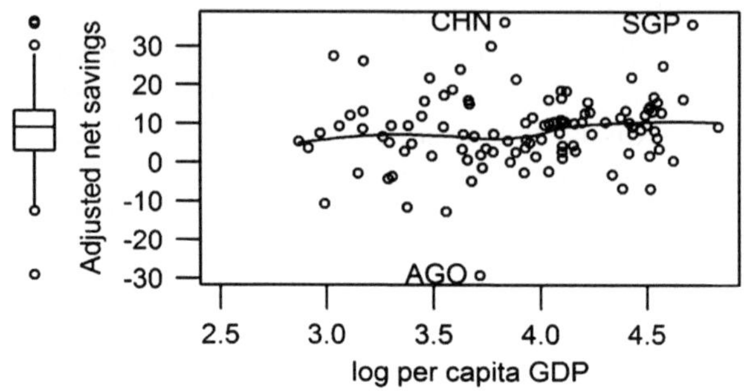

Fig. 1.26 Scatter plot of adjusted net savings versus logarithm of per capita GDP. No correlation. Worryingly, several countries have zero or negative levels of adjusted savings. *Source* World Development Indicators, World Bank (2012)

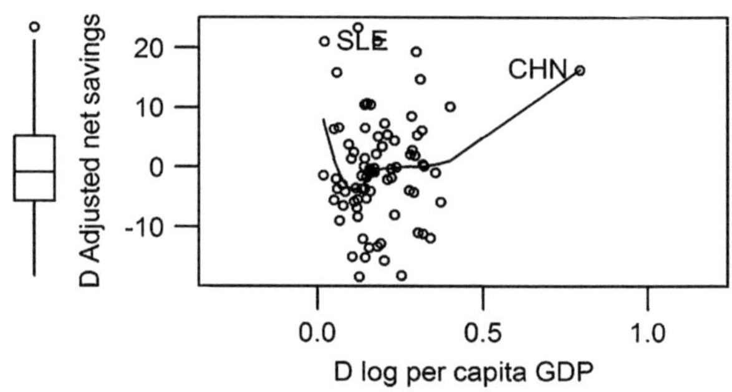

Fig. 1.27 Scatter plot of change in adjusted net savings versus change in the logarithm of per capita GDP. Adjusted net savings were adverse for several countries. *Source* World Development Indicators, World Bank (2012)

mineral resources undermine democracy? If sustainable development is about balancing poverty removal and the environment, how can we establish the causal effects of dams—those most controversial development projects—on poverty? We look at these issues in Chap. 7.

Before we examine different kinds of environmental issues from Chap. 3 onwards, we look at different kinds of models in Chap. 2.

References

Arrow K, Bolin B, Costanza R, Dasgupta P, Folke C, Holling CS, Jansson B-O, Levin S, Maler K-G, Perrings C, Pimentel D (1996) Economic growth, carrying capacity, and the environment. Ecol Appl 6(1):13–15

Berlin I (1953) The hedgehog and the fox: an essay on Tolstoy's view of history. Weidenfeld and Nicolson, London

Daly HE, Farley J (2010) Ecological economics: principles and applications. Island Press, Washington, DC

Dasgupta P, Maler KG (1997) The resource-basis of production and consumption: an economic analysis. In: Dasgupta P, Maler KG (eds) The environment and emerging development issues, vol 1. Oxford University Press, New York

Dryzek JS (2005) The politics of the earth. Oxford University Press, New York

Guha R (2005) The environmentalism of the poor. In: Dryzek JS, Schlosberg D (eds) Debating the earth: the environmental politics reader. Oxford University Press, New York
Hodgson GM, Maki U, McCloskey DN (1992) Plea for a pluralistic and rigorous economics. Am Econ Rev 82:xxv
Meadows DH, Meadows DL, Randers J, Behrens WH III (2005) The nature of exponential growth. In: Dryzek JS, Schlosberg D (eds) Debating the earth: the environmental politics reader. Oxford University Press, New York
Norgaard RB (1989) The case for methodological pluralism. Ecol Econ 1:37–57
Pandit MK, Sodhi NS, Koh LP, Bhaskar A, Brook BW (2006) Unreported yet massive deforestation driving loss of endemic biodiversity in Indian Himalaya. Biodivers Conserv 16(1):153–163
Stern DI (2004) The rise and fall of the environmental Kuznets curve. World Dev 32(8):1419–1439
Tetlock PE (2005) Expert political judgment. Princeton University Press, Princeton
Tietenberg TH, Lewis L (2009) Environmental and natural resource economics. Pearson, Boston
Vatn A (2005) Institutions and the environment. Edward Elgar, Cheltenham
World Bank (1992) World development report 1992: development and the environment. Oxford University Press, New York
World Bank (2012) World development indicators. http://databank.worldbank.org. Accessed 5 Oct 2012

Chapter 2
Models and Frameworks

Abstract I discuss theoretical and empirical models used in environmental economics in a basic manner. I discuss constrained optimization models with an example of a non-renewable resource that is depleted over two periods. I then briefly look at models that use game theory and differential equations. In the discussion of regression models, I use the idea of a causal graph to help distinguish between association and causality. I then briefly set out the institutions and development framework of Elinor Ostrom. I conclude with a framework for thinking about diverse models—both theoretical and statistical.

Keywords Models · Optimization · Game theory · Differential equation · Causality · Statistical

Modern economics uses theoretical and empirical models; in several economics journals, it is difficult to see research articles without a model. Theoretical models are typically mathematical while the empirical models are statistical. Environmental economists use constrained optimization models to capture the essence of choices made by firms or households; these choices have environmental implications. Often, game theory is used to see how actors interact. Theoretical models are often dynamic, using differential equations, which link today's actions to the world tomorrow. Empirical work in environmental economics uses econometrics—the adaptation of statistics by economists—extensively. Increasingly, empirical work aims to establish causality, which is vital to policy, but difficult to establish.

In this chapter I discuss these theoretical and empirical models in a basic manner, briefly, and separately. In the research published in environmental economics journals the models are far more complex, and theoretical and empirical models are often used together. While environmental economics seems to use models universally, it is possible to use alternative frameworks—Nobel Laureate Elinor Ostrom (2009) developed the Institutions and Development Framework, which I discuss briefly at the end of the chapter. I conclude this chapter with a framework to think about models.

V. Dayal, *The Environment in Economics and Development*,
SpringerBriefs in Economics, DOI: 10.1007/978-81-322-1671-1_2,

2.1 Constrained Optimization Models

Economists frequently use constrained optimization models. According to Screpanti and Zamagni (2005, p. 381), 'Samuelson's argument, that all the problems faced by economics (in the neoclassical approach) can be reduced to problems of constrained maximization, was very important.' An objective function is maximized subject to one or more constraints.

In dynamic optimization we consider problems where the choices we make today affect our choices tomorrow.

Consider the extraction of a stock of oil. This will benefit those who consume oil, but will be costly to extract.

Let the net benefits (i.e. benefits minus costs) of extracting Q units of oil be $a\,Q - b/2Q^2 - c\,Q$ and the total oil reserves = R.

We first examine the problem of maximizing net benefits from extracting oil without worrying about the total oil reserves; this gives us the static optimum. We then examine the extraction of oil over two periods, given that total extraction is limited by finite reserves.

If oil is extracted to maximize net benefits in a particular period, the optimal static quantity ($Q^{STATIC*}$) is given by taking the derivative of the net benefits (called marginal net benefits), and equating to zero

$$a - bQ^{STATIC*} - c = 0$$

$$\text{So } Q^{STATIC*} = (a - c)/b.$$

$$\text{If } a = 10,\ c = 2 \text{ and } b = 0.5,\ Q^{STATIC*} = 16.$$

We now consider the dynamic problem. Consider only two periods, now or later, indexed by 0 or 1. Let Q0 and Q1 denote extraction in periods 0 and 1. Then Q0 + Q1 cannot be more than R. If R is more than twice the static optimum extraction, i.e. $Q^{STATIC*}$, then choices now do not affect choices later. If $R < Q^{STATIC*}$, we have a dynamic optimization problem.

We use dynamic optimization to solve this problem. We have a discrete time optimization problem, and will use the Lagrange approach.

In the Lagrange approach, we use a methodological construct—we form an expression called the Lagrangian:

Lagrangian = Objective + Multiplier × Constraint, and then maximize the Lagarangian. This has the added benefit of yielding the multiplier that has an economic interpretation of a 'shadow price'.

In our situation the objective = net benefits in period 0 + net benefits in period 1. The constraint is that Q0 + Q1 = R. Therefore, the Lagrangian, L, is given by:

$$\begin{aligned} L &= \{aQ0 - \tfrac{1}{2}\,b\,Q0^2 - c\,Q0\} + \{[aQ1 - \tfrac{1}{2}\,b\,Q1^2 - c\,Q1]/(1+r)\}], \\ &- \lambda\,[Q0 + Q1 - R], \\ &= \left\{\sum [aQt - \tfrac{1}{2}\,b\,Qt^2 - c\,Qt]/(1+r)^t\right\} - \lambda\,[Q0 + Q1 - R] \end{aligned}$$

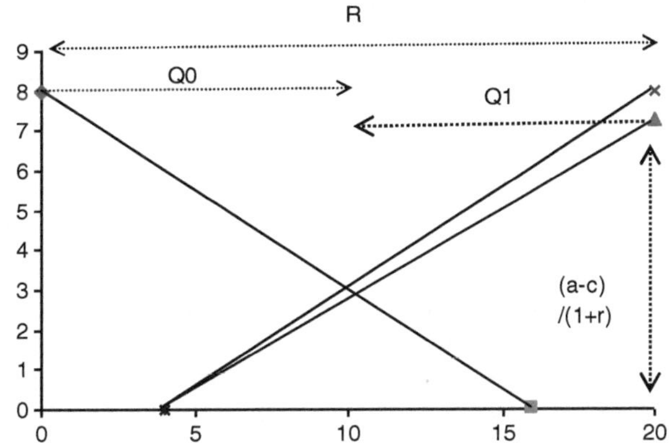

Fig. 2.1 Extraction of oil over two periods. Total resource available (R = 20) is represented on the *horizontal axis*, Q0 (extraction in period zero) goes from *left* to *right*, Q1 (extraction in period one) goes from *right* to *left*; marginal net benefits on the y axis

where λ is the multiplier.

The partial derivative with respect to Q0 $= a - bQ0 - c - \lambda = 0$

The partial derivative with respect to Q1 $= \{[a - bQ1 - c]/(1 + r)\} - \lambda = 0$

$$\text{So } a - bQ0 - c = \{[a - bQ1 - c]/(1 + r)\} \tag{2.1}$$

The marginal net benefit (in present value terms) across the two periods is equated.

This combined with the constraint, gives us the answer. About 10.3 units are used in the first time period and about 9.7 units in the second. Thus more than half the resource should be extracted in the first time period.

Figure 2.1 provides an intuitive feel for the problem. On the x axis we have quantity of oil. Total reserves are 20; moving rightwards from zero we have Q0 and moving leftwards from 20 we have Q1. On the y-axis we plot the marginal net benefits; with the discounted (i.e. divided by 1 + r) net benefit curve for the second period being lower than the undiscounted curve. Where the two net benefit curves for the two periods intersect we have the solution to Eq. 2.1. The higher is r, the more is Q0* relative to Q1*. In other words, we extract more now and leave less for later—a recurrent theme in resource economics. We shall encounter a dynamic optimization model in the Appendix of Chap. 6.

2.2 Game Theory Models

Game theory models help us model interdependent decisions for more than one person. If we consider two persons, each person's decision depends on the other's. While seeming like a purely technical extension of single person optimization, it often leads to quite different insights. Notably, game theory can show the tension between individual and social rationality and its resolution through collective action.

Table 2.1 Payoff matrix for a two player game

Player A	Player B	
	Left	Right
Up	(9, 27)	(3, 24)
Down	(0, 0)	(6, 3)

A game consists of: a set of players; a set of strategies for each player; and the payoffs to each player for every possible list of strategy choices by the players.

We will only study games in which there are two players, each of whom can choose between two strategies. Here, the players are called A and B. Player A has two strategies, called "Up" and "Down". Player B has two strategies, called "Left" and "Right". The table showing the payoffs to both players for each of the four possible strategy combinations is the game's payoff matrix (Table 2.1).

If A plays Up and B plays left then A's payoff is 9 and B's payoff is 27 (Table 2.1). A play of the game is a pair such as (U, L) where the first element is the strategy chosen by A and the second is the strategy chosen by B.

We examine which play is likely given the game's payoff matrix, by examining each cell in Table 2.1 in turn. Here, If B plays Right then A's best reply is Down rather than Up since $6 > 3$. So (U, R) is not a likely play.

If B plays Right then A's best reply is Down. If A plays Down then B's best reply is Right. So (D, R) is a likely play.

A play of the game where each strategy is a best reply to the other is a Nash equilibrium. Our example in Table 2.1 has two Nash equilibria: (U, L) and (D, R). A Nash equilibrium represents individual rationality—it may not be the best outcome for the players collectively; both may be better off with some other play. In Chaps. 3 and 4, we will see examples of the Prisoner's Dilemma where individual rationality is at odds with collective rationality.

2.3 Differential Equation Models

Differential equations are used commonly in the physical and natural sciences, and extensively in mathematical ecology.

In a differential equation, a variable is changing continuously with time, and the change in the variable is described by the equation.

An example is $y = dx/dt = x$; here the change in x is itself a variable and equal to x. Visualizing this gives us an insight into the evolution of x over time (Fig. 2.2).

If $x = 0$ then $dx/dt = 0$, i.e. x will not change. We say that $x = 0$ is an equilibrium. If $x = 1$ then $dx/dt = 1$, so x will increase. If $x = -1$, then $dx/dt = -1$, so x will decrease. Because a slight push to x from $x = 0$ will result in x moving further away, we say that $x = 0$ is an unstable equilibrium (Fig. 2.2).

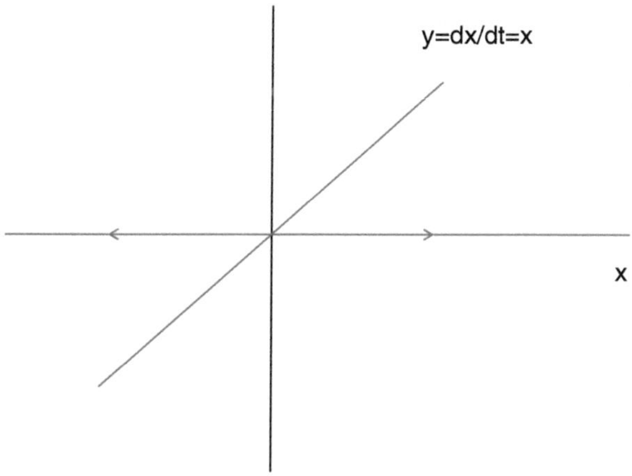

Fig. 2.2 Graph of y = dx/dt (= x) versus x. There is an unstable equilibrium at x = 0

If y = dx/dt = −x, then by similar reasoning, y = 0 will be a stable equilibrium (Fig. 2.3).

Stewart (2010) explains how mathematical models can help us probe beyond the surface. Non-linear dynamics can be complex. A graph of carbon (C) and temperature (T) over time (t) gives the impression that because temperature leads carbon, carbon dioxide emissions are not causing changes in temperature. We need to first model the natural process and Stewart uses non-linear differential equations to model the mutual dependence of carbon and temperature (Fig. 2.4), the equations are such that temperature leads carbon in a graph of their time series. The set of equations (Stewart 2010, p. 168) is: (1) $dT/dt = \sin t - 0.25\ C - 0.01\ T^2$, and (2) $dC/dt = 0.1\ T - 0.01\ C^2$.

To this natural process we can add the shock to the system because of high emissions of carbon dioxide by human beings (Fig. 2.5). In the resulting output

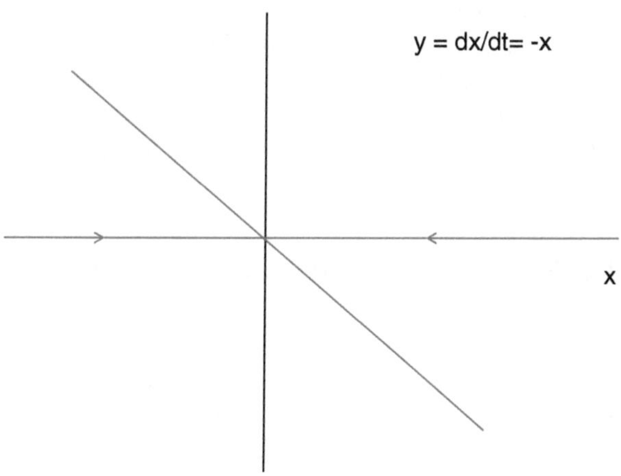

Fig. 2.3 Graph of y or dx/dt (= −x) versus x. There is a stable equilibrium at x = 0

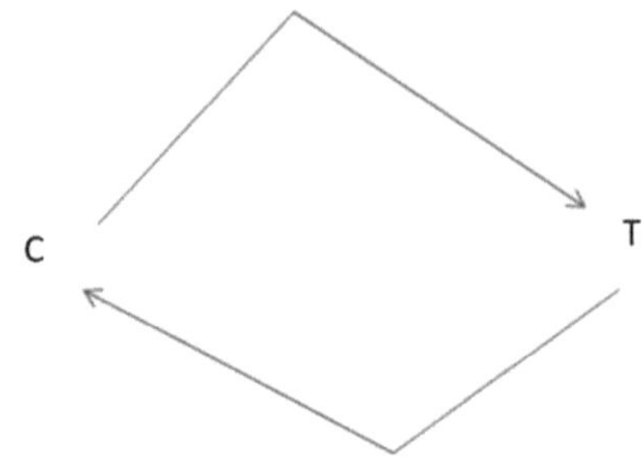

Fig. 2.4 Natural process (in which C and T cause each other) modeled by Ian Stewart; the resulting graph of time series of output of natural process shows T leading C

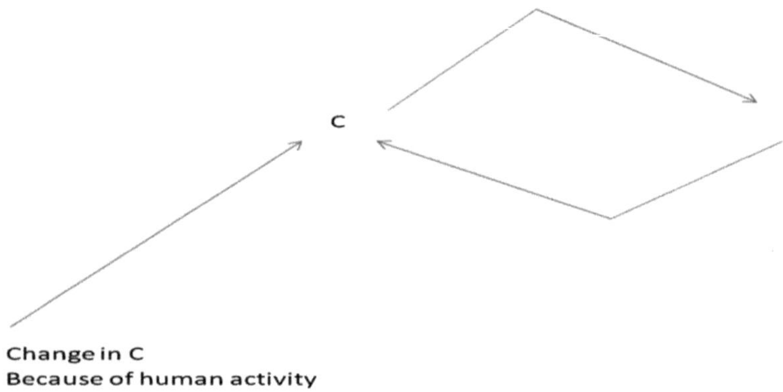

Fig. 2.5 Human intervention leading to increases in C, graph of time series still shows T leading C

from the model, although we have increased carbon dioxide from outside the system, temperature continues to lead carbon dioxide. However, if a change in temperature is plotted along with the change in carbon dioxide over time, we see that the temperature increases at the same time as the increase in carbon dioxide.

In other words, in the model Stewart (2010) created with non-linear differential equations, although carbon dioxide causes temperature, the appearance of the system as captured in time series graphs would lead to a superficial, and wrong, impression that temperature causes carbon dioxide emissions. Chapter 5 on complex ecology uses simple differential equations.

2.4 Regression Models and Causality

In a regression model we have observations on a dependent variable, say y, and one or more independent variables, say x. y is likely to be related to x, or we think it is, but not exactly, so we model this as

$$y = \beta 1 + \beta 2\ x + \varepsilon$$

where ε is a disturbance term.

Econometricians often use the notion of a data generating process—we observe data that has been generated in the world by some process and we hope to use regression to recover that. One of the key assumptions of the classical linear regression model, the specification assumption, is that we can estimate the dependent variable as a linear function of some independent variables plus a disturbance term (Kennedy 2003). For example, if the data generating process for example is $y = 0.2 + 20\ x$, then a regression of y on x helps us recover the equation—we use a formula to estimate $\beta 2$ so that we come as close to 20 (the true value) as possible.

Regressions may indicate correlation or association rather than causality.

Causality is important because it is implicit in assertions on, or advocacy of, policies. We can distinguish between regression that is predictive or descriptive (conditional expectation) and regression that is causal.

The difficulty in dealing with causal issues is related to the nature of the research questions and the complexity of the systems. For example, we can contrast the following two questions: (1) which of the following interventions has a greater effect on educational outcomes, school bag or blackboard, versus (2) what are the causes of deforestation in different countries? The causal issue is easier in the case of the effect of interventions on educational outcomes than in the case of the causes of deforestation. Pearl (1999) emphasizes the distinction between causal thinking and probability theory:

> The word cause is not in the vocabulary of standard probability theory. It is an embarrassing yet inescapable fact that probability theory, the official language of many empirical sciences, does not permit us to express sentences such as 'Mud does not cause rain'; all we can say is that the two events are mutually correlated, or dependent—meaning that if we find one, we can expect to encounter the other. Scientists seeking causal explanations for complex phenomena or rationales for policy decisions must therefore supplement the language of probability with a vocabulary for causality, one in which the symbolic representation for the causal relationship 'Mud does not cause rain' is distinct from the symbolic representation for 'Mud is independent of rain' (p. 1)

To summarize, we use probability for empirical work, but causal thinking requires us to put in a directional arrow: rain → mud. A regression $Y = a + b\ X1 + c\ X2 + e$ can be interpreted predictively or causally. Predictively, we say the regression gives us the conditional expectation of Y. If we interpret it causally, we have in mind an implicit causal graph (as in Fig. 2.6); the correctness of this causal interpretation depends on the correctness of the implicit causal graph for the situation that we are studying. If the causal pathways do not correspond with what appears in Fig. 2.6, then the causal interpretation is problematic.

If we want to explore the effect of X on Y, following Morgan and Winship (2007), we can list the key ingredients of causal graphs as follows:

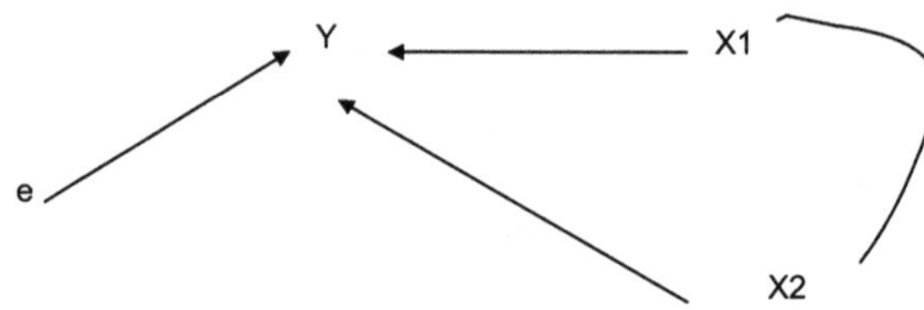

Fig. 2.6 Implicit causal graph for regression $Y = a + b\,X1 + c\,X2 + e$

- Common cause (controlling for M, the common cause, will block path): X ← M → Y. Here M causes X as well as Y.
- Mediator (controlling for Z, will block path): X → Z → Y. Here X causes Z and Z causes Y.
- Collider (controlling for B, opens path): X → B → Y. Here X and Y are both causes of B.

Whether we should control for a variable depends on whether it is a common cause, a mediator, or a collider. However, we need to see the causal graph as a whole. Figure 2.7 illustrates three specification options for studying the effect of X on Y, given the causal graph.

The intuition for excluding the collider is best given with an example. Assume a situation where a car fails to start in cold weather when there is petrol in the tank. While petrol in the tank of a car and very cold weather are uncorrelated, they can be common causes of a car failing to start in cold climates. The car not starting is the collider. Whether there is petrol in the car or not tells me nothing about cold weather. But if my car fails to start, and there is petrol in the tank, I would guess that cold weather is the cause.

If we wish to study the causal effect of X on Y, we can also experimentally vary X and see how the outcome of the experiment, Y, varies between the 'treatment' and the 'control' group. In this case we free X from the influence of M if our experiment is carefully designed. In the next chapter, we will look at John Snow's famous use of a 'natural experiment' to study cholera. In Chap. 4, we see how

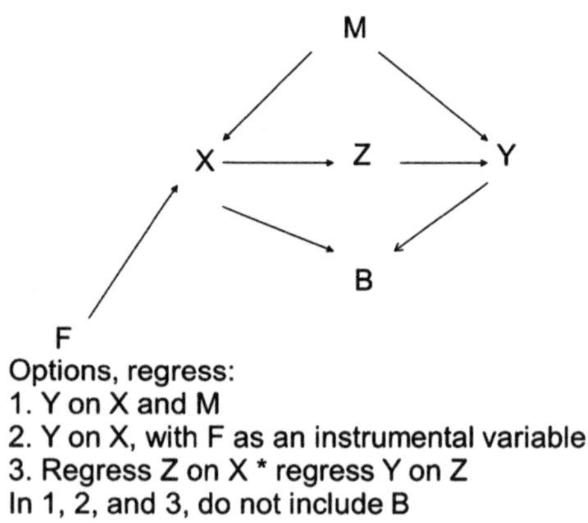

Fig. 2.7 Causal graph and regression options

Somanathan and co-authors used regression and matching to establish the effects of management regime on forest stock. In Chap. 6, we discuss the causal issues that arise while studying carbon storage and livelihoods. In Chap. 7, we see two applications that use the method of instrumental variables to overcome simultaneous causation bias.

2.5 The Institutions and Development Framework

Vatn (2005) distinguishes between three different kinds of institutions: conventions, norms and formally sanctioned rules. But Vatn (2005) sees a tension between the individualist and social constructivist positions in the social sciences with regard to the approach to institutions—a tension that can be plotted in terms of the direction of causality between individuals and institutions. As Hodgson (2000) puts it: “In the writings of Veblen and Commons there is both upward and downward causation; individuals create and change institutions, just as institutions mold and constrain individuals” (p. 326). Ostrom (2005) points out that institutional analysis requires “digging deeper than markets and hierarchies” (p. 819), the analyst has to recognize institutions that are often intangible, and not easily measurable. Alston (1996) also draws attention to the difficulty of observing institutions quantitatively:

> Institutional changes usually have some unique features limiting the data points and thus generally preventing conventional statistical analysis … Frequently, quantitative measures of the causes or consequences of institutional change are simply not available; even when they are available, better evidence may come from the qualitative historical record (pp. 29–30).

In this brief I focus on models. But we can think of frameworks—which are more general than models—and include more elements of reality. A framework may include more than one model. The Nobel Laureate Elinor Ostrom developed the Institutions and Development framework. In this framework, the context influences the action arena and interactions, which lead to outcomes (see Fig. 2.8). Outcomes can feedback into the context and the action arena and interactions. In the case of some action arenas and interactions, these may be represented by a game theory model. Among the contextual or exogenous variables are rules or institutional arrangements. Thus, we have a more inclusive view—institutions can help resolve social dilemmas represented by game theory models. Rules and

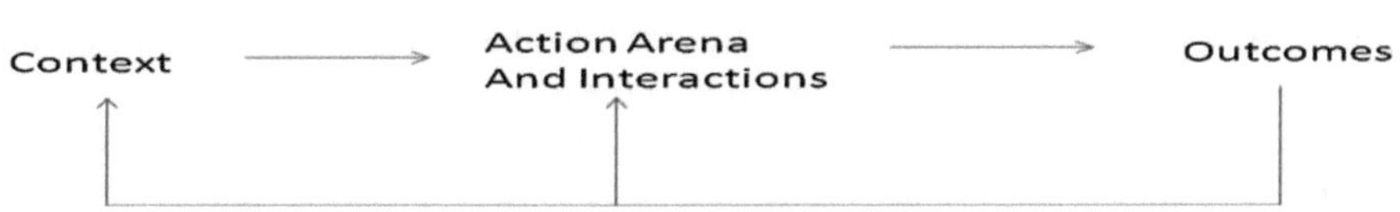

Fig. 2.8 The institutions and development framework

Table 2.2 Four-fold classification of goods

	Excludable	Non-excludable
Rival	Private goods, e.g. coffee cup	Common-pool resources, e.g. forests, fisheries
Non-rival	Club goods, e.g. cable TV	Public goods, e.g. reducing greenhouse gases

institutional arrangements can be examined at multiple levels—operational and collective choice (rules for making rules) levels.

Although Ostrom (2009) worked with experiments to study game theory models in the laboratory, she also documented the immense variety of rules that are used by people in the world. The framework was also used when she and her co-workers conducted a meta-analysis—to systematically learn from diverse studies of the commons.

In her Nobel lecture, Ostrom (2009) said that she and her colleagues found that the focus on two organizational forms—the state and the market—did not do justice to the wide variety of institutional arrangements that humans design. They found that the assumption of rational individuals worked well in certain market situations, but was inadequate in diverse social dilemmas. They rejected Samuelson's two-fold classification of goods—private and public. James Buchanan had developed the concept of club goods, and Ostrom and her colleagues added a fourth type of good, common pool resources (Table 2.2). Common pool resources like forests and fisheries, which are non-excludable and rival, affect millions of people in developing countries. Reducing greenhouse gases is a global public good—it is non-excludable and non-rival (Table 2.2).

2.6 Conclusions and Pointers: A Framework for Thinking about Diverse Models—Both Theoretical and Statistical

Dasgupta (2002), responding to critics of modern economics, said that most economists go ahead and do economic analysis. I think there is an element of truth in the observation that modern economists aim to master sophisticated techniques in their training and then use them, and don't spend their time on philosophical reflection. However, Bromley (2006, p. 87), who could be regarded as a critic of standard economics, reflects on how economists fix belief: 'The standard approach to economics is embedded in the hypothetico-deductive method. On this approach, primitive axioms (covering laws) inform the search for particular assumptions and applicability postulates that will then suggest hypotheses to be tested against data from the "real" world. The axioms entail postulates of rationality, self-interest, stable preferences, and the alleged desire to maximize utility. Indeed, the core axioms of economic theory are rarely subjected to tests of their veracity.'

Bromley's discussion is deep and sophisticated, requiring repeated study. He does not explicitly discuss statistical models. He does, however, distinguish between mechanical cause and reason—if a man switches on a light, the switch is the mechanical cause of the light coming on, but not the reason.

King (1998) attempted to unify the methodology of political science, but he does so under a general theory of statistical inference. King et al. (1994) aimed to include even qualitative inquiry under such a theory. The purpose here is not to unify like the hedgehog, but to consider plural extensions of core economic models, like the fox. In this framework I identify elements of diverse models.

In this brief, while discussing statistical models, I pay attention to issues of causality, and I use informal causal graphs, thus drawing on Pearl's pioneering formal work on causal graphs. I view a causal graph as implicit in a statistical model, with a theoretical model helping us think about a causal graph. Here, I think of environment and development economics as resulting from an interplay between theoretical and statistical models.

We make use of models (M) in environment and development economics; both theoretical models (M^T) and statistical models (M^S).

2.6.1 Theoretical Models

A theoretical model (M^T) can be thought of as having the following list of attributes, listed below:

M^T: $Tech^T$, A^T, V^T

where $Tech^T$ represents a technique (for example, game theory); A^T denotes assumptions and axioms; and V^T denotes variables. The technique used could be mathematical or verbal. Assumptions and axioms are to some extent tied to the technique—constrained optimization techniques in neoclassical microeconomics use the axiom of rationality (Bromley 2006). Over a long period, the average economist invests in such techniques, so such axioms may become part of the economist's mental reflexes. The set of variables V^T varies from problem to problem. In neoclassical economics V^T is usually prices and quantities.

2.6.2 Statistical Models

A statistical model, M^S, can be thought of as having the following list of attributes: a set of variables V^S, a causal graph CG, a set of parameters that are to be estimated θ, a technique T^S, and statistical assumptions A^S. We would have data on the variables V^S, which may be seen to be connected with an implicit, default causal graph or an explicit causal graph (see Figs. 2.6 and 2.7). When we use regressions, the parameters we estimate would include the coefficients and their standard errors. Often attention is centred on the 'significance' (often equated with statistical significance) of θ, A^S, and not so much on CG.

A particular economic analysis addresses a specific problem, by harnessing elements of a theoretical model (M^T) and/or elements of a statistical model (M^S). A problem may be framed in a new way by mapping a model used for a different purpose to the phenomenon being studied—we may use models of investment not just for the stock of machinery but also investment in human capital (education), or nature (forest preservation). We may go from the output of a regression of sulphur dioxide on per capita income to the metaphor of the Environmental Kuznets Curve, and develop a theoretical model—i.e. go from M^S to M^T. Or we may go from a theoretical model of monetary valuation of air pollution to a statistical model—i.e. go from M^T to M^S.

References

Alston LJ (1996) Empirical work in institutional economics: an overview. In: Alston LJ, Eggertson E, North DC (eds) Empirical studies in institutional change. Cambridge University Press, New York

Bromley DW (2006) Sufficient reason. Princeton University Press, Princeton

Dasgupta P (2002) Modern economics and its critics. In: Maki U (ed) Fact and fiction in economics. Cambridge University Press, Cambridge

Hodgson GM (2000) What is the essence of institutional economics? J Econ Issues 34(2):317–329

Kennedy P (2003) A guide to econometrics. The MIT Press, Cambridge

King G (1998) Unifying political methodology: the likelihood theory of statistical inference. The University of Michigan Press, Ann Arbor

King G, Keohane R, Verba V (1994) Designing social inquiry. Princeton University Press, Princeton

Morgan SL, Winship C (2007) Counterfactuals and causal inference. Cambridge University Press, Cambridge

Ostrom E (2005) Doing institutional analysis: digging deeper than markets and hierarchies. In: Menard C, Shirley MM (eds) Handbook of new institutional economics. Springer, Dordrecht

Ostrom E (2009) Beyond markets and states: polycentric governance of complex economic systems. Nobel Prize Lecture, Stockholm

Pearl J (1999) Graphs, causality and structural equation models. In: Ader HJ, Mellenbergh GJ (eds) Research methodology in the social, behavioral and life sciences. Sage University Press, London

Screpanti E, Zamagni S (2005) An outline of the history of economic thought. Oxford University Press, New Delhi

Stewart I (2010) Professor Stewart's Hoard of mathematical treasures. Profile Books, London

Vatn A (2005) Institutions and the environment. Edward Elgar, Cheltenham

Chapter 3
Traditional and Modern Pollution

Abstract Pollution is a key concern in environmental economics, and economists have used their models to argue that this market failure can be overcome by harnessing market signals. The simple model of pollution control makes the argument clear, but in practice, developing countries use diverse instruments to control industrial pollution. In developing countries traditional pollution is a major cause of disease. We want to reduce pollution because we think it has harmful effects, but how do we establish our knowledge of its effects? Establishing the causality convincingly is difficult, but was done by John Snow in the middle of the nineteenth century in the case of cholera. The simple model of pollution control suggests that we consider the benefit of pollution control, but how do we establish them? For many, environmental economics is synonymous with monetary valuation. Monetary valuation is achieved by using a theoretical model along with an econometric one. In a developing country context, if we dig deeper, we may recognize the role of norms.

Keywords Pollution · Valuation · Norms

3.1 Introduction

People in developing and developed countries face different environmental risks. In developing countries traditional forms of pollution—indoor air pollution from burning solid fuels and unsafe water and sanitation—are greater environmental risks than modern air and water pollution. According to the Global Health Risk report of the WHO (2009), in low and middle income countries in 2004, the following percentages of deaths were attributable to different risk factors: 3.9 % to indoor smoke from solid fuels, 3.8 % to unsafe water, sanitation and hygiene and 1.9 % to urban outdoor air pollution. In contrast, in high income countries, urban outdoor air pollution is the main environmental risk—with 2.5 % of deaths attributable to it (WHO 2009).

V. Dayal, *The Environment in Economics and Development*, SpringerBriefs in Economics, DOI: 10.1007/978-81-322-1671-1_3,

The core economic model of pollution is a theoretical model that asks us to weigh the costs and benefits of pollution not absolutely (pollute or not)—but in terms of an extra unit (at the margin). Although the core economic model suggests that we should use economic instruments, in practice, diverse instruments have been used, as we see in the first extension. In the next extension we see that we can use statistical models to establish the effects of pollution and intervention programmes. In the third extension, we examine physical and social complexities related to the economic framework for understanding air pollution. In the appendix we compare different aspects of two theoretical models of pollution.

3.2 Core Economic Model: Balancing Costs and Benefits of Pollution Control

The economics of pollution control is one of the key areas of environmental economics. In the economic approach we examine the benefits and costs of controlling pollution (Fig. 3.1).

We want to maximize: total benefits (B), total costs (C) of reducing pollution (R). We can think of B–C as the surface of a hill, and its maximum is like the top of a hill, where the slope of the hill is zero. In other words, B–C will not change with a very small change in R, or more precisely in the language of calculus, the derivative of B–C with respect to R is zero. It follows that MB = MC or marginal benefit = marginal cost, or the change in benefit from a small change in R is equal to the change in cost from a small change in R when we are maximizing benefits. In Fig. 3.2 the optimum abatement of pollution is at q* (Fig. 3.2). However, if the polluter has no legal requirement to reduce pollution, we are not likely to see any significant reduction in pollution.

We could examine the pollution reduction issue somewhat mathematically with an emphasis on 'marginal' and 'optimal'; and undoubtedly there is great merit in seeing the benefits and the costs of pollution. Yet, another way of framing the issue is to put the label 'polluter' next to marginal abatement cost, and the label 'victim' next to marginal damage cost. The polluter may be a giant factory, and the victim may be a powerless villager; we are then likely to be indignant. We are then thinking of equity as a criterion for policy. Bromley and Anderson (2012) emphasize that legal recognition of the rights of the victim is an important

Fig. 3.1 The economic approch to pollution

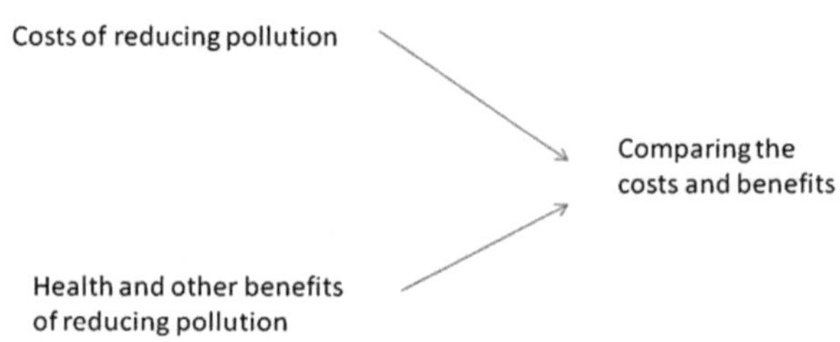

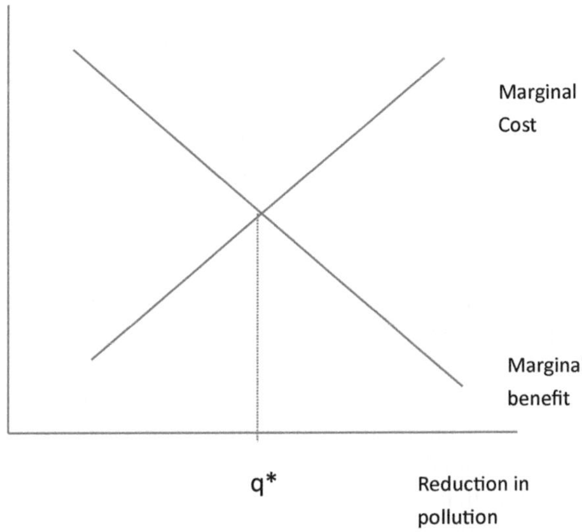

Fig. 3.2 Marginal benefit and marginal cost of reducing pollution; the optimal level of reduction is q*

prerequisite to the management of pollution. This, they assert, is likely to follow a change in society's attitude to pollution.

Once the rights of the polluter are recognized, how should pollution be reduced? Should the pollution agency lay down guidelines for factories, or mandate the use of particular technologies for reducing pollution? An alternative is to use the analogy of prices that signal information to market participants—the government can impose a tax on pollution. If the tax rate is suitably calibrated it leads the polluter to compare the costs of reducing pollution with the tax rate; it also rewards a factory that finds new ways of reducing pollution.

3.3 Extension 1: Implementing a System of Market Signals for Cost-Effective Pollution Control

The core externalities model has the germ of an idea, a way of looking at the issue of pollution. It is not a detailed manual for implementation. Implementation in the real world is often context specific with path dependencies, learning by doing, and interactions between regulators, polluters and society in general. In the core externalities model we ignore the issue of monitoring and enforcement, the capacity of the pollution-regulating agency, or where information will be generated on the costs of damage and abatement.

Sterner and Coria (2012) discuss the experience in developing countries of using policy instruments for industrial pollution. They emphasize the role of institutions, in particular, for monitoring and enforcement. They also stress that apart from efficiency, 'Considerable attention must be paid to distributional, informational and political criteria as well as to the process of policy implementation itself.' (p. 397). Sterner and Coria (2012) provide examples of the implementation of instruments for pollution control in China, Indonesia and Mexico, which I summarize below.

In 1979, China enacted legislation enabling the use of pollution levies, and actual implementation began a few years later. Fees were paid only if emissions were more than a certain level. Most of the fees were used to finance abatement by industry. Fees were low and less than what was necessary to bring about compliance with standards.

According to Sterner and Coria, developing countries used voluntary agreements to overcome poor enforcement of environmental regulations. In Mexico, ten voluntary agreements with about 600 firms were signed during the 1990s. In 1992, the Clean Industry Programme was created. It was an auditing programme—plants paid for an environmental audit. If necessary, they cleaned up. Eventually, once they complied with regulations, they were certified as clean. In Mexico, it appeared that dirty firms were attracted to this programme to get good publicity and avoid penalties by regulators. In contrast, in developed countries already clean firms used voluntary agreements to establish their credentials.

According to Sterner and Coria (2012), in Indonesia, 'the risks of ineffective monitoring, weak enforcement, and even corruption were obvious'(p. 385). The regulatory agency chose to use a rating system: Programme for Pollution Control Evaluation and Rating (PROPER). Simple and clear labels were used. The best rating was gold, and this indicated world-class clean technology and waste-minimization and pollution prevention efforts. The worst was black, which indicated serious environmental damage and no pollution-control effort. In 1995, 187 plants were covered, and two-thirds of them were not complying with regulations. These ratings began to be disclosed publicly and over time, more firms were included in the programme.

3.4 Extension 2: Causal Analysis for Pollution

In the core economic model of pollution, we had a curve representing the marginal benefits of reducing pollution. In practice it is hard to establish the effects of pollution. This may also be crucial in the courts, which cannot act without evidence. It is instructive to go back in time in a currently developed country—to London in the middle of the nineteenth century. John Snow studied the cause of cholera, showing that it was spread by water and not by a miasma as was then believed. Some statisticians like Freedman (1991) have warned us about the pitfalls of using regression analysis for causal inference. However, Freedman (1991) praised John Snow's careful work on cholera, which used 'shoe leather and logic' (p. 300) (i.e. field work and logic) rather than statistical techniques to arrive at causal inferences.

When cholera broke out in the Broad Street area of London in 1854, John Snow carefully mapped the location of victims and community pump-wells, and found that the victims tended to be close to the Broad Street pump. John Snow suspected that the pump on Broad Street was contaminated, but failed to establish that. However, the discovery of the bacterium Vibrio cholerae only came in 1886 (Tufte 1997).

It was Snow's use of a natural experiment that anticipated one of the important ways of establishing causality today (Freedman 2009). In a natural experiment, units of study are assigned to treatment or control not by the analyst but by nature. Snow made a comparison between the houses served by two water companies—(1) Southwark and Vauxhall, and (2) Lambeth—that differed in where they sourced their water (Fig. 3.3). The Southwark and Vauxhall company sourced its water from a contaminated stretch of the Thames and the death rate per 10,000 among the households was 315. In contrast, the Lambeth company had moved its source to a cleaner part of the river upstream and the death rate per 10,000 among the households it serviced was 37. Snow argued that the houses serviced by the two companies only differed in terms of the water supplied, and not in any other way.

To establish the effects of such interventions as the effect of improved stoves we have to grapple with causal issues (Pattanayak and Pfaff 2009). If households that adopt improved stoves differ systematically from households that do not, then the estimation of the causal effect has to account for this. Social interactions may also be important. On the basis of a review of empirical research, Pattanayak and Pfaff suggest that community coordination and public information are important along with programmes aiming to help households adopt technologies and practices that overcome the problems of indoor air pollution and water and sanitation.

3.5 Extension 3: Physical and Social Complexities Related to the Economic Framework for Understanding Air Pollution

The economic models that have been developed in developed countries to examine the benefits of reducing air pollution are really aimed at modern pollution. Often, however, developing countries experience the worst of both traditional air pollution resulting from the use of biomass fuels for cooking, and the air pollution resulting from industry and transport.

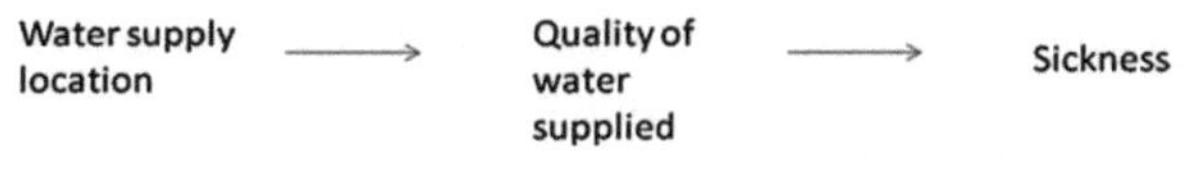

Fig. 3.3 Snow used the difference in water supply location as a natural experiment to find the cause of cholera

In the case of air pollution, in addition to exposure to outdoor and indoor air pollution, workplace exposure could pose a potential risk to health. Ideally, economic analysis should use an integrated framework because it is cumulative exposure over time and space that results in poor health, irrespective of whether it originates in a stove or mine. In the economics literature, Pitt et al. (2005) stressed the importance of gathering data on the person specific exposure to air pollution, and the related data on time allocation across different micro environments and used survey data to examine health effects of cooking on rural Bangladeshi women. Das et al. (2009) considered other micro environments—outdoor, work, and other indoor space besides the kitchen. The exposure to work related pollution includes a source of pollution not studied often, namely, mining.

The key contribution of Das et al. (2009) was that they conceptualized and estimated the simultaneous exposure to both outdoor and indoor air pollution, factors relating to time allocation, and the resulting effects on health. In their paper, they developed a model drawing on health production models (Harrington and Portney 1987), agricultural household models (Singh, Squire and Strauss 1986), and a branch of environmental health sciences, 'Total Exposure Assessment' (Smith 1993). The empirical implementation of this framework incorporating both indoor and outdoor air pollution required the use of a household questionnaire which included time budget questions, measurement of air pollution concentrations in different micro-environments, and included clinical measurements of respiratory health.

Das et al. (2009) aimed to understand and evaluate the total exposure to air pollution in the mining regions of Goa, India. Total exposure is the result of people spending time in different micro-environments (indoors, in the kitchen, and outdoors, for example) with different levels of air pollution concentration levels. The exposure is cumulative and over time leads to greater susceptibility to respiratory problems. They studied this process in different mining clusters, with different levels of cumulative exposure among the population. Pollution was not only caused by mining and associated transport but also from combustion of fuels for cooking—indoor air pollution.

Their study area was the iron ore mining region of the state of Goa in India. For the study, they divided the mining region of Goa into five clusters, including a control cluster with no mining activity. These clusters had varying levels of mining activity, vintage of mining and air pollution. Cluster 1 was the mining region with the earliest mining activity and Cluster 2 was the most intensively mined cluster during the study. Cluster 3 was the region where mining activity was at its inception. Cluster 4 consisted of the mining corridor, which was the region where trucks transported the ore from the mines to the barges on the coast. Cluster 5 was the control region that was away from the mining region.

Cluster 4 (mining corridor, trucking) had only 8 % of its households using only biomass for cooking, and an ambient concentration as high as 528 (Table 3.1), in contrast with cluster 5 (control, away from mining), where though the outdoor concentration was low, the proportion of households using only biomass for cooking was the highest in all the clusters. The concentrations of indoor air

Table 3.1 Average outdoor and indoor concentration of PM10, and proportion of households using only biomass for cooking, by cluster

Cluster	Concentration of PM10 outdoors	Proportion of households using only biomass for cooking
1 (mining region with the earliest mining activity)	294	0.35
2 (most intensively mined)	389	0.26
3 (mining activity beginning)	301	0.20
4 (mining corridor, trucking)	528	0.08
5 (control, away from mining)	71	0.37
Total	323	0.25

pollution in biomass fuel using households are even higher than the high levels of urban outdoor air pollution. The typical 24 h average concentration of PM10 (particulates smaller than 10 microns in diameter) in homes using biofuels may range from 200 to 5,000 $\mu g/m^3$ or more, depending on the type of stove, fuel and housing (Ezzati and Kammen 2002).

Das et al. (2009) found age and gender to play significant roles in time allocation. The results of the study revealed that only those households that used biomass fuels alone were likely to experience indoor concentrations of air pollution that were greater than outdoor concentrations. The factors affecting fuel choice were education, wealth and availability of commercial fuels. After accounting for endogeneity and measurement errors, the researchers found biomass fuel and smoking to be statistically significant factors in explaining chronic respiratory symptoms, even after factoring in exposure to air pollution indoors, outdoors and in the workplace.

I now offer a re-interpretation of the instrumental variable that was meant to unpack causality using the air pollution study by Das et al. (2009). The authors of the study had worked several summers trying to examine the effect of total exposure to air pollution (i.e., indoor plus outdoor pollution, etc., weighted by the time spent). They struggled because it was not 'right' in their judgment since they knew they had measurement error and they suspected endogeneity (simultaneous causation). As seen in Fig. 3.4a, exposure is a cause of sickness which is a cause of the inability to work, which in turn affects the allocation of time to different activities and exposure to air pollution. In Fig. 3.4b, the disturbance term is the common cause of both exposure and sickness. However, the paper by Pitt et al. (2005) on the health effects of indoor air pollution, which uses female hierarchy as an instrumental variable, helped them establish the causal effect of exposure on sickness as evident in Figs. 3.4a and b. In the theoretical model that they used, as with Pitt et al. (2005), they assumed that the household was optimizing utility, which guided the empirical research. Since this assumption solved the problem at hand, they were able to conclude the research on a triumphant note.

However, in a detailed discussion, Agarwal (1997) points out that while economists have improved on unitary models by developing bargaining models of

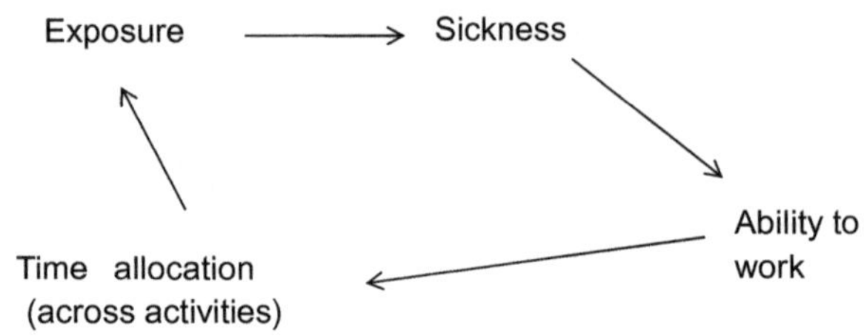

Fig. 3.4a Endogeneity of exposure and sickness

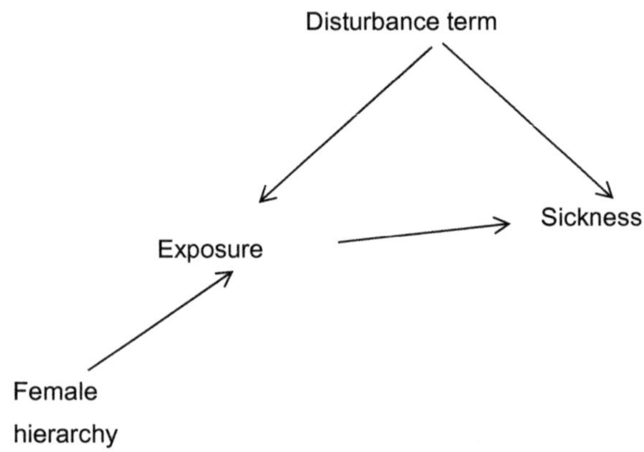

Fig. 3.4b Causal graphs for exposure, sickness and female hierarchy

the household, they have left out social norms from the account. Social norms, Agarwal (1997) maintains, are exogenous in the short run but endogenous in the long run and, therefore, (1) set limits to the domain of bargaining, (2) determine bargaining power, and (3) influence the conduct of bargaining. However, Agarwal (1997) offers a methodological suggestion to the perceived problem:

> I both use and emphasize the usefulness of what I term 'analytical description' for capturing the complexity and historic variability of gender relations in intra- and extra-household dynamics. By analytical description I mean a formulation that seeks to comprehensively spell out both qualitative and quantitative factors that might impinge on outcomes, without being pre-constrained by the structure that formal modeling imposes, or by data limitations. (p. 2)

The disadvantage of analytical description is that we may be uncomfortable about its validity. Therefore questions of validity should inform the design of further studies that seek to go beyond analytical description although this may be difficult. Akerlof and Kranton (2010), who argue that gender matters in the workplace in the United States, suggest that careful observations rather than statistical tests are more enlightening in studying identity. However, in contrast to Agarwal, they seek to modify, rather than abandon, formal theoretical models. Following Friedman's (1953) ideas about "The Methodology of Positive Economics" broadly, Das et al. (2009) did not worry much about whether the household was actually optimizing; what mattered to them most was the prediction or getting the regression 'right'. But the efficacy of the instrumental variable—female hierarchy, in this instance—should make us pause because it lends support to a view of the household which is in tune with the role of norms and identity. Pattanayak and Pfaff stress the importance of social interactions and the difficulty in identifying them empirically (2009).

Appendix

In this appendix I compare a few features of the basic theoretical model used to value reductions in morbidity due to air pollution (Freeman 1993) with the theoretical model used by Das et al. (2009) (discussed in Extension 3).

In Freeman sickness S = S (C, a, b) where C is concentration, a is averting activity, and b is mitigating activities. On the other hand, in Das et al., sickness of an individual depends on total exposure to pollution of that individual (which can vary between persons in a household) E, consumption of cooked food (CF), doctor-visits (D), individual characteristics (Z_i), and household characteristics (Z_{hh}): $S_i = S_i(E_i, CF_i, D_i; Z_i, Z_{hh})$. Total exposure incorporates time spent in different micro-environments, but unlike in some western cities where people may avoid going outdoors on bad days, here the concentration indoors, particularly in the kitchen, may be high. Here the only mitigating activity is doctor visits.

A marked contrast between Freeman and Das et al. is the more detailed treatment of total exposure, E_i, by Das et al.:

$E_i = t_o^i\ C_o + t_k^i\ C_k + t_w^i\ C_w + t_{in}^i\ C_{in}$ where d denotes time, i indexes individuals, o is for outdoor, k for the kitchen, w for work, in for indoor and C denotes concentration. So Co, i.e. outdoor concentration is not assumed to be the dose as in Freeman, but is only one component of total exposure.

Another difference in the two models is the utility functions: in Freeman, this is U(X, f, S) where X, f and s are consumption, leisure and sickness respectively. In Das et al., $U = U(S^C, S^{AM}, S^{AF}, X^{NF})$ where S is sickness and X denotes consumption. The key difference is that in Das et al. children (C), adult males (AM) and adult females (AF) are distinguished.

Finally, in Freeman, time spent working is a choice variable, but in Das et al. there is a choice between time spent in several activities and associated micro-environments, including, in the case of adult females, cooking and gathering biomass for fuel.

References

Agarwal B (1997) 'Bargaining' and gender relations, within and beyond the household. Feminist Econ 3(1):1–51

Akerlof GA, Kranton RE (2010) Identity economics: how our identities shape our work, wages, and well-being. Princeton University Press, Oxford

Bromley D, Anderson G (2012) Vulnerable people, vulnerable states: redefining the development challenge. Routledge, New York

Das S, Dayal V, Murugesan A, Uma R, Sehgal M, and Chhabra SK (2009) An integrated empirical model of health effects of air pollution: the case of mining in Goa, India. IEG discussion paper, Institute of Economic Growth, Delhi
Ezzati M, Kammen DM (2002) The health impacts of exposure to indoor air pollution from solid fuels in developing countries: knowledge, gaps and data needs. Resources for the Future, Washington, DC [Discussion Paper 02–24]
Freeman AM (1993) The measurement of environmental and resource values: theory and methods. Resources for the Future, Washington
Freedman DA (1991) Statistical models and shoe leather. Sociol Methodol 21:291–313
Freedman DA (2009) Statistical models: theory and practice. Cambridge University Press, New York
Friedman M (1953) The methodology of positive economics. In: Friedman M (ed) Essays in positive economics. University of Chicago Press, Chicago
Harrington W, Portney PR (1987) Valuing the benefits of health and safety regulation. J Urban Econ 22:101–112
Pattanayak SK, Pfaff A (2009) Behavior, environment, and health in developing countries: evaluation and valuation. Ann Rev Resour Econ 1:183–217
Pitt MM, Rosenzweig MR, Hassan MN (2005) Sharing the burden of disease: gender, the household division of labor and the health effects of indoor air pollution. CID working paper No. 119, center for international development, Harvard University, Boston, MA
Singh I, Squire L and Strauss J (eds) (1986) Agricultural household models: extensions, applications and policy. Johns Hopkins University Press, Baltimore
Smith KR (1993) Fuel combustion, air pollution exposure, and health: the situation in developing countries. Annu Rev Energy Env 18:529–566
Sterner T, Coria J (2012) Policy instruments for environmental and natural resource management. RFF Press, New York
Tufte ER (1997) Visual explanations. Graphics Press, Connecticut
WHO (2009) Global health risks. Mortality and burden of disease attributable to selected major risks. World Health Organization, Geneva

Chapter 4
Livelihoods and the Commons

Abstract Some public and microeconomics textbooks present Hardins' Tragedy of the Commons and the Prisoner's Dilemma Game and stop there, signaling the inevitable tragedy. However, a more satisfactory treatment by Wydick uses game theory to explain how the Prisoner's Dilemma of the commons can be overcome. Somanathan et al.'s study of Van Panchayats is important both for its result (community management is more cost-effective than management by the forest department), and for its method (establishing causality carefully). Agricultural household models help us incorporate diverse linked production and consumption activities of the household related to biomass extraction. However, community attributes and ecology may have co-evolved historically, influencing patterns of biomass extraction.

Keywords Commons · Biomass · Livelihoods · Game theory

Dasgupta and Maler (2009, p. 21) stress the importance of the commons in developing countries: 'In studying nature's roles in rural life and the rural institutions that have emerged to better meet those roles, investigators have drawn attention to local resource bases, which comprise such assets as ponds and streams, water holes and aquifers, swidden fallows and threshing grounds, woodlands and forests, grazing lands and village tanks, and fisheries and wetlands.'

In the core economic model of the tragedy of the commons, individual rationality compels each person to plunder. However, a simple theoretical model by Wydick (2008) shows that successful collective action changes the game. Since in theory, both tragedy and its avoidance are possible, we need to study the question empirically. A statistical model used by Somanathan et al. (2009) established the cost-effectiveness of village council management in Uttarakhand, India. Dayal (2006) had used a theoretical model with a statistical model to study the extraction of biomass in Ranthambhore National Park. The statistical results led him to ponder the role of social norms, missing from his theoretical model. In the appendix, I see how harnessing mathematical and statistical techniques lead to greater cohesion between the theoretical and statistical model in Dayal (2006).

V. Dayal, *The Environment in Economics and Development*,
SpringerBriefs in Economics, DOI: 10.1007/978-81-322-1671-1_4,

4.1 Core Economic Model: Tragedy of the Commons

Garett Hardin (see Hardin 2005) portrayed the overexploitation of the commons as an inexorable tragedy, a portrayal that was very influential. One way of capturing the essence of the idea of the tragedy of the commons is to model the use of the commons as a Prisoner's Dilemma game with two players, who could conserve or plunder (Wydick 2008).

In Table 4.1, we have two players who can conserve or plunder. We can see in the above game that no matter whether player 2 plays conserve or plunder, it pays player 1 to plunder. Plundering the commons dominates conserving the commons. Hence, both players will plunder the commons, and will get a payoff of 3 each, though they could have got more if both had conserved.

4.2 Extension 1: Ways of Overcoming the Prisoner's Dilemma

In the Hardin story, the tragedy is almost inevitable and the actors are trapped in the Prisoner's Dilemma. However, the essence of collective action is transforming the game itself. If either the state or the community imposes a fine of 2 whenever an actor plunders, the game in Table 4.1 is transformed to the game in Table 4.2. Now the Nash equilibrium is where both actors conserve—the game is no longer a Prisoner's Dilemma.

The fine of 2 units could be levied by a government agency or by the community itself. In Chap. 2 we had seen the Institutions and Development Framework of Elinor Ostrom (2009). There, the context (with such elements as biophysical and community attributes, and rules) affected the action arena and interactions. The action arena and interactions could be represented as games. The Institutions and Development framework was used by Elinor Ostrom to synthesize studies of 47 irrigation systems and 44 fisheries. She found that farmer managed irrigation systems performed better than government irrigation systems, and informal fishery groups allocated space, time, and technology to reduce over-harvesting.

Table 4.1 Prisoner's Dilemma game for tragedy of the commons

		Player 2	
		Conserve	Plunder
Player 1	Conserve	(4, 4)	(2, 5)
	Plunder	(5, 2)	(3, 3)

Table 4.2 Transformed game for conserved commons

		Player 2	
		Conserve	Plunder
Player 1	Conserve	(4, 4)	(2, 3)
	Plunder	(3, 2)	(1, 1)

4.3 Extension 2: Evaluating the Effect of Management Regimes on Forest Stock

How do we compare the efficacy of state and community forest management? Somanathan et al. (2009) studied the long-run effects of transfer of management of some areas of state-managed forest to local communities in the central Himalayas of India. This study is important not only for its result but also its method. The authors found that village council-management cost an order of magnitude less per unit area and did no worse in terms of conservation than state management.

Separating out the effects of decentralization from other factors affecting forests is difficult (Somanathan et al. 2009). The authors compared the costs of managing state forests with village council forests. They used government data for state forest costs and survey data for the costs of village council forests. The costs of managing state forests were at least 7 times more per hectare compared to the costs of managing village council forests.

The authors used the percentage of crown cover to compare state and village council managed forests. Since the devolution of state forests to council management was done in 1930 the authors went through historical records; they found that the areas kept as state forests were systematically different from those devolved to village councils. To account for this initial difference in assignment of areas, the authors controlled for aspect and population density in their regressions (Fig. 4.1).

As a check on their results, they also used the method of matching—comparing satellite image polygons of village council lands and state forests that were as close to each other as possible (Fig. 4.2). They concluded that state forests did not have greater forest cover than comparable village council forests.

Such a careful statistical study establishes the credentials of community management of forests

4.4 Extension 3: Role of Social Ecology in the Dependence on the Commons

In Chap. 2 I discussed the Institutions and Development framework, in which community attributes can affect the action arena and interactions. Dayal (2006) focused on the extraction of forest biomass by village households around

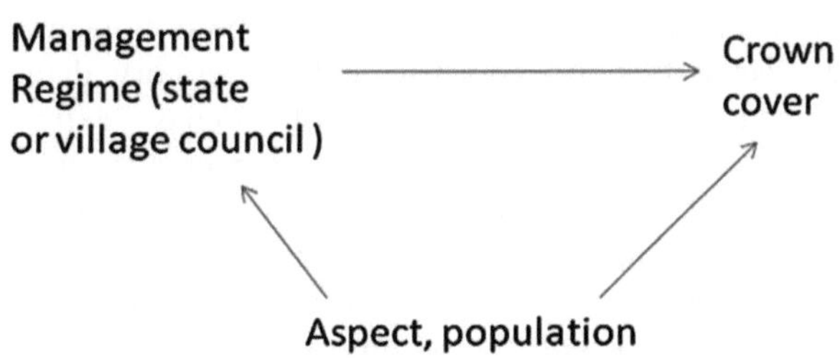

Fig. 4.1 Causal links between key variables in the study of forest management by Somanathan et al. (2009)

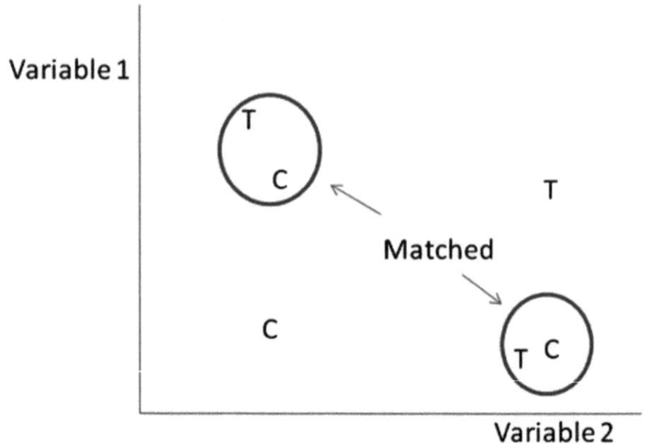

Fig. 4.2 An intuitive depiction of matching—treatment (*T*) and control (*C*) units are matched so that they resemble each other closely in terms of covariates (here, Variables 1 and 2)

Ranthambhore National Park in India and developed a microeconomic model of the decisions regarding levels and sources of extraction of forest biomass. The objective of this model was to study biomass extraction, including grazing, fuelwood and fodder. Biomass extraction from the park was a product of the level of extraction and share of biomass extracted from the park. When households both produce and consume a good, a household model is appropriate (Singh, Squire and Strauss 1986; Sadoulet and de Janvry 1995).

In the first model of how much, the village household maximizes utility subject to time and budget constraints. The village household balances the allocation of labour to get maximum benefits. When it allocates labour to grazing, it also gains a by-product in the form of fuelwood. Agricultural labour yields greater grain, and agricultural residue that can be used to feed livestock and used for energy. The village household is likely to gather biomass because the opportunity cost of time may be lower than the price of the fodder or fuelwood available in the market, at least at several points in the year.

In the second model of where to extract from, the village household minimizes costs of gathering biomass from different types of land: public, private and the park. Given that biomass growth and opportunity costs of time follow a seasonal pattern on forest and agricultural land, the household is likely to extract from different patches of land.

The models of how much and where lead to reduced form equations of biomass extraction as functions of exogenous variables. A household survey of 227 households in 4 villages around Ranthambhore—Gopalpura, Indala, Ramsinghpura and Fariya—was conducted. These villages have different locations and characteristics. Econometric and exploratory data analysis of the survey data helped reveal different facets of biomass extraction by households. A key improvisation was examining the percentage share of the park as a source of grazing, fuelwood and fodder for village households. The study found village location, ownership of biogas, and caste to be key explanatory variables of forest biomass extraction. Does the household model do full justice to the phenomenon under study? I will discuss this with respect to the fuelwood analysis.

Dayal (2006) regressed the fraction of fuelwood sourced from Ranthambhore National Park on the following explanatory variables:

- Caste dummy (Brahmin), statistically significant at 1 % level;
- Village dummy (Indala), also statistically significant at 1 % level;
- Quantity of land, statistically significant at 10 % level;
- House type (a proxy for wealth), household size, fraction of males, cattle owned, and goats owned, which were not statistically significant.

These results encourage us to examine the role of caste in biomass extraction more closely. As the above study shows, an economist using a microeconomic model and econometric analysis is not at ease with the bewildering variety of castes encountered in the field—the multivariate regression analysis used a dummy for only one or two castes (here Brahmin and low caste). In consequence, the analysis was coarse in its treatment of the variety of castes in a given Indian village. In another paper, however, Dayal (2008) conducted a non-parametric small sample investigation of diverse castes in one village. In this paper where the investigator did not have a formal model and did not use sophisticated econometrics, he showed that there was a great deal of heterogeneity among the different castes in their biomass extraction patterns, i.e., fuelwood, fodder and grazing (see Table 4.3).

Conversations that I had in the field with key respondents confirmed the important role caste plays in bio-mass extraction. One respondent asserted that Gujjars were very comfortable with rearing goats while a Brahmin respondent thought that he knew more than the other castes about cattle-rearing because his cows gave him high yields. But while caste has no role in the theoretical model of Dayal (2006), it plays a role in the statistical model because applied economists control for 'household characteristics'. But it is a slow moving variable, with zero measurement error, in contrast to other variables, and that partly explains its statistical significance. With the econometric evidence goading me, I ventured into social ecology, and found Gadgil and Malhotra's (1998) fascinating case study set in the Western Ghats of India, which provides a functional interpretation of caste and its ecological significance:

> The relatively simple society of the high-rainfall tracts near the crest of the Western Ghats is largely made up of small, often single-clan settlements of Kunbis and Gavlis. Here the Kunbis lived … in the lower valleys, while the Gavlis lived … on the upper hill terraces. … Thus, the cultivation of valleys and lower hill slopes was restricted to Kunbis and that of hill terraces to Gavlis; maintenance of livestock and use of fodder and grazing resources was largely with Gavlis, while Kunbis had the monopoly of hunting wild animals (Gadgil and Malhotra 1998 p. 31).

Table 4.3 Forest biomass extraction indicators (%) by caste (Fariya village)

	Gujjar	Nai	Berwa	Koli	Brahmin
Used park for fodder	32	17	14	10	0
Used park for grazing	68	8	21	30	13
Used park for fuelwood	60	33	71	70	13

The quote above shows how caste and ecology have co-evolved over centuries in much of India and the dominant role that caste as a social norm plays in the traditional rural economy. As Dasgupta (2012) says, "Social norms are not constructed out of thin air; they evolve" (p. 186). In the case of caste, he suggests that "exploitation can masquerade as cooperation" (p.180). These reflections on caste help us appreciate the tension in the social sciences between the individualist and social constructivist positions (Vatn 2005) and to recognize the role that caste plays as an institutional norm.

Appendix

In this appendix I draw attention to the match between the theoretical model (MT; see appendix of Chap. 2) and statistical model (MS) of Dayal (2006), discussed in Extension 3 of this chapter. One way theory can guide empirical work is by identifying a variable for which data can then be gathered. Also the mathematical technique in the theoretical model may facilitate analysis of a feature of the problem being studied, and this feature can also be studied by use of an appropriate statistical technique in the statistical model.

The quantity of interest in Dayal (2006) is biomass (fuelwood, fodder, and grazing) collected from the park:

Collection of biomass from the park = collection of biomass (q) * fraction of biomass collected from the park (θ) $=$ qθ.

Dayal did not assume that $\theta = 1$, as was implicit in the papers by Bluffstone (1995) and Bardhan et al. (2001), and collected data on θ in a survey, along with q. Dayal formulated a theoretical model of extraction of biomass from Ranthambhore National Park, consisting of two sub-models: (1) decisions regarding q,. and (2) decisions regarding θ, given q.

Since both θ and q are ≥ 0, the theoretical model explicitly (Dayal 2006) treated the possibility of corner solutions (θ and q can be zero) using the mathematical technique of deriving Kuhn-Tucker conditions; and the statistical model used the technique of Tobit regressions.

References

Bardhan P, Baland J, Das S, Mookherjee D, Sarkar R (2001) Household firewood collection in rural Nepal: the role of poverty, collective action and modernization. Working Paper. University of California, Berkeley

Bluffstone RA (1995) The effect of labor market performance on deforestation in developing countries under open access: an example from Nepal. J Environ Econ Manag 29:42–63

Dasgupta P (2012) Dark matters: exploitation as cooperation. J Theor Biol 299:180–187

Dasgupta P, Maler K-G (2009) Environmental and resource economics: some recent developments. In: Chopra K, Dayal V (eds) Handbook of environmental economics in India. Oxford University Press, New Delhi

Dayal V (2006) A micro-econometric analysis of household extraction of forest biomass goods in Ranthambhore National Park, India. J Forest Econ 12:145–163

Dayal V (2008) Inter- and intra-village diversity among forest dependent households in Ranthambhore National Park, India. Int J Ecol Econ Stat 10:27–39

Gadgil M, Malhotra KC (1998) The ecological significance of caste. In: Guha Ramachandra (ed) Social ecology. Oxford University Press, New Delhi

Hardin G (2005) The tragedy of the commons. In: Dryzek JS, Schlosberg D (eds) Debating the earth: the environmental politics reader. Oxford University Press, New York

Ostrom E (2009) Beyond markets and states: polycentric governance of complex economic systems. Nobel Prize Lecture, 8 December 2009, Stockholm, Sweden

Sadoulet E, de Janvry A (1995) Quantitative development policy analysis. The Johns Hopkins University Press, Baltimore

Singh I, Squire L, Strauss J (1986) Agricultural household models. The Johns Hopkins University Press, Baltimore

Somanathan E, Prabhakar R, Mehta BS (2009) Decentralization for cost-effective conservation. PNAS 106(11):4143–4147

Vatn A (2005) Institutions and the environment. Edward Elgar, Cheltenham

Wydick B (2008) Games in Economic Development. Cambridge University Press, Cambridge

Chapter 5
Complex Ecology

Abstract The starting point for modeling biological resources is using a model of fish growth represented with a logistic equation and seeing the effects of different levels of harvest. Protected areas in developing countries represent interactions between ecological systems, the modern tourist industry, and the traditional rural economy. A predator prey model with multiple stakeholders was used to model wildlife in Ranthambhore National Park. Models can be extended with scenario analysis if we cannot control the system easily or it is less predictable. Valuation estimates of natural sites use static economic models; Kanchan Chopra argued that such short run economic values are based on long run ecological dynamics. In nonlinear dynamic systems it is possible to get an environmental regime shift; econometric techniques to detect structural breaks may detect such regime shifts, given suitable data. A non-linear equation can generate 'deterministic chaos'—apparently random behavior that is not random.

Keywords Ecology · Valuation · Regime shift

How we think of Nature influences our models in environmental economics. Natural systems often experience sudden, catastrophic changes. According to Scheffer et al. (2001, p. 591), 'Nature is usually assumed to respond to gradual change in a smooth way. However, studies on lakes, coral reefs, oceans, forests and arid lands have shown that smooth change can be interrupted by sudden drastic switches to a contrasting state.' Ecology is complex—it is nonlinear, dynamic, and often not easily controlled or predicted.

The core economic model in this chapter focuses more on the ecology (growth of a biological resource) than the economics (harvest). It lays the base for the first extension that discusses a dynamic simulation model of a national park in India and related scenarios. Extension two discusses the scenario analysis by the Millenium Ecosystem Assessment. Extension three discusses a paper that combined a short-term model of monetary value and a long-term ecological model. In the next extension, we see that statistical models can help us study regime shifts. The appendix is a brief and elementary foray into deterministic chaos exhibited by a logistic difference equation.

V. Dayal, *The Environment in Economics and Development*, SpringerBriefs in Economics, DOI: 10.1007/978-81-322-1671-1_5,

5.1 Core Economic Model: Logistic Fish Growth with Harvest

A starting point for examining the issue of biological resources is to think of a general equation that might be used to model the growth of living resources like fish.

Change in fish stock = growth of fish − harvest of fish = G − H

Biology and the environment shape growth (G) and the harvest (H) is determined by the fisherman. We shall not model H but look at the implications of different levels of H. In Chap. 4 we had examined different ways of managing common pool resources and the extraction of forest biomass. In the Institutions and Development framework in Chap. 2, biophysical attributes are part of the context, affecting the action arena and interactions. Here we focus on the biological factors reflected in G.

G is often assumed to be logistic, i.e.

$$G = rX(1 - (X/K))$$

where r is the instantaneous rate of growth and K is the carrying capacity. If we multiply the expression out we see that G is quadratic, and $G = 0$ if either $X = 0$ or $X = K$. Figure 5.1 shows a graph of G.

We first see what will happen if $H = 0$. If $X > 0$ and $X < K$, G is positive, and X will grow; if $X > K$ G will be negative and X will fall. $X = K$ is a 'stable' equilibrium (see Chap. 2).

The logistic equation is a simplified view of complex ecology. A biological resource can grow but if it is harvested at a very high level it can get extinct.

We now see the effects of H (Fig. 5.2). The level of the fish will not change over time if $G = H$, i.e. growth = harvest. If $G > H$ then the level of the fish will

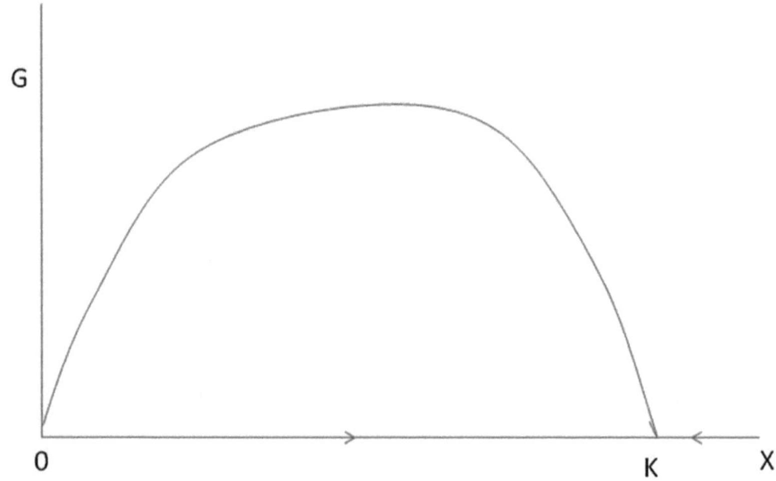

Fig. 5.1 Logistic growth of fish

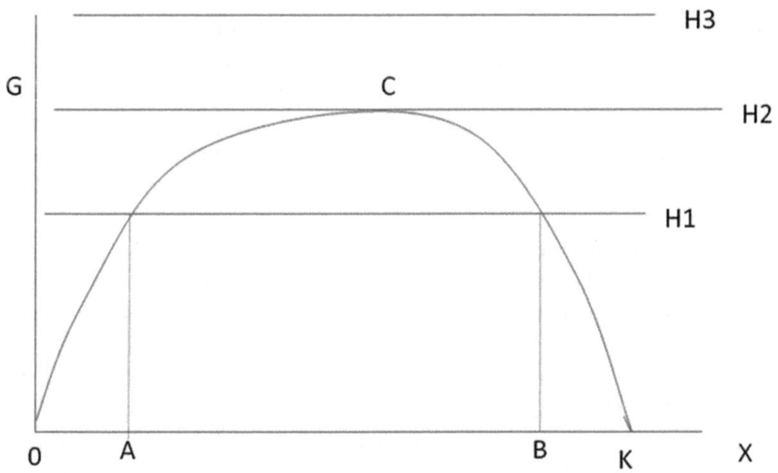

Fig. 5.2 Seeing the effects of different levels of harvest (*H1*, *H2*, and *H3*) on fish stock

increase, and if G < H the level of the fish will decrease. In Fig. 5.2 we see that if the stock is more than A but less than B with harvest H1 the stock will increase. If X < A, G − H1 will be negative and X reaches zero.

With the logistic equation we see that we can get the same growth of the resource with a low or a high stock. So, if we are in equilibrium—i.e. the stock is not changing—we can have the same harvest with a low or a high stock. If the costs of harvest depend on the stock, then we might favour having a high stock. If the stock itself has a nonuse value, then we might favour having a high stock.

We could increase the harvest until it just touches the growth curve and this would be the maximum sustained yield (H2 in Fig. 5.2). If H is more than this (H3 in Fig. 5.2) we will be in a situation where the fish stock will die out eventually. Since the G curve is not known and there can be stochastic disturbances, we have to be cautious.

5.2 Extension 1: A Model for Wildlife in Ranthambhore National Park

The core economic model ignores interaction between different species and ecological processes, nor does it consider multiple stakeholders. Here we shall see a model with these two features. Dayal (2007) studied how an exotic tree would affect people and wildlife in Ranthambhore National Park in India, famous for its tigers. A number of villages surround the park. Villagers go into the park to collect fuelwood and fodder, and graze their livestock.

An important cause of resource mismanagement is ignorance of ecological processes, and underestimating the effect of present practices on the future state of the resource (Baland and Platteau 1996). In Ranthambhore, park managers planted *Prosopis juliflora* because it was productive and grew quickly in poor conditions. They felt that it would help meet the fuelwood and fodder needs of villagers, and therefore help reduce the 'incredible pressure' on the park. However, *Prosopis juliflora* is a biologically invasive species and will harm the ecology of the park in the long run. Therefore, we see that a well-intentioned intervention could have an adverse impact.

Ecological economic modeling is difficult. Ecosystems consist of several species with nonlinear relationships (Sterner 2003). With several species and nonlinear relationships, the analyst has to rely on numerical simulation (Costanza et al. 1993).

In what follows I will follow an intuitive, step-by-step view of the somewhat technical model of Dayal (2007). The bioeconomic simulation model is a predator–prey model with logistic growth of prey, and a non-linear predation response. The carrying capacity of the prey depends on vegetation cover. There are four kinds of prey: cattle, goats, wild herbivore grazers and wild herbivore browsers. There are three key ecological interactions in the model: predator–prey, prey–prey, and *Prosopis juliflora*-prey. There are four economic agents: the wildlife manager, who is assumed to be interested in having the maximum number of tigers over time, the cattle owner who gets revenue from selling milk or cattle, the goat owner who gets revenue from selling goats, and the wood gatherer.

There are four scenarios. In scenarios 1 and 2, *Prosopis juliflora* is not removed, while in 3 and 4 it is removed. In scenarios 1 and 3 tigers are maximized, while in 2 and 4 cattle owner and goat owner benefits are maximized (Table 5.1).

In scenarios 4 and 3, *Prosopis juliflora* is removed in the 15th and 60th years, but grows back. However, in these two scenarios it never grows too much (Fig. 5.3). We conjecture that ecological succession is a possibility—as *Prosopis juliflora* adds nutrients to the soil, it cumulatively sows the seeds of its own destruction. In scenario 2, the turning point comes about the 80th year. In scenario 2, *Prosopis juliflora* is not removed and goats are not checked, so they help it spread fast. In scenario 1, goats are checked so *Prosopis juliflora* spreads at a slower rate, and the turning point is not reached, even by the 100th year. As described before, *Prosopis juliflora* affects the competing prey, and the prey compete with each other. Finally prey interact with the tiger.

Tiger levels in the scenarios with cattle and goat feeding in the park are much lower than those without, illustrating the tradeoff between tigers and villager resource dependence. In addition, in the scenarios where nothing is done about

Table 5.1 Model scenarios for Ranthambhore national park

	Prosopis juliflora removed	*Prosopis juliflora* not removed
Tigers maximized	Scenario 3	Scenario 1
Cattle owner and goat owner benefits maximized	Scenario 4	Scenario 2

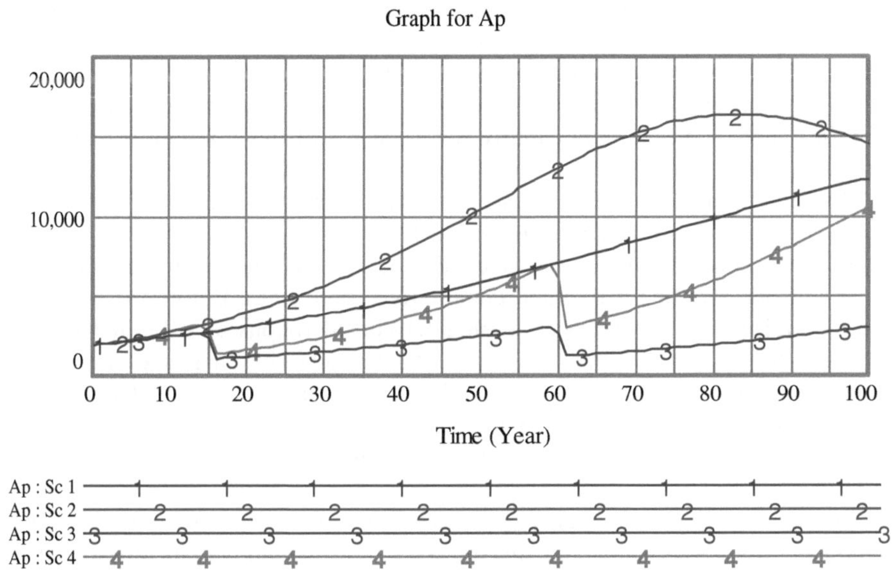

Fig. 5.3 Spread of area under *Prosopis juliflora* in the park over time

Prosopis juliflora the tiger paths are lower, or the probability of tiger extinctions are higher.

Now, for the ranking of the four scenarios. The four agents have rather different rankings of the four scenarios. Of all four agents, the wood gatherer is the most indifferent between the four scenarios. For the goat owner and cattle owner, being able to use the park makes a big difference. For the goat owner the scenario with *Prosopis juliflora* is slightly better, and vice versa for the cattle owner. Finally, for the park manager, it is clear that in addition to the traditional task of containing livestock, there is a need to handle *Prosopis juliflora*.

Dayal (2007) suggested adaptive management of the park with experimentation, monitoring, and learning with respect to *Prosopis juliflora*. The learning process will involve aiming to see how the tree is best cleared, what effect it is having on the native flora and fauna, and how best to get the greatest economic benefits from the *Prosopis juliflora* tree.

5.3 Extension 2: Millenium Ecosystem Assessment Scenarios

Scenarios are explorations into an uncertain future. Scenarios are difficult to assess since they are often deliberately imaginative and exploratory; nevertheless, it is well known that they have been used with profit by many organizations. Shell, for instance, used them very successfully in the context of the unprecedented rise in oil prices in the 1970s. To elaborate, ‘Scenarios are plausible, provocative and relevant stories about how the future might unfold. They can be told in both words and numbers. Scenarios are not forecasts, projections or recommendations, though model projections may be used to quantify some aspects of the scenarios' (MA 2005, p. 36). A mix of quantitative and qualitative techniques is the dominating feature of scenario analysis. It is because of this characteristic that scenario exercises carry a special applicability for problems of the environment and ecosystems and for system analysis in general.

The Millenium Ecosystem Assessment (MA) work on scenarios was probably the most detailed scenario exercise related to ecosystems undertaken in recent times. The scenarios exercise was conducted by an interdisciplinary team of experts, using both qualitative and quantitative approaches. Before the MA, scenario exercises had incorporated ecological considerations to a limited degree. Although they included direct environmental impacts, they neglected ecological dynamics. In the MA, ecology is central to the scenarios. 'The Millenium Ecosystem Assessment scenarios break new ground in global environmental scenarios by explicitly incorporating both ecosystem dynamics and feedbacks' (MA 2005, p. 147).

The MA developed four alternative scenarios. Two kinds of considerations, significant from socio-economic perspectives were paramount in differentiating between these scenarios: (1) the magnitude and nature of global interconnectedness, and (2) proactive or reactive approaches to the environment (Cork et al. 2006).

The globally connected scenarios were 'Global orchestration' and 'TechnoGarden', while the environmentally proactive scenarios were 'Adapting Mosaic' and 'TechnoGarden'. The regionalized scenarios were 'Order from strength' and 'Adapting Mosaic'. The dominant approach for sustainability in each scenario is listed below:

- Global orchestration: sustainable development, economic growth, public goods.
- Order from strength: reserves, parks, national-level policies, conservation.
- Adapting mosaic: Local–regional co-management, common property institutions.
- Techno garden: Green-technology, eco-efficiency, tradable ecological property rights.

The MA scenarios are addressed at a global scale, and do not address policy in a clear fashion. This recognizes the fact that most policy is determined at the national government level. As MA (2005, p. 60) itself points out, 'The appropriateness of a given approach to ecosystem management depends largely on the degree of uncertainty about a system's behaviour and the degree to which the system can be controlled' (Table 5.2).

Table 5.2 Controllability, uncertainty and suggested approach to ecosystem management by MA (2005)

Controllability	Uncertainty	
	Low	High
Uncontrollable	Resilience building	Scenario planning
Controllable	Optimizing command and control	Adaptive management

5.4 Extension 3: Incorporating Ecological Dynamics while Valuing a National Park

Chopra and Adhikari (2004) simulated ecology-economy interactions in the Keoladeo National Park. They argued that wetlands give rise to a variety of values. To value an ecosystem service we need to identify the (1) physical or environmental linkages which result in the supply of the service and (2) the economic links which help the ecosystem service contribute to human welfare. Alternative methods of valuation have been used: revealed and stated preference. The valuation can be static or dynamic.

In traditional recreational valuation, the number of trips is a function of travel cost incurred and household characteristics; in Chopra and Adhikari (2004) the number of trips is a function also of ecological health of the park. The ecological health of the park can be parametrized only by using medium-or long-run time series data and by modelling the wetland system. Upstream demand for water influences the ecological health of the wetland. The state of the wetland is determined by changing stocks of water, biomass, and birds in it. Thus, the short-term value is linked to the long-term value (Fig. 5.4).

The simulation model used by Chopra and Adhikari (2004) has the following modules:

- Water. Water storage is the stock variable.
- Biomass. Examines factors impacting biomass and changes in it.
- Birds. Number of birds is the main stock variable.
- Net income. Income from tourism and resource extraction is influenced by preceding modules.

Chopra and Adhikari (2004) made projections for key variables for 23 years on a monthly basis. They found that (from the travel cost model) the visits by tourists were not responsive to private costs. The direct and indirect income from the park depended on ecological health indices. Further, the response or elasticity of income was more at high values of the ecological health indices. In other words, not only was the ecological health a significant determinant of income from the park, the relationship was marked by a non-linearity as the ecological health indices varied over time.

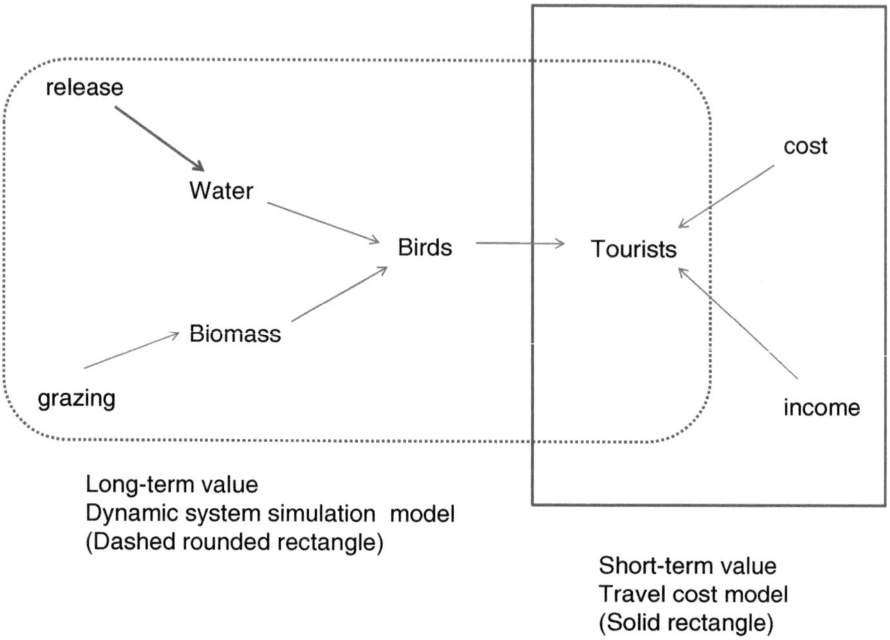

Fig. 5.4 The link between static value and ecological dynamics in Chopra and Adhikari (2004)

5.5 Extension 4: Regime Shifts and Detecting them

According to Scheffer et al. (2001), we often witness regime shifts in nature. Mathematical models of regime shifts are technical, but I will use the core model of fish growth and harvest of this chapter metaphorically to convey the main idea.

Let $G = 0.1 * X(1 - (X/100))$, i.e. $r = 0.1$ and $K = 100$. Let the initial value of $X = 60$. Initially, $H = 2$, for 50 time periods, and then H is increased to 3. We simulate this with the Vensim software, and this gives us the following graphs:

In the Figs. 5.5 and 5.6, there is a step up in the harvest (driver) level in the 50th year which leads to a change in X (state).

Andersen et al. (2008) suggest that ecologists would do well to draw on other disciplines when they statistically test for regime shifts. For example, they can draw on developments in econometrics that have lead to tests of structural breaks.

Since 1990, econometric tests of deterministic versus stochastic trends, and structural breaks have been developed. A trend is a persistent long-term movement of a variable over time. Modern econometrics distinguishes between stochastic and deterministic trends. A deterministic trend is a nonrandom function of time (e.g. a clearly visible steady growth of 5 % year). A stochastic trend is random and varies over time (Stock and Watson 2003). In addition to a stochastic or a deterministic trend, a time series variable may have a structural break. A structural break is a change in the parameters of a model characterizing the variable (e.g. slope or

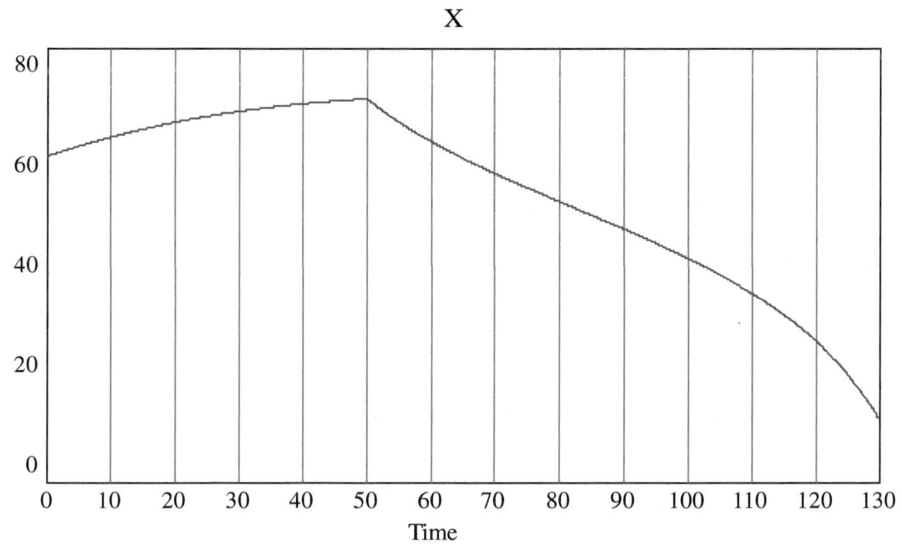

Fig. 5.5 Levels of X over time

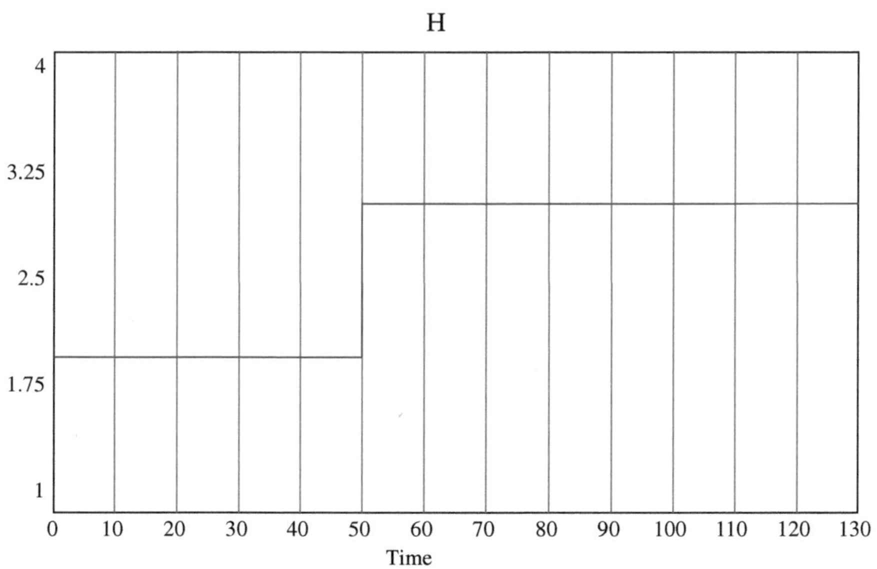

Fig. 5.6 Levels of H over time

level). The distinction between a stochastic and a deterministic trend break is based on how frequent the shocks to the trend are (Hansen 2001). In a stochastic trend, shocks occur frequently while in the case of a deterministic trend with a break, shocks occur at the break. The statistical tests for a stochastic trend are sensitive to the presence of structural breaks. Hence, both stochastic trends and breaks should be tested.

Niraj et al. (2012) studied temporal patterns in poaching and illegal wildlife trade on eighteen legally protected or regulated species or categories—15 of wild fauna and three of wild flora of India, and carried out tests for the presence of stochastic trends and structural breaks. The dashed line in Fig. 5.7 shows the recorded detected poaching data for the tiger, while the solid line shows the linear prediction based on the detected structural break. The break date detected is the third quarter of 2001; prior to that detected tiger poaching was increasing, thereafter it was falling.

5.6 Concluding Remarks on Complexity

To say that something is complex may imply that it is difficult to understand. We get further than this banal statement by contrasting a linear equation and a non-linear difference equation.

The deterministic component of a simple regression equation is

$$Y = a + bx$$

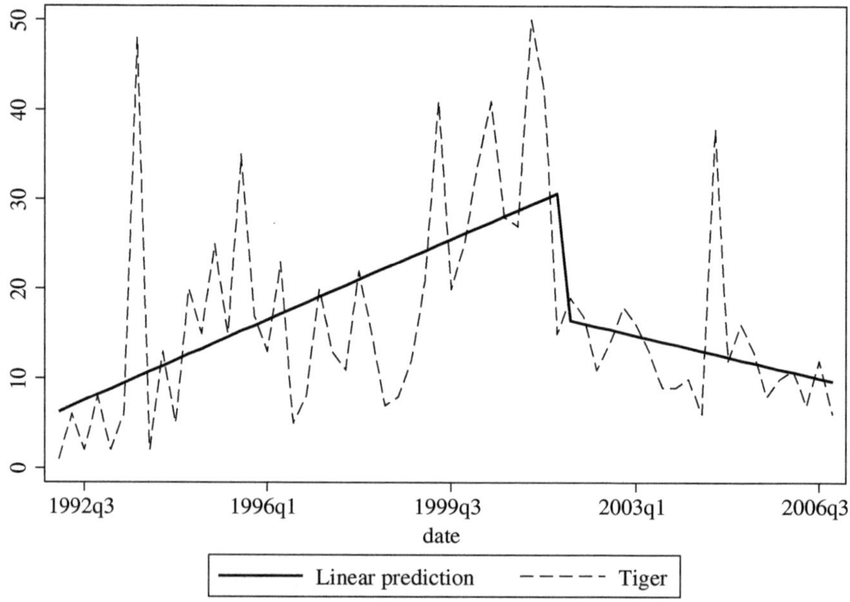

Fig. 5.7 Detected tiger poaching in India over time

So a value of x is associated with a value of y. We could control x, and perhaps predict y in this neat, ordered world. Double x and y doubles.

With a non-linear difference equation, say a logistic one, we can get a dramatic change in the behavior of the system when a parameter changes.

If we take the logistic difference equation:

$$\Delta y_t = r\, y_t(1 - y_t/k) = r\, y_t - \left(y_t^2/k\right)$$

We find two steady states: 0 and k. The left hand side is zero when either y_t is zero or y_t is k. We say that y is in a steady state—it does not change. $y_t = k$ is the stable steady state.

Thus with nonlinear dynamics we can have multiple equilibria. When we see the world governed by nonlinear dynamics then we may try to see how we can go from a bad equilibrium to a good equilibrium. Also, there may be sudden changes beyond thresholds.

We can examine the behaviour of the logistic equation by taking k = 100, and varying r from say 0.1 upwards. We see below (Fig. 5.8) that when r = 0.3 there is a smooth approach to the equilibrium. However, when r = 2.7 we see what appears to be a complex, random pattern that is actually deterministic, i.e. we have chaos (mathematically).

Linear models may be large, with over 100 equations, but their complexity may be low in comparison with models of non-linear difference or differential equations with just a small number of equations.

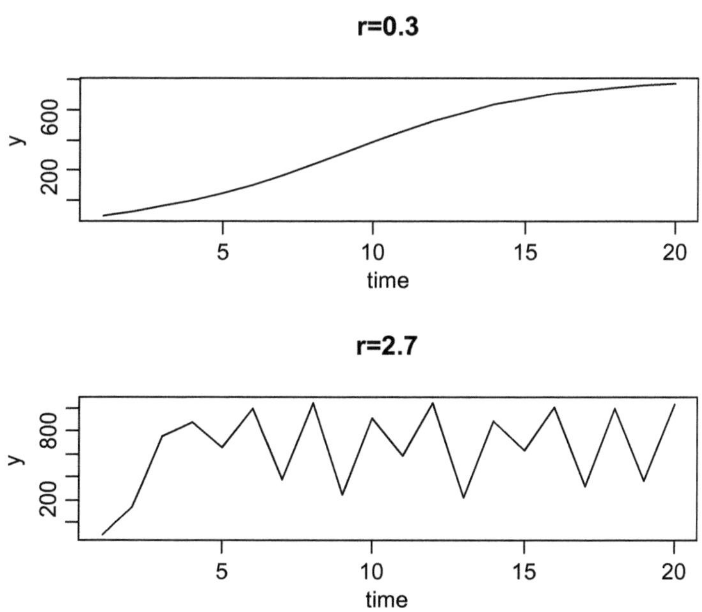

Fig 5.8 Evolution of y over time with a logistic equation, with r = 0.3 and r = 2.7

References

Andersen T, Christensen J, Hernandez-Garcia E, Duarte CM (2008) Ecological thresholds and regime shifts: approaches to identification. Trends Ecol Evol 24(1):49–57
Baland J, Platteau J (1996) Halting degradation of natural resources: is there a role for rural communities?. Oxford University Press, Oxford
Chopra K, Adhikari SK (2004) Environment development linkages: modelling wetland system for ecological and economic value. Environ Dev Econ 9:19–45
Cork SJ, Peterson GD, Bennett EM, Petschel-Held G, Zurek M (2006) Synthesis of the storylines. Ecol Soc 11(2):11. http://www.ecologyandsociety.org/vol11/iss2/art11/
Costanza R, Wainger L, Folke C, Maler KG (1993) Modeling complex ecological economic systems. Bioscience 43(8):545–555
Dayal V (2007) Social diversity and ecological complexity: how an invasive tree could affect diverse agents in the land of the tiger. Environ Dev Econ 12:1–19
Hansen BE (2001) The new econometrics of structural change: dating breaks in US labor productivity. J Econ Perspect 15:117–128
MA (2005) Ecosystems and human well-being: scenarios, vol 2. Island Press, London
Niraj SK, Krausman PR, Dayal V (2012) Temporal and spatial analysis of wildlife seizures in India from 1992 to 2006. Int J Ecol Econ Stat 24(1):79–109
Scheffer M, Carpenter S, Foley JA, Folke C, Walker B (2001) Catastrophic shifts in ecosystems. Nature 413(11):591–596
Sterner T (2003) Policy instruments for environmental and natural resource management. RFF Press, Washington DC
Stock JH, Watson MW (2003) Introduction to econometrics. Pearson Education, Delhi

Chapter 6
Global Public Goods

Abstract Global public goods affect people all over the earth. Sandler stresses the aggregation technology of different global public goods; the mitigation of carbon dioxide is a summation public good while checking biological invasions is a weakest link public good. Simple game theory models of summation and weakest link public goods are considered. While climate change is widely perceived to be the major environmental issue for humanity, Perrings claims that biological invasions are one of the most important challenges. I consider the ingredients of a model where global change consists of climate change and linked biological invasions; the formal model is in the Appendix. A key issue in climate change is the discount rate, and Partha Dasgupta argues that if climate change is truly disastrous the discount rate could be negative, strengthening the case for acting to avoid the disaster. Chhatre and Agarwal investigated the following question: if we have an interest in sequestering carbon in the forests of developing countries, how are livelihoods likely to be affected; this involves some conceptual and empirical issues.

Keywords Global public goods · Game theory · Carbon · Biological invasions · Discount rate

According to Stern (2008), 'Greenhouse gas emissions are externalities and represent the biggest market failure the world has seen'. Although biological invasions are relatively less well known, Perrings et al. (2010) suggest that 'the problem of invasive species makes all other environmental problems pale into insignificance'. Biologically invasive species include pests and pathogens, plants and animals, which invade and take over ecological systems, harming the production of ecosystem services.

Climate change is a global public good, and a simple game theory model helps illustrate the divergence between individual and social rationality. Although the prevention of the spread of biological invasives is a global public good, we need to model it differently from climate change because it is a weakest-link public good. Our problems may be compounded by the interaction of climate change and biological invasives—discussed in extension two, and a formal model is set out in the appendix. Because climate change is a long-term phenomenon, the choice of

V. Dayal, *The Environment in Economics and Development*,
SpringerBriefs in Economics, DOI: 10.1007/978-81-322-1671-1_6,

the discount rate is a key issue. Theoretical arguments guide the choice of the discount rate and illustrate implicit equity issues. In the next section we see how livelihoods and carbon storage are related.

6.1 Core Economic Model: Game Theory Model of Public Goods

Reducing greenhouse gases is a public good—it is characterized by non-rivalry and non-excludability. A simple game theory model illustrates the issue of free riding. Table 6.1 illustrates the payoff matrix for a public good with a cost of 10 and per person benefit (non-excludable) of 8. Not contributing dominates contributing to the public good. The game leads to each person not contributing. Thus, the Nash equilibrium is not Pareto optimal—both players would have been better off if both of them had contributed.

6.2 Extension 1: Distinguishing Between the Aggregation Technology of Different Public Goods

Apart from non-rivalry and non-excludability, public goods have a third dimension: aggregation technology—how do units of input add up (Sandler 2004)? Examples of aggregation technologies are summation (above) or weakest-link public goods. According to Perrings et al. (2002) biological invasives are a weakest-link public good.

In a weakest-link public good, benefits can only be enjoyed if both players contribute. Table 6.2 shows the payoff matrix for a weakest-link public good with cost of a unit being 5, benefits of 8 will be received by each only if both players

Table 6.1 Payoff matrix of a public good

		Player B	
		Do not contribute	Contribute
Player A	Do not contribute	(0, 0)	(8, −2)
	Contribute	(−2, 8)	(6, 6)

Table 6.2 Payoff matrix for a weakest link public good

		Player B	
		Do not contribute	Contribute
Player A	Do not contribute	(0, 0)	(0, −5)
	Contribute	(−5, 0)	(3, 3)

contribute. There are two Nash equilibria—(1) both players contributing and (2) both not contributing.

6.3 Extension 2: Interlinked Global Change with Climate Change and Biological Invasions

As Howarth and Norgaard (1995) point out, we now confront a world with interacting global change, which means that our earlier specific and separate models, while providing useful insight are probably incomplete—here we consider interlinked climate change and biological invasions. It is feared that climate change would lead to ecological disturbance and thereby help exotics from becoming biologically invasive (Dukes and Mooney 1999). According to Sutherst (2000), "Climate change influences all invasive species by affecting their spread and colonization of new habitats. (p. 217)" Carlton (2000) discusses the role of global climate change (along with other drivers) on ocean biodiversity. For instance, exotic species suited to warmer water could expand their ranges to occupy higher latitudes. McMichael and Bouma (2000) warn that climate change could foster the spread of pests and pathogens. "Warmer conditions would tend to extend the geographic range (elevation and latitude) and the seasonality of many vector borne infectious diseases (VBDs) such as malaria and dengue fever, while curtailing the range of others (e.g., schistosomiasis) (p. 201)". McMichael and Bouma say that although there is empirical evidence for the association between climate conditions and infectious diseases, there is less evidence for causality. There is some evidence that the range of malaria extended to higher altitude areas in Pakistan between 1924 and 1990 (McMichael and Bouma 2000), possibly associated with an increase in temperature in critical months. The combination of climate and biological invasives could be deadly—Batrachochytrium dendrobatitis, a fungal skin pathogen is believed to have caused the extinction of two-thirds of harlequin frog species in the New World tropics (Thomas and Ohlemuller 2010).

In the appendix I develop a formal optimal control model that is meant to provide a conceptual framework to examine key features of linked climate change and biological invasives.

Although climate change is seen to be driven by aggregate greenhouse gases, and these are estimated for different countries, which means that there is an aggregate source, in the case of invasives there are multiple invasive species, and one species can have a variety of effects. For example, in Hawaii, feral pigs have harmful effects on a variety of ecosystem services—for example, they contribute to soil erosion and create habitat for disease.

Ostrom (2009) argued, in the case of climate change, that we should not wait for a single optimal global solution to emerge, but use a more polycentric approach with action at several levels. Dasgupta (1982) points out the implications of nonconvexities. These complexities might be viewed as strengthening the case for such fairly well understood measures as fuel taxes, which Sterner (2007) advocates. In the case of biological invasives, a case can be made for adaptive management.

In the model (see Appendix) I assumed there is an abatement function that reduces the impacts of the damage function. Both are not known, and solutions have to be found and learnt. According to Zavaleta (2000), although there is substantial evidence about the damage caused by invasive species, most efforts to control such species have been localized and restricted, rather than widespread. Because the expenditures for control of Tamarix (a weed) occur in the early years while benefits from its removal are enjoyed in a wider period, the economic case for its removal is sensitive to the discount rate.

According to Babu et al. (2010) who report on a restoration programme in Corbett National Park in India, 'any restoration programme for … invasive species would … need to be informed by an understanding of the biology of the invader, the local soil and micro climatic conditions, the status of the ecosystem, the larger landscape matrix, and most importantly, the requirements of the stakeholders'.

6.4 Extension 3: The Discount Rate in Climate Change and Equity

The discount rate can change which project or policy is good or bad—Fig. 6.1 shows how the present value of 1,000 units at 50 time periods in the future is affected by the discount rate. The Stern Review of Climate Change has been debated a lot. A key issue is what should the discount rate be?

In his fundamental treatment of human well-being and the environment, Dasgupta (2001) sets out some basic ideas. Essentially, the social welfare at time t can be represented by

$$W_t = \sum \left[1/(1+\delta)^t\right] U(C_t)$$

Here δ is the discount factor and is 'the rate of pure time preference'. It is discounting utility. If we are discounting consumption, and call that discount factor ρ, what is the relationship between ρ and δ?

Fig. 6.1 Present value of 1,000 units 50 years from now versus the discount rate

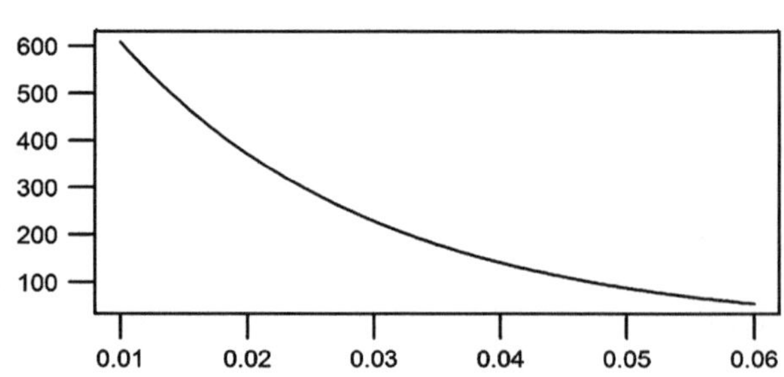

It can be shown that

$$\rho = \delta + \eta\, g$$

In words, consumption discount rate = pure rate of time preference (impatience) + elasticity of marginal well being * rate of growth of consumption

η accounts for the fact that if consumption is higher, marginal utility will be lower, but η can also be interpreted as a social preference for equality of consumption among generations

If $\delta = 0.002$, η is 2, the per capita growth rate is say, 2 %, then $\rho = 4.2$ %.

We see that the discount rate could be negative, if we forecast consumption to be declining. The forecast of consumption will determine the discount rate, which will affect the case for acting to prevent climate change. So if climate change is going to be so disastrous that it affects growth negatively, the discount rate will reinforce the need to act now.

Although CO_2 emissions have increased over the last few decades, on the whole, a consensus has emerged that emissions should be reduced. But who should cut emissions? The answer depends on notions of equity (Rose and Kverndokk 1999). Do nations have equal rights, so should nations cut emissions proportionately; or do people have equal rights, so should nations cut emissions according to per capita emissions? Or should we equalize abatement costs across nations?

And how does the discussion of the discount rate connect with the questions of equity? η above reflects the notion that a rich person would have less marginal utility for money than a poor person (Sterner and Persson 2008). Critics of the Stern Review have argued that Stern used too low a value of η, but a high value has two implications: (1) it makes the action on climate change hinge much more on growth forecasts, and (2) rich countries, or rather, people, should bear more of the costs of reducing greenhouse gases.

6.5 Extension 4: Livelihoods and Carbon Sequestration in Developing Countries

Chhatre and Agrawal (2009) focused on factors that affected tradeoffs and synergies between the level of carbon storage in forests and their contributions to livelihoods. The authors found that larger forests were more effective in enhancing both carbon and livelihoods outcomes, particularly when local communities also had high levels of rule-making autonomy. Their study drew on data from different countries gathered by the International Forestry Resources and Institution's (IFRI) research program, and used regression analysis. I discuss their relevant and interesting study with respect to two aspects: (1) institutional variables, and (2) causal graphs.

6.5.1 Institutional Variables

Chhatre and Agrawal (2009) aimed to study institutions using variables such as rule-making autonomy and ownership. Since rule-making autonomy is difficult to observe quantitatively, Chhatre and Agrawal (2009) used perceptions of rules by users and assumed that when it was "about the right level of conservation", the variable "AUTONOMY" equaled one whereas it was zero otherwise. However, Ternstrom et al. (2010) have objected to the use of the term "autonomy" for this perceived phenomenon, arguing instead that the variable underlying autonomy appeared to reflect sustainability. In their response to this objection, Chhatre and Agrawal (2010) recognized the underlying variable to be the perception of rules, which I consider to be a crucial variable. However, the debate between Tersntrom et al. (2010) and Chhatre and Agrawal (2010) also draws attention to a feature in regression analysis where we are often forced to collapse something varied and complex into something binary. Hence, when analyzing institutions quantitatively, we often translate a subtle social process into a variable whereas if prior thought about institutions goes into the research design a more nuanced approach is possible. For example, Chopra and Gulati (1998) captured the evolution of institutions over time by making distinctions in dummy variables.

6.5.2 Causal Graphs

Chhatre and Agrawal (2009) appear to be using a causal interpretation of regression since they make reference to causal pathways. Heuristically, a causal graph can help us see what difficulties we face when, like Chhatre and Agrawal (2009), we use cross-section data to model a dynamic, path-dependent process. Although Ternstrom et al. (2010) raise the issue of the dynamics of the resource, Chhatre and Agrawal, as evident from their response (2010), are quite aware of the issue, pointing to data limitations such as the lack of panel data that are common to quantitative studies of the commons. Carbon storage and livelihoods have a dynamic element in that carbon storage and livelihoods can both be high today but fall tomorrow (Ternstrom et al. 2010). Even with a very simplistic causal graph of carbon storage and livelihoods, which abstracts from such biophysical details as fire and grazing and institutional details, the causal graph brings out our difficulties (Fig. 6.2).

We only observe values for the last time-period in a long process with path dependence. However, a cross-section will sometimes have a large variation in a slow-moving variable while high frequency time series will give us variation in fast-moving variables. And institutions are usually slow-moving variables. We can use such cross-sectional data in descriptive regression and speculate about possible causal mechanisms, aware that the regression is only a shadow of these.

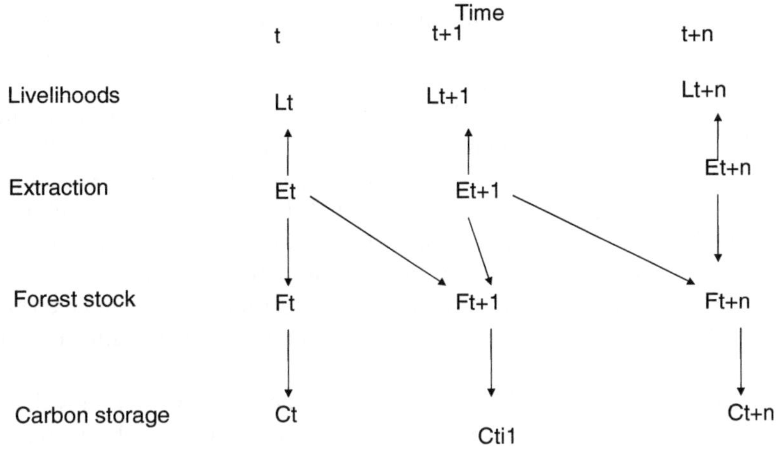

Fig. 6.2 Causal graph of carbon storage and livelihoods

In an empirical enquiry we could think of a causal graph, but where would that come from? It could be from a microeconomic model or theory. However, different disciplines have different styles of theorizing, each discipline concentrating more often than not on certain kinds of causal pathways. Nevertheless, scholars from different disciplines could brainstorm and think about possible pathways. Again, by way of illustration, I refer to the paper by Chhatre and Agrawal (2009), my paper (Dayal 2006), and to my knowledge of similar economic studies (for example, Pattanayak et al. 2004), while drawing also on Gibson et al. 2000. As Fig. 6.3 makes evident, there are different categories of pathways: institutional, economic, sociological, contextual and biophysical. The causal link (I1 in Fig. 6.3) between rules in use and extraction and, thereby, forest stock is one of the key insights of the volume titled People and Forests edited by Gibson et al. (2000).

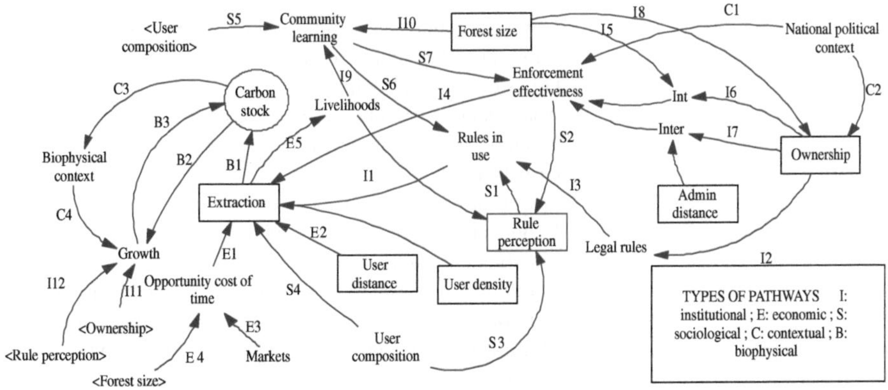

Fig. 6.3 Causal pathways for carbon stock and livelihoods

Schweik (2000) found that institutional factors—such as the caste system and the status of rule monitoring—along with factors such as distance and geographical barriers played a role in the spatial distribution of shorea robusta in the Chitwan District of Nepal while Agrawal (2000), who engaged in an empirical study of village forest councils in Almora district in India, found that smaller forest councils were less successful in collective action than larger forest councils—suggesting the causal paths I5 and I6 in Fig. 6.3. Economic studies such as those by Pattanayak et al. (2004) and Dayal (2006) emphasize the causal pathway E1. The variables that are enclosed in Fig. 6.3 are observed in the Chhatre and Agrawal (2009) dataset. We could focus on how carbon stock is affected by rule perception. So carbon stock is in a circle. We can then focus on pathways relating to these variables.

Apart from the number of causal pathways, there are other issues that need attention such as the issue of complicated feedbacks, the possibility that some causal arrows might be time- and context-specific, and the fact that there might be path dependence and evolution.

Appendix

In this appendix I develop a model for interlinked climate change and biological invasions. It combines the considerations considered separately in different sections of this chapter (Table A.1) .

Table A.1 Symbols and variables in the model

Symbol	Variable
R	Rich country
P	Poor country
U	Social utility
C	Aggregate consumption
ρ	Utility discount rate or rate of pure time preference
M	Emissions of greenhouse gases
Q	Gross or potential output
A	Abatement of greenhouse gases or exotic invasives
G	Stock of greenhouse gases
F	Growth of exotic invasives
S	Spread of exotic invasives
δ	Depreciation of man-made capital
K	Man-made capital
λ	Multiplier or co-state variable for stock of greenhouse gases
ω	Multiplier or co-state variable for stock of exotic invasives
μ	Multiplier or co-state variable for man-made capital
D	Damage
O	Outlay

I establish a conceptual framework using an optimal control model. Two countries, one rich (R) and another poor (P) confront the issue of exotic invasives (E) and greenhouse gases (G). Both countries get together to maximize utility (U)—a function of aggregate consumption (C)—over time; so they seek to maximize

$$\int_0^\infty [U(C^P(t)) + U(C^R(t))]e^{-\rho t}dt \tag{6.1}$$

subject to several dynamic constraints, relating to the capital stock (K), and G and E.

Output is determined solely by capital, K. Apart from consumption and depreciation (δ), some potential output is lost due to damages (D) because of greenhouse gases and exotic invasives. Some output is used as an outlay (O) to abate (A) greenhouse gases and exotic invasives. Suppressing time notation, we thus have

$$dK^P/\,dt = Q^P(K^P) - D^P_G(G) - D^P_E(E^P) - C^P - O^P_E(A^P E) - O^P_G(A^P_G) \tag{6.2}$$

where the superscript P stands for poor country and the subscript E and G stand for exotic invasives and greenhouse gases. The equation of motion for K^R, is symmetric to Eq. (6.2).

The stock of greenhouse gases increases with emissions (M) which are a function of output. Emissions are reduced by abatement (A) and there is some absorption (γG). Hence, dG/dt is assumed to be

$$dG/dt = M^P(Q^P(K^P)) - A^P_G + M^R(Q^R(K^R)) - A^R_G - \gamma G \tag{6.3}$$

Eiswerth and Johnson (2002) had modeled an alien invasive species following its establishment using a logistic growth function. Following them, we think of an aggregate stock of invasives (E) whose growth is density-dependent and also increased by the stock of greenhouse gases. There may also be some spread (S) from the other country, and growth of invasives may be abated. Hence, we assume that

$$dE^R/dt = F^R(E^R, G) + S^R(E^P) - A^R_E \tag{6.4}$$

The current value Hamiltonian is:

$$H = U^R(C^R) + U^P(C^P) + \lambda\, dG/dt + \omega^R dE^R/dt + \omega^P dE^P/dt + \mu^R dK^R/dt + \mu^R dK^P/dt$$

where λ, ω and μ are co-state variables. The current value Hamiltonian can be interpreted as a performance indicator, balancing the flow of consumption benefits with the value of increases in man-made capital, the value of the increases in stock of bad greenhouse gases, and the value of exotic invasives.

Our control variables are consumption and the abatement of greenhouse gases and exotic invasives (three controls for each country).

Assuming an interior solution, there are three static efficiency conditions for the rich country, and symmetric conditions for the poor country. These are as follows:

$$\partial U/\partial C^R = \mu^R \tag{6.5}$$

$$\mu^R * \partial O_G^R/\partial A_G^R = -\lambda \tag{6.6}$$

$$\mu^R * \partial O_E^R/\partial A_E^R = -\omega^R \tag{6.7}$$

In Eq. (6.5) we see that the marginal value of consumption from output needs to be balanced against the marginal value of an addition to the stock of man-made capital. Equations (6.6) and (6.7) are marginal cost should be equal to marginal damage conditions. The stocks will change, so will the marginal values and so will the shadow prices. We have dynamic efficiency or portfolio balance conditions as follows.

$$\begin{aligned} d\mu^R/dt = {} & \rho\mu^R - \mu^R * \partial Q^R/\partial K^R + \delta\mu^R \\ & - \lambda * \partial M^R/\partial Q^R * \partial Q^R/\partial K^R \end{aligned} \tag{6.8}$$

$$\begin{aligned} d\lambda/dt = {} & \rho\lambda + \mu^P * \partial D^P/\partial G + \mu^R * \partial D^R/\partial G \\ & + \gamma\lambda - \omega^P * \partial F^P/\partial G - \omega^R * \partial F^R/\partial G \end{aligned} \tag{6.9}$$

$$\begin{aligned} d\omega^R/dt = {} & \rho\omega^R + \mu^R * \partial D^R/\partial E^R - \omega^P * \partial S^P/\partial E^R \\ & - \omega^R * \partial F^R/\partial E^R \end{aligned} \tag{6.10}$$

Equation (6.10) shows that the optimal rate of growth of the shadow price of the exotic invasive stock in the rich country depends on the instantaneous marginal damage caused by the exotic invasive species in the rich country, the marginal value of the spread of the invasive in the poor country due to the rich country exotic invasive stock, and the marginal value of the change in growth due to a stock size change. Equation (6.10) has a symmetrical counterpart for the poor country. Equation (6.10) and the equation of motion for the exotic invasive reflect the fact that exotic invasives are weakest-link public goods. Similarly Eq. (6.9) and the equation of motion for G reflect the summation public good nature of abatement of greenhouse gases. In Eq. (6.9) the evolution of the shadow price of G depends on marginal damages in both the rich and poor country plus the marginal values of increased exotic invasive growth in the two countries.

References

Agrawal A (2000) Small is beautiful, but is larger better? forest-management institutions in the Kumaon Himalaya, India. In: Gibson GC, McKean MA, Ostrom O (eds) People and forests: communities, institutions and governance. MIT Press, London

Babu S, Love A, Babu CR (2010) Resolution to restore. Curr Conserv 4(1):6–10

Carlton JT (2000) Global change and biological invasions in the oceans. In: Mooney HA, Hobbs RJ (eds) Invasive species in a changing world. Island Press, Washington

Chhatre A, Agrawal A (2009) Trade-offs and synergies between carbon storage and livelihood benefits from forest commons. PNAS 106(42):17667–17670

Chhatre A, Agrawal A (2010) Reply to Ternstrom et al.: challenges of studying multiple outcomes simultaneously. PNAS 107(14):E53–E53

Chopra K, Gulati SC (1998) Environmental degradation, property rights and population movements: hypotheses and evidence from Rajasthan (India). Environ Dev Econ 3:35–58

Dasgupta P (1982) The control of resources. Harvard University Press, Cambridge

Dasgupta P (2001) Human well-being and the natural environment. Oxford University Press, Oxford

Dayal V (2006) A micro-econometric analysis of household extraction of forest biomass goods in Ranthambhore National Park, India. J For Econ 12:145–163

Dukes JS, Mooney HA (1999) Does global change increase the success of biological invaders? Tree 14(4):135–139

Eiswerth ME, Johnson WS (2002) Managing nonindigenous invasive species: insights from dynamic analysis. Environ Resource Econ 23:319–342

Gibson GC, McKean MA, Ostrom E (eds) (2000) People and forests: communities, institutions and governance. MIT Press, London

Howarth RB, Norgaard RB (1995) Intergenerational choices under global environmental change. In: Bromley DW (ed) The handbook of environmental economics. Blackwell, Oxford

McMichael AJ, Bouma MJ (2000) Global changes, invasive species, and human health. In: Mooney HA, Hobbs RJ (eds) Invasive species in a changing world. Island Press, Washington

Ostrom E (2009) A polycentric approach for coping with climate change. World Bank, Washington

Pattanayak SK, Sills E, Kramer R (2004) Seeing the forests for the fuel. Environ Dev Econ 9(2):155–179

Perrings C, Williamson M, Barbier EB, Delfino D, Dalmazzone S, Shogren J, Simmons P, Watkinson A (2002) Conserv Ecol 6(1):1. URL: http://www.consecol.org/vol6/iss1/art1

Perrings C, Burgiel S, Lonsdale M, Mooney H, Williamson W (2010) Globalization and bioinvasions: the international policy problem. In: Perrings C, Mooney H, Williamson M (eds) Bioinvasions and globalization: ecology, economics, management and policy. Oxford University Press, Oxford

Rose A, Kverndokk S (1999) Equity in environmental policy with an application to global warming. In: van den Bergh JCJM (ed) Handbook of environmental and resource economics. Edward Elgar, Cheltenham

Sandler T (2004) Global collective action. Cambridge University Press, Cambridge

Schweik CM (2000) Optimal foraging, institutions, and forest change: a case from Nepal. In: Gibson GC, McKean MA, Ostrom O (eds) People and forests: communities, institutions and governance. MIT Press, London

Stern N (2008) The economics of climate change. Am Econ Rev: Pap Proc 98(2):1–37

Sterner T (2007) Fuel taxes: an important instrument for climate policy. Energy Policy 35:3194–3202

Sterner T, Persson UM (2008) An Even Sterner review: introducing relative prices into the discounting debate. Rev Environ Econ Policy 2(1):61–76

Sutherst RW (2000) Climate change and invasive species: a conceptual framework. Global change and biological invasions in the oceans. In: Mooney HA, Hobbs RJ (eds) Invasive species in a changing world. Island Press, Washington

Ternstrom I, Mukhopadhyay P, Ghate R (2010) Sustainability, autonomy, and benefits from forest commons. Proc Nat Acad Sci—PNAS 107(14):E52–E52

Thomas CD, Ohlemuller R (2010) Climate change and species' distributions: an alien future? In: Perrings C, Mooney H, Williamson M (eds) Bioinvasions and globalization: ecology, economics, management and policy. Oxford University Press, Oxford

Zavaleta E (2000) Valuing ecosystem services lost to Tamarix invasion in the United States. In: Mooney HA, Hobbs RJ (eds) Invasive species in a changing world. Island Press, Washington

Chapter 7
Sustainable Development and Institutions

Abstract The World Bank now publishes estimates of adjusted savings for the world's countries to keep track of sustainable development; the environment is seen as a gigantic capital asset. I explore these estimates for different countries. Dasgupta and Maler, who have worked on theoretical models of environmental accounting, initially used optimal control models but have shifted to modeling imperfect economies, in which institutions can affect resource allocation. Sneddon et al. suggest the importance of deliberative democracy for sustainable development, and Vatn describes the use of deliberative processes, which can build on structured information. Duflo and Pande statistically estimate that on average, dams in India increased poverty.

Keywords Sustainable development · Accounting · Dams · Democracy

In 2010, the conventional measure of net national savings for the economy of Egypt was 7.8 % of gross national income, but the broader measure of 'adjusted savings' for the economy of Egypt was 3.6 % of gross national income (World Bank 2012). The measure of 'adjusted savings' is an attempt by economists to measure progress in sustainable development. In this chapter I discuss sustainable development from different perspectives, with institutions as a common theme.

The core economic model (Dasgupta and Maler 2009) treats the environment as a capital asset and derives the appropriate measure of sustainability. The first extension looks at estimates of adjusted net savings for some select economies. The next extension is about deliberative democracy and sustainable development. Then I discuss a verbal theoretical model and a statistical model used by political scientists to examine the effects of oil on democracy. Next, I describe a statistical model used to evaluate dams. Two appendices (A.1) compare two theoretical models of resource accounting, and (A.2) discuss the statistical assumptions of the instrumental variables technique used to overcome simultaneous causation bias.

V. Dayal, *The Environment in Economics and Development*,
SpringerBriefs in Economics, DOI: 10.1007/978-81-322-1671-1_7,

7.1 Core Economic Model: The Environment is a Gigantic Capital Stock

We want to sustain human well-being. Human well-being has constituents and determinants, and in the economic model of sustainable development we sustain consumption—a determinant of human well-being—over time. To sustain consumption over time it is necessary to maintain levels of wealth intact—we can track wealth by examining levels of our assets or net investments in them. It is important to include not merely things like factories and machines but also natural capital (e.g. forests) and human capital (e.g. education).

Dasgupta and Maler (2009; see the Appendix of this chapter) derive the following condition for sustainability

$$\Sigma p_{it} dK_{it}/d_t \geq 0 \tag{7.1}$$

where p is the shadow price of the ith capital asset (K) at time t. A shadow price is the social value of one more unit of the asset.

Essentially, we see that in Dasgupta and Maler's (2009) theoretical model, the economy will be able to sustain the well-being of people if the sum of the changes in different assets weighted by the shadow price of each asset is positive. This sum could be carried out over the time period of a year for an economy as a whole, in which case we have a measure of what could be called net saving or adjusted saving, or the change in assets brought about by a project could be examined, in which case we have a measure of the net benefits of the project (see Dasgupta 2012). In the appendix we see how Dasgupta and Maler's (2009) theoretical model incorporated the role of institutions, in contrast to most theoretical models of sustainability, (including Dasgupta et al. 1997), which leave out institutions.

7.2 Extension One: 'Adjusted Savings' Estimates

The World Bank has been computing adjusted savings (corresponding to Eq. (7.1) above) for different countries on an annual basis. In the following equation for adjusted net savings, all the values are expressed as a % of gross national income:

Adjusted net savings = gross savings − consumption of fixed capital + education expenditure − energy depletion − mineral depletion − carbon dioxide damage − particulate emission damage. One important qualification in interpreting this indicator is that it is ignoring demographic changes, or the rate of population growth (see Dasgupta 2012). I now turn to an examination of these estimates for a few economies (Table 7.1).

All the economies listed in Table 7.1 have positive adjusted net savings, though the US has a very low level. China's adjusted net savings level was high, even though it had the highest level of particulate emission damage and carbon dioxide damage, because its gross savings was so immense. The table shows that Egypt

Table 7.1 Adjusted net savings and components for select economies in 2010

Indicator name (% of GNI)	Brazil	China	Egypt	India	Indonesia	Kenya	Mexico	Russia	United States
Gross savings	16.8	52.7	18.2	34	32.9	16	24.6	28.6	10.9
Consumption of fixed capital	12.2	10.8	10.3	9.3	10.5	7.3	12	12.4	14
Net national savings	4.6	41.9	7.8	24.7	22.3	8.7	12.6	16.2	–3.1
Education expenditure	5.2	1.8	4.4	3.1	4.3	5.9	4.8	3.5	4.8
Energy depletion	1.6	3.7	6.8	2.5	5.3	0	5.4	13.2	0.8
Mineral depletion	1.7	1.4	0.2	1.3	1.3	0.1	0.3	1.1	0.1
Carbon dioxide damage	0.2	1.1	0.8	0.9	0.5	0.3	0.3	0.9	0.3
Particulate emission damage	0.2	1.2	0.7	0.7	0.8	0.1	0.4	0.1	0.1
Adjusted net savings	6.1	36.3	3.6	21.8	18.8	13.1	11	4.5	0.4

Source World Bank (2012)

and Russia had low net savings and high rates of energy depletion. At a macroeconomic level economies with a large reliance on energy may not save enough. Several countries—Sudan, Kazakhstan, Syrian Arab Republic, Yemen and Mongolia had adjusted net savings levels that were negative and levels of energy depletion that were high (>10 %) (World Bank 2012). Yemen and Mongolia had levels of adjusted net savings that were less than –10 % (World Bank 2012).

In the case of non-renewable energy, and other mineral resources, it is important to invest the revenue from extraction in other forms of wealth. According to the World Bank report, The Changing Wealth of Nations (World Bank 2010), Botswana, known for transparency and good governance, did well in investing its mineral revenues, and so saw its real wealth and GDP per capita grow. In contrast, Botswana's neighbor Namibia was less successful in using mineral assets to build national wealth.

In thinking of the use of environmental and natural resource accounting, I think it is vital to distinguish between management and scorekeeping. Having good estimates of poverty is scorekeeping; they tell us where poverty is greater, and when it has gone down and when it has gone up. But to manage poverty one needs research which examines the determinants of poverty, and its response to different policies that are implemented. Similarly, environmental and natural resource accounting has a scorekeeping and a management function; in my opinion, its major function is scorekeeping. Even today, a substantial proportion of economists and policy makers tend to think of the environment as a 'luxury', if it enters their thinking at all. Environmental economists need to communicate not only with physical scientists and social scientists, but also with economists and policy makers, and environmental accounting speaks to them in a language they understand easily.

I would be cautious about the prospects for environmental and natural resource accounting to inform environmental management directly. A key issue is that of scale. Pollution or natural resource, and especially, ecosystem, issues have a natural scale at which they need to be addressed—the airshed or urban conglomeration for air, the river basin or sub-basin for a river, the aquifer for groundwater, and so on. Moreover, there are non-linearities and site-specific details. The water that is 'pumped' out by forests is greatest at an intermediate age, low when the forest is young or old. Grassland may be more conducive to ecosystem services than forest in certain locales.

7.3 Extension 2: Value Articulating Institutions in a Deliberative Democracy

According to Sneddon et al. (2006, p. 264) 'notions of deliberative democracy … are crucial to any discussion of sustainable development policies and sustainability politics.' This argument for democracy is echoed by Paehlke (2005, p. 173) who writes that 'environmentalism has in practice widely and consistently led to (or at least sought) an expansion of democratic opportunities and an opening of administrative decision making to public participation.' In discussing institutions for high quality growth, the development economist Rodrik (2008) stresses the importance of democracy as a meta-institution. In his well known book, Development and Freedom, Sen (2000) had said that 'no substantial famine has ever occurred in any independent country with a democratic form of government and a free press,' but also added, 'India's success in eradicating famines is not matched by that in eliminating regular undernutrition.' According to Gutmann and Thompson (2004), in a democracy, leaders should give reasons for their decisions, to promote collective decisions and help correct mistakes made.

I now turn to a discussion of what Vatn (2005) terms 'value articulating institutions'—valuation is not seen only as a technique that we get right by employing the right models in the right way, but the outcome of a social process shaped by the specific value articulating institution. While at one time economists saw project evaluation primarily as a technical exercise, some economists now advocate deliberative methods. Economists can use such techniques as multi-criteria analysis to foster deliberative democracy in the consideration of projects and programmes.

Multi-criteria analysis can be explained with an example. I may want to buy a vehicle or rent a home. I can think of criteria: for the vehicle, cost, speed, safety etc.; for the home, number of rooms, view, light etc. I can then think of alternative vehicles and homes and rank them within each criterion. I can then weight the different criteria and arrive at a decision.

A cost-benefit analysis can be thought of as a specific form of multi-criteria analysis, i.e. multi-criteria analysis can be thought of as a more general form of cost-benefit analysis, with more flexible ways of aggregation. However, the philosophies are quite different—cost-benefit analysis draws on welfare economics theory, whereas multi-criteria analysis doesn't need that.

Vatn describes some deliberative value articulating institutions, three of which are briefly listed below:

- Citizen's juries: small group of citizens—10 to 20 jurors—normally selected at random; especially successful in Germany, being used since 1970s.
- Consensus conferences: originated in Denmark in the 1980s; developed by the Danish Board of Technology; 10–16 lay citizens in a 4-day inquiry.
- Focus groups: small randomly selected citizen's discussion group (about 10), led by a moderator; used in market research.

Vatn suggests that multi-criteria methods can be used with deliberative processes.

7.4 Extension 3: How Resources May Curse Democracy

If we carry out resource accounting we may find that an economy that is very dependent on mineral extraction will have lower adjusted savings. But if we agree with Sneddon et al. (2006) that deliberative democracy is important for sustainable development, we may have more reason to worry—there is a substantial literature on how abundant natural resources may curse democracy. In his book on the oil curse, Ross (2012) formulates a verbal model of how oil can affect democracy.

I will summarize Ross's (2012) verbal model in this paragraph, hoping to do justice to it. Citizens care about their economic benefits from public goods relative to the cost of what they pay as taxes. Their well being leads to political support. If they are unhappy, they will support democracy rather than an autocrat in power. With oil, taxes can be lower, if accompanied by a lack of transparency, then revenues can be used for patronage and thus lead to greater political support for the ruler in power.

Ross used a variety of evidence, carefully harnessed in the form of tables, graphs and statistical models. Ross (2012, p. 63) asserts:

> from the late 1970s to the late 1990s, a wave of democracy swept across the globe, bringing freedom to countries in virtually every region—except the petroleum-rich countries of the Middle East, Africa, and the former Soviet Union. From 1980 to 2011, the democracy gap between the oil and non-oil states grew ever wider … oil has kept autocrats in power by enabling them to increase spending, reduce taxes, buy the loyalty of the armed forces, and conceal their own corruption and incompetence.

Such studies as that by Ramsay (2011) support the findings by Ross (2012). Ramsay argues that there is simultaneous causation between oil income and democracy. To overcome this he uses an innovative instrumental variable in his

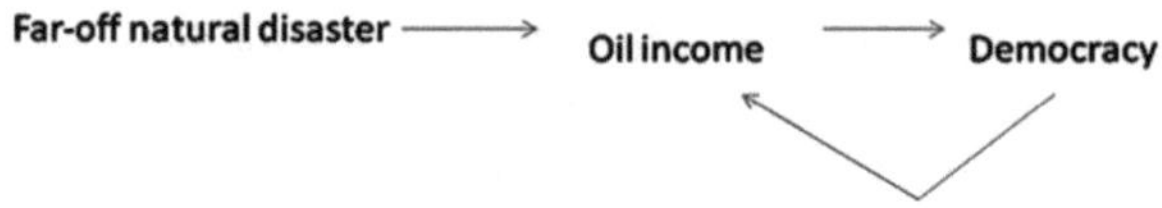

Fig. 7.1 Ramsay (2011) used damage due to far-off natural disasters as an instrumental variable for examining the effect of oil income on democracy

statistical analysis—damage due to far off natural disasters—that can affect oil income directly but not political institutions (Fig. 7.1).

Ramsay (2011, p. 508) finds that 'increasing oil income exerts a negative, statistically significant, and much larger impact on democracy than ordinary least-squares regression analyses imply.'

7.5 Extension 4: Statistical Evaluation of Dams and Poverty

Dams are controversial development projects. Environmentalists often criticize dams. Advocates suggest that they help growth and therefore are needed in developing countries to alleviate poverty. And yet, protests by those who will lose control over natural resources because of a dam are a part of what Guha (2005) calls the 'environmentalism of the poor.' How would we assess the effect of dams?

A comprehensive cost-benefit analysis would look at the costs (for e.g. displacement) and the benefits (for example, increased agricultural production). Usually the project agency will have prepared a document suggesting diverse effects. Typically the analyst will use this and other information to guess at the effects; such an exercise is a bundle of implicit causal claims. However, in statistical evaluation, the outcome of some intervention is assessed statistically, with careful attention to causality. Instead of implicit causal claims though, we make statistical assumptions that are often subtle (see Appendix A.2 of this chapter).

According to Duflo and Pande (2007), by 2000, 19 % of the world's electricity and 30 % of its irrigated area were accounted for by dams. But, dams had displaced over 40 million people. There was no systematic empirical evidence on how the average large dam affected the poor. They study this question for India.

Duflo and Pande's paper is notable for harnessing the combined power of several datasets for different variables—dam location, river gradient, agricultural production, and rural poverty. Duflo and Pande paid careful attention to biophysical features of dams, and used this knowledge to estimate the causal effects of dams. The unit of analysis is districts, which are parts of states in India. They distinguish between districts upstream of a dam and those downstream of a dam.

Duflo and Pande argue that dams and agricultural production simultaneously influence each other—dams can affect agricultural production, but states with high agricultural production can build more dams. Duflo and Pande use river gradient as

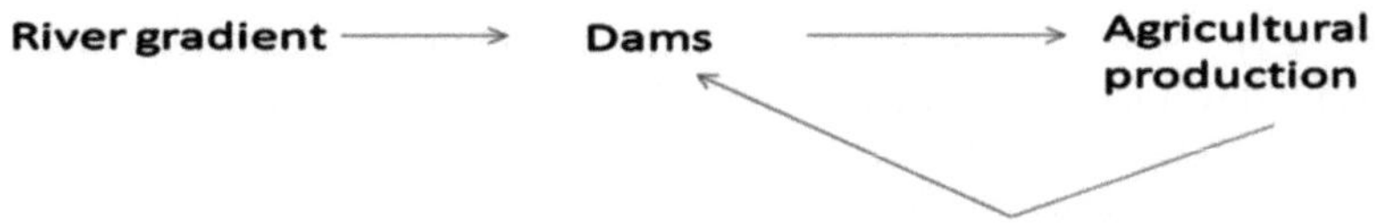

Fig. 7.2 Duflo and Pande (2007) used river gradient as an instrumental variable

an instrumental variable to overcome simultaneity (Fig. 7.2). They find that dam construction significantly increases agricultural production (0.34 %) and yield (0.19 %) in the downstream districts. However, each dam is associated with a significant poverty increase (headcount ratio) of 0.77 % in its own district. Although poverty decreases in downstream districts, the poverty reduction in downstream districts is insufficient to compensate for the poverty increase in the dam's own district.

Duflo and Pande (p. 637) state that 'The inability or unwillingness of those who benefit from dams to compensate groups of losers, or of the state to require them to do so when both groups are clearly identifiable ex-ante, suggests poorly functioning institutions of redistribution.' We thus see that they too point to institutions as constituents of what Dasgupta and Maler (2009) term resource allocation mechanisms. In Duflo and Pande and Dasgupta and Maler (2009) institutions are part of underlying mechanisms at work, but implicit. In World Bank (2010), Ross (2012) and Ramsay (2011), the analysis deals explicitly with institutions. In Vatn (2005) there is an appeal to building the institutions of deliberative democracy.

Appendix A.1

I compare two models: DM2 (Dasgupta and Maler 2009) with DKM1 (Dasgupta et al. 1997); we can use mathematical techniques innovatively to frame an issue differently.

In both DM2 and DKM1, welfare over time is very similar. In DM2 welfare at time t is

$$W_t = \int_t^{\infty} U(C_\tau)e^{-(\tau-t)}d\tau$$

where C is aggregate consumption. In DKM1 current social welfare, U is a function not only of C, but also of the environment and labour.

The key difference between DKM1 and DM2 is the use of α—a resource allocation mechanism—by DM2. The co-evolution of institutions and the state of the economy is reflected in α. This means that C, resource flows R, and capital stocks K, are functions of α. DM2 write the value function V can as

$V(K_t, \alpha,_t) = W_t$, where W_t is given by the expression above. DM2 define sustainable development as a path where $dV_t/dt \geq 0$. By using the value function directly, and assuming that α is autonomous, DM2 show that $dVt/dt = \Sigma p_{it}\, dK_{it}/dt = I \geq 0$ on a sustainable development path.

In contrast, DKM1 use optimal control theory to derive the adjustments that should be made to get net national product—this is common in theoretical models dealing with this issue—and the model is silent about institutions.

DM2 argue that sustainable development requires examining wealth and not GNP or even NNP; whereas DKM1 derive results for adjustments to NNP.

Appendix A.2

In this appendix I briefly discuss the statistical assumptions behind using instrumental variables.

Let our regression equation be

$$Yi = \beta 0 + \beta 1\ Xi + ui,\ i = 1, \ldots, n$$

And let Xi be correlated with ui because of simultaneous causality (i.e. X and Y cause each other).

We could use an instrumental variable Z to estimate the effect $\beta 1$ of X on Y.

The conditions for a valid instrument are: (1) instrument relevance: the correlation between Z and X should not be zero and should be high; and (2) instrument exogeneity: the correlation between Z and u should be zero.

We can test for instrument relevance statistically. Exogeneity is subtle—we need to use thinking and judgement. If we have more than one instrument, we can use a statistical test to aid our thinking and judgement, but it is 'incumbent on both the empirical analyst and the critical reader to use their own understanding of the empirical application to evaluate whether this assumption is reasonable' (Stock and Watson 2011, p. 454).

References

Dasgupta P (2012) Inclusive national accounts: introduction. Working paper no 67–12. SANDEE, Kathmandu

Dasgupta P, Maler KG (2009) Some recent developments. In: Chopra K, Dayal V (eds) Oxford handbook of environmental economics in India. Oxford University Press, New Delhi

Dasgupta P, Kristrom B, Maler KG (1997) The environment and net national product. In: Dasgupta P, Maler KG (eds) The environment and emerging development issues, vol 1. Oxford University Press, Oxford

Duflo E, Pande R (2007) Dams. Q J Econ 122(2):601–646

Guha R (2005) The environmentalism of the poor. In: Dryzek JS, Schlosberg D (eds) Debating the earth: the environmental politics reader. Oxford University Press, New York

Gutmann A, Thompson D (2004) Why deliberative democracy?. Princeton University Press, Princeton

Paehlke R (2005) Democracy and environmentalism. In: Dryzek JS, Schlosberg D (eds) Debating the earth: the environmental politics reader. Oxford University Press, New York

Ramsay KW (2011) Revisiting the resource curse: natural disasters, the price of oil, and democracy. Int Organ 65(03):507–529

Rodrik D (2008) One economics, many recipes: globalization, institutions, and economic growth. Princeton University Press, Princeton

Ross ML (2012) The oil curse: how petroleum wealth shapes the development of nations. Princeton University Press, Princeton

Sen A (2000) Development as freedom. Oxford University Press, Delhi

Sneddon C, Howarth RB, Norgaard RB (2006) Sustainable development in a post-Brundtland world. Ecol Econ 57:253–268

Stock JH, Watson MW (2011) Introduction to econometrics. Addison-Wesley, Boston

Vatn A (2005) Institutions and the environment. Edward Elgar, Cheltenham

World Bank (2010) The changing wealth of nations: measuring sustainable development in the new millennium. World Bank, Washington, DC

World Bank (2012) World development indicators. http://databank.worldbank.org. Accessed 5 Oct 2012

Index

V. Dayal, *The Environment in Economics and Development*, SpringerBriefs in Economics, DOI: 10.1007/978-81-322-1671-1, © The Author(s) 2014

MIX
Papier aus verantwortungsvollen Quellen
Paper from responsible sources
FSC® C105338

If you have any concerns about our products,
you can contact us on
ProductSafety@springernature.com

In case Publisher is established outside the EU,
the EU authorized representative is:
Springer Nature Customer Service Center GmbH
Europaplatz 3, 69115 Heidelberg, Germany

Printed by Libri Plureos GmbH
in Hamburg, Germany